FOURTH EDITION

The Professional Cosmetologist

*Written to assist students taking state or national licensing tests written by individual states, the National Interstate Council of State Boards of Cosmetology, or Educational Testing Service.

FOURTH EDITION

The Professional Cosmetologist

John W. Dalton

West Publishing Company
St. Paul   New York   Los Angeles   San Francisco

Copyediting: Patricia A. Lewis
Text Design: John Edeen
Dummy Artist: David Farr, Imagesmythe, Inc.
Illustrations: Scientific Illustrators and Paula Cheadle
Cover Image: ''Nina'' by Michel Canetti
Cover Design: Kristen Weber
Index: Patricia A. Lewis
Prepress, printing, and binding by West Publishing Company

West's Commitment to the Environment

In 1906, West Publishing Company began recycling materials left over from the production of books. This began a tradition of efficient and responsible use of resources. Today, up to 95 percent of our legal books and 70 percent of our college texts are printed on recycled, acid-free stock. West also recycles nearly 22 million pounds of scrap paper annually—the equivalent of 161,717 trees. Since the 1960s, West has devised ways to capture and recycle waste inks, solvents, oils and vapors created in the printing process. We also recycle plastics of all kinds, wood, glass, corrugated cardboard, and batteries, and have eliminated the use of styrofoam book packaging. We at West are proud of the longevity and the scope of our commitment to our environment.

Photo Credits

xxvii, xxix, xxx @ David Young-Wolff/PhotoEdit; **2** Courtesy of Scruples Professional Salon Products; **3** (a-c) Tony Evans, (d) @ Andre Gallant/The Image Bank; **6** (top) @ Tony Freeman/PhotoEdit, (middle) @ Tom McCarthy/The Picture Cube, (bottom) @ David Young-Wolff PhotoEdit; **7** (top) @ David Young-Wolff/PhotoEdit, (margin) @ Sam Zarember/The Image Bank; **8,9** @ David Young-Wolff/PhotoEdit; **10** @ MARVY! Advertising Photography; **12** @ Sobel/Klonsky/The Image Bank; **13** @ Maria Taglienti/The Image Bank; **16, 17** @ David Young-Wolff/PhotoEdit; **24** Courtesy of Scruples Professional Salon Products; **25, 26, 27, 29, 30** @ David Young-Wolff/PhotoEdit; **32** Courtesy of Scruples Professional Salon Products ; **42, 43, 44, 45, 49, 51** Tony Evans; **62** Courtesy of Scruples Professional Salon Products; **67** Courtesy

Credits continued following subject index

610 Opperman Drive
P.O. Box 64526
St. Paul, Minnesota 55164–0526

Printed in the United States of America

99 98 97 96 95 94 93 92   8 7 6 5 4 3 2 1 0

Library of Congress Cataloging in Publication Data

Dalton, John W., 1942–
    The professional cosmetologist / John W. Dalton. — 4th ed.
        p.   m.
    Includes bibliographical references and index.
    ISBN 0-314-73042-7 (NASTA).—ISBN 0-314-78706-2 (soft).
    1. Beauty culture. I. Title.
TT957.D27 1992
646.7′2—dc20
                                 9131043
                                 CIP ∞

To my wife Judy
for her patience, support, and love

Contents

CHAPTER 21
Chemical Hair Relaxing   408

CHAPTER 22
Thermal Pressing   430

CHAPTER 23
Recurling the Hair (Soft Curl Perm)   446

CHAPTER 24
Describing the Skin   464

CHAPTER 25
Facial Treatments   490

CHAPTER 26
Applying Makeup   512

CHAPTER 27
Nail Anatomy, Disorders, and Diseases   530

CHAPTER 28
Manicuring and Pedicuring   546

CHAPTER 29
Wigs and Hairpieces   572

CHAPTER 30
Shaving   582

Part III

Salon Management and Retailing

CHAPTER 31
Planning a Salon   592

CHAPTER 32
Salon Operations   604

CHAPTER 33
The Psychology of Interpersonal Skills and Retailing   626

Preface ▓▓

How to Use The Professional Cosmetologist

To the Instructor ▓▓▓▓▓▓▓▓▓▓▓▓▓▓▓▓▓▓▓▓▓▓▓▓▓▓▓▓▓▓▓▓▓▓▓▓▓▓▓

Since the first edition of THE PROFESSIONAL COSMETOLOGIST was published 15 years ago, the field of cosmetology has undergone many changes as new technologies have developed and new issues have emerged. This fourth edition of the text has been thoroughly revised to include the most up-to-date information available to cosmetologists as well as new supplementary materials for the student and instructor. In addition, this new edition incorporates recommendations from state boards of cosmetology, classroom instructors, cosmetology school owners, and manufacturers. Their helpful suggestions will make learning easier for students, simplify teaching for instructors, ensure greater success for students taking the state board examinations, and provide greater protection for salon clients.

To keep the book as current as possible, many new topics have been added. For example, THE PROFESSIONAL COSMETOLOGIST is one of the first cosmetology texts to address the issue of the prevention of acquired immune deficiency syndrome (AIDS) in the workplace. Technical material regarding the prevention of skin cancer has also been included as well as information about the role of Retin-A in reducing wrinkles.

Another important and current topic addressed by the book is the preservation of the environment. A special section on ecology and the need for recycling has been included at the beginning of the book. While the ecological problems we face cannot be solved by a single textbook, we can make students more aware of their environment and the role they can play in protecting it. Here we hope to raise students' level of concern and provide them with information that will help them develop healthful, environmentally sound practices both in the salon and in their personal lives. Given the proper information, something can be done about environmental issues *today*. As technology changes, we will continue to provide the most current information in future revisions.

A topic of considerable interest to students is their own success as cosmetologists. Certainly, interpersonal communications and sales techniques play an important part in the overall success students will enjoy in the salon. Therefore, to assist students in achieving their personal career goals, we have added a new chapter on the psychology of interpersonal communications and retail sales techniques.

In addition to these changes in content, this edition also has a completely new appearance. For the first time, THE PROFESSIONAL COSMETOLOGIST uses full color throughout, a feature that will make the text more appealing to students and easier to use. The photographs and drawings, which are entirely new, not only make use of color, but have been reworked to update the steps in the procedures and make them even clearer. A new design with an easy-to-read format also adds to the appeal of the text. In addition, theory objectives and practical objectives have been abbreviated and clearly labeled, and the answers to the end-of-chapter questions have been removed from the text to provide instructors with more flexibility in using the questions.

Finally, the supplementary materials have also been revised and expanded. The following materials are available for instructors and students:

- **The Instructor's Manual.** The Instructor's Manual has been revised and contains a plethora of materials to assist instructors in organizing and teaching their courses in cosmetology. Included in the manual are final test questions, student performance checklists, supply checklists, lesson plans, and cross-references to the text.

- **Transparency Acetates.** A package of full-color transparency acetates consisting of figures from the book is available.

- **State Board Review Book.** The **State Board Review Book** now has 2,200 questions that can be used to measure the competency of each student. The multiple-choice questions have been combined with pictorial situation questions. In type and style, these questions closely follow the guidelines prescribed by state boards of cosmetology and national testing organizations.

- **Theory and Practical Workbook.** The study guide for THE PROFESSIONAL COSMETOLOGIST has been totally revised. It is now called the Theory and Practical Workbook and includes material on both the theory and practical objectives. Combining these materials into one book is more cost effective for your students. Several new features have been added to the workbook, including artwork, a final test, and progress tracking charts. The tracking charts were developed with the assistance of Don Pierson and Lin Patterson (instructors I work with), then modified according to recommendations from reviewers in different states. The progress charts will make it easier for you to track student progress and decide when to give additional assignments. These charts are perforated for easy removal, or they may be left in the workbook for reference.

Each objective in the Theory and Practical Workbook is referenced to the corresponding page in the textbook, to enable you and the student to identify the exact source of the information.

■ **On-Line Computer Study, Testing, and Reporting.** Using this carefully written computer study program and either a Macintosh or IBM computer, your students will be able to attempt to answer a question and then view the correct answer. They can also take tests on the computer, and their test scores will be automatically recorded for you to review or print out later. These test results are password protected so that only the instructor can view and report (print) them later.

To the Student

Introduction to the Professional Cosmetologist Learning System

This short section, which has been designed around a series of questions you might ask, will help you use "performance-based learning" effectively. This introduction will serve several purposes:

1. Define important terms.
2. Identify the resources in this system.
3. Explain the Dalton MASTER PLAN for using these resources.
4. Give hints for preparing for state board exams.

The Dalton MASTER PLAN provides the key to effective use of THE PROFESSIONAL COSMETOLOGIST LEARNING SYSTEM, which has been practiced successfully for many years in schools and training facilities throughout the country.

What is a Performance-Based Learning System?

We refer to this as a "performance-based" system because the skills you learn are the ones you must do on the job as a cosmetologist. The services emphasized here are those performed by successful cosmetologists, as determined by studies conducted by cosmotology schools, state boards of cosmetology, universities, and the author.

Notice that we call this a "learning system"—not just a textbook. A textbook is only one of the many resources that you will use in learning cosmetology. The following are some of the other resources that are available:

- Your instructors
- Fellow classmates
- Audiovisual materials
- Workbooks
- Computers
- Lectures/demonstrations

All these resources combine to form a "learning system" that has been carefully designed to help you develop the "performance" skills required of cosmetologists.

What Resources does the Professional Cosmetologist Learning System Include?

The following major resources make up the learning system:

- You, the student
- This textbook
- Your instructor
- The Theory and Practical Workbook
- The questions in the State Board Review Book
- The computer study and testing program

How Do I Begin to Use the Professional Cosmetologist Resources to Learn Cosmetology?

Your first step is to learn what these resources can offer. Begin by becoming acquainted with your textbook:

1. Turn to the table of contents at the front of the book. The chapter titles indicate the skills you must master and the knowledge you must learn in order to become a cosmetologist. Look the contents over carefully.

2. Select any chapter in the contents and read through the list of performances. After instruction and practice, you should "know" the information described here and should be able to "do" these activities. These performances are called "theory objectives" and "practical objectives," respectively, depending on whether they emphasize information or activities; they will act as the stepping stones by which you advance your skill.

3. Page through the text, glancing at the illustrations and becoming familiar with the basic layout of the book.

What Is the Dalton Master Plan?

The plan consists of six steps: motivate yourself, analyze, study, take time, emphasize practice, and review.

Motivate Yourself

Successful use of this system requires your active, interested participation. Make up your mind from the beginning to concentrate, work hard, and use all available resources. Renew your self-motivation at the beginning of each chapter and whenever you need a little attitude boost. Start each chapter by reading the title and learning objective carefully. These items explain what the chapter is about and why it is important.

Analyze

The learning, theory, and practical objectives are an important part of the plan. Take time to analyze them carefully:

1. Read and study each learning objective. This tool tells exactly what you must do at the end of instruction and practice to perform the skill discussed in the chapter.

2. Analyze the level of acceptability statement carefully. This statement identifies the conditions under which you must perform the skill and indicates at least how well you must perform it for mastery.

3. Read and study the theory and practical objectives. They explain the precise steps you must take to perform the learning

objective. Accomplishing these objectives will be the main part of your work in each chapter. Your instructor may add information or examples to these objectives.

Study

Once you have analyzed the introductory material in each chapter, begin studying to achieve each objective:

1. Read the instructional material in the theory objectives carefully. Notice that each objective is printed conveniently in the margin at the beginning of the material. Refer back to this statement whenever necessary so you always know what performance you are working to master.

2. Look up unfamiliar words in the glossary at the end of each chapter.

3. After you have studied the materials in the book carefully, do the activities for the theory objectives in the Theory and Practical Workbook. Check your answers immediately and ask your instructor to explain any points you do not understand.

4. Read the instructional material in the practical objectives. Study the procedures, including the figures, carefully.

5. Complete the activities for the objectives in the workbook. Again, check your answers immediately and clear up any questions, keeping in mind that your instructor will have the "most right answer."

Take Time

Clarify any confusion or misunderstanding about the skill you are learning:

1. Ask your instructor for help in problem areas.

2. Review the procedures for the practical objectives.

3. Gather the supplies necessary to practice this skill.

Emphasize Practice

Practice each skill using the following steps:

1. Walk through the procedure step by step using your text.

2. Ask your instructor for clarification and assistance.

3. Try doing the performance with little or no help from the text, your instructor, or other resources.

4. Perform the task (job) for evaluation with no help from resources.

Review

Once you complete each performance to the level of acceptability, review the entire chapter:

1. Try answering the questions in the State Board Review Book that accompanies this learning system.

2. Team up with a few of your classmates and ask each other study questions. Doing this will also provide a good review.

This simple Dalton MASTER PLAN is the key to your successful use of the learning system!

How Should I Prepare for the State Board Exams?

Here are a few suggestions for preparing for your licensing examinations:

- Use this entire learning system as described in the Dalton MASTER PLAN.

- Review all workbook activities for theory and practical objectives.

- Review study questions at the end of each chapter.

- Answer the sample questions in the State Board Review Book which is part of the system.

- Follow all directions given by your intructor.

Putting It All Together

You are about to benefit from the use of a "performance-based learning system." Each skill is divided into specific performances or activities you must complete to become a successful cosmetologist. Instructions are organized into a "learning system" composed of various resources. As the figure illustrates, you, the student, are the center of this system. As the center of this learning system, you must use the system effectively, so let's review how the Dalton MASTER PLAN will guide you to success:

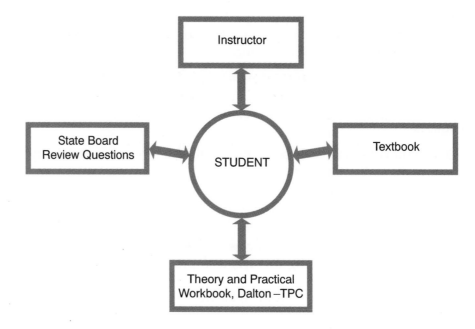

- **Motivate yourself.**

  - Take charge of your learning.
  - Begin each chapter by reading the title and learning objective.

- **Analyze.**

  - Study the learning objective.
  - Make sure you understand the level of acceptability.
  - Read the theory and practical objectives.

- **Study.**

  - Study the theory objective instructional materials, and do the workbook activities.
  - Study the practical objective instructional materials, and do the workbook activities.

- **Take time.**

  - Clarify all problem areas.
  - Review the procedures for the practical objectives in the textbook.
  - Gather the supplies needed to practice this skill.

■ **Emphasize practice.**

- ■ Walk through the procedures in the text.
- ■ Ask your instructor for assistance when necessary.
- ■ Do the performance with minimal help from resources.
- ■ Do the performance with no help from resources.

■ **Review.**

- ■ Look over each chapter.
- ■ Answer the questions in the State Board Review Book.
- ■ Try the study questions in the text.

Following this plan will enable you to master the skills of a licensed cosmetologist. Good learning!

Acknowledgements

In every step during the preparation of this text vital assistance was provided by a number of people whose existence is acknowledged with gratitude (with apologies to anyone inadvertently omitted). The most important expertise, guidance, and support was provided by my wife Judy. Others that gave their support and expertise are West Publishing Company Editor, Denise Simon; Editorial Assistant, Bridget Neumayr; and the Production Editors, Sharon Kavanagh and Nancy Roth. New and improved artwork was done by George Morris, Scientific Illustrators.

The author also wishes to express his appreciation to Ann Music Streetman for her contributions to each edition of this book. I would also like to thank Idella Biggs-Nemo, R. C. I., for her material on "Hair Cutting for the Black Clients' Hair" and "Makeup Techniques for the Black Woman."

Special thanks are due to Frank Jacobi of Citrus College/ El Camino College, California, for his generous support of this project. I would also like to thank the following individuals and companies for their contributions to this book: Myrtle Aase, State Board, Florida; Nellie Basone, Citrus Community College, California; Candace Kay Caro, Cutters Hair Beauty School, Arizona; Della Condon, Riverside City College, California; Mary Crosby, Sacramento City College, California; Dennis Danilak, Northern Alberta Institute of Technology, Canada; Dudley Products, Inc., Greensboro, North Carolina; Barbara Funk, St. Lawrence College, Ontario, Canada; G. Pat Hark, San Jacinto College, North Texas; Linda Harris, Central Carolina Community College, North Carolina; Florian Harvat, Minnesota; Faye Hoffman, College of Albemarle, North Carolina; Richard L. Jones, Oklahoma Institute of Hair Design, Oklahoma; Bill C. Knaak, Convergent Systems, Inc., Minnesota; Carole Laubach, Texas; Linnea Lindquist, Minneapolis Technical College, Minnesota; Robert Mager, California; Barbara McKinney, Trinity Valley Community College, Texas; Sandy Monahan, John A. Logan College, Illinois; National Beauty Supply, New Hope, Minnesota; Dianna Pfaff, Parkersburg Beauty College, West Virginia; Lynn Phillips, Douglas MacArthur State Technical College, Alabama; Nancy (Chism) Powell, Brevard Community College, Cocoa, Florida; Rosario Sciortino, New Jersey; Scruples, Inc., Lakeville, Minnesota; Sol Major, California; Spectrums of Minnesota: Susan Martin, Kim Giles, Alex Almen, Jane Haapala; Judy Stewart, Joseph's College of Beauty, Nebraska; Doris A. Thomas, North Florida Beauty Academy, Florida.

Special thanks to Michael Cole and the Salon Development Corp. of St. Paul, Minnesota, for their assistance with the material in the Psychology of Retail Sales chapter. The material used was based on Mr. Cole's book "A LITTLE OFF THE TOP".

The author gratefully acknowledges the following individuals and schools who kindly responded to our survey questionnaire. Their comments and suggestions were invaluable in the preparation of this 4/e: ALABAMA: Douglas MacArthur State Technical College–Lynn Phillips; ARIZONA: "Cutters Hair Beauty School"–Candace Kay Caro, DeVae College of Beauty, Yuma School of Beauty; ARKANSAS: Searcy Beauty College–Dan Seaton; CALIFORNIA: Career Academy of Beauty, Elegante Beauty College, Palomar Institute of Cosmetology, Sacramento City College–Mary Crosby; CANADA: St. Lawrence College–Barbara Funk; COLORADO: Highland Hills Beauty Academy–Linda C. Purdy; CONNECTICUT: Sampieri School of Hair Design; FLORIDA: Manhattan Beauty School, North Florida College of Cosmetology–Doris Anita Thomas, Sheridan Vo-Tech Center, Suncoast Beauty School; GEORGIA: Athens Area Technical Institute, Academy of Hair Arts and Design–Elizabeth Wendel; IDAHO: Razzle Dazzle College; ILLINOIS: Alvareita's College of Cosmetology, Du Quoin Beauty College, Granite City School of Beauty Culture, Hair Professional Beauty College–Joanne Guthrie, John A. Logan College–Sandy Monahan, John Amico School of Hair Design, Pivot Point Beauty School–Roberta D. Scholz, Cathy Schmidt Meckley, Jay Kemplin, Suzanne Theuns, D. Osborne, Steven Lai; INDIANA: P.J.'s College of Cosmetology–Betty Fields; IOWA: Iowa School of Beauty–Jane Brown; LOUISIANA: Alexandria Academy of Beauty, Moler Beauty College–Sherry Castillion, Stevenson's Academy of Hair Design; MICHIGAN: Kirtland Community College, Michigan College of Beauty–Barbara A. Nicaise, Taylortown School of Beauty; MINNESOTA: Cosmetology Training Center, Hess Hair Milk Laboratories, Robinson Beauty School; NEBRASKA: Bahner College of Hairstyling, College of Hair Design–Karen Stroman, Joseph's College of Beauty–Judy Stewart; NEVADA: Silver State Beauty College; NEW YORK: Shear Ego Intel School of Hair Design, Wilfred American Education Corporation–Dorothy Soressi; NORTH CAROLINA: Beaufort County Community College–Sharon L. Everett, Central Carolina Community College–Linda Adams-Harris, College of Albemarle–Faye Hoffman, Edgecombe Community College, Isothermal Community College; OHIO:

Skelly Beauty Academy, Inc.; OKLAHOMA: Oklahoma Institute of Hair Design–Richard L. Jones; OREGON: Beau Monde College of Hair Design, La Grande College of Beauty & Barbering, The Dalles School of Beauty–Peggy Jennings; PENNSYLVANIA: Lancaster School of Cosmetology–Carol Micciche, Lansdale School of Cosmetology; SOUTH CAROLINA: Farah's Beauty School; TEXAS: Guthrie's Beauty College, San Jacinto College, North–G. Pat Hark, Shear Cuts Beauty Academy–Shirley A. White; VIRGINA: Potomac Academy; WASHINGTON: Karen's Beauty School, Shoreline Community College; WEST VIRGINIA: Parkersburg Beauty College.

Special Report: Ecology in the Salon

Theory Objectives

1. List ecologically sound practices that can be put into effect in the salon.
2. List resource conservation practices that can be put into effect in the salon.

Introduction

The **environment** around us—the air we breath, the water we drink, the food we eat—is being threatened by the chemicals we use and the trash we put in our garbage cans. Ideally, anything we put into the trash should be biodegradable. **Biodegradable** products decompose (break down) through natural decaying processes. If they are discarded in a landfill, biodegradable products become part of the soil as a natural process. Plants can grow in this soil without absorbing harmful chemicals from the trash. If the trash is not biodegradable, it may not decompose at all, or even worse it may break down into harmful elements that contaminate (pollute) the soil and are absorbed by plants.

All of us should be concerned with how fast our landfills are filling with garbage. We are soon going to run out of places to put our trash. We should also be concerned with what kind of trash we are putting there, since some of it is contaminating not only the soil where we grow our food, but also the rivers and underground aquifers (underground lakes) that give us drinking water.

Theory Objective 1
Ecological Practices in the Salon

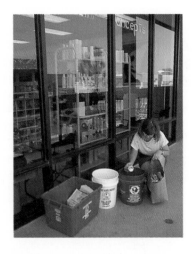

Despite the concern about **ecology** (the science that studies the relationship of living things to each other and to their environment), science and technology cannot immediately solve all the problems threatening our *environment*. It takes time to develop substitutes for some of the professional products used in the home, school, and salon. While long-term solutions are being sought, however, cosmetologists can do some things to slow down the landfill and air-quality problems:

- Separate your aluminum cans, glass, plastic, and newspapers into individual paper bags for **recycling** (reuse).
- Mix chemicals, such as those for hair coloring, accurately. Mix only the amount needed for the hair length of the client. It is better to mix a little more if you need it than to mix too much at the beginning of the service.
- Use **nonaerosol,** pump-type hair sprays.

- Drink from reusable, easily sanitized cups rather than plastic or styrofoam ones.

- Use sanitized cloth neck strips that can be relaundered rather than the disposable type.

- Purchase products such as shampoo in larger rather than smaller containers—for example, quart, gallon, or even 5-gallon (liter, 4-liter, or 20-liter) containers. Use metered pumps for dispensing products.

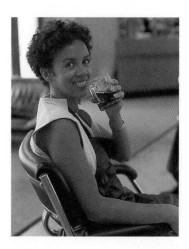

- Request products that are packaged in **recycled** paper. Use paper bags for selling retail items, and avoid plastic bags unless they are the **recyclable** type.

- Request synthetic, biodegradable products when possible, instead of plastic or animal-derivative products.

- Use cardboard displays rather than plastic ones (unless the plastic is recyclable).

- Select implements that can be reused and easily sanitized.

- Purchase containers made from recyclable plastic.

- Use only enough of a product to complete your service.

- Eliminate wasteful practices.

- To protect yourself as well as the clients you serve, learn as much about the chemicals and products that you use as is practically possible. In the United States, ask your supplier for the Materials Safety Data Sheet (MSDS), which describes the safe use, toxicity, and safe disposal of products used in schools and salons. In Canada, ask for the Workplace Hazard Materials Information Standards (WHMIS) Sheet for the same type of information.

Theory Objective 2
Resource Conservation
Practices in the Salon

As cosmetologists, you can do your part to conserve energy and water by following these practices:

- If the client's hair dries faster than you expected under the hair dryer, turn off the timer so that the dryer will stop running.

- To conserve electricity, unplug thermal irons when they won't be used for long periods of time. Remember to turn them off at night.

- To conserve water, put an aerator on the nozzle of your shampoo hose; with the aerator, you will use half as much

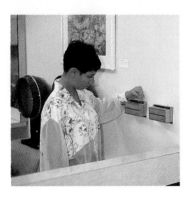

water pressure when giving services at the shampoo bowl. (Also, leave the nozzle of the hose resting against the drain basket so that any water left in the hose will go down the drain rather than onto the floor.)

- Place a brick in the reservoir tank of the toilet(s) to limit the amount of water flushed down the drain, or use a toilet designed to save water.
- Use high-efficiency, energy-saving water heater.
- Use a high-efficiency, energy-saving lighting (fluorescent) where possible.
- Where practical, use room air conditioners rather than central air conditioning to put the cool air only where you need it.
- Where practical, use lower heat settings and higher cooling settings to conserve energy.

Glossary

Biodegradable Capable of decomposing (breaking down) through natural decaying processes.

Ecology The science of the relationship of living things to each other and to their surroundings (their environment).

Environment The surroundings of living things, such as the air and water.

Nonaerosol hair spray A hair spray that has a pump instead of a gas propellant.

Recyclable A product that can be broken down into its original materials, which then can be reused.

Recycle To break down a product into its original materials and then reuse those materials.

Questions

1. Are styrofoam cups biodegradable?
2. Can aluminum cans be recycled?
3. What is a landfill?
4. What is the environment?
5. List four ecological practices for the salon.
6. List four resource conservation practices that can be used in the salon.
7. What type of water heater should be used?

8. Where practical, what type of lighting should be used in the salon?
9. Can glass and paper be recycled?
10. From an ecological standpoint, what is the best way to dispense hair spray?

FOURTH EDITION*

The Professional Cosmetologist

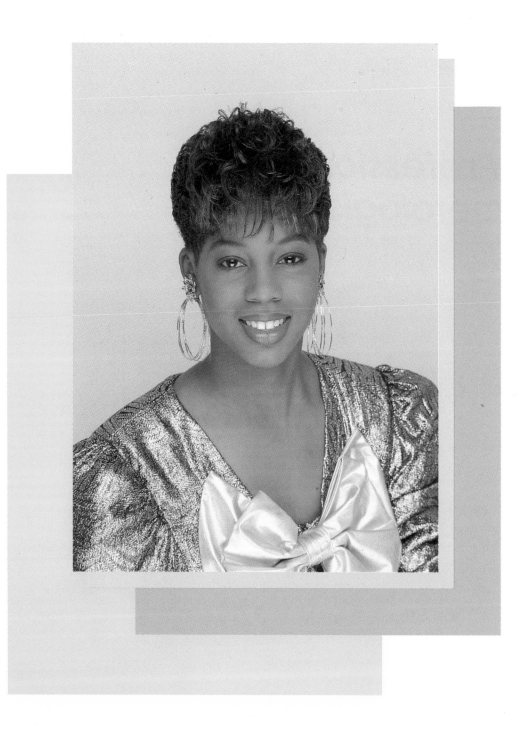

Careers in Cosmetology

General Requirements

Several personal grooming and hygiene practices are especially desirable for all people working in cosmetology. Some of them might seem rather obvious, but you should keep them in mind.

Personal Grooming

Personal grooming refers to one's daily appearance and cleanliness (Figure 1.1). Your clothing should be freshly laundered, your shoes should be polished, your nails should be neatly manicured, your

Figure 1.1
Personal grooming and hygiene are particularly important for a cosmetologist.

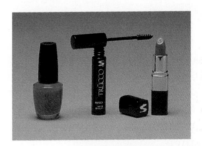

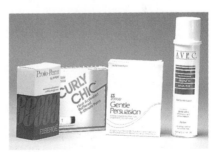

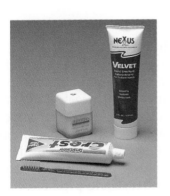

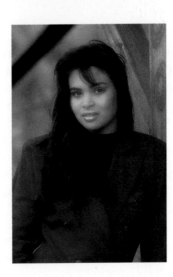

As a beginning student in cosmetology, you have probably thought about your career as something in the distant future. Actually that career is not very far away. You have already taken the first step, and before you know it, a wide range of exciting and challenging opportunities will be yours.

Cosmetology is the art and science of beauty care. A person who is licensed to perform these services is a **cosmetologist.** One of a cluster of health-related occupations, cosmetology involves care of the skin, hair, scalp, and nails. Because cosmetology is both an art and a science—as well as a business—it offers a particularly wide variety of opportunities. If you have a flair for the artistic, you will be able to find positions that emphasize this kind of skill. Many business opportunities are also available to experienced cosmetologists. As a beginning student, you may not be thinking far ahead, but knowing what opportunities are available if you wish to advance may help you start planning for the future.

This chapter explains the basic requirements for different careers in cosmetology and offers a number of suggestions that will help to make your student life successful. Figure 1.2 lists some of the career options available to you and shows how they may lead to higher positions.

skin should be properly cleansed and cared for, and your hair should be arranged neatly. Cosmetologists deal directly with the public every day, and an attractive appearance is very important. Although people shouldn't be judged by appearances, the fact remains that they often are. First impressions can be powerful and are difficult to change.

Personal Hygiene

Maintaining an effective daily **personal hygiene** schedule is as important to you as it is to your clients. You probably know about the basic elements of personal hygiene, such as bathing or showering, brushing and flossing your teeth, and using a mouthwash every day to prevent **halitosis** (hal-eh-TOH-siss), or bad breath. However, there are other aspects of personal hygiene that many people do not practice. They are very important, and you should remember them. A good place to start is with this working definition of personal hygiene: the daily routine you follow to preserve and promote your health.

Nutrition. In these days of fast-food restaurants, we often fail to eat properly. We have a cup of coffee and a roll for breakfast, grab a

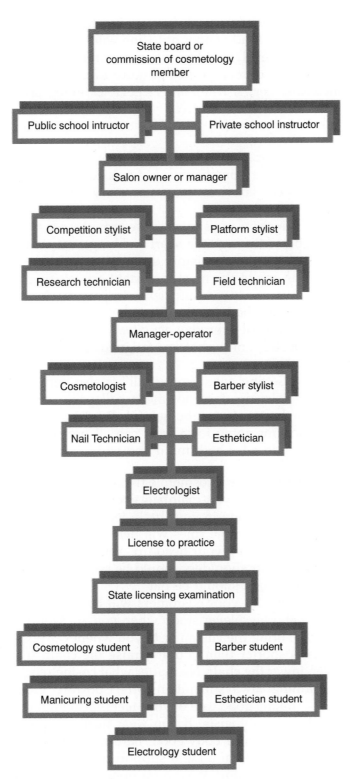

Figure 1.2
*Careers in cosmetology
provide many opportunities for
advancement.*

State board or
commission of cosmetology
member

Public school intructor

Private school instructor

Salon owner or manager

Competition stylist

Platform stylist

Research technician

Field technician

Manager-operator

Cosmetologist

Barber stylist

Nail Technician

Esthetician

Electrologist

License to practice

State licensing examination

Cosmetology student

Barber student

Manicuring student

Esthetician student

Electrology student

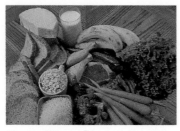

Figure 1.3
Eat a balanced diet.

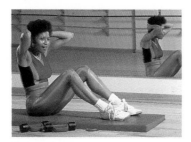

Figure 1.4
Exercise is important.

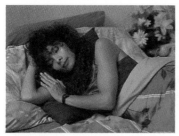

Figure 1.5
Do you get enough sleep?

cheeseburger and french fries for lunch, and have fried chicken for dinner. This kind of poor **nutrition** will keep you from performing at your peak level. Good nutrition depends on the **balance** as well as the **amount** of food you eat (Figure 1.3). Eating a proper balance of meat, fish, eggs, fruits and vegetables, milk, and cereal daily will make you look better, feel better, and work better. If you are uncertain about your diet, ask your doctor or a nutritionist.

Exercise, Sleep, and Relaxation.   There is nothing wrong with working hard, but sometimes we work too hard. Exercise, sufficient sleep, and relaxation are as necessary as work for a healthy (and happy) life.

Vigorous physical exercise provides a fast, continuous pumping of blood through the heart and lungs, refreshing the entire body and keeping the circulatory system in good working order (Figure 1.4). It is one of the most important aspects of good health.

We also need sufficient sleep and relaxation for both our mind and our body's sake. Sleep helps relieve us of the frustrations and tensions of everyday activity. Most of us need seven or eight hours of sleep, or we become fatigued and cannot function properly (Figure 1.5).

"Getting away from it all" is also very important for good health. Relaxing does not mean collapsing into a deep sleep, although short naps can be helpful. Reading a good book, watching television, or going for a walk can all provide the change of pace necessary to relax both mind and body.

Good Posture.   As a cosmetologist, you will be on your feet much of the time. Unless you maintain good body **posture,** you will feel a great deal of strain in your back, legs, and feet.

A few simple rules will help you to maintain good posture (Figure 1.6). Keep your head up. Your chin should be parallel with the floor. Your shoulders should be relaxed, and your stomach and lower abdomen should be flat.

Some of your customers will be taller than you are; others will be shorter. Never stoop when you are working. Keep this rule in mind: bring the customer to you whenever possible. If your customer is shorter than you are, **raise the chair.** If your customer is taller, **lower the chair.** No matter what cosmetology services you are performing, always maintain correct posture, erect but relaxed.

Taking good care of your feet is also important, especially for female cosmetologists. If you wear heels, they should be low and broad to give your body good, natural support. High, skinny heels will cause foot strain. Light support hosiery can also provide added support and comfort. Wearing support hosiery now may also prevent or reduce future problems with your legs. If you have any special problems, consult a foot doctor.

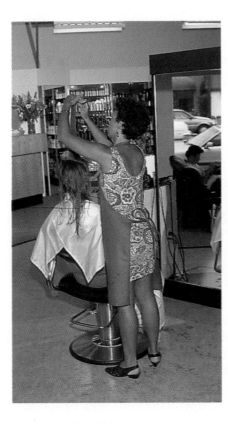
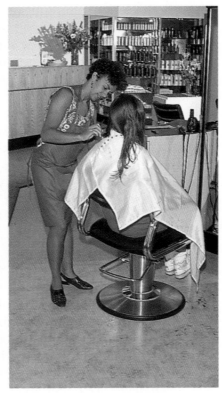

Figure 1.6
How is your posture?

Communicating with Others

Because careers in cosmetology are people-oriented, they require good communications skills—the ability to convey one's thoughts and attitudes in a pleasant manner, both verbally and nonverbally.

Verbal Communication. **Verbal communication** involves what is said and how it is said. A client will always appreciate a courteous response or question and will always resent an impolitely phrased one (Figure 1.7). But **verbal communication concerns how** you say something as well as **what** you say. A cheerful tone and proper inflection (emphasis) in your voice let a client know that you are enthusiastic and ready to help. A cheerful voice is important on the telephone, too. Also remember to speak distinctly so that the client has no trouble understanding you. Being careful about your verbal communications doesn't cost a thing, and it often means the difference between success and failure.

Nonverbal Communication. Imagine walking up to a counter in a store where two clerks are standing. One slinks over to you, slouches, looks all around the store, and then finally asks you what you want. The other walks directly over to you, stands erect but relaxed, looks you straight in the eye, and asks the same question.

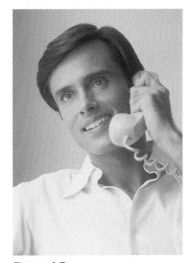

Figure 1.7
Verbal communications are very important for a successful salon.

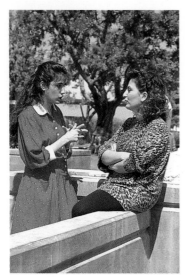

Figure 1.8
*Body language communicates
an attitude.*

Both clerks communicated an attitude to you before they spoke a word. You probably felt that the first clerk couldn't care less and that the second clerk was interested in serving you. Yet they may have said exactly the same words in the same tone of voice. The first clerk, in fact, may even have been more anxious to serve you than the second clerk, but didn't communicate that attitude.

This is an important point to remember. Nonverbal communication, sometimes called **body language,** tells a client that you are interested even before you speak (Figure 1.8). Much of **nonverbal communication involves being a good listener.** Eye contact is also very important. By looking directly at the client when you are speaking and listening, you show that you are interested in what he or she has to say.

Requirements for a Student

Although a person usually can enter a cosmetology program at any age, most state boards (or commissions) of cosmetology (or beauty culture) require that a student be sixteen or seventeen years old before applying for the state's written and demonstration examinations. But, remember, your state's requirements may be different.

Whatever your age, you will be well on your way to success as a student and, later, as a cosmetologist if you develop the personal qualities of dependability, reliability, and congeniality (getting along with people) (Figure 1.9).

Educational requirements vary from state to state, but generally a student must have at least an eighth-grade education. Although courses in science (anatomy, physiology, chemistry, biology), business (economics, accounting, law), psychology, and art are not required, they are helpful. Additional education, later in life as well as now, is often needed to progress.

If you cannot meet the financial requirements of a cosmetology student, ask your instructor for information on how to obtain financial aid. Remember that cosmetology students cannot earn money, except tips, from their experience in a school or salon.

Health Requirements

You may be required to have a complete physical examination by a doctor before you are accepted as a student. In addition, it is good practice to have a checkup every six months. Be sure to ask your doctor to examine you for allergic reactions and color blindness.

Since cosmetologists should not work when they have a contagious disease such as influenza or strep throat, it is important to **stay healthy.** Be sure to consult your doctor whenever you are in doubt about your health.

Allergies. You will be exposed to cosmetic products, such as shampoo, makeup, lipstick, hair spray, and the like. People who are extremely sensitive to cosmetics may suffer **allergies,** or severe reactions, to them or become ill if they breathe the fumes from cosmetics in a beauty salon or school.

Cosmetologists are more concerned about allergies than the average person. Ask your doctor to watch for any problems in this area. Being alert to signs of trouble is especially important since you can develop an allergy suddenly, even though you have never had one in the past.

Color Blindness. **Color blindness** is the partial or total inability to see colors. Some types of color blindness will keep a person from becoming a cosmetologist. While blindness to red and green is permitted, blindness to browns and blonds could keep the student from performing hair coloring tasks. You can be tested for color blindness by your family eye doctor (see Figure 1.10).

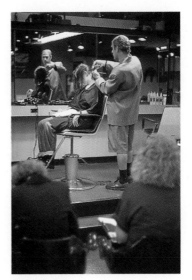

Figure 1.9
All cosmetology students should develop the ability to get along well with people.

Requirements for a Licensed or Registered Cosmetologist

A licensed or registered cosmetologist has successfully completed the written and practical examinations given by the state. Various terms are used to describe this person, including the following:

- Licensed Cosmetologist, L.C.
- Registered Cosmetologist, R.C.
- Registered Beauty Culturist, R.B.C.
- Hairstylist
- Operator
- Coiffeur (male cosmetologist)
- Coiffeuse (female cosmetologist)
- Hairdresser
- Beautician

Hair fashions change as rapidly as clothing fashions. Thus, most cosmetologists find it necessary to attend local workshops and seminars to keep pace with the ever-changing hairstyles and new products and techniques. These seminars are sponsored by **Hair America (Official Hair Fashion Committee),** which is the educational arm of the **National Cosmetologists Association.** Private and public cosmetology schools also offer seminars that should be attended whenever possible. Full-service beauty supply dealers and manufacturers also conduct educational seminars that feature current hairstyling techniques and new products.

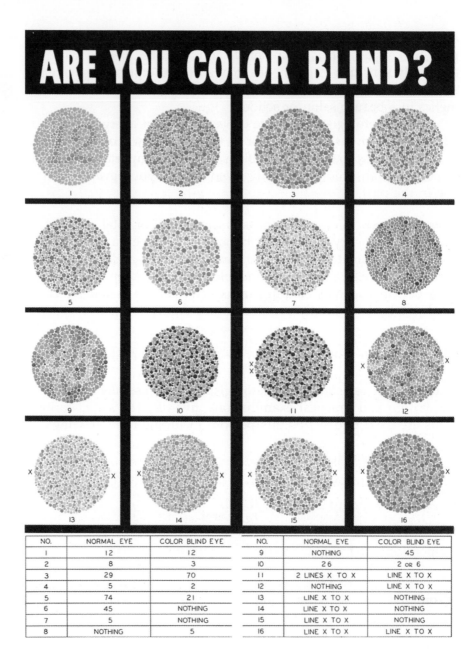

Figure 1.10
Color blindness chart.

NO.	NORMAL EYE	COLOR BLIND EYE	NO.	NORMAL EYE	COLOR BLIND EYE
1	12	12	9	NOTHING	45
2	8	3	10	26	2 OR 6
3	29	70	11	2 LINES X TO X	LINE X TO X
4	5	2	12	NOTHING	LINE X TO X
5	74	21	13	LINE X TO X	NOTHING
6	45	NOTHING	14	LINE X TO X	NOTHING
7	5	NOTHING	15	LINE X TO X	NOTHING
8	NOTHING	5	16	LINE X TO X	LINE X TO X

Guarantee

Experienced cosmetologists earn money in proportion to the volume
and type of services they render for their clientele. New graduates,
however, have not developed a clientele yet, so they are paid the
minimum hourly wage required by the state or federal **minimum
wage law.** The amount of money the salon owner **must** pay full-time
employees (those who work **40 hours per week**) is sometimes referred to as the "**guarantee.**"

For example, suppose you are a newly licensed cosmetologist who begins working for My Fair Lady Beauty Salon as a full-time employee. You can expect to make the minimum wage times 40 hours per week. If the minimum wage is $6 per hour, therefore, you would earn $240 per week ($6 × 40 hours).

The weekly rate of $240 will continue until your yearly receipts (the amount you earn for the salon) double. To put this another way, the salon owner's break-even point occurs when the amount of money a new employee brings in for services is twice as much as the employee is being paid at an hourly rate. Thus, in our example, you would have to bring $480 (2 × $240) into the salon. Until you bring in $480 per week, the salon owner is losing money. This is true because you must be paid the $240 whether you have five clients, ten clients, or no clients at all. Oftentimes, if an employee has not developed a basic clientele in three to six months, he or she should consider additional training or employment in a different salon.

Commission

An experienced hairdresser with an established clientele usually receives a **commission,** which is a percentage (%) of the money the salon takes in for the services performed by the employee. For example, if you agreed to work in the salon for a 50 percent commission and brought in $600 during the week, your commission would be $300 (0.50 × $600) less all taxes.

The usual job steps for the newly licensed hairdresser are to (1) work in a salon for the minimum wage, or guarantee, and then (2) develop a clientele. When the services the employee performs bring in twice as much money as the guarantee, he or she receives a commission on the amount that is over the guarantee.

As an operator's clientele increases, it is reasonably easy to exceed the base pay. As with other jobs, skills and salesmanship in cosmetology increase with experience, producing a larger clientele over time.

Barber Stylist

A **barber stylist** is a person who has graduated from an approved school of barbering and successfully passed a licensing test. The duties of a barber stylist are difficult to define because the laws regulating this practice vary from state to state. For example, some states license barbers and cosmetologists together. Other states have a "crossover" licensing arrangement that permits a licensed barber or cosmetologist to obtain the other license with a minimum of additional schooling or, in some cases, none at all. In one state, a barber stylist is not licensed to give permanent waves or manicures. Nevertheless, the tendency does seem to be toward the merging of barbering and cosmetology licensing, and this trend will probably continue over the next ten years. The term **tonsorial,** which means pertaining to barbering, is sometimes used in reference to barber stylists.

Manicurist (Nail Technician)

The manicuring business is more popular today than it has ever been (Figure 1.11). Many states have a separate license for **manicurists.** Manicuring became "big business" with the introduction of new products and services to strengthen and beautify the fingernails and, in some cases, the toenails. Nail wrapping and the application of artificial nails have been added to the services offered in beauty salons and also in some barber salons (where permitted by law). In many states, manicuring salons are licensed as separate and different businesses from beauty salons.

Esthetician

Esthetics involves the **preservation** and **beautification of the skin on the face and neck.** It is becoming a very lucrative business due to today's emphasis on looking young. Esthetics involves the use of specially formulated products, vitamins, facial procedures, and facial appliances to clean, stimulate, and preserve the texture of the skin. Facial salons have been successful in many parts of the country. A practitioner of esthetics is called an **esthetician.**

Figure 1.11
Manicuring has become "big business" today.

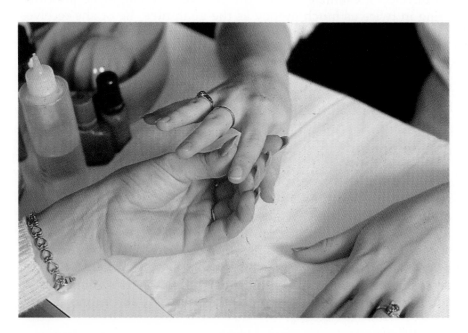

Electrologist

In **electrology,** electrical current traveling through a very fine needle is used to **remove unwanted facial and body hair permanently.** A practitioner of electrology is called an **electrologist.** Licensing laws vary considerably from state to state, and some states do not license electrologists at all. With the ongoing concern about consumer protection, it seems likely that more and more states will license electrologists to ensure that the consumer (client) will receive a service from a competent and trained electrologist. Currently, electrology is usually taught by the manufacturer rather than a licensed cosmetology school.

Research and Field Technicians

A **research technician** works for a cosmetics manufacturer, usually in the research salon, testing new products for quality, safety, and marketability (Figure 1.12). The research technician's clients are persons who come into the salon for *free* services. They are required to sign release forms because of the experimental nature of those services.

    Field technicians travel extensively throughout an area (one or several states) to demonstrate a manufacturer's products in salons, schools, and educational seminars.

    Research and field technicians must be of legal age, eighteen to twenty-one years old, depending on the state in which they work. In addition to being mature, poised, and observant, they should be able to speak effectively before small or large groups of people.

    Most state laws require that any technician who is practicing cosmetic sciences on another living person must be a licensed or registered cosmetologist or an instructor. Manufacturers may also require one or two years of experience in a salon.

    The base salary for both a research technician and a field technician is usually between the salary of the average salon operator and that of a manager-operator in a given area. A research technician's salary is usually increased at six-month intervals, while raises for field technicians are often part of a bonus program that is based on increases in the dollar volume of sales. The field technician's traveling expenses are also paid by the company.

Competition and Platform Hairstylists

Hairstylists who have a creative flair and enjoy the challenge of competing or performing before large audiences often become **competition** or **platform hairstylists** in addition to working in a salon (Figure 1.13).

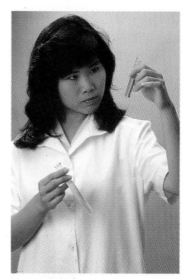

Figure 1.12
The research technician does experimental work.

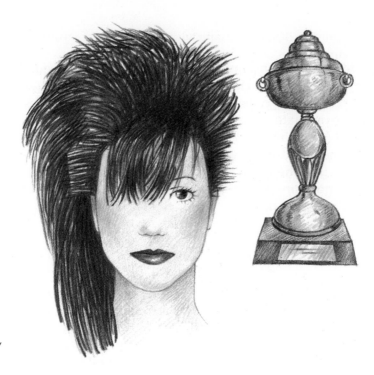

Figure 1.13
Those with a creative flair may enjoy competition hairstyling.

A hairstyling contest is an event in which cosmetologists challenge each other's hairdressing skills. Hairstylists are judged on the basis of several qualities:

- Originality
- Execution
- Adaptability
- Trend

Originality refers to the general design of the style. **Execution** refers to how well the design was set and combed into the hair. **Adaptability** refers to the suitability of the hairstyle: did the hairstyle improve the appearance of the model? **Trend** is the basic silhouette and design from which the contestants work. Most contests have specific rules of their own that are distributed before each contest.

Contests are sponsored by the National Cosmetologists Association or one of its local affiliates as well as by manufacturers and beauty supply dealers. Newly licensed or registered cosmetologists enter contests along with very experienced practitioners. Many contests also encourage student participation on the local, state, and national levels.

Trophies, plaques, cups, and cash prizes are awarded. Many different types of contests are available: student, novice, and women's daytime, evening, and fantasy hairstyling as well as air waving and men's hairstyling.

Cosmetologists who repeatedly win these contests are often offered jobs as platform hairstylists, which means they conduct hairstyling demonstrations at educational seminars for manufacturers. These seminars usually take place on Sundays and Mondays in the fall and spring. The audience can vary in size from five to two hundred persons. Platform artists are paid a daily rate in addition to all expenses for travel, meals, and lodging. Favorable publicity can help increase the platform stylist's clientele.

Manager-Operator

In some salons, the **manager-operator** merely supervises the work of other operators, while in others he or she also serves clients. In either case, the manager-operator usually must be legally an adult and have obtained a manager-operator's license from the state board (commission) of cosmetology. Licensing requirements vary from state to state.

A manager-operator needs several special skills. In addition to being a registered cosmetologist who has a basic education and is skilled in all of the salon's basic services, the effective manager of an average-size salon (three or four operators) should have two or three years' work experience. He or she should also be able to assist the owner in managing the salon. Having the personality and the patience to supervise workers is an essential characteristic. Bookkeeping training and knowledge of other management tasks, such as purchasing supplies, can be helpful; attending management seminars on the MBO (management by objectives) system can be a good way to acquire management skills.

The pay range for a manager-operator varies from salon to salon. Some of the usual methods of compensation are (1) an additional weekly commission of 5 percent over the operator's commission (for a total of 55 percent); (2) an additional commission of 5 percent at the end of the year; or (3) an additional percentage above the total dollar figure for the salon.

The knowledge and experience that a manager-operator gains can prepare him or her for salon ownership.

Salon Owner

A **salon owner** usually is a working cosmetologist who has developed **business skills** as well as professional cosmetology skills (Figure 1.14). He or she should be an expert technician who has developed a large clientele and should also possess the personal

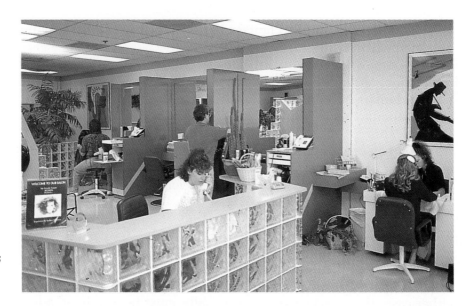

Figure 1.14
A successful salon owner earns more in the long run than an operator.

qualities necessary for dealing with a wide variety of customers and employees.

Although a person can become a salon owner as soon as he or she is legally an adult, most salon owners have had at least one year's experience as a manager-operator. Such experience is invaluable for operating one's own business—for everything from advertising to bookkeeping. In addition, an owner is wise to take advantage of educational opportunities such as seminars on management and staff-training programs.

The working salon owner gets a 58 percent commission on the work he or she performs. (This percentage equals the operator's 50 percent plus, the manager-operator's 5 percent plus another 3 percent.) The money leftover after expenses have been paid is the owner's profit. The owner takes all of the financial risk and must have an excellent credit rating plus enough money (capital) to make down payments for the purchase of supplies, equipment, and salaries to open the salon. In the long run, a successful owner makes more money than an operator.

Public and Private School Instructors

Instructors are licensed, registered, or certified to teach by the state board (commission) of cosmetology and the state's department of education. Some state departments of education require college courses, including human relations, philosophy of vocational education, teaching methods and practices, tests and measurements, and course construction. State boards (commissions) of cosmetology require successful completion of a written and practical exam. Some

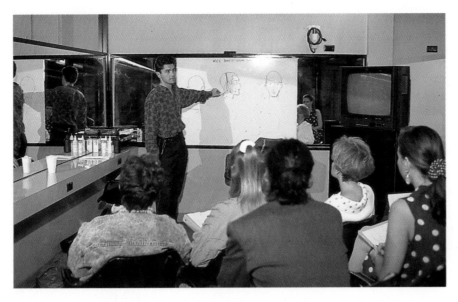

Figure 1.15
An instructor should have an interest in students as individuals.

states require instructors to take yearly physicals. The instructor is generally an expert in most aspects of cosmetology. Age requirements vary from state to state.

The successful instructor has exceptional patience and an interest in students as individuals and potential professionals (Figure 1.15). At times an instructor will have to function as a counselor, friend, or even parent to students.

Preparing a Resumé

Whatever cosmetology career field you choose, you will need a **resumé**—a document that provides an overview of your education and a brief summary of your professional qualifications and experience.

Therefore we will briefly examine the elements of an effective resumé and cover letter. A sample cover letter and resumé appear in Figures 1.16 and 1.17.

Elements of a Resumé

There is no single ideal format for a resumé, simply because the likes and dislikes of potential employers vary considerably. One employer may want a complete, precise history of your entire life. Another may be bored by all that and want just a brief outline of your experience in the industry. Another may be more interested in your appearance or your technical ability and will not even look at your resumé. Nevertheless, there are some guidelines for preparing an effective resumé. Keep in mind that the purpose of a resumé is to gain a personal interview.

October 14, 1992

Sam Tabrucko
My Fair Lady Beauty Salon
827 Belmont Avenue
Center City, AR 71805

Mr.Tabrucko:

Debi Sandstrom, one of your stylists at your Countryside Mall salon told me that you will soon be hiring stylists for your new salon that will be opening in Timberbrook Center. Because I am currently located only eight blocks from Timberbrook and have been looking for an opportunity to join your organization for the past year, I would like to introduce myself.

As the enclosed resumé indicates, I have had only a year and a half of on-the-job experience. However, as you will note, besides having graduated from the most prestigious cosmetology school in the area, I have had extensive advanced training in all areas of this profession. Much of my advanced training, as well as my cosmetology school work, emphasized the importance of client handling and sales. I would be pleased to meet with you to demonstrate the impact that training has had on my personal sales skills.

I would be grateful if you would consider me as an applicant for a stylist position in your Timberbrook location.

Cordially,

Mary Ann Colesky

Figure 1.16
A sample cover letter.

Length.   Your personality will be reflected in the length of your resumé. You may choose to describe your education and work experiences in significant detail, or you may prefer to summarize everything in as few words as possible. Whichever method you choose, or any in between, it is important to include a **cover letter** that provides a brief synopsis of your experience and education.

Completeness.   Most employers will check carefully to discover any "holes" or irregularities in your employment record. If you were out of work for six months at one point, or had five jobs in two years, or changed your residence several times in a short span, an alert employer may suspect that something is amiss. If you do not include an explanation of such discrepancies in your resumé, you should be prepared to respond to possible questions.

Contents.   The resumé should include the following features:

1. **Vital statistics.** Include your name, address, and telephone number.

2. **Educational background.** Primary emphasis should be placed on any postsecondary education you may have had with a focus on your training in the area in which you want to work. For example, the resumé in Figure 1.17 was prepared by a woman who is looking for a job as a hairstylist.

3. **Past experience.** Include all the jobs you've had in the past, not just those connected with the industry in which you want to work. That experience should receive the most emphasis,

Figure 1.17
A sample resumé.

Resumé
Mary Ann Colesky
2781 Timberbrook Court
Center City, AR 71805
(668) 555-2210

Education
Secondary–Graduate of Ames High School
Postsecondary–Arizona Community College (one year)
High Prestige Beauty College–Graduated 1985
Advanced Classes and Courses
   Michael Cole's SET Training (1985)
   Scruples Advance Perm Class (1985)
   Scruples Color Class (1986)
   Scoey Mitchell Sales Course (1986)
   Color Line Color Class (1986)

Previous Employment
Divine Hair (November 1986–Current)
   Duties: Hairstylist, color consultant, assistant manager, in charge of
      merchandising lobby
Hair by Joe Salon (November 1985–November 1986)
   Duties: Hairstylist in charge of retail products, activating inactives,
      assistant to the station merchandiser
The Dill Pickle (Novermber 1982–August 1984)
   Duties: waitress, hostess, assistant manager

References
Dan Shabo, Instructor
High Prestige Beauty College
2172 Apple Street
Dorington, AR 71302
(688) 555-7227

Sylvia Bodacious, Manager
Hair by Joe Salon
1672 Grand Avenue
Dorington, AR 71302
(688) 555-2121

Obidia Spindel, Owner
Divine Hair
210 Center Street
Center City, AR 78105
(688) 555-8888

Please feel free to contact any of these people concerning this resumé.

however. List your most recent job first. In addition to the name of the place where you worked, you should also describe any special duties you were required to perform (i.e., color consultant, new-stylist orientation, inventory control, assistant manager, and so forth).

4. **References.** Include the names of three **references**—people who have given you permission to use their names in your resumé. Be sure to give the current address and telephone number for each of your references. You should also include a statement giving the potential employer permission to contact these people. Some resumés even contain letters of recommendation from the references. Immediate family members should not be used as references.

5. **Cover letter.** The cover letter may be your only opportunity to impress the employer. Consequently, a letter that is short, to the point, interesting, and assertive may give you an advantage. The cover letter should highlight the quality of your training and experience along with a brief statement of your career goals and how they seem to fit the job opportunity the employer has available. Although you may send the same resumé to several potential employers, you should write a new cover letter for each job for which you apply; each letter should explain how you meet the specific requirements of that particular employer.

Neatness and Accuracy.   Neatness counts. Resumés should always be neatly typed and carefully checked to be sure that they do not contain spelling or grammatical errors. Some employers automatically eliminate any resumés that have even the most minute flaw. Although you may not choose to go to the extreme of having your resumé typeset and keylined, bear in mind that employers often believe that the quality of your work as a cosmetologist is reflected in the way you prepare your resumé.

What to Avoid.   Your resumé should not specifically mention your sex, race, creed, religion, national origin, age, or marital status. Many employers will not even accept a resumé that includes such information because of the potential for civil rights action.

Glossary

Allergy Extreme sensitivity to a factor or substance in the environment.

Barber stylist A person who has graduated from an approved school of barbering and successfully passed a licensing test.

Body language Communication through eye contact, facial expression, posture, and other nonverbal means.

Color blindness A partial or total inability to see or differentiate colors.

Commission A percentage of the money taken into the salon for the services performed by the employee.

Competition hairstylist A hairstylist who enters hairstyling contests to win trophies, plaques, cups, or cash prizes.

Cosmetologist A person licensed to perform the services of cosmetology or beauty culture.

Cosmetology The art and science of beauty care involving care of the skin, hair, scalp, and nails.

Cover letter A brief synopsis of your experience and education, to be used with a resumé.

Electrology The removal of unwanted facial and body hair by electric current. A practitioner of electrology is called an **electrologist.**

Esthetics The preservation and beautification of the skin of the face and neck. A practitioner of esthetics is called an **esthetician.**

Field technician A cosmetologist who travels extensively throughout an area to demonstrate a manufacturer's products in salons, schools, and educational seminars.

Guarantee The amount of money a salon owner must pay a full-time employee; it is governed by the state or federal minimum wage law.

Halitosis (hal-eh-TOH-siss) Stale or foul-smelling breath.

Instructors Persons who are licensed, registered, or certified to teach cosmetology by the state board or commission of cosmetology and the state's department of education.

Manager-operator A person of legal age who is a registered cosmetologist and who is licensed to manage and operate a salon.

Manicurist (nail technician) A practitioner who specializes in the care of hands and fingernails; sometimes feet and toenails are included.

Nonverbal communication Communication of one's thoughts and attitudes without words; the use of body language.

Nutrition The process of maintaining good health by eating a balanced diet and the proper amount of food.

Personal hygiene The daily routine followed to preserve and promote one's health.

Platform hairstylist A hairstylist who is paid to conduct demonstrations before an audience, such as at educational seminars.

Posture The way you hold your body. In good posture, the head is up, the chin is level with the floor, the shoulders are relaxed, and the stomach and lower abdomen are flat.

References Persons listed in your resumé who have agreed to comment on your qualifications and work experience.

Research technician A cosmetologist who works for a cosmetics manufacturer testing new products and comparing them to determine their quality, safety, and marketability.

Resumé A document that provides an overview of your educational and professional qualifications and experience.

Salon owner A working cosmetologist who has developed business as well as professional skills and owns a beauty salon.

Tonsorial Pertaining to barbering; a barber is a tonsorial artist.

Verbal communication Communication of thoughts and attitudes through spoken words and through the tone and inflection used in speaking.

Questions

1. Define cosmetology.
2. Name three general areas in which the cosmetologist is licensed to perform services.
3. Define personal hygiene.
4. Does good posture have anything to do with taking care of your feet?
5. What is it called when a client has a reaction to a cosmetic product used in the salon?
6. According to law, what is the least amount of money that a full-time beginning cosmetologist can be paid?
7. To be considered a full-time employee, how many hours per week must you work?
8. What term is used for a licensed person who specializes in the preservation and beautification of the skin of the face and neck?
9. What is the technical name for the person who permanently removes hair using an electrical device?
10. What is halitosis?
11. What document goes with a resumé?
12. Is it necessary to get permission to list a person as a reference?
13. Should your age be given in a resumé?

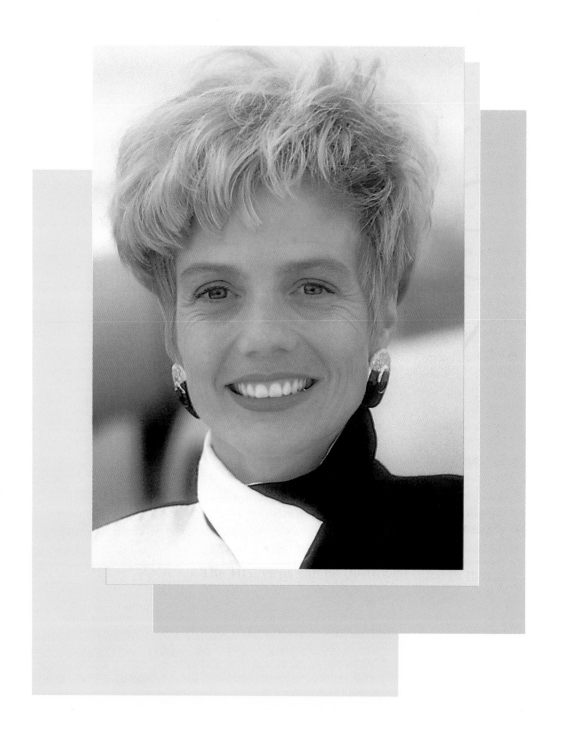

Ethics in Cosmetology

Professional Ethics

Professions usually have boards or commissions that establish **codes of ethics. Professional ethics** are systems of rules that tell professionals how they should act when they offer their skills to the public. The boards or commissions may function on a state or national level, or both (as in the case of the state and national bar associations and medical associations). The codes apply to all members of a profession. Thus, as a cosmetologist, you should be familiar with the code of ethics established by the cosmetology boards or commissions in your state. You should always comply with your state's laws and regulations.

Professionals have special knowledge and skills that their clients do not have (Figure 2.1). Therefore, in a sense, members of the general public are at the mercy of the professionals from whom they seek services. A code of ethics not only protects the public but also helps the professionals to whom it applies, since it gives the public a reason to have faith in that profession.

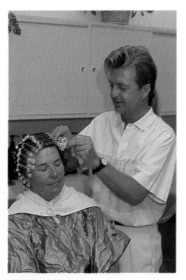

Figure 2.1
Ethical behavior means that you do not undertake to perform a service unless you can do it competently.

Applying Professional Ethics to Cosmetology

Your client will expect three things from you as a professional cosmetologist. The first is **competence.** Your client will expect you to have the necessary knowledge and skill to provide services effectively. Since cosmetology is a fast-moving profession, you will need to add to the information you learned as a student (Figure 2.2). What was a new style five years ago might not even be used today. The best product in today's market might be considered hopelessly old-fashioned ten years from now. Or five years from now, scientists may discover that a chemical that they thought was safe has harmful side effects. Thus, you must keep up with advances in cosmetology.

Just think how difficult life would be if you couldn't trust anyone! You can buy a burglar alarm to protect your house from robbers and count your change in the store to be sure that the cashier doesn't shortchange you. But how can you make sure your doctor will give you the best medical treatment possible, or that the pilot will do a good job of flying the plane that you are on? At one time or another, all of us need to have faith that other people will act **ethically,** that is, **honestly** and with **good intentions.**

Ethical behavior involves voluntary acts performed in a climate of knowledge and freedom of choice. You may have heard people say that someone has followed the "letter of the law" but not the "spirit of the law." Such a person has not behaved ethically. In practice, **ethics** means that when you choose to perform a service for a client, you should make sure you have the knowledge and skill to perform it properly.

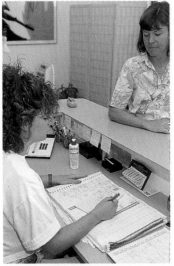

Figure 2.2
To remain competent, a cosmetologist should keep up with new techniques and products.

Indeed, by presenting yourself as a professional cosmetologist, you are saying that your knowledge and skills are up-to-date.

Secondly, your clients will expect you to have a sense of **responsibility.** This can be expressed as the Golden Rule: Do unto others as you would have them do unto you. You want people to be reliable and to have integrity in dealing with you, so you should do the same for your clients. Be honest with them, and have a sincere concern for their welfare.

Your clients will also expect you to enjoy **working with the public.** This expectation requires dedication and discipline. "The customer is always right" is one way of expressing dedication, but it might be even more important to think of your client as your friend. If your friend were "in a pinch" and needed help or a favor at the last minute, you would do everything possible to help. You should do the same thing for a client who may need an appointment at a bad time or on short notice (Figure 2.3). Most clients will appreciate this kind of consideration and, like good friends, will be with you for a long time.

Remember, however, that being a client's friend does not mean being chatty, gossipy, or too familiar. Don't pry into your client's personal life, and if he or she mentions something personal, keep it to yourself. Being discrete is part of being a friend. Furthermore, by being a good friend to others, you will discover that you are your own best friend.

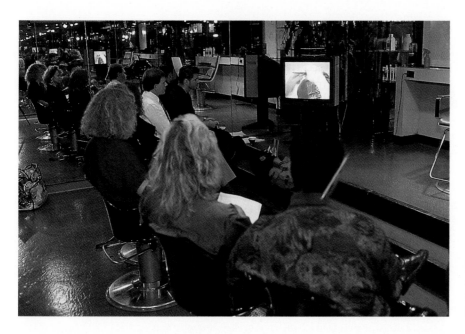

Figure 2.3
A professional will find time for a client who needs help on short notice.

The Ethical Responsibilities to the Client and Public in General

The following guidelines will help you maintain professional standards and ethics toward your clients and the general public.
Your responsibilities to clients include the following:

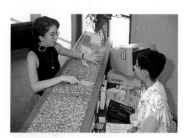

Figure 2.4
A professional will not make any unfair or unwarranted charges.

- Give a full measure of service in the best interests of the client.

- Learn new methods, accept new ideas, and always look for ways to improve techniques.

- Make no charges for services that you cannot prove by valid evidence are fair (Figure 2.4).

- Refrain from false representation of services and misleading advertising.

- Refrain from misrepresenting the type, quality, and manufacturer of products used in services.

- Give the client, where possible, the benefit of the doubt when differences of opinion arise.

- Observe the rules of public sanitation and personal hygiene set forth by law.

- Refrain from discussing with one client the type of service rendered to another.

■ Refrain from discussing with anyone personal matters confided to you by a client.

■ Never render service in such a manner that a charge of gross negligence, incompetency, or misconduct would be warranted.

You have the following **responsibilities to the general public:**

■ Place dedication to service before financial reward or other personal gain.

■ Stand ready to volunteer your special skills, knowledge, and training for the public welfare.

■ See that those admitted to the practice of cosmetology are properly qualified by character, ability, and training, and that those who thereafter prove unworthy of these privileges are deprived of them.

■ Carry malpractice and professional liability insurance.

Standards among Professionals

You owe your colleagues and your employer the same ethical conduct you owe your clients. Remember that you are part of a "team." Your work contributes to your salon's success or failure and thus to the livelihood of your co-workers. If you are an employer, creating a pleasant atmosphere in your salon encourages your employees to work well (Figure 2.5). Even if you work all by yourself, you are in a "partnership" with other cosmetologists—including the one on the other side of town. By running down the "competition" or charging ridiculously low or rediculously high prices, you can cause the entire profession to lose a client. If you hurt other cosmetologists, you usually hurt yourself as well.

The following guidelines concern **ethical conduct toward others in your profession:**

■ Conduct yourself in a spirit of fair dealing, cooperation, and courtesy toward other cosmetologists.

■ Refrain from soliciting clients by offering services, through advertising or other means, at a price below the range charged for similar services by other professionals in the community.

■ Refrain from directly or indirectly offering employment to an employee of another salon unless that person responds to your public advertisement on his or her own initiative.

■ Refuse to endorse or permit your name to be used in publicity or advertising for cosmetic products made primarily for consumption outside salons.

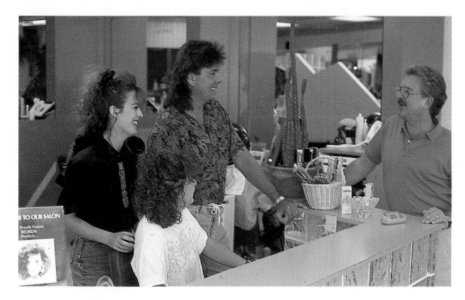

Figure 2.5
Creating a pleasant work atmosphere is one of the salon owner's responsibilities.

- Refrain from lending your talents to industry trade events that are not in the best interest of the profession.

- Refrain from directly or indirectly, falsely or maliciously discrediting the ability of a fellow cosmetologist or injuring his or her reputation.

- Keep private any information given in confidence by a fellow cosmetologist in any matter of business and refrain from using it to his or her detriment.

- Refrain from using an office on a professional cosmetology commission or board for personal gain.

- Refrain from performing any act designed to promote your own interests at the expense of the profession or professional co-workers.

The following guidelines deal specifically with the **responsibilities of the employer to the employee:**

- Set as your goal the mutual benefit of one another.

- Assume responsibility for the services rendered by the employee.

- Instill professional pride in the employee regarding the quality of performance.

- Observe all wage and hour regulations—federal, state, and local (Figure 2.6).

- Establish salon charges that will permit both you and the employee to receive a fair reward.

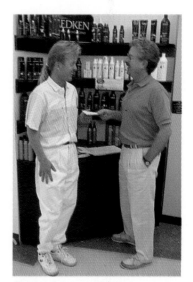

Figure 2.6
The employer is responsible for observing state and federal minimum wage laws.

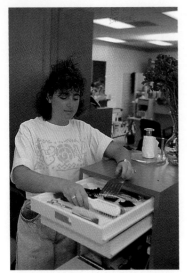

Figure 2.7
An employee is responsible for helping to maintain an attractive workplace.

■ Provide financial incentives for the employees to increase their abilities (since this will result in a gain for both you and the employee).

■ Exert reasonable effort to assist an employee who has not been dismissed "for cause" in securing employment elsewhere.

■ Encourage employees to participate in civic, cultural, social, political, and religious organizations.

These guidelines, in turn, deal with the **responsibilities of the employee to the employer:**

■ Work with management and co-workers to maintain an attractive and sanitary establishment (Figure 2.7).

■ Take pride in maintaining a good reputation for the establishment.

■ Participate in training sessions provided by the employer.

■ Refrain from misrepresentation when accepting a position.

■ Give reasonable notice when employment must be terminated.

■ Volunteer to help with salon duties if needed.

Finally, every individual **cosmetologist has responsibilities to the profession at large:**

■ Uphold the dignity and honor of the profession.

■ Affiliate with a unit of a recognized organization of the profession and contribute your time, energy, and ability to maintaining the standards of the profession.

■ Safeguard the profession by allowing only those qualified by education and good moral character to be admitted into it (when you have that authority).

■ Understand and comply with the laws, rules, and regulations of cosmetology. This way you will be contributing to the public health, welfare, and safety of the community. Refrain from helping others evade these laws.

Glossary

Code of ethics Systems of rules that tell members of a profession how they should act when they offer their skills to the public.

Ethics Moral values concerning voluntary acts performed in a climate of knowledge and freedom of choice.

Professional ethics Ethics that apply to the performance of one's job.

1. If you dislike someone you work with, is there anything wrong with telling your clients?
2. Would it be reasonable for your employer to insist that you arrive for work 15 minutes before your first appointment?
3. Should you attend continuing-education workshops even though you have to pay the admission charge?
4. Is there anything wrong with telling your clients that you dislike your boss?
5. Is it against professional ethics to sell your clientele services they do not necessarily need?
6. How are you acting when you treat others honestly and with good intentions?
7. Is ethical behavior voluntary or mandatory?
8. What is the system of rules telling professionals how they should act when they offer their skills to the public?
9. True or false? It is a part of professional ethics to learn new methods, accept new ideas, and improve techniques.
10. True or false? Carrying malpractice insurance is a part of professional ethics.
11. True or false? There is nothing unethical about gossiping.
12. Should you advertise cut-rate prices for services?
13. As a salon owner, should you set your prices so both you and your employees receive a fair reward?
14. True or false? Breaking laws formulated by your local city council has nothing to do with the professional ethics of cosmetology.

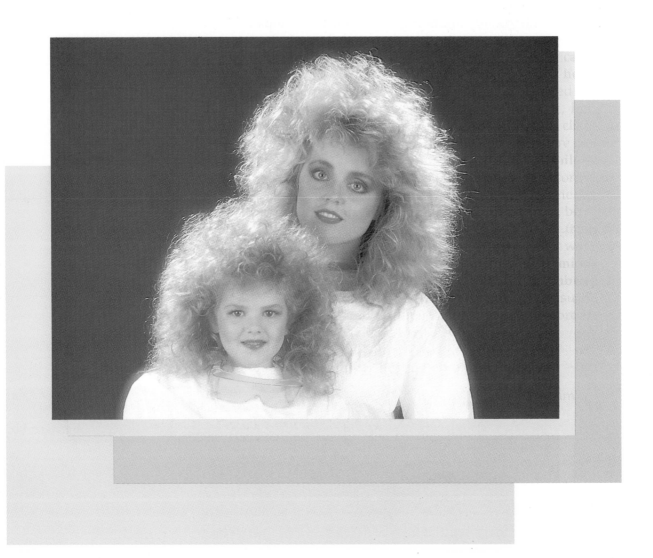

Sanitizing and Sterilization

With the sanitation supplies described in this chapter, use chemical agents and ultraviolet rays to sanitize implements and equipment in the salon. Follow the proper steps to sanitize the setting, combing, and cutting implements contained in your implement kit within 20 minutes. Score 85 percent or better on a multiple-choice exam on the information in this chapter.

In order to achieve the above level of competence, you should master the following chapter objectives.

Theory Objectives

1. Define the terms used to describe and classify bacteria.
2. Define viruses, the immune system, and infection control.
3. Describe the five methods of sanitation.
4. Describe the measures used to sanitize the service area.
5. Describe the safety measures for the use and storage of chemicals, fire safety, and first aid in schools and salons.

Practical Objective

6. Sanitize implements and equipment.

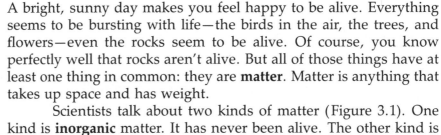

Introduction

Promoting and protecting good health in the community is called **public hygiene** or **sanitation** (san-eh-TAY-shun). Everyone who provides services to the public has a responsibility to help protect the health of the community. Since, as a cosmetologist, you will perform services on the hair, scalp, and other parts of a client's body, you must keep the salon clean and sanitary by following certain procedures to destroy harmful germs that can contaminate working implements and equipment and spread disease.

Theory Objective 1
Terms Used to Describe
and Classify Bacteria

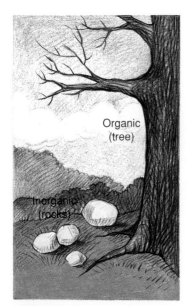

Figure 3.1
The two kinds of matter

A bright, sunny day makes you feel happy to be alive. Everything seems to be bursting with life—the birds in the air, the trees, and flowers—even the rocks seem to be alive. Of course, you know perfectly well that rocks aren't alive. But all of those things have at least one thing in common: they are **matter**. Matter is anything that takes up space and has weight.

Scientists talk about two kinds of matter (Figure 3.1). One kind is **inorganic** matter. It has never been alive. The other kind is **organic** (awr-GAN-ik) matter, which includes all things that are living or have been alive in the past. A living tree is organic matter, but so is a dead tree. Unlike inorganic matter, organic matter can be food for other living things after it dies. (For instance, when leaves die and fall from a tree, they provide food for the grass around the tree and for the tree itself.

Organic matter comes in many shapes and sizes. The basic units of organic matter are called **cells**. (Smaller units exist, but you don't need to be concerned about them here.) Any independent group of cells is called an **organism**. We see many organisms around us every day. Some of them are rather simple, while others are very complicated and are described by scientific formulas. But another kind of organism exists as well. Some people aren't even aware of these organisms. They look right at the organisms every day without seeing them. These are **microorganisms** (migh-kroh-OR-gehn-iz-uhmz). Humans can see microorganisms only by using a microscope. Some of them are made up of only a few cells or sometimes just a single cell.

One group of microorganisms that cosmetologists must know about are **bacteria** (bak-TIR-ee-ah). The scientific study of bacteria is called **bacteriology**. Bacteria are one-celled microorganisms, sometimes called **microbes** (MIGH-krohbs). They are also called germs. Bacteria are everywhere—in the air, on the ground, and even inside our bodies. Scientists only discovered them a little more than a hundred years ago. Before that time, people lived in constant fear of diseases and epidemics like the Black Death, which killed over one-third of all the people living in Europe six hundred years ago. Although people today sometimes talk about "epidemics," no one living in a modern country like the United States needs to worry about an epidemic like the Black Death unless he or she ignores the rules of good personal and public hygiene.

The reason is very simple: public health, or sanitation. After scientists discovered that some bacteria cause disease (pathogens [PATH-ah-jenz], or **pathogenic** [path-ah-JEN-ik] bacteria), governments began to make and enforce laws to improve sanitation and thus protect the health of the community. This is why knowledge of bacteria and sanitation is so important for the cosmetologist.

There are two basic kinds of bacteria: **pathogens** and **nonpathogens**. **Pathogenic bacteria** can **cause disease**. They are commonly called **germs**. **Nonpathogenic bacteria** do not cause disease. Actually, most of them are very helpful (one particular type—**saprophytes** [SAP-roh-fightz]—causes dead organic matter to decay and thus helps enrich the soil). The bacteria in yeast cause bread to rise, and other bacteria create the alcohol in wine.

Pathogenic bacteria are divided into three types: **cocci** (KOK-sigh), **spirilla** (spigh-RIL-ah), and **bacilli** (bah-SIL-igh). Each has a different **shape**, which can be seen through a microscope. Cocci are **round**, spirilla have **spiral** shapes, and bacilli are shaped like **rods**. (Figure 3.2).

Cocci (round) usually cause pus-forming diseases such as boils, abscesses, and pustules. There are three forms of cocci: staphylococci (staf-eh-low-KOK-sigh), streptococci (strep-tah-KOK-sigh), and diplococci (dip-low-KOK-sigh).

- **Staphylococci** (Figure 3.2d), usually grow in clusters, generally produce **local** infections (those found in a small area on or in the body). Hospitals have found that this type of infection can spread very easily unless all objects that come in contact with patients are sterilized properly.

- **Streptococci** (Figure 3.2e), usually cause **general infections** (those caused by the spread of bacteria through the bloodstream to a large part of the body). Rheumatic fever is an example of a general infection caused by streptococci.

- **Diplococci** (Figure 3.2f), which occur in pairs, cause bacterial pneumonia.

- **Spirilla** (spiral) cause cholera and syphilis, while **Bacilli** (rod-shaped) cause such serious diseases as diphtheria, leprosy, tuberculosis, and

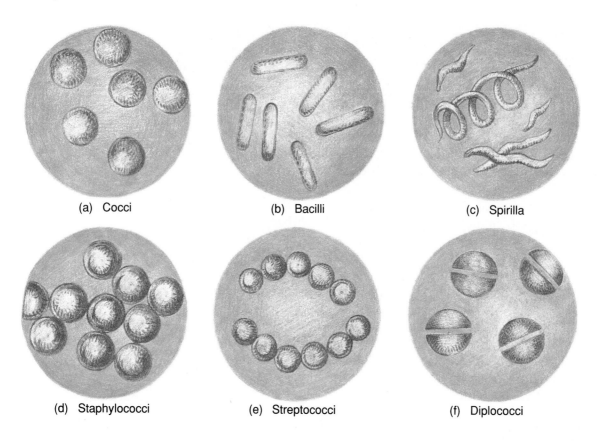

(a) Cocci   (b) Bacilli   (c) Spirilla

(d) Staphylococci   (e) Streptococci   (f) Diplococci

Figure 3.2
Pathogenic bacteria

typhoid fever. Both bacilli and spirilla have **flagella** (fleh-JELleh) or **cilia** (SIL-ee-ah), which are whiplike extensions (tails) that enable the cell to move in a liquid (Figure 3.3).

Pathogenic bacteria must have **favorable conditions to grow and cause disease**. Among other things, they need **heat, moisture, and the absence of direct sunlight**.

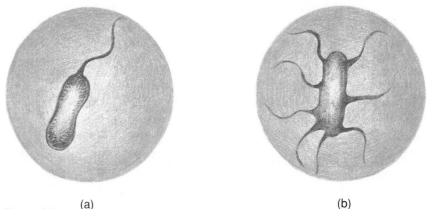

(a)   (b)

Figure 3.3
Bacilli (a) with one extension (tail); (b) with many extensions (tails).

All forms of bacteria multiply (reproduce) by division. As the cell is nourished, it grows larger. When it has grown as large as it can, it divides itself into two cells that are the same size (Figure 3.4). These are called **daughter** cells. This process of cell division is called **mitosis** (migh-TOH-sis). Mitosis can happen as often as once every 20 minutes.

When bacteria are growing and multiplying in favorable conditions, they are in an **active cycle.** When the conditions are unfavorable for bacteria, the cells die or become **inactive**. Some bacteria, including bacilli, can live through an inactive cycle by forming spherical **spores.** These spores, which move easily through the air, are much more **resistant** to heat, chemicals, and sunlight in this inactive state. The bacteria live as spores until their surrounding conditions improve. Then they change back to their original form and return to the active cycle. Although spore formation is not very common among bacteria, it is a factor you should consider when keeping the salon sanitary. Some spores can survive for a long time in extreme heat (water boils at 212° Fahrenheit) and cold (liquid helium freezes at −507° Fahrenheit).

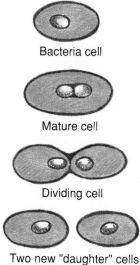

Bacteria cell

Mature cell

Dividing cell

Two new "daughter" cells
Figure 3.4
Cell division (mitosis)

Theory Objective 2
Viruses, the Immune System, and Infection Control

Viruses are especially important kinds of pathogens. They differ from bacteria in size, characteristics, and activity. Viruses are called **ultramicroscopic** because they cannot be seen unless they are magnified up to one million times by a scanning electron microscope.

A **virus** (VIGH-ruhss) **is essentially a parasite** (an animal or plant that lives in or on another organism without helping it to live). Viruses can enter many kinds of cells, reproduce, and then destroy the cell (Figure 3.5). This is called a viral infection. When this happens, thousands of viruses are able to infect other cells.

Viruses probably cause more than half of the diseases affecting humans, animals, and plants. Influenza, chicken pox, the common cold, and acquired immunodeficiency syndrome (AIDS) are caused by viruses.

Normally, most **illnesses are caused by pathogenic bacteria** that enter the **mouth, nose, ears, broken skin, or eyes.** Therefore, the cosmetologist must be especially concerned about bacteria that affect the head, arms, and feet. Disease-causing bacteria are often sent into the air by a person who has a disease. These bacteria are also transferred to other people by hands, food, drinking glasses, or other objects touched by a person who has an **infection.** An infection occurs when pathogenic bacteria or viruses have entered a body and multiply to the point of interfering with its normal state. Infections may or may not be **contagious** (kuhn-TAY-juhss). If a disease is contagious, it can be transmitted to another person through touch

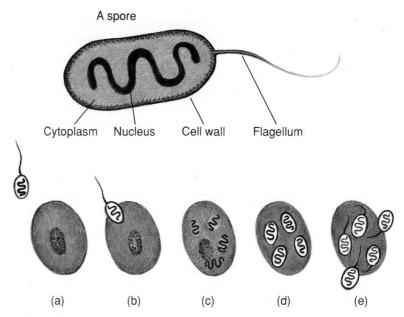

A spore

Cytoplasm   Nucleus   Cell wall   Flagellum

(a)   (b)   (c)   (d)   (e)

Figure 3.5
Viral infection: (a) virus approaches cell; (b) virus attaches itself to cell; (c) virus multiplies inside cell; (d) virus matures; (e) virus bursts from destroyed cell and spreads to new cells.

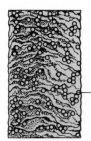

—Fungus spore

Figure 3.6
Microscopic view of a hair that has been infected with ringworm.

or through the air. Another term used to mean contagious is **communicable** (koh-MYOO-ni-kah-behl).

Persons who have a contagious disease (such as influenza, ringworm, or head lice) should **isolate** (separate) themselves from others (Figure 3.6). It is very important for cosmetologists who have contagious diseases to isolate themselves since they can infect clients through close contact and handling of implements and equipment. It is just as important for practitioners to refuse service to clients who have contagious diseases.

A **susceptible** person is one who is likely to become ill from direct or indirect contact with disease-causing bacteria or viruses. For example, a person in poor health is more likely to become ill from such contact than a healthy person.

Immunity (ih-MYOO-neh-tee) is the ability of the body's defense mechanisms to fight off disease. The body fights bacterial infections in two basic ways: **active immunity (natural)** and **passive immunity (acquired).** The body defends itself in the following manner:

1. **Active (natural) immunity** occurs when the body makes **antibodies** (also called white blood cells), which destroy harmful bacteria in the blood. In addition, when certain poisons (**toxins**) develop in the blood, the body produces **antitoxins,** which destroy the poison.

The outermost layer of the skin (**epidermis** [ep-eh-DER-mis]) protects the body from bacteria. When this layer of skin is punctured or cut, bacteria can enter, and an infection may develop if the wound is not treated.

When the active immunity systems are fighting disease, they produce waste products in the same way that a fire produces ashes. The body discards these waste products through the lungs, sudoriferous glands (sweat glands), intestines, and urinary tract.

2. **Passive (acquired) immunity** occurs when antibodies from another person or animal are injected into the body. The most common form of passive immunity comes from shots, such as polio or flu shots.

3. **Acquired immunodeficiency syndrome (AIDS)** is a disease caused by a virus that interferes with the body's natural immune system and causes the immune system to break down. This virus is called the **HIV virus** (Human Immunodeficiency Virus).

AIDS is a life-threatening disease. Once you have become infected with the disease, there are only a very limited number of drugs that will help you feel better. There is no known cure for AIDS at this time. Three important factors to keep in mind are how the disease is transmitted, the common routes of transmission (Figure 3.7), and, perhaps most important, how the virus is destroyed. AIDS is transmitted from one person to another from contact with bodily fluids:

- Blood

- Semen

- Vaginal secretions

The following are the four main routes by which the virus is transmitted from one person to another:

1. **Sexual contact.** Sharing of semen and/or blood via heterosexual or homosexual activity. Sexual contact should include the use of a condom for "safe sex." Injury to the mucous membrane of the rectum may cause this sharing of fluid to occur. Because of this, anal intercourse is considered a high-risk activity. Abstinence is 100 percent safe.

2. **Injection.** Sharing of needles and syringes via illegal or accidental activity.

3. **Maternal.** Child transplacental transfer; perinatal transmission (the mother is infected through sharing needles for intravenous drugs or through sexual contact and then transmits the virus to her child before it is born).

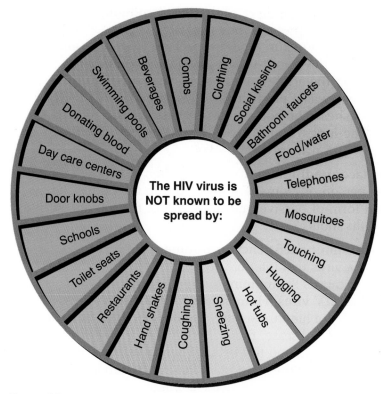

Figure 3.7
The HIV virus is NOT known to be spread by...
Source: U.S. Department of Health and Human Services/Minneapolis Health Department

4. **Transfusion of blood or blood products.** Now, all blood is screened for the AIDS virus, so this form of transmission has become quite rare.

The HIV virus can be destroyed outside the body in four ways:

- Exposure to air and heat
- 70 percent ethanol/isopropyl/alcohol
- 1:10 to 1:100 dilution of household bleach
- Use of at least 3 percent hydrogen peroxide solution (6 percent in some states)

Hepatitis B, a viral infection that attacks the liver, is also a health concern requiring careful sanitation procedures to protect the cosmetologist and the client.

Therefore, it is very important to remember these rules:

- Be very thorough when you are sanitizing implements that penetrate the skin, such as ear-piercing devices and needles used in electrolysis. These devices should be discarded in a puncture-proof container or carefully cleaned and disinfected between uses.

■ The same procedures should be followed for other implements, such as razors, haircutting scissors, electric clippers, and cuticle scissors.

■ Cosmetologists with open or weeping sores should not come in direct contact with a client, until their sores have healed. Therefore, it is advisable to wear gloves whenever possible, so that your hands do not become injured when working with chemicals.

Infection Control Procedures

To prevent infections, when a client or student is exposed to blood by a scissors cut, razor cut, needle prick, laceration, or other exposure to broken skin or mucous membrane, the student should take the following steps:

1. Put on disposable rubber gloves.

2. Thoroughly wash the exposed area or wound with soap and water.

3. Disinfect the area with a topical disinfectant using one of the methods described above.

The ultimate authority for prescribing procedures to prevent the spread of HIV infection and hepatitis B lies with state regulatory bodies. Consult your state health department and state board or commission of cosmetology for current regulations and guidelines regarding AIDS and hepatitis B.

Theory Objective 3
Methods of Sanitation

Now that you have read about the various forms of bacteria, there are two terms that you will want to learn and keep in mind as you clean your working area.

The process of **sterilization** (stehr-il-eh-ZAY-shun) is used to kill all bacteria (pathogenic and nonpathogenic) on an implement. The process of **sanitation** destroys pathogenic bacteria. Although sterilizing kills all bacteria and is, really, the ideal way to clean, it is almost impossible to make implements sterile and **keep** them that way. Bacteria are everywhere, including in the air around us. So, even if an implement is sterilized, as soon as it hits the air in the salon, it is no longer sterile. But it will be sanitary—**aseptic** (ay-SEP-tik) or free from pathogenic bacteria—if the entire school or salon

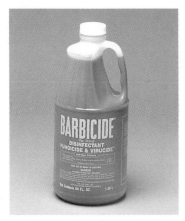

Figure 3.8
A chemical sanitizing agent

has been cleaned thoroughly. This is why it is very important to keep everything in the salon sanitary. If pathogenic bacteria are in the salon or school, the implements used there will be toxic (unsanitary), also called **septic** (SEP-tik) (from sepsis).

Public health or sanitation refers to the set of procedures used to stop the spread of communicable diseases and the development of other infections caused by pathogenic agents. Under rules and regulations issued by public health departments and state boards of cosmetology, salons and schools are required to keep their equipment and implements, working areas, and building in a sanitary condition at all times.

The beauty school or salon uses two basic types of agents in sanitizing implements and equipment: **chemical** agents and **physical** agents.

Five kinds of **chemical** sanitizing agents are used (Figure 3.8):

1. Antiseptics
2. Disinfectants
3. Fumigants
4. Bactericides
5. Germicides and fungicides

Antiseptics (an-teh-SEP-tiks) halt or prevent the growth of pathogenic bacteria. They are often used to maintain the sanitary condition of implements already sterilized. Doctors often use **3–5 percent hydrogen peroxide** solution as an antiseptic to cleanse the skin.

Disinfectants (dis-in-FEK-tahnts), **fumigants** (FYOO-migahnts) or **vapors**, **bactericides** (bak-TIR-eh-sighdz), and **germicides** (JER-meh-sighdz) are chemicals that destroy pathogenic bacteria. You should use these cleaners very carefully. These chemicals are very useful for sterilizing implements, but they are very strong and usually are caustic, which means that they can burn your skin.

Antiseptics, on the other hand, are not disinfectants. They do not destroy all bacteria. They can be used on the skin. In addition, most disinfectants can be diluted with water and used as antiseptics.

Whenever you use any of these cleaners, you should also remember that sanitizing methods **do not kill bacteria instantly.** Complete destruction of bacteria always requires some time, depending on the agent or method used.

Numerous chemical cleaners are available. Sanitizing chemical agents come in different strengths and forms, including liquids, tablets, capsules, and powders. Many cleaners sold by full-service beauty suppliers are ready to use and require no mixing or diluting. **In choosing a disinfectant, you should consider the following:**

1. Which chemical agent is recommended by the state board of cosmetology or state health department?

2. Is the chemical agent easy to buy and inexpensive?

3. Is the chemical agent easy and safe to use, or will it cause serious skin or respiratory irritation?

4. Is it noncorrosive (made so that it does not harm plastic or metal implements) and does it work quickly?

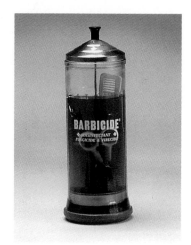

Figure 3.9
A dry sanitizer

Always follow all safety precautions, directions for diluting, and other procedures recommended by the manufacturer. Chemicals should be poured carefully to avoid waste and damage.

Combing and setting implements are ordinarily sanitized with **quaternary ammonium** (KWOT-er-ner-ee ah-MOHN-ee-um) (**"quats"**) or **formalin**, which is a **formaldehyde** (for-MAL-deh-highd) solution. Note: Not all states permit the use of formaldehyde. Check with your regulatory board or agency for a list of approved chemicals. Metal implements, such as blow-comb attachments, curling irons, manicure implements, electric clippers, scissors, and shapers (razors), are sanitized with **70 percent ethyl alcohol or 99 percent isopropyl alcohol**. Equipment such as shampoo bowls and fixtures in the dispensary and bathroom is sanitized with Lysol or diluted forms of formaldehyde (Figure 3.9).

Use of quaternary ammonium compounds varies from state to state. To be effective, a quats solution must be as strong as **1 part quats to a 1,000 parts water**. For safety, it should not be mixed any stronger. A solution of 2/3 ounce of quats in 1 gallon of water (20 milliliters quats in 3.8 liters of water) yields a 1:1,000 sanitizing solution. Mixed to this strength, a formula will kill all of the following:

- Herpes simplex virus

- Influenza A

- Adenovirus type 3

- Staph bacteria

- Fungus

- Vegetable bacteria

ALWAYS FOLLOW THE MANUFACTURER'S DIRECTIONS. WEAR GLOVES WHEN REMOVING IMPLEMENTS from a wet sanitizer containing this solution. The ordinary quats formula is one part quats to **1,000 parts water** (1:1000). Some salons use formalin as a disinfectant. It is basically 37 percent formaldehyde, 6.5 percent methanol, and 56.5 percent water.

The use of quats and formalin brings us to an important point you should remember whenever you use any chemical. The

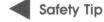 Safety Tip

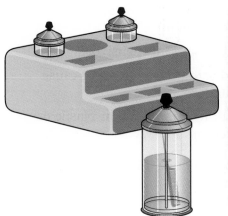

Figure 3.10
A wet sanitizer

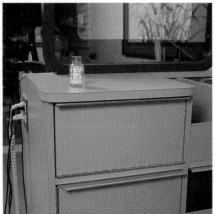

Figure 3.11
A dry sanitizer

kind of disinfectant that is required will vary from state to state (for instance, some states prohibit the use of formaldehyde), so it is very important to **follow the directions on the label of whatever disinfectant you are using, follow the requirements of your state board of cosmetology or state health department, and consult your instructor or manager before you mix a disinfectant**.

Chemical agents are used in two kinds of sanitizing containers: **wet sanitizers** and **dry sanitizers**. The **wet sanitizer** sterilizes the implements, and the **dry sanitizer** keeps them sanitized until they are used.

The **wet sanitizer** uses water and a chemical agent. The wet sanitizer must be **nonmetal**, large, and deep enough so that combs, brushes, rollers, and other items can be covered by the chemical solution (Figure 3.10). It also must have a cover to prevent contamination.

The **dry sanitizer** is an airtight cabinet or drawer that has a chemical agent in it (Figure 3.11). The unit can be made of wood, metal, or plastic. It must be large enough to hold combing, setting, or cutting implements after they have been removed from the wet sanitizer. A germicide called a **fumigant**, which emits bacteria-destroying vapors, is used in the dry sanitizer. The vapors are effective only if the drawer or door of the unit is closed. A capped saltshaker containing a solution of borax and formaldehyde can make an excellent fumigant. The shaker is placed so that it stands upright in the bottom of a dry sanitizer. The solution should contain one tablespoon of borax and one tablespoon of formaldehyde. Ready-to-use tablets are also available and are preferred to using a

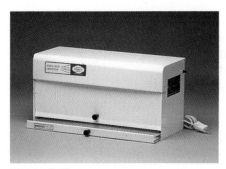

Figure 3.12
An ultraviolet dry sanitizer

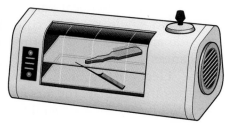

Figure 3.13
*An ultraviolet dry sanitizer with
a blower-heater*

shaker. Formaldehyde packets are also effective. Not all states recommend the use of fumigants, however.

Ultraviolet rays are the sanitation method involving **physical** agents most often used by salons. These rays have a germicidal effect; that is, they kill most bacteria and some viruses (Figure 3.12). One type of ultraviolet sanitizer has a small blower-heater that dries the combing and setting implements while the rays sterilize them (Figure 3.13). Although they are expensive, ultraviolet sanitizers are used in some schools and salons.

Two other physical methods for sterilization, **moist heat** and **dry heat,** are not ordinarily used in beauty schools or salons. Moist heat, for example, is not used because it takes too long and can damage setting and combing implements.

Theory Objective 4
Measures Used to
Sanitize the Service
Area

Sanitary measures must be used for the care of: (1) all implements used in performing a service, (2) personal habits, and (3) in maintaining the area in which the service is performed.

This objective will discuss the procedures used to keep the beauty school or salon building in sanitary condition. The discussion will include air purification, plumbing, furnishings, floors, and lighting. The procedures used to sanitize implements will be discussed in the chapters in which the implements are used. Personal habits will be discussed where they apply to the job.

The number of products used daily by the practitioner has increased dramatically. Tiny chemical particles from cold waving solutions, chemical relaxers, hair sprays, oxidizing permanent hair colors, bleaches, and other solutions are in the air. To a certain extent, this air pollution is an occupational hazard, but the school or salon

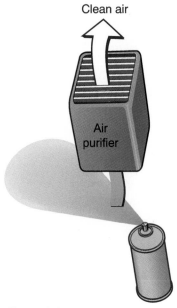

Figure 3.14
An air purifier

owner who is aware of this problem can reduce or eliminate the bad effects of these chemical particles and pathogenic microorganisms.

No single piece of equipment is economically practical to provide air purification for the salon or school. A combination of appliances seems to be the best solution.

Electronic air precipitators (air purifier or air cleaner) remove particles and circulate the air (Figure 3.14). These appliances usually are rated by their CFM (cubic feet per minute). They vary in their capacity to circulate a **cubic foot** of air per **minute**.

Most electronic air precipitators filter the air by drawing air through cellulose and/or charcoal filters. Then the air is drawn toward electrodes, and the impurities are deposited onto another filter. The cleaned air is then blown back into the salon. Although these appliances are small, they do a good job of removing viruses, bacteria, and chemicals from the air inside the building.

Air conditioners cool, dehumidify (remove moisture), and cleanse pollutants from air coming into the building from the outside. Air conditioners ordinarily use a fiberglass filter to cleanse the air and then circulate it through the building, but the air purifier cleans the air better.

Forced-air furnaces heat and, to some extent, cleanse the air. As air inside the building cools, it returns to the furnace where it is drawn through a fiberglass filter and heated. Then it is blown back into the working area. **Exhaust fans** (ventilation fans) also can help circulate the air, although they do not clean it. Exhaust fans blow the unhealthy air outside.

The level of humidity in a room is related to the degree of heat needed for comfort. Adjusting the humidity level with a humidifier or dehumidifier, with the advice of an appliance dealer, can make the salon more comfortable. **Humidifiers** add moisture to the air, preventing excessive drying of the skin and reducing static electricity that may be generated during hair combing. **Dehumidifiers** remove excessive moisture from the air.

Schools and salons with good air-sanitation programs generally lose fewer workdays to illnesses caused by bacteria.

All schools and salons must have **continuous hot and cold water.** Most public health departments also require a **vacuum breaker** for each shampoo bowl (Figure 3.15). This fixture prevents the reverse flow of contaminated water and keeps it from backing up into the fresh-water supply system.

Bathroom plumbing fixtures must be sanitized and kept in good working order. Clean, individual hand towels must also be provided.

School and salon furnishings and floors must have surfaces that can be washed and sanitized regularly. Sanitizing chairs and other equipment is discussed in the procedures section of this chapter. Curtains should be washable and must be kept clean.

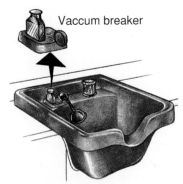

Figure 3.15
A vacuum beaker stops unclean water from mixing with fresh water.

Adequate lighting is necessary because of the nature of the services offered in the beauty school and salon. Any reputable lighting dealer can provide advice.

An important part of preparing to be a licensed cosmetologist is recognizing the importance of safety. Knowing how to work safely and maintain a safe environment is an important part of the licensing requirements. Making the school/salon a safe place to give and receive services is everybody's job—not just the job of the instructor/manager. Everyone has to BE AWARE OF SAFETY and practice hairdressing skills in the manner that is safest for everyone in the school/salon. Everyone has to "pitch in."

This objective will explain what you can do to make the school/salon a safe place to work and what you should do if a certain kind of accident happens. The paragraphs that follow will describe safety precautions when using certain chemicals; how to store chemicals safely and why; fire safety measures; and first aid for minor cuts and burns.

Hazardous Chemicals

Many products that are used in the school/salon could be dangerous to you or the client. For example, formaldehyde is suspected of causing cancer, so many states have prohibited its use for sanitizing purposes. Since each state has different laws, you will need to check with your instructor to determine whether formaldehyde (formalin) is allowed in your state. If it is permitted, you should take extra care when using it.

Safety Precautions for Sanitizing Chemicals.   Whenever you use sanitizing chemicals, you should take the following precautions:

1. Read mixing instructions before use.

2. Mix exactly according to the manufacturer's directions.

3. Wear gloves or use forceps when removing combs, brushes, or other implements from a wet sanitizer containing formalin.

4. Keep formalin fumes away from your eyes and nose and try not to inhale any fumes, which may irritate the delicate tissues of the eyes and nose.

5. Store formaldehyde (formalin) in a safe place well out of the reach of children, who may not know that it is poisonous.

6. Whenever you pour any product from its original container into another container, carefully label the new container so that anyone picking up a bottle will be able to see clearly what product he or she is about to use.

Other Hazardous Products.   **Alcohol, nail polish remover, some instant conditioners, and hair spray** are other examples of potentially hazardous products, in that they are very **flammable.** Whenever possible, flammable products should be stored in **metal cabinets**, and they should be **kept away from** sources of extreme **heat.** For example, these flammable products should **not** be stored near a water heater, furnace, or other appliances where a spark, heat, or flame might ignite them and cause a fire. Do not allow clients to smoke cigarettes, pipes, or cigars when these products are in use.

As a student, you probably would not think that **soiled towels** are very hazardous, but they are—if they are not stored in a **closed, fireproof container.** The problem arises because the ammonia used to tint hair sticks to a towel. That towel may then be put in a container with towels saturated with sodium bromate from the neutralizer used for cold waving. Mixing towels saturated with ammonia and sodium bromate causes the formation of **bromine gas.** This gas is likely to ignite spontaneously (**spontaneous combustion**); that is, a fire starts without an outside source of flame such as a match or spark. Storage of these towels in a covered, fireproof container is very important.

Storage of Chemicals

Light, temperature, moisture, and air are the four most important things to consider when storing products.

Light.   Light, particularly ultraviolet light from the sun, changes the chemical makeup of products. Have you ever noticed that some products used in the school, salon, or home are packaged in dark-colored amber bottles? The dark container protects the contents from light. As additional protection, these products should probably be stored in a closed cabinet, rather than displayed in the front window of the salon.

Temperature.   Heat in any form also changes the chemical makeup of products. A school or salon is likely to contain a number of sources of heat: the hot sun shining through an undraped window; furnace; hot water heater; hair dryers; wig dryers; towel dryer; and curling irons. All professional products should be stored away from any form of heat in a cool, dry area of the salon.

Moisture.   Moisture from an extremely damp basement may cause a product to become moldy. Store supplies in a DRY AREA. If beauty supplies are contaminated with water from too much moisture, they may become inactive and will not work.

Air.   Air will dilute (water down) most products or allow the active chemicals in a product to escape. Keeping all products tightly capped and in their original box or package will allow you to keep the chemicals in their active state much longer than if you left the products uncapped. Tightly cap all products after use! Clean air makes for a **safe work environment.**

Never store any salon supplies or chemicals in the same area where food is stored. For example, do not store sanitizing chemicals alongside breakfast cereal or any other food product.

Fire Safety

Most state, province, county, local, or municipal laws require that any public service business have at least one **fire extinguisher** conveniently located in the school or salon (Figure 3.16). The fire extinguisher must be regularly inspected and serviced at **least once a year** to make sure it will work in the event of a fire. A large business may be required to have several fire extinguishers. In the event of a fire, be sure that your clients leave the school or salon. Call your **local emergency phone number**. Many areas use the "911" emergency phone number, but the number may vary from area to area. Check with your instructor to determine the phone number used in your area. If any client is injured as the result of a fire or injured elsewhere on the salon/school premises, **seek medical assistance!**

First Aid for Minor Cuts and Burns

A **first aid kit** available at all times for minor injuries.

Minor Cuts.   From time to time accidents do happen, so it is important to know what to do if you or the client should receive a minor cut from scissors, cuticle nippers, electric clippers, or a shaper (razor). You will find the following procedure helpful:

1. Wear gloves to protect yourself from blood-borne contamination.
2. Stop the bleeding using a clean towel or cotton and apply pressure on the cut.
3. Sanitize the wound with a good antiseptic. (Gently wash the area with soap and water before applying the antiseptic.)
4. Apply **Mycitracin ointment** to prevent infection (available over-the-counter in drugstores). Better penetration of the skin is achieved if a bandage is applied at night; however, the bandage should be removed during the day. Mycitracin is

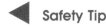
Safety Tip

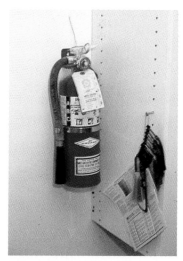

Figure 3.16
Schools and salons are required by law to have a fire extinguisher. It must be in working order, and you should know how to use it.

advised because it has the widest range of antibiotic content to prevent infection.

If you or your client receives a severe cut, **seek medical assistance** from a physician or hospital. **Take the client to a doctor!**

Chemical Burns.   Many of the chemicals used to curl, straighten, and bleach or color hair could burn your skin or the skin of the client. When these products are used **carelessly**, burns often occur in the areas around the client's front hairline, on the neck, and behind the ears. You will learn how to prevent chemical burns when your instructor assigns those chapters. If you should happen to give one of these services to an overly sensitive client who develops a chemical burn, you will find the following procedure helpful:

Safety Tip ▶

1. Thoroughly flush (rinse) the burned area with cool water. Or, saturate a towel with cool water, wring out the towel, and apply it to the burned area of skin.

2. Apply a thin layer of Mycitracin ointment with a clean cotton swab to prevent infection.

3. Cover with a bandage at night to allow for better penetration of the ointment, but uncover during the day.

If the burn is open and seeping fluid, advise the client to go to a physician.

Another effective antibiotic ointment that can be purchased over-the-counter is **Neosporin ointment**™. **Do not use** Gentian Violet Jelly (New York permits use) as this is only available with a doctor's prescription and stains the client's skin and clothes purple. If you used it on a client, you would actually be practicing medicine, which is against the law.

If any irritating chemicals drip into the client's eye(s), gently flush the area with cool water immediately and contact a physician. **Do not apply anything other than cool water to the eye(s).**

Physical Burns.   Physical burns are injuries to the skin that result from touching the skin with a mechanical device, such as a curling iron, pressing comb, or other hairstyling implement used carelessly. The following procedure will be helpful if such burns occur:

1. Apply a cold compress (a clean towel saturated with cold water and then wrung out) to reduce pain and swelling.

2. Apply Mycitracin™ ointment to prevent infection. Cover with a bandage at night for better penetration. Uncover during the day.

For severe burns, take the client to a physician.

Supplies

- soap (Dreft) and water (Figure 3.17)
- (fumigant) tablets or packets
- 70 percent alcohol
- quats (or formalin)
- comb and brush cleaner
- paper towels
- ammonia
- sponge
- wet sanitizer
- laundered towels
- cotton
- Lysol (optional)
- sodium hypochlorite (household bleach)

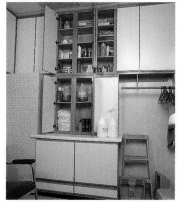

Figure 3.17
A supply dispensary

The basic procedure for sanitizing soiled implements is as follows:

1. Remove foreign material, such as hair, from combs and brushes.
2. Wash in hot soapy water.
3. Rinse with hot water and place in a wet sanitizer.
4. Rinse with water, dry, and place in a dry sanitizer.
5. Change the chemical sanitizing solution regularly.

Preparation and Mixing

Procedure

1. Remove only the combing and setting implements (clips, combs, brushes, rollers) from your kit.

2. Close the sink drain, add comb and brush cleaner to the sink **according to the directions on the label**, and turn on the **hot** water until the desired level is reached.

3. Select a rectangular container with a tight-fitting cover to use as a wet sanitizer; it should be large enough (about gallon-size) to hold clips, combs, brushes, and rollers (Figure 3.18).

Rationale

1. Combing and setting implements are usually sanitized with the **same** soaps and chemicals, but cutting implements require a different process.

2. Cleaning excess hair, hair spray, and oil from implements makes it easier to sanitize them. Cleaners dissolve hair spray and oil better in hot water.

3. The cover is necessary to prevent contamination of the sanitizing solution, which will be mixed in the container. This container and its solution will be the wet sanitizer.

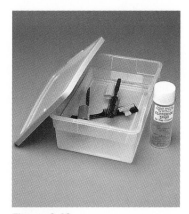

Figure 3.18
A wet sanitizer

4. Fill this container almost to capacity with **cold** water.

5. Mix a 25 percent formalin solution with cold water or mix a quats solution, carefully following the label instructions.

4. Cold water works better with formalin than hot water does.

5. Formalin is **poisonous** and flammable and can irritate your skin. The first time you use it, ask the instructor or manager to be sure that you are using it safely. **Do not smell** any disinfectant because doing so can injure mucous membranes in your nose. Keep formalin away from your eyes! If some does get into your eyes, flush with clean water for 15 minutes! **Call a doctor immediately**.

Sanitizing Solutions

Chemical	Form	Strength	Use
Formalin	Clear liquid	25% solution	Wet sanitizer; immerse for 10 minutes
Formalin	Clear liquid	10% solution	Wet sanitizer; immerse for 20 minutes
Alcohol	Clear liquid	70% solution	Immerse sharp cutting implements for at least 10 minutes

6. Cover the solution in the wet sanitizer and return it to the dispensary cabinet.

6. The chemical should be covered and properly stored when not being used.

Sanitation Practices

Procedure

1. Comb all visible hairs from the brushes before putting them in the solution. The hair should be discarded into a closed refuse container.

2. Immerse combs, clips, and brushes in comb and brush cleaning solution in the sink. Scrub combs and brushes against each other until all have been cleaned.

Rationale

1. This helps the sterilizing solution destroy bacteria more easily. To maintain sanitary conditions, the hair must be put into a **closed refuse container.**

2. The scrubbing helps the cleaner remove accumulated oil, hair spray, and soil, but does not destroy bacteria.

3. Rinse all implements with hot water; place them in the sanitizing solution (completed in step 6) and cover.

3. Rinse implements to remove cleaner residue. Covering the container prevents contamination of the solution.

4. Implements should be immersed for 10 minutes.

4. It takes about 10 minutes to destroy bacteria completely. Clips rust easily, so do not leave them immersed for longer than 20 minutes, or add a rust inhibitor such as sodium nitrite or glycerine.

5. Fill the sink with hot water and cleaner again.

5. This is the best way to clean hair spray and oil from the rollers and rack.

6. Immerse rollers and rack or tray in the cleaning solution in the sink and stir the solution with your hand. Then drain the sink and rinse the rollers with hot water.

6. This cleaner will dissolve setting lotions and remove temporary hair colors from the rollers. Swishing the solution in the sink speeds cleaning. Rinse the cleaner thoroughly from the rollers.

7. Remove combs, brushes, and clips after they have been in the sanitizer for 20 minutes.

7. Use the rubber gloves or tongs to remove these implements. The solution could burn or remove the top layer of skin.

8. Dry all combs, brushes, and clips individually with a clean towel and put the combs and brushes in either an ultraviolet or a dry sanitizer.

8. Using a damp comb or brush in final styling can straighten the hair and ruin the hairstyle. Also, clips rust easily. So all implements must be dried thoroughly. An ultraviolet or dry sanitizer will keep implements sanitary.

9. Place the clips in the implement kit, which contains a fumigant. (Fumigant tablets should be placed in a salt shaker-type container inside the kit. Fumigant packets also work well.)

9. This will keep the implements sanitary.

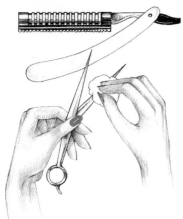

Figure 3.19
Sanitizing metal scissors with 70 percent alcohol.

10. Follow the same steps to sanitize the rack and rollers or tray. Thoroughly dry them and put them in a dry sanitizer.

11. Wet a small piece of cotton with 70 percent alcohol and carefully wipe the cutting edges of the scissors and shapers (razors) (Figure 3.19). Wiping the blades also helps keep them sharp. Then, put them in a dry sanitizer.

12. Using fine steel wool, remove oils, hair sprays, and setting lotions from curling irons and pressing combs. Wipe them with a ball of cotton dampened with alcohol, and place them in a dry sanitizer.

13. Close and return all cleaners to the proper place. Dispose of used cotton in a closed refuse container.

14. Clean all shampoo capes and aprons with an ammonia solution.

Sanitizing Equipment

Procedure

1. Follow label directions to mix a 5 percent formalin solution.

2. Obtain clean paper towels from the dispensary; using the solution mixed in step 1, wipe the back, seat, arms, and hood of each

10. Standard procedure. Rollers are dried because bacteria can grow quickly in moist places. Fumigant vapors inside the kit will keep the rollers and rack sanitary.

11. This sanitizes metal hairdressing implements. The fumigant will keep them sanitary (see page 52).

12. Remove the buildup from implements before sanitizing them. Electrical implements must not be placed in a wet sanitizer. Electrical shock or damage could result.

13. Exposure to air contaminates and evaporates alcohol. Keep all chemicals well out of a child's reach.

14. This solution works best on plastic and vinyl.

Rationale

1. A solution of this strength usually will not damage upholstery fabrics or counter surfaces as it sanitizes.

2. Since formalin may stain clothing fabrics or cause them to deteriorate, each unit should be dried. Although the formalin

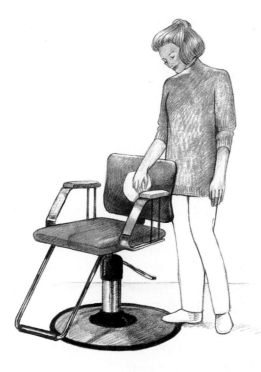

Figure 3.20
Sanitizing salon equipment with quats.

dryer-lounge unit. Also wipe the reception chairs, the desk, and the hydraulic styling chairs, including their bases (Figure 3.20).

3. Drain used solution from the sink and place soiled paper towels in a closed refuse container.

4. Mix 2 ounces of ammonia in 1 quart of tepid water (60 milliliters of ammonia in 0.95 liter of water) to clean soil and hair spray from mirrors, windows, sinks, and so forth (Figure 3.21).

solution sterilizes the unit, drying with a paper towel puts some bacteria on it again. The units are not sterile, but they are sanitary.

3. This maintains sanitary conditions.

4. Ammonia dissolves soil and hair spray on mirrors, windows, sinks, and so forth.

Sanitation Rules for Salons and Schools

1. All schools and salons should be well lighted, heated, and ventilated. Air filters should be changed at the time recommended by the manufacturer.

2. Floor coverings should be washable. If carpeting is used, it should be a commercial grade and fire resistant. Carpet only the areas permitted by your state's law.

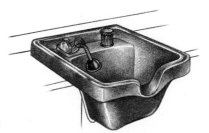

Figure 3.21
Sanitize the neck of the shampoo bowl after each use.

3. Walls and wall coverings should be washed and kept clean.
4. Pets, such as birds and cats, are not permitted (although a seeing eye dog for the blind is allowed).
5. No area of the school or salon may be used for residential purposes, such as sleeping quarters for owners, students, or employees.
6. Hair should be swept up immediately after the haircut and disposed of in a closed receptacle.
7. Implements should not be stored in uniform pockets. For example, combs, brushes, clips, hair nets, and permanent wave rods should not be carried in uniform pockets.
8. Separate male and female bathrooms are required by most states. They must be in working order, sanitized regularly, and have hot and cold water, soap, and a system that provides clean towels for each individual.
9. Beauty supplies and cosmetics should not be shared. For example, eye liner, lip color, powder puffs, emery boards, cheek color, combs, and brushes should not be in common use by the students and their clients. Remember that your eyes, mouth, ears, and nose are openings that could permit disease-causing bacteria or viruses to enter your body.
10. Drinking water faucets must be in working order; individual cups must be provided in some states.
11. Label all containers indicating the contents of the container and its strength.

Glossary

Active (natural) immunity The ability of the body's defense mechanisms to fight off disease by making antibodies (white blood cells) that destroy harmful bacteria in the blood.

AIDS A life-threatening disease caused by the HIV virus, which interferes with the body's immune system, causing it to break down; AIDS stands for acquired immunodeficiency syndrome.

Antibodies Substances in the blood that destroy harmful bacteria.

Antiseptics (an-teh-SEP-tiks) Substances that halt or prevent the growth of pathogenic bacteria.

Aseptic (ay-SEP-tik) Free from pathogenic bacteria.

Bacilli (bah-SIL-igh) Rod-shaped pathogenic bacteria that produce such serious diseases as diphtheria, leprosy, tuberculosis, and typhoid fever.

Bacteria (bak-TIR-ee-ah) One-celled microorganisms, sometimes called microbes.

Bactericides (bak-TIR-eh-sighdz) Chemicals that destroy pathogenic bacteria.

Bacteriology The study of bacteria.

Bromine gas A gas formed when ammonia and sodium bromate combine.

Cells The basic units of living matter.

Cilia (SIL-ee-ah) Whiplike extensions that cause a cell to move in a liquid. Also called flagella.

Cocci (KOK-sigh) Round pathogenic bacteria that usually cause pus-forming diseases such as boils, abscesses, and pustules.

Communicable (koh-MYOO-ni-kah-behl) See **Contagious.**

Contagious (kuhn-TAY-juhss) Capable of being transmitted to another person through touch or the air.

Dehumidifiers Devices that remove excessive moisture from the air.

Diplococci (dip-low-KOK-sigh) Round bacteria that usually appear in pairs and cause bacterial pneumonia.

Disinfectants (dis-in-FEK-tahnts) Chemicals that destroy pathogenic bacteria.

Dry sanitizer An airtight cabinet or drawer containing a chemical agent; it is used to store sanitized implements until they are used.

Electronic air precipitators Electric air cleaners.

Epidermis (ep-eh-DER-mis) The outermost layer of the skin.

Flagella (fleh-JEL-leh) Whiplike extensions that cause a cell to move in a liquid. Also called cilia.

Formaldehyde (for-MAL-deh-highd) A chemical that is used in some preparations to sanitize combing and setting implements.

Formalin A disinfectant composed of 37 percent formaldehyde, 6.5 percent methanol, and 56.5 percent water.

Fumigants (FYOO-mi-gahnts) Chemicals that destroy pathogenic bacteria.

Germ A common name for any pathogenic agent (bacteria or virus) that causes disease.

Germicides (JER-meh-sighdz) Chemicals that destroy pathogenic bacteria.

Hepatitis B A viral infection that attacks the liver.

HIV The virus that causes AIDS.

Humidifiers Devices that add moisture to the air, preventing excessive drying of the skin and reducing static electricity.

Immunity (ih-MYOO-neh-tee) The ability of the body's defense mechanisms to fight off disease.

Inorganic matter Matter that has never been alive.

Microbes (MIGH-krohbs) One-celled organisms, sometimes called bacteria.

Microorganisms (migh-kroh-OR-gehn-iz-uhmz) Organisms that can be seen only by using a microscope.

Mitosis (migh-TOH-sis) A process of cell division.

Nonpathogenic bacteria Bacteria that do not cause disease.

Organic (awr-GAN-ik) matter All things that are living or have been alive in the past.

Passive (acquired) immunity The ability of the body's defense mechanisms to fight disease upon injection of antibodies from another person or animal.

Pathogenic (PATH-ah-jen-ik) bacteria Bacteria that cause disease; commonly called germs.

Public sanitation The set of procedures used to prohibit the spread of communicable diseases and the development of other infections.

Quaternary ammonium (KWOT-er-ner-ee ah-MOHN-ee-um) ("Quats") A chemical used in solution for sterilizing combing and setting implements.

Saprophytes (SAP-roh-fightz) Bacteria that cause dead organic matter to decay and thus help enrich the soil.

Septic (SEP-tik) Toxic, unsanitary.

Spirilla (spigh-RIL-ah) Spiral-shaped pathogenic bacteria that cause cholera and syphilis.

Spontaneous combustion Process by which a fire starts without an outside source of flame such as a match or spark.

Spores (sporz) A spherical state in which some bacteria can survive for long periods of extreme heat and cold.

Staphylococci (staf-eh-low-KOK-sigh) Round, pathogenic bacteria, usually growing in clusters, that generally produce local infections.

Sterilization (stehr-il-eh-ZAY-shun) The process of killing all bacteria (pathogenic and nonpathogenic).

Streptococci (strep-tah-KOK-sigh) Round pathogenic bacteria that usually cause general infections.

Susceptible Especially likely to become ill from direct or indirect contact with disease-causing bacteria or viruses.

Toxins Poisons.

Ultramicroscopic Refers to things so small they can be seen only when magnified up to one million times by a scanning electron microscope.

Vacuum breaker A fixture that prevents the reverse flow of contaminated water and keeps it from backing up into the fresh water supply system.

Virus An ultramicroscopic parasitic pathogen.

Wet sanitizer A large, covered, nonmetal container that holds water and a chemical agent to sterilize implements.

1. What two-word term is used to refer to practices that promote and protect good health in the community?
2. Name the term given to anything that takes up space and has weight.
3. What term is used to refer to all basic units of organic matter?
4. What are the small organisms that cannot be seen without a microscope?
5. Which microorganisms are studied by cosmetologists?
6. What is the scientific study of bacteria called?
7. Are pathogenic bacteria harmful to humans?
8. Are nonpathogenic bacteria harmful to humans?
9. List the three types of bacteria and describe their respective shapes.
10. What conditions must exist for bacteria to grow?
11. Using your own words, explain the difference between sterilization and sanitation.
12. Describe the actions of antiseptics, fumigants, and disinfectants.
13. If you drank a large amount of a disinfectant, would it be harmful?
14. Name two disinfectant chemicals used by cosmetologists.
15. What liquid is used to sanitize metal implements, e.g., scissors?
16. What percentage hydrogen peroxide solution is an effective antiseptic?
17. Is 70 percent ethyl alcohol the same strength as 70 percent isopropyl alcohol?
18. What strength quats is needed to kill stubborn viruses such as the herpes simplex virus?
19. Is it necessary to wear gloves to remove combs and brushes from a wet sanitizer filled with quats?
20. Does the filter in an air conditioner clean the air as well as an air purifier?
21. Where should soiled towels be stored?
22. When ammonia fumes and sodium bromate fumes mix together, what hazard will result?
23. Where should flammable beauty products be stored?
24. What over-the-counter medicine will prevent infection from a chemical burn?
25. If a client is burned by a curling iron, should you apply Gentian Violet Jelly?
26. If an irritating chemical drips into a client's eye(s), what should you apply?
27. True or false? You can become infected with the AIDS virus by hand shakes.

28. True or false? AIDS is a disease solely of male homosexuals.
29. True or false? A mother with AIDS can transmit the virus to her unborn child.
30. True or false? AIDS is spread when a person infected with the virus shares body fluids with another person.
31. True or false? AIDS is a communicable disease.
32. True or false? You can get AIDS by sitting next to someone with AIDS.
33. True or false? The AIDS virus attacks the body's immune system.
34. True or false? Intravenous drug users are at risk for contracting the AIDS virus.
35. True or false? People get AIDS by donating blood.
36. True or false? There is no complete cure for AIDS.

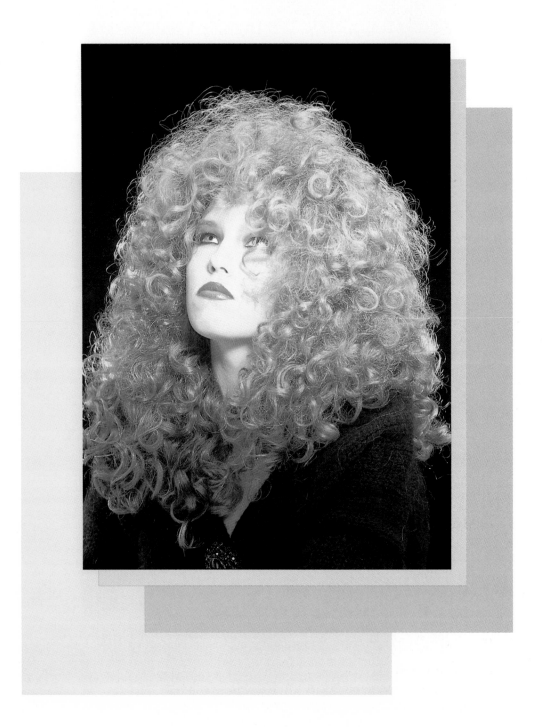

Describing the Hair

Learning Objective

With the information in this chapter and help from your instructor, define, identify, describe, and analyze the hair, its structure, function, composition, diseases, disorders, and condition. Score 85 percent or better on a multiple-choice exam on the information in this chapter.

In order to achieve the above level of competence, you should master the following chapter objectives.

Theory Objectives

1. Define hair and describe its function, location, composition, and types.
2. Describe the basic histology of the hair and surrounding structures.
3. Describe hair growth.
4. Identify the factors involved in analyzing hair condition.
5. Describe the abnormal conditions, diseases, and disorders of the hair and scalp.
6. Describe the removal of superfluous hair.

Theory Objective 1
Hair Function, Location, Composition, and Types

Hair performs **two functions: cosmetic** and **protective.** Hair **adorns** the body to improve the appearance of the individual. On certain parts of the body, it protects the skin from friction.

Although the hair of many animals covers larger areas of their bodies and provides better protection than human hair, we also have hair over most parts of our bodies, except for the palms of the hands, soles of the feet, lips, and a few other very small areas. But human hair is not easy to see, except on the scalp, face, arms, and legs.

Introduction

Trichology (tri-KOL-eh-jee) is the scientific study of the hair and its diseases. People who specialize in studying the hair and diseases related to the hair are called **trichologists** (tri-KOL-eh-jists). They are highly educated scientists, and as specialists, they constantly read and study all new information about the hair and diseases related to the hair.

You are studying to become a cosmetologist, not a trichologist. However, most services offered in a beauty school or salon are directly related to the hair. To perform services safely and effectively for your client, you will need to know the composition, structures, function, disorders, diseases, and condition of the hair. Although this chapter will give you the knowledge you will need, you should keep in mind that it covers only the basics.

The ability to recognize diseases of the hair and scalp has become increasingly important in recent years. More and more people are using over-the-counter hair products and appliances. As a result, cosmetologists are seeing more complex hair problems today than at any time in history. To cope with these problems, manufacturers have researched and developed many new preparations to help the professional cosmetologist. When should you use which product? The answer to this question is complicated, but it begins in this chapter. Other units will help complete the answer.

There are two basic types of hair: **lanugo** (lan-OO-goh) **(vellus) hairs** and **terminal hairs.** Lanugo (vellus) hairs are all over the body. They are fine and lightly pigmented (colored). Terminal hairs are **coarser, thicker,** and more pigmented (colored). Terminal hairs are found on the scalp, face, and extremities.

Making general statements about hair is difficult because its length, strength, and rate of growth vary on different parts of the body. Hair is grouped in six types: (1) scalp, (2) eyebrow and eyelash, (3) beard, (4) body, (5) pubic, and (6) underarm (axillary). The technical names for hair involved in salon services are (1) **capilli** (cah-PIL-igh), which is scalp hair; (2) **supercilia** (soo-per-SIL-ee-ah) and **cilia,** which are the eyebrows and eyelashes, respectively; and (3) **barba,** which is beard hair (Figure 4.1).

Scalp hair provides a cushion that helps the skull protect the brain. The eyebrows and eyelashes shield the delicate tissues of the eyes (for instance, from a speck of dirt or dust). Beard hair protects the face. Both men and women have beard hair, but male hormones make men's beard hair much coarser than women's. Pubic hair protects the genital region, and axillary hair shields the soft underarm skin.

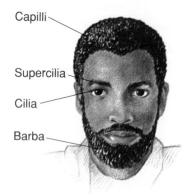

Capilli

Supercilia

Cilia

Barba

Figure 4.1
Types of facial hair

Hair is a slender, threadlike **appendage** (ah-PEN-dij), or extension of the skin. It is made of hard, keratinized protein. **Keratin** (KER-eh-tin) is a protein found in the human skin. It is located in the **epidermis** (the outer layer of skin, which is made of soft keratin that protects the body—you will hear more about the layers of the skin in Chapter 22). There are two kinds of keratin: soft and hard. Hard keratin forms the chemical basis of hair. Hair is made up of approximately 51 percent carbon, 7 percent hydrogen, 18 percent nitrogen, 5 percent sulfur, and 19 percent oxygen. Hair is nourished (fed) by protein that comes from food. The protein is carried to the hair by blood vessels.

A **molecule** (MOL-eh-kyool) is the smallest possible unit of any compound. It is made up of two or more atoms chemically combined. These atoms are joined, or connected, by bonds. The building blocks of protein molecules are organic substances called **amino acids.** Healthy hair has 18 or more of these amino acids.

As a cosmetologist, you will be especially interested in two amino acids: **cystine** (SIS-teen) and **tyrosine** (TIGH-rah-seen). Cystine is important for cold waving and chemical relaxing, while tyrosine is involved in hair coloring.

Hair is made beneath the scalp where amino acids form proteins. As this happens, chemical reactions that produce **peptide** (PEP-tighd) **linkages** take place. These peptide linkages are held together by cross-bonds. The hair has three types of cross-bonds: cystine, hydrogen, and salt (the salt bonds are less important). When these cross-bonds are joined together in the hair, they are called **poly** (many) **peptide bonds.** During hair-care services, the polypeptide bonds are broken and re-formed by both physical and chemical actions. Hydrogen bonds are broken physically when the hair is stretched while it is still wet and wound around a roller. The bonds re-form as the hair dries in a curled position or shape.

Cystine bonds (also called disulfide or sulfur bonds) are broken chemically by applying reducing agents to the hair (Figure 4.2). Then the bonds are re-formed by oxidation. In cold waving, for example, the bonds are broken by ammonium thioglycolate (waving lotion) and re-formed by hydrogen peroxide (the neutralizer).

Theory Objective 2
Basic Histology of the Hair and Surrounding Structures

Hair histology (his-TAHL-eh-jee) involves the study of the microscopic structures of the hair. As was mentioned in Theory Objective 1, hair is like a thread. This thread is called the hair shaft.

The **hair shaft** is the dead portion of a hair that is above the skin. Starting from the inside and working out, the basic layers of the hair shaft are the medulla, cortex, and cuticle (Figure 4.3). The part of the hair below the skin is called the **hair root.**

Figure 4.2
The effect of chemical action on sulfur bonds.

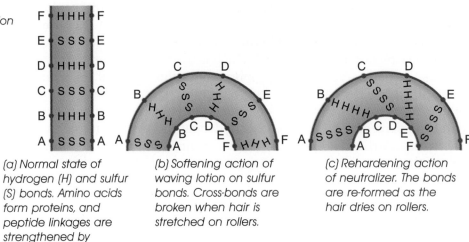

(a) Normal state of hydrogen (H) and sulfur (S) bonds. Amino acids form proteins, and peptide linkages are strengthened by cross-bonds.

(b) Softening action of waving lotion on sulfur bonds. Cross-bonds are broken when hair is stretched on rollers.

(c) Rehardening action of neutralizer. The bonds are re-formed as the hair dries on rollers.

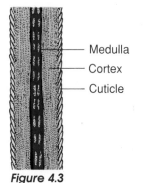

— Medulla
— Cortex
— Cuticle

Figure 4.3

Cross section of a hair shaft

The **medulla** (med-DUHL-ah) is the innermost layer of the hair shaft. It may contain soft keratin. The medulla is the least important layer of the hair. Some hair, such as lanugo hair (the short, soft hair found on some parts of the body, such as the arms), does not have a medulla (Figure 4.4).

The **cortex** (KOR-teks), or middle layer, is the largest layer of the hair. It makes up about 75 percent of a single hair and contains the coloring pigment (melanin). Natural hair colors have one or a combination of the following pigments: yellow, red, brown, and black.

The **cuticle** (KYOO-ti-kehl) is the outside layer of the hair; it consists of clear, horny cells that overlap (imbricate) to form the outer layer of the hair shaft (Figure 4.5). The density of the cuticle varies from 5 to 15 layers of cells, depending on a person's race. Caucasians usually have fewer than 7 layers; Orientals usually have from 7 to 10 layers; and blacks may have as many as 15 cuticle layers.

The hair grows through the **follicle** (FAHL-i-kehl), which encases the root. The follicle is a long, slender, pocketlike depression in the skin. Two glands and one muscle are located near the follicle. The two glands are an apocrine sweat gland and a sebaceous gland. (A **gland** is cell or group of cells that removes material from the blood, changes the material in some way, and secretes it either to another part of the body for further use or eliminates it from the body.) These glands empty into the follicle through ducts.

The **arrector pili** (ah-REK-tehr PIGH-ligh) **muscle** is attached to the follicle below these two glands (Figure 4.6). Changes in skin temperature cause this muscle to contract (become shorter), resulting in **"goose bumps."** Sudden fright also causes contraction. During this contraction, the hair stands straight up. The contraction of this muscle also forces sebum into the follicle, where it lubricates the hair and skin.

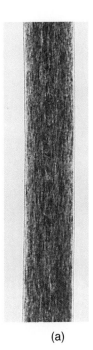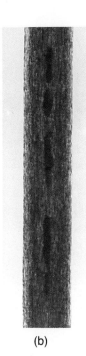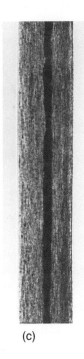

(a)   (b)   (c)

Figure 4.4
Microscopic photo of (a) a hair without a medulla; (b) a hair with intermittent medulla; and (c) a hair with continuous medulla.

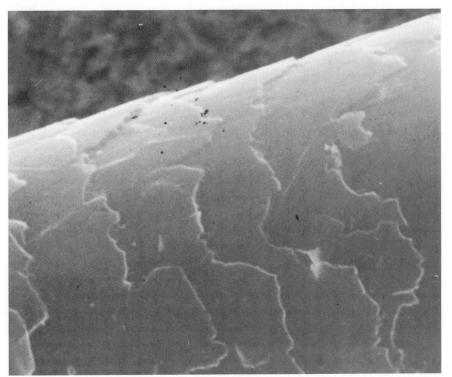

Figure 4.5
Cuticle layers (imbrications) of a hair seen under the scanning electron microscope.

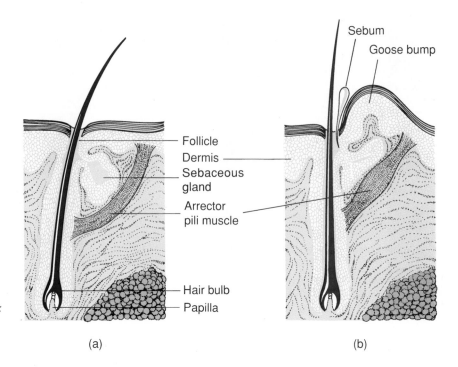

Figure 4.6
*(a) Arrector pili muscle relaxed;
(b) arrector pili muscle
contracted.*

At this point, you have traced the hair backwards, in a sense, from the hair shaft to the follicle. The glands and the muscle are at the top of the follicle. Hair is made farther down, at the other end of the follicle.

The **hair bulb** is the bottom part of the follicle. The hair bulb almost completely surrounds a small, nipplelike projection called the **papilla** (pap-PIL-ah), which grows from the dermis (the layer of the skin just below the epidermis). The papilla contains a nerve and the blood supply (one capillary—a very small vessel) needed to form hair and keep it growing.

In the middle and upper parts of the hair bulbs are **melanocytes** (MEL-an-oh-sights) that make melanin and cells for making hard keratin (Figure 4.7). **Melanin** (MEL-eh-nehn) gives hair its

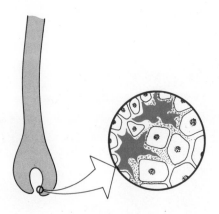

Figure 4.7
*Detail of the hair bulb, showing
melanocytes forming pigment.*

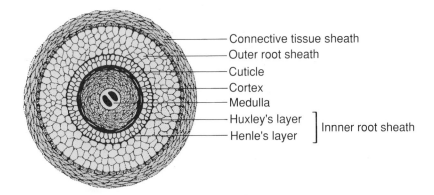

- Connective tissue sheath
- Outer root sheath
- Cuticle
- Cortex
- Medulla
- Huxley's layer ⎤
- Henle's layer ⎦ Innner root sheath

Figure 4.8
Horizontal cross section through a hair and root sheath.

color. When the melanocytes cannot make melanin, a person's hair turns gray. Cosmetologists call gray hair **canities.**

Have you ever seen a child with gray hair? His (or her) gray hair is probably **congenital** (since birth). This is one type of gray hair. The other type, **acquired gray hair** (canities), often occurs by the early forties, although it can occur at almost any age. Whether and when your hair will turn gray are usually determined by **heredity.**

The keratin that is made in the hair bulb is actually turned into keratinized protein just above the hair bulb in two layers of the follicle called Henle's layer and Huxley's layer (Figures 4.8 and 4.9).

The process of keratinization (changing keratin into hard protein) is slow. It occurs in stages, but when the hair comes out of the follicle, it has been completely changed into hard protein.

Figure 4.9
Vertical cross section through a hair and root sheath.

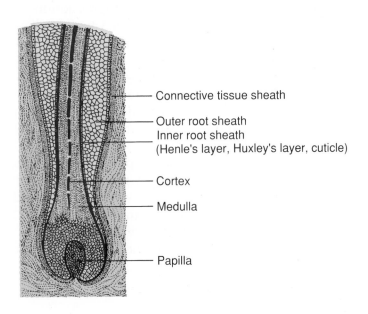

- Connective tissue sheath
- Outer root sheath
- Inner root sheath
  (Henle's layer, Huxley's layer, cuticle)
- Cortex
- Medulla
- Papilla

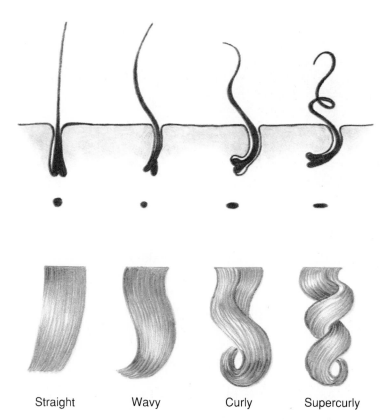

Figure 4.10
The angle of the follicle and the shape of the shaft affect the curliness of the hair.

Straight   Wavy   Curly   Supercurly

The possibility of infection at the mouth of the follicle (right next to the skin, where the hair emerges) is a good example of why personal hygiene is important. There is a depression in the skin at the mouth of the follicle. This depression is a perfect place for bacteria, sebum, and dirt to collect. If this happens, it can cause either a minor infection or a serious disease.

As you know, hair can have different shapes and degrees of curliness. You often can see the four different categories by looking at cross sections of hair shafts under a microscope. A **flat** hair shaft is supercurly; a **semi-oval** one is curly; an **oval** one is wavy; and a **round** one is straight (Figure 4.10).

The **angle** at which the follicle approaches the surface of the skin can affect the shape of the hair. A follicle that is curved and parallel to the skin produces a supercurly hair shaft. A follicle that approaches the skin at a slight angle forms a wavy shaft. The angle of the follicle for a curly shaft is in between that for a supercurly and a wavy shaft. A follicle that is perpendicular to the surface of the skin produces a straight hair.

Figure 4.12 shows various aspects of hair at high magnifications.

Hair appears very early on the human body. In fact, it appears on a human embryo near the eyebrows by the sixth or seventh week after conception (in other words, even before birth). Other hairs appear after the twelfth week.

All human hair grows in cyclical periods that differ from one region of the body to another. **Scalp hair,** for example, grows for **two to five years** before it goes into a resting phase. Hair growth on the trunk, limbs, and other areas occurs in periods of four to six months.

Hair goes through three recognized cycles of growth: **anagen, catagen,** and **telogen** (Figure 4.11).

The **anagen** (AN-ah-jen) **stage** is the **growth period.** The length of the anagen stage determines the length of the hair shaft. The anagen stage has two phases. During the first phase, the hair bulb stretches itself out into the follicle. During the second period, hard keratin is synthesized in the follicle. Although the anagen stage normally lasts from 2 to 5 years, periods of 25 years have been recorded. In the anagen stage, **scalp hair grows** at a rate of about **half an inch per month.**

During the **catagen** (KAT-eh-jen) **stage,** hair growth slows and club hairs form. Keratinization does not take place during this stage.

The **telogen** (TEL-oh-jen) **stage** is a resting period that continues until the next anagen stage begins. Although scientists do not know exactly how long the telogen stage lasts, they think it is short—three or four months.

The number of hairs on normal scalps varies according to hair color: **90,000** for **red** hair; **105,000** for **black** hair; **110,000** for **brown** hair; and **140,000** for **blonde** hair.

During the telogen stage, the hairs are removed easily by vigorous brushing. Under normal conditions, 85 to 95 percent of the terminal (coarse) scalp hairs are in the anagen stage; 1 percent are in the catagen stage; and from 4 to 14 percent are in the telogen stage.

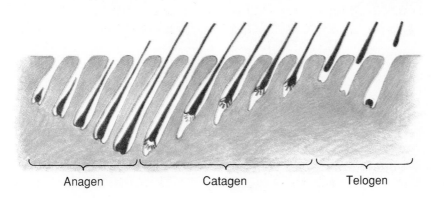

Figure 4.11
The three stages of hair growth

Anagen   Catagen   Telogen

Figure 4.12
Highly magnified views of hair

(a) Magnified 1,000 times, the hair cuticle is composed of overlapping layers.

(b) Using a magnification of 15,000×, this micrograph indicates that the cuticle layers are held together with a gluelike substance, appearing as a white membrane between cuticle layers. When this substance is damaged, for instance, by chemicals, environmental causes, and excessive heat from curling irons and blow dryers, it deteriorates, allowing the layers to separate. This causes the hair to lose luster and sheen.

(c) A knotted hair magnified 400× shows severe damage with the cuticle layers separating, particularly in the area of the knot. The loose cuticle causes the hair to feel rough and become tangled during styling.

(d) A hair magnified 1,000× shows a break (split from using brush rollers).

(e) This cross section of a hair, magnified 2,000× shows the medulla at the center, the color pigmented cells of the cortex, and the cuticle as one layer.

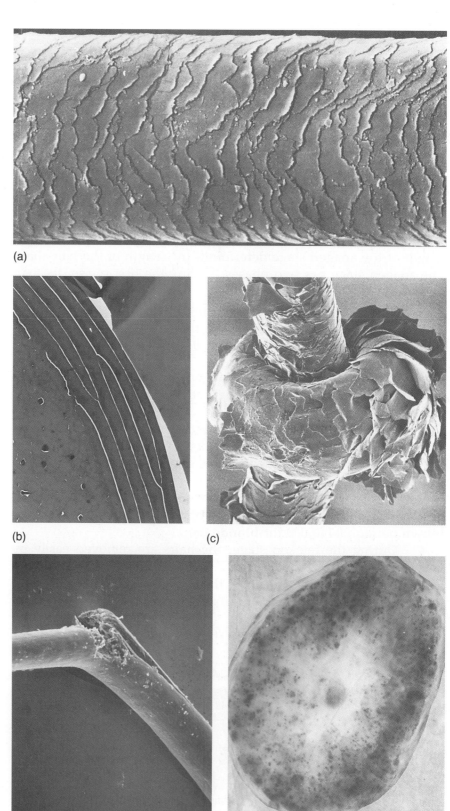

(a)

(b)

(c)

(d)

(e)

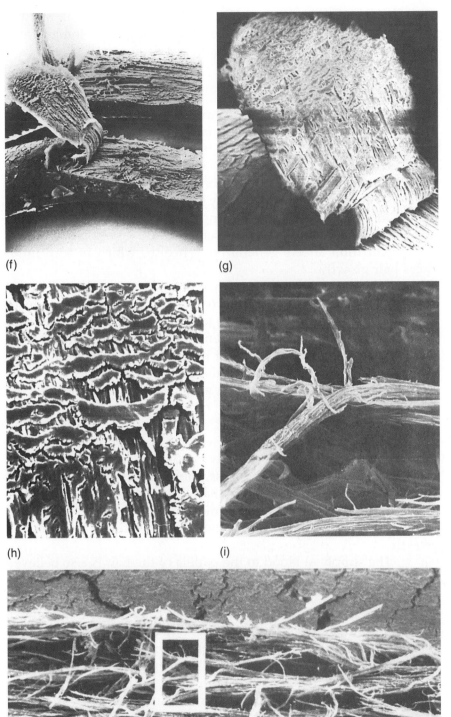

(f)

(g)

(h)

(i)

(j)

(f) When hair wound around a pin is nicked with a razor blade, a split is clearly visible at a magnification of 200×. When the split section is torn, the longitudinal fibers of the cortex are revealed.

(g) At 400×, the flap shows that where the hair is cut, the details of the fibers of the cortex are obscured by a plastic-like or adhesive coating. Where the hair is torn, the structural details of the fibers are visible.

(h) At 2,000×, the coating now believed to be a micropolysaccharide (carbohydrates bound to protein and mucoproteins that form a cement substance) is apparent where the long fibers have been cut.

(i) At 2,000 ×, more detail of the fibers' development into a cable is visible.

(j) This scanning electron micrograph at 200× shows the fibers from the cortex that have been pulled from the split hair by adhesive tape. The fibers do not lie parallel but are twisted and often cross each other. They also form a cable, similar to spun sewing thread. The entanglement of the individual fibers gives the hair its strength and elasticity.

Thus, hair grows almost continuously. However, nearly all the tiny vellus hairs on the scalp are in the telogen stage. On the average, humans lose between 50 and 75 hairs per day.

Influences on Hair Growth

Hair is affected mainly by **climate** and the **seasons** of the year. Hair grows faster in warmer climates than in colder ones and faster in summer than in winter.

Hormones increase hair growth on the scalp. Since women generally have proportionately more female hormones than men have male hormones, women rarely become bald. In contrast, many men gradually lose their hair. During menopause, women may find that their vellus hairs have a coarser texture.

Nutrition affects general body health, which in turn influences hair growth.

Stimulation may promote hair growth, although this has not been proved. For instance, trauma (shock) such as nail biting causes nails (also appendages of the skin) to grow faster. Hair growth similarly might be stimulated by frequent (more than once a week) scalp massages. However, the hair shaft is a **dead** structure, and the papilla, where growth begins, is at the base of the follicle; therefore, close shaving, trimming, tweezing, cutting, or singeing (burning the ends of the hair) and creams, gels, or ointments will not make hair grow faster.

Hair seems to grow faster when it is cut short because any growth is noticeable, but it actually is not growing faster.

As part of the aging process, most men naturally lose some hair. This is called **male pattern hair loss** (baldness). Figure 4.13 shows how hair loss progresses as men become older. As mentioned earlier, male hormones (testosterone) are also thought to affect hair growth.

The supply of blood to the papilla of the hair is also believed to affect hair growth. Currently, one drug is available that increases this blood flow. This drug, a clear liquid named **Minoxidal** (Rogaine), is being prescribed by dermatologists for the treatment of hair loss in men (and sometimes women).The drug was originally called Loniten and, in pill (tablet) form, was used to treat persons with high blood pressure. Doctors discovered that persons taking these pills grew extra hair on the face, scalp, arms, and so forth. The hair also grew out longer and darker than normal.

Minoxidal is a very powerful drug and potentially dangerous. Both the liquid and the pill forms of this drug have had serious undesirable side effects. For example, the directions that come in the package of Loniten warn that it may cause the following:

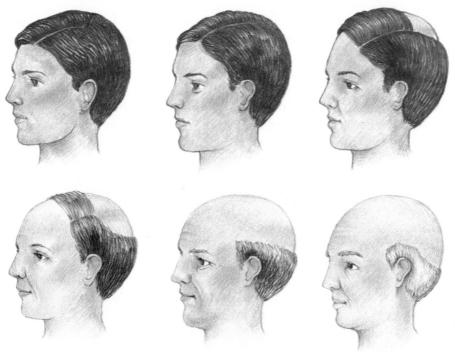

Figure 4.13
Male pattern hair loss

- Increased heart rate.
- Rapid weight gain.
- Increased difficulty breathing.
- New or worsening pain in the chest, arm, or shoulder or signs of severe indigestion.
- Dizziness, lightheadedness, or fainting.

The diluted (watered down) liquid form of Minoxidal has had some limited success in stopping hair loss. It will also cause hair to grow in a certain percentage of people. Usually the younger the person is, the better the results will be. This drug should be taken only on the written prescription of a doctor.

Theory Objective 4
Factors Involved in Analyzing Hair Condition

As a student and later as a practicing cosmetologist, you will learn to watch for certain signals or signs when you prepare treatments for a client. The condition of a client's hair shaft—indicated by its texture, porosity, elasticity, appearance, and feel—will rank high on your list of concerns.

Hair texture is related to its **diameter. Fine** hair has a smaller (thinner) diameter than **medium** hair, and **course** hair has a larger diameter than medium hair. At least two structures can influence the diameter of the hair: the medulla and the cuticle.

As was pointed out earlier in the chapter, some hair does not have a medulla (see Figure 4.4a). You can see whether a hair has a medulla or not by looking at it under a microscope. (The medulla also can be distributed unevenly through a hair.) Overall, whether a hair has a medulla or not is not particularly important. Hair without a medulla may have a smaller diameter than hair that has a medulla.

For many years, scientists thought that the cuticle protecting the cortex was made up of only one layer. In recent years, however, scientists, aided by the scanning electron microscope, have learned that hair has from 5 to 15 imbricated (overlapping) cuticle layers.

You must consider hair texture when selecting products. Products are made in strengths that are best for various hair conditions. Fine hair ordinarily does not have as much **tensile strength** (the ability to stretch without breaking) as medium hair, and coarse hair has greater tensile strength than medium hair.

Hair **porosity** (poh-RAHSS-eh-tee) refers to the amount of moisture that can be absorbed by the cuticle layers. There is a direct relationship between porosity and the number of cuticle layers in the hair. Porosity is also affected by the acidity or alkalinity of the products used. **Alkaline** (AL-kah-lin) preparations cause the overlapping cuticle scales to "open," or stand away from the cortex, to a certain extent. **Acid** preparations have a tendency to "close" the overlapping cuticle layers, causing them to lie tightly against the cortex.

You can test the porosity of the hair by the following procedure (Figure 4.14). Hold a strand of dry hair one inch square straight out from the scalp between the middle and index fingers of your left hand. Slide the middle and index fingers of your right hand along the strand toward the scalp. The more the strands pile up or slide toward the scalp, the more porous the hair is. This occurs because the fingers of the right hand will "catch" the cuticle scales of the hair that are not closed. If the cuticle scales are tightly packed against the cortex, the hair is **not porous.** Nonporous hair is considered resistant to certain services because its cuticle is difficult to penetrate.

The **elasticity** of the hair refers to its ability to stretch without breaking and return to its original form. **Dry hair** with good elasticity can normally be stretched one-fifth, or **20 percent,** of its length, while **wet hair** can be stretched two-fifths, or **40 percent (sometimes 50 percent),** of its length without breaking. Some companies make instruments that measure the tensile strength of hair. Your instructor may wish to demonstrate one of these instruments in class.

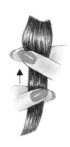

Figure 4.14
Porosity test

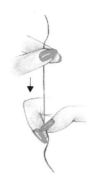

Figure 4.15
Elasticity test

Although small machines are sold to determine the exact **tensile strength,** or elasticity of the hair, you can perform a simple manual test that is quick and very accurate (Figure 4.15). Pluck one hair from your client's head. Holding the hair between the middle and index fingers of your left hand, slide the hair between the thumbnail and index finger of your right hand in the direction of the cuticle scales. This action produces a "ribboning" effect; the hair will spiral like a piece of wrapping ribbon. The number of spirals the hair makes indicates its elasticity. The more the hair spirals, the stronger it is. Few spirals indicate that the hair is weak or fragile. Hold the hair at each end in a straight position for three seconds and then release one end. If the hair hangs straight with very little or no curl, its elasticity is not very good.

The **appearance** of the hair should be lustrous and shiny. The **sebaceous gland secretes oil (sebum)** into the hair follicle (Figure 4.16). The sebum works its way to the scalp, where it is transferred onto the hair shaft by brushing and gives the hair sheen and luster. The sebum seals moisture in the hair and protects it from sun, wind, and weather. Without sebum, the hair appears dry and lusterless.

The **feel** of the hair is another indicator of its condition. In some cases, touching the hair is the only, or best, way to check hair texture and to detect certain conditions, such as color buildup. There is no "magic formula" for learning how hair should "feel." This is a sense that you can develop only through experience and help from your instructor or manager.

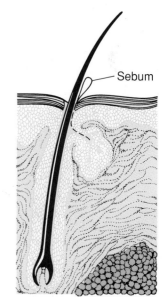

— Sebum

Figure 4.16
Sebaceous gland secreting sebum

Theory Objective 5
Abnormal Conditions, Diseases, and Disorders of the Hair and Scalp

As a student and later as a cosmetologist, you will probably see abnormal conditions (maybe even very serious disorders and diseases) of the hair. Although you will not—in fact, cannot—treat these diseases, you should be able to recognize them. **Trichosis** (tri-KOH-siss) is any diseased condition of the hair.

Conditions of Overgrowth

Hypertrichosis (high-per-trik-OH-siss)—excessive growth of unwanted hair—is also called **superfluous** hair or **hirsutism** (HIR-soot-iz-uhm) (Figure 4.17). **Congenital** hypertrichosis is considered hereditary.

    Localized hypertrichosis takes two forms. Sometimes it appears as two or three hairs growing in a mole or as considerable growth over large areas of the body. Refer persons with hypertrichosis to a dermatologist. Electrolysis may be necessary to treat this condition, but it should be done only on a doctor's recommendation. If moles are not involved, it is all right to bleach or tweeze a few hairs on a small area of skin. Removal of excess hair will be treated in the next theory objective (see page 81).

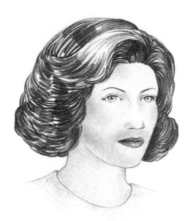

Figure 4.17
Superfluous hair

Classification of Hair Loss

Alopecia (al-ah-PEE-shee-ah) means hair loss (Figure 4.18). There are many kinds of alopecia and many reasons for it. The most familiar is probably alopecia of the scalp. It is particularly important in beauty-care services because it is so noticeable, but there are many other forms.

    There are two categories of alopecia of the scalp: (1) diffuse (scattered) and (2) patchy. Patchy alopecia also comes in two varieties: one causes scars; the other does not. In the scarring variety, hair cannot grow because the papilla of the follicle has been destroyed.

    There are five types of **diffuse hair loss:**

1. Male pattern hair loss.
2. Female pattern hair loss.
3. Temporary hair loss in females.
4. Hair loss due to trauma caused by physical or chemical interference with natural growth.
5. Hair loss due to disorders of the body.

Each type has its own characteristics:

1. **Male pattern hair loss** is a receding hairline caused by heredity, aging, or a decrease in hormones. Young clients should consult a dermatologist for preparations that may at least slow the hair loss.

2. **Female pattern hair loss** occurs in women over 50 as a result of a relative increase in the male hormone. There is no effective treatment, but maintenance of a healthy scalp is important.

3. **Temporary hair loss in females** can follow childbirth, nervous upset, or the use of anesthetics or may occur for no apparent reason. During pregnancy, hair growth increases, but after delivery, hair loss occurs until the body returns to its normal state. Baldness seldom results from childbirth.

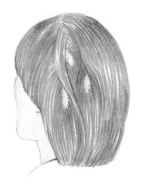

Figure 4.18
Alopecia areata (oval bald patches)

4. **Different kinds of trauma,** both physical and chemical, can cause hair loss. Accident, injury, or infection (such as pneumonia) can cause hair loss because of the shock to the nervous system. Some chemicals used to treat certain diseases and conditions can also cause hair loss.

5. Some **disorders of the body** also can cause loss of hair. Diseases of the endocrine system of the body, such as an underactive thyroid or pituitary gland, can lead to loss of hair. Some congenital (birth) defects can cause loss of nails as well as hair. Treatments for different kinds of cancer can also cause hair loss. When treatment stops, the hair grows back.

There are two types of **patchy nonscarring hair loss:**

1. **Alopecia areata** (ay-reh-AT-ah) refers to an **oval bald patch** usually caused by bodily disorders (see Figure 4.18). There may be one or several patches, but there is no scaling or infection. Alopecia areata usually affects the scalp, eyebrows, eyelashes, and beard, but it can occur in any area. In 6 to 12 months, the hair is usually (though not always) restored.

2. **Tinea** (TIN-ee-ah) **capitis** (of the scalp) is characterized by broken-off hairs, scars and occasionally infection (Figure 4.19). This is a ringworm infection. The scales on the surface of the scalp are very white or gray. Do not serve a client with tinea of the scalp; advise the client to see a doctor.

Although they do not fall into the category of patchy nonscarring hair loss, four other types of alopecia exist. Total loss of scalp or body hair is called **alopecia totalis** (toh-TAL-iss); it is usually permanent. Its cause is unknown, but it may be linked to infections

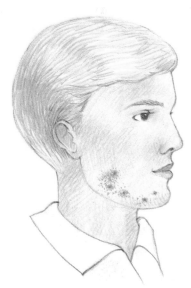

Figure 4.19
Tinea barba

(teeth, prostate, sinuses, gallbladder, and so forth) and emotional problems. Heredity is also involved. **Alopecia universal** is a loss of hair all over the body. **Alopecia senilis** (seh-NIL-iss) refers to loss of hair occurring in old age, and **alopecia prematura** refers to hair loss early in life.

Three types of patchy hair loss cause scars:

1. Rare tinea of the scalp.

2. Bacterial infection of the scalp.

3. Damage to skin from third-degree burns, overdose of X-rays, trauma, caustics, and other severe skin injuries.

Diseases and Disorders of Hair Other Than Loss

In many cases, you will be able to recognize hair diseases or disorders quickly and easily because you will notice that the client has lost a considerable amount of hair.

Trichorrhexis nodosa (tri-koh-REK-siss no-DOH-sah), or **knotted hair,** is an uncommon disease of the beard and pubic hair of adults; it is characterized by nodular swelling along the hair shaft (Figure 4.20a). If you look at hair having this disease under a microscope, you will see a definite pattern of breaks across the hair.

Monilethrix (mon-i-LETH-riks), or **beaded hair,** involves rhythmic, alternating constrictions along the hair shaft that look like nodes or beads (Figure 4.20b). Hairs with this disease are usually

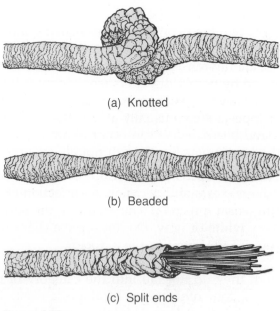

(a) Knotted

(b) Beaded

(c) Split ends

Figure 4.20
Examples of hair disorders

coarse, dry, and dull. They eventually break off at the constrictions, leaving a stubble either over the entire scalp or in localized areas. Alopecia does not result from this condition. The cause of monilethrix is unknown, but both the hair shaft and the follicle are involved, and obviously the keratinization process is affected.

Pili (PIGH-ligh) is a general term that means pertaining to the hair. It appears in the names of many hair disorders.

Pili annulati (PIGH-ligh an-nyoo-LAY-tigh), or **ringed hair,** is characterized by dark and white bands in some or all of the scalp hair. If a client has this condition, you will be able to spot it easily in ordinary light. This hair may appear to lack pigment, but actually pigment is present. Heredity seems to be a factor in the development of this condition. There is no treatment.

Pili incarnati (PIGH-ligh in-CAR-nay-tigh), or **ingrown hair,** occurs in individuals who have short, bristly, recurved hairs. This disorder affects facial areas that are shaved every day. The hair simply reenters the skin, irritates it, and causes a pimple. This irritation can be complicated further if the disease does not stop when the hair is allowed to escape through an opening in the skin.

Trichoptilosis (tri-kop-ti-LOH-siss), or **split ends,** also known as **fragilitas crinium (fragile hair shaft),** is characterized by splitting along the length of the hair shafts (Figure 4.20c). This is not a disease, and its cause is not known. Professional conditioning treatments should improve this disorder.

Theory Objective 6
Removal of Superfluous Hair

Many of your clients will want superfluous hair removed. Two basic processes are used to remove unwanted hair temporarily: **epilation** (pulling the hair from the follicle) and **depilation** (removing part of the hair shaft at skin level).

1. **Tweezing** (plucking or epilation) involves pulling the hairs from the follicle in the areas of the eyebrows, upper lip, chin, and neck (Figure 4.21).

2. Cutting (depilation) involves applying shaving cream and cutting the hair with a safety razor (Figure 4.22). Some people, feeling that shaving cream is unnecessarily messy, use an electric razor instead.

3. Waxing removes hair by using a wax solution that has a strong chemical base—the same chemicals that are used in cold waving solution. **After a predisposition test** to ensure that the client will not react to the chemicals, the wax is heated to a **comfortable** temperature. Always remember these rules:

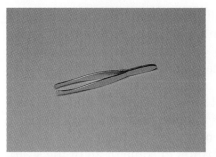

Figure 4.21
Tweezers (epilation)

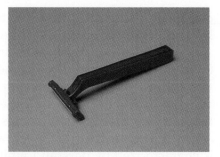

Figure 4.22
Razor (depilation)

Safety Tip ▶

- Test the temperature of the wax **before** applying it to a client.

- Avoid using wax on tender or diseased skin, such as red or irritated skin, moles, or warts.

- Be careful not to allow wax to run into the client's ears or eyes or onto sensitive areas that could cause harm.

- **Remember—wax can burn!**

When the wax is ready, it takes on a creamy appearance. It is applied with the natural growth of the hair and covered with gauze or a similar kind of wrapping (Figure 4.23).

This preparation softens the hair, and the gauze can be peeled off safely in about two minutes (Figure 4.24). If you follow the label directions, you will find that this type of depilatory is simple to use and leaves the skin soft and pliable.

4. A variety of over-the-counter foam and liquid depilatories (depilation) are available. However, **always give a skin test** (allergy test) on a hairless part of a client's arm **before using a depilatory.** Use depilatories very carefully because they are very strong and may irritate the skin (do not use on client's arms). Their basic ingredient, thioglycolate, dissolves hair. Be sure to wash the area where the depilatory was used with warm water to remove the chemicals.

All temporary measures are just that; the hair will soon grow out again, and the procedure will have to be repeated.

The only permanent way to remove hair is through **electrolysis** (eh-lek-TRAHL-eh-siss). The licensed or registered person who performs electrolysis is called an **electrologist.** In some states, any licensed cosmetologist may remove hair by electrolysis; in others, a separate license is needed. Because of the possibility of contracting AIDS, **disposable, puncture-resistant gloves** should be worn for the entire service. (Check with your state board, department of health,

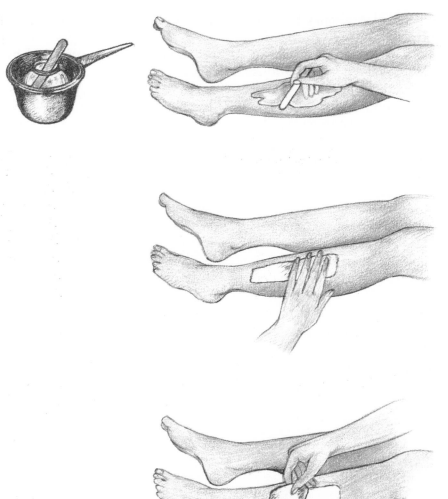

Figure 4.23
Removal of superfluous hair by hot waxing method

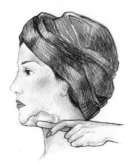 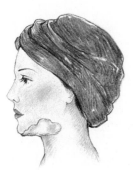 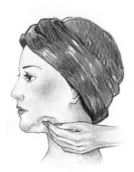

(a) Apply wax   (b) Allow wax to cool   (c) Remove wax

Figure 4.24
Hot wax works in about two minutes.

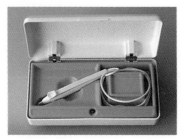

Figure 4.25
Electrolysis machine

or other state agency to learn about other requirements.) Dispose of gloves and needles properly.

The electrologist uses a **short-wave machine,** approved by the Federal Communications Commission, to remove hairs **only** in the hairline, eyebrows, cheeks, lips, chin, underarms, arms, legs, and so on (Figure 4.25).

The electrologist follows several steps to remove the hair. He or she inserts a new or thoroughly sterilized short-wave needle ⅛ to ¼ inch into the hair follicle, following the angle of the follicle with respect to the scalp (Figure 4.26). The operator inserts the needle manually and steps on a foot pedal that starts the machine, but once started, the machine works automatically. The current stops and starts according to the selection set on the time and intensity controls. The current destroys the papilla of the hair follicle. The hair then slides easily from the skin. The strength of the current and the length of time it runs are determined by the texture of the hair, e.g., fine, medium, or coarse (coarser hair may require more current and time), the type of machine, and the electrologist.

Safety Tip ▶

An electrologist **never** removes hair from eyelids or ears, from inside the nose, from moles or warts, or from inflamed or diseased skin. Clients who have diabetes cannot be treated. If the electrologist is unsure of the client's health, he or she should request written permission from the person's doctor prior to giving the service. The electrologist always maintains a sanitary work area and

Figure 4.26
Inserting electric needle to destroy the papilla of the hair follicle

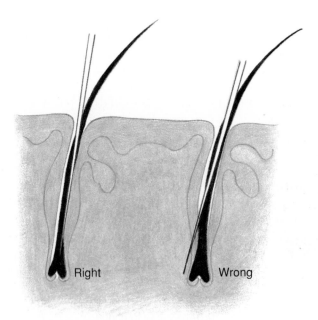

Right   Wrong

implements. Additional information about electrology will be presented in the electricity chapter.

Superfluous hair can be bleached instead of removed. Lightly pigmented hair on the arms, legs, and face can be bleached, but hair growing from moles or warts must **not** be lightened. Handle bleaches carefully to protect the skin and eyes.

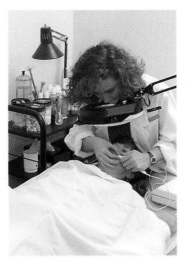

Figure 4.27
Electrologist removing hair.

Glossary

Acid preparations Products that cause the cuticle layers of the hair to "close" or lie tightly against the cortex.

Alkaline (AL-kah-lin) preparations Products that cause the cuticle layers of the hair to "open" or stand away from the cortex to a certain extent.

Alopecia (al-ah-PEE-shee-ah) A hair loss or baldness of temporary or permanent nature. Some of its forms are **alopecia areata** (ay-reh-AT-ash), an oval bald patch; **alopecia prematura,** hair loss occurring before middle age; **alopecia senilis** (seh-NIL-iss), hair loss due to age; **alopecia totalis** (toh-TAL-iss), a permanent total hair loss; and **alopecia universal,** hair loss all over the body.

Amino acids Organic substances that are the building blocks of the protein molecule.

Anagen (AN-ah-jen) stage The growth period of hair.

Appendage (ah-PEN-dij) The extension of something; used in this chapter to refer to hair as an appendage of the skin.

Arrector pili (ah-REK-tehr PIGH-ligh) A muscle attached to the follicle that contracts with changes in skin temperature.

Barba Beard hair.

Canities Gray hair.

Capilli (cah-PIL-igh) Scalp hair.

Catagen (KAT-eh-jen) stage The period in which hair growth slows and club hairs form.

Cilia (SIL-ee-ah) Eyelashes.

Congenital Existing since birth.

Cortex (KOR-teks) The middle and largest layer of hair; contains the coloring pigment.

Cuticle (KYOO-ti-kehl) The outside layer of clear horny cells that overlap to form the outer layer of the hair shaft.

Cystine (SIS-teen) An amino acid found in hair; important in cold waving and chemical relaxing.

Cystine bonds Chemical bonds in the hair that are broken by applying strong alkalies and acids to the hair. They are re-formed during oxidation or by applying a chemical neutralizer. Also called disulfide or sulfur bonds.

Elasticity The ability of the hair to stretch without breaking and return to its original form.

Electrologist A person trained to remove hair by destroying the papilla at the base of the hair root by electrolysis.

Electrolysis (eh-lek-TRAHL-eh-siss) Permanently removing the hair by destroying the papilla at the base of the hair root with an electric needle.

Follicle (FAHL-i-kehl) A long, slender, pocketlike depression of the skin from which hair grows.

Gland A cell or group of cells that removes material from the blood, changes that material, and secretes it to another part of the body or eliminates it.

Hair bulb The bottom part of the follicle surrounding the papilla.

Hair histology The study of microscopic structures of the hair.

Hirsutism (HIR-suh-tiz-uhm) An excessive growth of hair in unwanted places.

Hypertrichosis (high-per-trik-OH-siss) Excessive unwanted growth of the hair; also called superfluous hair or, in extreme cases, hirsutism.

Keratin (KER-eh-tin) A protein found in the human skin and its appendages: hair and nails.

Lanugo (lan-OO-goh) hairs Fine, lightly pigmented hairs occurring all over the body; also called vellus hairs.

Male pattern hair loss The loss of hair due to the aging process in males.

Medulla (meh-DUHL-ah) The innermost layer of the hair. Some hairs do not have a medulla.

Melanin (MEL-eh-nehn) A kind of pigment that gives hair its color.

Melanocytes (MEL-an-oh-sights) Cells that make melanin.

Minoxidal (MIN-ox-idal) A clear liquid preparation being prescribed by dermatologists for the treatment of hair loss, particularly in men, but sometimes for women.

Molecule (MOL-eh-kyool) The smallest possible unit of any compound, made up of two or more atoms chemically combined.

Monilethrix (mon-i-LETH-riks) A condition in which hair appears to have nodes or beads along the shafts.

Peptide (PEP-tighd) linkages Amino acid combinations held together by cross-bonds that form the hair. These bonds are broken and re-formed by physical and chemical actions during hair-care services.

Pigment A substance that gives hair its color.

Pili (PIGH-ligh) A prefix that means pertaining to the hair.

Pili annulati (PIGH-ligh an-nyoo-LAY-tigh) A condition characterized by dark and white bands in some or all of the scalp; also called ringed hair.

Pili incarnati (PIGH-ligh in-CAR-nay-tigh) Ingrown hairs.

Porosity (poh-RAHSS-eh-tee) The amount of moisture that can be absorbed by the cuticle layers of the hair.

Porous Capable of absorbing moisture.

Short-wave machine A machine used by an electrologist to remove superfluous hair.

Supercilia (soo-per-SIL-ee-ah) Eyebrows.

Superfluous (soo-PER-fluh-wuhs) hair Unwanted hair.

Telogen (TEL-oh-jen) stage The resting period of hair growth.

Tensile strength Elasticity.

Terminal hair Coarse, thick, pigmented hair found on the scalp, face, and extremities.

Tinea capitis (TIN-ee-ah) of the scalp A condition of broken hairs, scaliness, and, occasionally, infection caused by bacteria. Ringworm—a vegetable parasite.

Trichology (tri-KOL-eh-jee) The scientific study of the hair and its diseases.

Trichologists (tri-kOL-eh-jists) People who specialize in studying the hair and diseases related to the hair.

Trichoptilosis (tri-kop-ti-LOH-siss) Hair that splits along the length of the hair; commonly called split ends.

Trichorrhexis nodosa (tri-koh-REK-siss no-DOH-sah) An uncommon disease of beard and pubic hair characterized by nodular swelling along the hair shaft.

Trichosis (tri-KOH-siss) Any diseased condition of the hair.

Tyrosine (TIGH-rah-seen) An amino acid found in the hair that is involved in hair coloring services.

Questions

1. What is the technical name for the scientific study of the hair and its diseases?
2. Aside from protection, what is the function of hair?
3. Briefly define lanugo hair.

4. What is a threadlike appendage of the skin called?
5. What is the outer layer of the skin?
6. What is the smallest unit of a compound?
7. The basic building block of the protein molecule has a two-part name. What is the name?
8. What are the other names for cystine bonds?
9. Using your own words, write a definition for hair histology.
10. Using the text, write definitions for the following terms: hair shaft, medulla, cortex, cuticle.
11. What is the hair follicle?
12. What muscle causes "goose bumps" on the skin?
13. Where is the papilla located, and what does it do?
14. What is melanin?
15. What is a simple two-word definition for canities?
16. What is the technical term for the process that changes soft keratin to hard protein (keratin)?
17. What are the three growing cycles of the hair?
18. What are the four types of hair on the head?
19. Does hair grow faster in summer or winter?
20. What is the technical name given to an oval, bald patch on the head?
21. What is another name for ringworm of the scalp?
22. Before giving a service to a client using a depilatory, what should you do?
23. Why do you have to be extremely careful when using hot wax on a client?

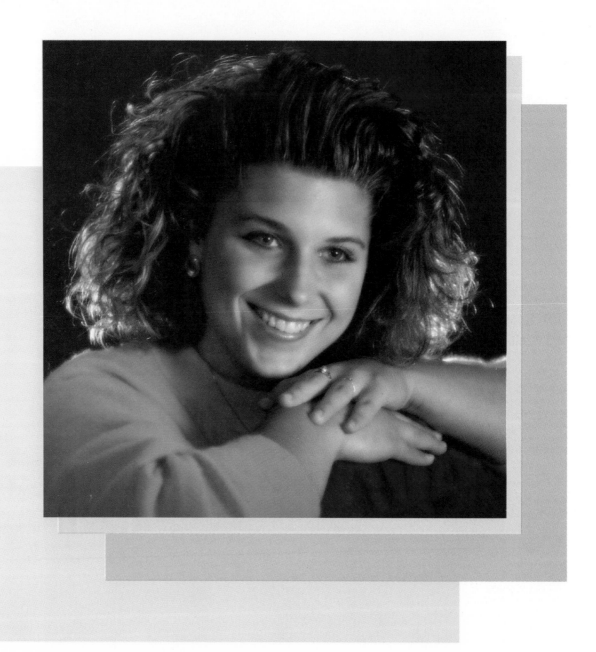

Shampooing

Learning Objective

Use shampoo supplies to cleanse the scalp and hair following the proper steps given in this chapter. Perform the service within 10 to 15 minutes. Score 85 percent or better on a multiple-choice exam on the information in this chapter.

In order to achieve the above level of competence, you should master the following chapter objectives.

Theory Objectives

1. Describe the physical and chemical actions of shampooing, including the effects of alkaline shampoos and acid rinses.
2. Describe the characteristics and contents of the various kinds of shampoos and identify appropriate products for conditioning the client's scalp and hair.
3. Recognize scalp and hair irregularities and suggest corrective measures.

Practical Objectives

4. Drape the client and prepare the hair and scalp for shampoo.
5. Shampoo the hair.

Introduction

Shampooing cleanses the scalp and hair of dust, dirt, hair spray, sebum (oil), and other residue. How often the hair is shampooed depends on the hairstyle and its appearance. It also depends on how much oil is secreted from the client's scalp onto the hair. A very oily scalp will require shampooing more often than a normal scalp. While many clients will have their hair shampooed daily, others will wait a few days or perhaps even a week.

Because shampooing is a vital preliminary step for many services, it is performed frequently in the school or salon. Clients enjoy this service because effective shampooing manipulations relax the body and are good for the hair and scalp. Therefore, you must master this task early in the training program.

Theory Objective 1
Physical and Chemical Actions of Shampooing and the Effects of Alkaline Shampoos and Acid Rinses

The Physical and Chemical Actions of Shampooing

Shampooing involves both **physical** and **chemical** actions (Figure 5.1). The cosmetologist physically spreads the shampoo and exposes all surface areas of the hair for cleaning. Particles of oil, dirt, and other foreign substances are chemically attracted to shampoo molecules. These particles are then attracted to molecules of rinse water flowing along the hair shaft and are washed away. The rinse water uses both chemical action (attraction) and physical action (washing away) to complete the cleansing.

pH Ratings of Shampoos

It is important to understand the pH factor of shampoos so that you will know a product's chemical effects and its proper use (Figure 5.2). The term **pH (potential hydrogen)** indicates the concentration of hydrogen in a solution. This concentration determines a shampoo's pH rating; that is, whether a shampoo is **acid** or **alkaline** (AL-kah-lin). The pH scale shows the various degrees of acidity and alkalinity. The middle of the scale, 7, is the **neutral point.** At 7, the acidity and alkalinity balance each other so that the solution is neutral. Distilled water has a neutral pH, 7. The numbers 0 to 6.9 on the scale indicate acidity; the numbers 7.1 to 14 represent alkalinity.

Skin and hair are acid. They have a pH of **4.5–5.5.** Salon products that have the same pH as skin and hair are **acid-balanced.** This means that they do not change the natural pH of the skin or hair.

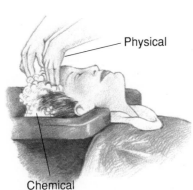

Physical

Chemical

Figure 5.1
Shampooing the hair

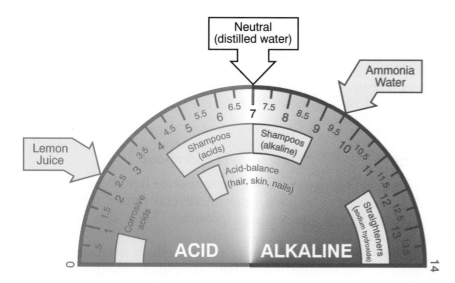

Figure 5.2
Knowing the pH factors of hair-care products is important.

Shampoos are either alkaline (pH of 7.1–8.5) or acid-balanced (4.5–5.5). If a client undergoes many hair services using alkaline products, you should recommend an acid-balanced shampoo; many styling lotions have a pH higher than 5.5, making an acid-balanced shampoo especially important. Alkaline shampoos are powerful cleansers, but they should be neutralized by an acid rinse, which brings the hair back to its natural pH.

The Effects of Alkaline Shampoos and Acid Rinses

To realize the importance of neutralizing an alkaline shampoo, you must understand the shampoo's chemical effects on the hair. Alkaline products, and water with a high alkaline content, cause the cuticle of the hair to swell and the hydrogen bonds to **soften.** In the process, the overlapping layers of cuticle scales, called **imbrications** (im-breh-KAY-shunz), open (Figure 5.3). This causes the hair to become more porous and reduces its tensile strength, or elasticity. In addition, natural oils are removed and moisture evaporates from the cortex.

Acid products shrink and harden the swollen cuticle. The imbrications close, which reduces the hair's porosity and enhances its luster. In addition to neutralizing the alkalinity of shampoos and some water, an acid rinse also eliminates soap curds produced by the interaction of hard water with fatty acids contained in some shampoos.

When you use an alkaline shampoo, you should explain to the client why an acid rinse is needed; otherwise, the client may think you are insisting on unnecessary products and expense.

Both natural acids and formulated products may be used as neutralizing rinses after you have used alkaline shampoos or other alkaline products. Effective natural acids include apple cider vinegar

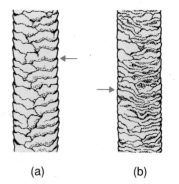

(a)   (b)

Figure 5.3
Imbrications of the hair shaft: (a) open and (b) closed.

(acetic acid), white vinegar (acetic acid), and lemon juice (citric acid). Neutralizing products are also made by cosmetic manufacturers. These products are marketed under many names, including normalizing creams, creme rinses, stabilizing conditioners, and instant conditioners.

Theory Objective 2
Characteristics and Contents of Shampoos and Products for Conditioning the Client's Scalp and Hair

The Characteristics and Contents of Shampoos

The three kinds of shampoos used in salons are liquids; semiliquids, and solids. These shampoos come in several forms: thin liquids, gels, creams, foams, pastes, and powders. They also come in a variety of containers.

Some shampoos are ready to use; others are concentrates that must be mixed with water. For example, 1 pint (0.47 liter) of concentrate might make 1 gallon (3.8 liters) of shampoo. Some superconcentrates make as much as 5 gallons (19 liters) from 1 pint (0.47 liter) of base. **Always read the manufacturer's directions** before mixing shampoos and **follow** the instructions carefully.

The fragrances added to shampoos serve two purposes. They mask unpleasant chemical odors and provide pleasant ones of their own that complement perfume or cologne. Although fragrances may be pleasant, they may also be a problem. Some individuals are allergic to the substances that create these fragrances. For example, **orrisroot,** which is found in many products, may irritate the skin and scalp and/or cause sneezing and coughing. Because of the possibility of allergic reactions, you should take particular care to dilute superconcentrates according to the directions on the label.

Some shampoos produce more lather than others. Many cosmetologists prefer to use a shampoo that lathers or foams heavily. Many people think that lather is a sign of cleansing power, but this is **not necessarily** true. Some shampoos that produce little lather **cleanse the scalp and hair very well.**

Salons usually use shampoos containing surface-active, complex detergents that have more cleansing power than shampoos based on plain bar soap. These detergents are more effective than soaps in emulsifying (breaking up) soil and unwanted substances. Another **advantage** is that they leave little or no residue (film) like the kind formed by the interaction of soaps and hard water. The final test for any shampoo is its effect on hair and, in particular, how well you and your clients like its effect on their hair.

Classifying Shampoos

Shampoos can be classified according to their special uses. These categories include nonstripping, medicated, all-purpose, conditioning, herbal, acid-balanced, powder-dry, and liquid-dry shampoos.

Nonstripping shampoos (non-strip shampoos) are formulated to cleanse without removing permanent hair coloring or toning colors used on prelightened hair. Always use a nonstripping shampoo on bleached hair.

Medicated shampoos contain ingredients for treating scalp and hair problems or disorders. Some medicated shampoos are available from your beauty supply dealer; others can be obtained only by prescription from the client's doctor. In addition, **demedicating shampoos** are available that may remove traces of medications being taken by the client.

Most shampoo manufacturers produce one or more **all-purpose shampoos.** These shampoos do not strip color, and they have a lower alkaline content than some specialty products. Some even include antifungus and antidandruff agents, in addition to ingredients that are very mild for hands. If an all-purpose shampoo meets the needs of the client, both the client and the salon can save considerable expense by avoiding **product duplication.**

Conditioning shampoos have small amounts of animal, vegetable, or mineral additives that improve the tensile strength and porosity of the hair. Some of these additives are proteins, which may go into the cortex or attach themselves to the cuticle of the hair shaft. Proteins in the better conditioning shampoos usually remain in the hair for more than two or three salon visits.

The water in certain areas contains minerals, such as iron and calcium. If these minerals are present, the water is called **hard water.** When these minerals are absent or are present only in very small quantities, the water is said to be **soft water.** If your salon has hard water, you will notice that shampoo does not lather as well as it would with soft water. Hard water can also create problems when chemicals, such as hair coloring and permanent waving, are used on the hair. A **water softener** can solve the hard water problem by removing unwanted minerals from the water.

Herbal shampoos contain natural ingredients and are intended to appeal to the "back-to-nature" trend. Although these natural ingredients may be helpful, the products are often expensive. Their performance should be judged carefully and compared with that of less expensive products.

Acid-balanced shampoos, as already mentioned, have about the same pH (4.5–5.5) as hair, so they do not change the hair's natural pH.

Powder-dry shampoos are designed for clients who cannot wet their hair. These shampoos are particularly helpful for bedridden persons. Powder-dry shampoos consist of powder or granules that absorb soil and oil as they are brushed through the scalp and hair.

Liquid-dry shampoos are also used on clients whose hair cannot be wet in a regular shampooing service. The solution is applied on cotton to small strands of hair. It loosens soil and residue, which can then be removed by towel-blotting immediately after the shampoo has been applied. The remaining solution then evaporates. Liquid-dry shampoos are used mainly on hand-tied hairpieces, such as wigs and wiglets, because ordinary shampoos cause the wefting (base material to which the hair is sewn) of hairpieces to deteriorate.

Safety Tip ▶

Because liquid-dry shampoos may be very **flammable** or **combustible** (one of their ingredients is benzene, a highly flammable product), the following precautions must be taken:

1. **Never** use liquid-dry shampoo near an open flame or gas or electric appliances.

2. **Never** smoke cigarettes or allow clients to smoke when liquid-dry shampoo is being used on them.

3. **Always** use liquid-dry shampoos in an open, well-ventilated area. Fumes from these products can irritate your lungs and eyes.

Theory Objective 3
Scalp and Hair Irregularities and Corrective Measures

Prior to shampooing (or any other service), you must examine the scalp and hair to (1) check for disease and (2) analyze their condition so appropriate products can be selected. If a **communicable disease** (one that can be transmitted from one person to another) is present, **do not serve the client. Do not shampoo the hair vigorously before giving a permanent wave, chemical relaxer, or other chemical service.** In most cases, a shampoo before chemical services is performed with very gentle manipulations. If you are not sure, ask your instructor.

As a cosmetologist, you will be concerned about recognizing communicable diseases. A **congenital disease** is a disorder that has existed since birth. (A person born with a heart condition has a congenital disease.) A **chronic** (KRON-ik) **disease,** such as emphysema, is a **long-term** or recurring disorder. A **short-term** condition, such as a common cold, is called an **acute disease.**

In examining the scalp and hair, you should watch for **skin diseases** (infections of the skin). Probably the most common skin disorder observed in the beauty salon is **dandruff.** It is characterized by an excessive number of small or large white flat scales shed from the outermost layer of the skin of the scalp. This layer is the **epidermis.**

The medical term for dandruff is **pityriasis** (pit-i-RIGH-ah-siss). There are two forms of pityriasis. **Pityriasis capitis simplex** (KAP-eh-tis SIM-pleks) is characterized by dry, flaky, white scales and may be treated by using a nonprescription medicated shampoo.

Pityriasis steatoides (stee-ah-TOI-deez) is characterized by yellow, oily, or waxy scales located close to the scalp. **Sebaceous** (see-BAY-shuhs) **glands** in the scalp produce a lubricating substance called sebum. If the sebaceous glands become overactive when dandruff is on a person's scalp, the scales stick together and become attached to the scalp and hair. Ordinary shampoos will not remove these scales, flakes, and oil deposits. This condition may require a medicated shampoo, or a shampoo prescribed by a doctor.

About two out of every three persons in the United States have dandruff (Figure 5.4). Although its cause has not been determined, scientists have developed several theories. According to one theory, dandruff is caused by nervous disorders related to high blood pressure (hypertension) and emotional stress. People living in cities get dandruff more often than people who live in small towns or on farms. Thus, dandruff may be related to the difference in life-styles.

Psoriasis (sah-RIGH-eh-siss) is a skin disease that can be chronic or acute. It is characterized by inflamed (red) patches and overlapping yellow or white scales. It is **not** contagious, and although the crust will bleed if disturbed, clients with psoriasis may receive cold waves and use hair colors. You should ask the client to give you a letter from a doctor stating that hair treatments are permissible.

Herpes simplex (HEHR-peez-SIM-pleks) is a viral infection (from a virus) characterized by inflammation of the skin and mucous membranes, especially those of the face and lips. Such inflammations are called **cold sores.** Exactly how this condition develops is not known, but it usually clears up in 6 to 10 days. It is a contagious condition, so facials and makeup applications are not recommended.

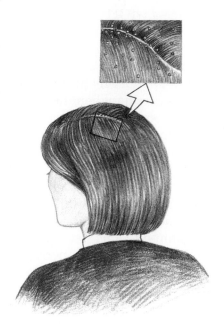

Figure 5.4
Dandruff

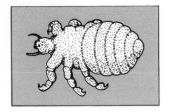

Figure 5.5
Head louse (pediculosis)

Pediculosis (pi-dik-yah-LOH-siss) is an animal parasitic condition. (A parasite is an organism or microorganism that lives on another organism.) Pediculosis involves **head lice** that lay their eggs on the scalp and hair shafts (Figure 5.5). Because of improved personal hygiene in the United States, head lice were not a common problem during the last few decades. Recently, however, the growing popularity of long hair and the failure of some people to shampoo their hair as often as they should have led to an increase in the occurrence of head lice. Since **pediculosis is contagious,** a client with this condition **cannot be served** in the school or salon. Effective treatment, including a medicated shampoo prescribed by a doctor or simply purchased over-the-counter at a pharmacy, can eliminate the condition in three or four days.

Safety Tip ▶

Scabies is another animal parasitic condition. It is an infestation of **itch mites,** which burrow into the scalp and cause irritation, leading to the scratching of the scalp. Scabies is very contagious. **Refuse service** to a person with this condition and refer him or her to a doctor.

Tinea (TIN-ee-ah), a skin infection caused by a fungus (vegetable parasite), is **very contagious.** This condition, which is commonly called **ringworm,** appears as circular inflamed areas of little blisters. A person with tinea **cannot be served** and should be advised to see a doctor.

Seborrhea (seb-ah-REE-ah) is a disorder of the sebaceous glands, which causes an **excessively oily scalp and hair. Hyper**activity (**over**activity) of the **sebaceous glands** causes this excessive secretion of **sebum,** which is transferred from the scalp to the hair (Figure 5.6). Seborrhea can be controlled by using a medicated shampoo for oily hair. Daily shampoos may be needed.

Asteatosis (as-tee-ah-TOH-siss) is caused by **hypo**activity (**under**activity) of the sebaceous glands. The glands produce too little sebum, which results in dry, scaly skin and/or hair that lacks luster. This is an unusual condition that is seldom seen in the salon.

A **steatoma** (stee-ah-TOH-mah), or **wen,** is a subcutaneous (beneath the skin) cyst occurring when the duct from the sebaceous gland to a hair follicle becomes clogged or blocked. Sebum accumulates and hardens beneath the skin until the duct is open again. This condition is not considered contagious.

Acne (AK-nee) is an eruptive skin disease caused by inflammation (irritation) of the sebaceous glands. It usually appears on the face, chest, and back. The condition can be controlled by a dermatologist. Clients having acne can be served in the salon and school.

Comedones (kahm-eh-DOH-neez), also called **blackheads,** occur when the skin is not cleansed properly and regularly. Sebum hardens around a speck of dirt or dust, clogging a pore and creating a slightly raised area.

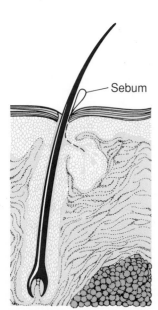

— Sebum

Figure 5.6
A sebaceous gland secreting sebum

Milia (MIL-ee-ah), also called **whiteheads,** are cysts that contain sebum trapped in a sebaceous duct.

Miliaria rubra (mil-ee-AR-ee-ah ROOB-rah) is an acute irritation below the top layer of skin. It is an inflammation of the sudoriferous (sweat) glands. Commonly called **prickly heat,** this disorder usually occurs during hot weather. It is not communicable.

Practical Objective 4
Drape and Preparation of Scalp and Hair

The three draping methods used in the beauty salon are the **dry drape, shampoo drape,** and **chemical drape.** Which of the three is used depends on the service requested by the client since each drape provides a different degree of protection. The following describes each draping method and explains when it is used:

1. **Dry drape.** A towel and/or a neck strip is placed around the client's neck, and a nylon or cloth cape may be used (Figure 5.7). This method is used for combouts, dry hair cutting, tweezing, and other dry services (Figure 5.8).
2. **Shampoo drape.** A towel is placed around the client's neck, and a plastic cape is secured over the towel. This method is used for all wet services.

Figure 5.7
Dry Drape

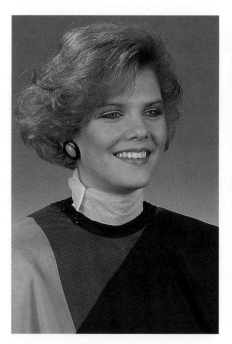
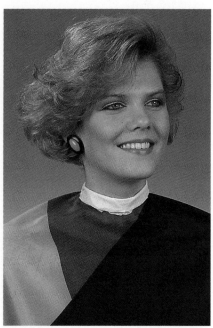

After folding the collar out of the way, place sanek strip around neck, then drape cape across front of client and secure velcro fastener or hooks at back of neck.

Fold sanek strip downward around edge of cape.

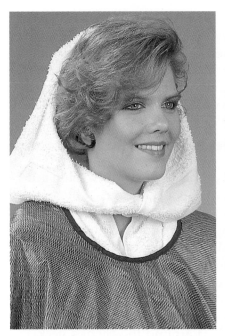 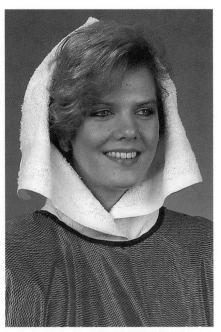

Turn the collar inward, place towel on crown of head, and slide bottom corners of towel around in front of the neck.

Drape cape across front of client, and secure fasteners at back of neck.

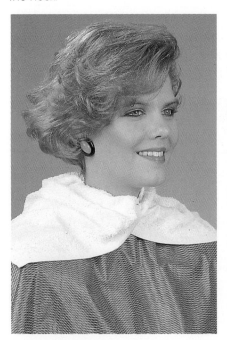 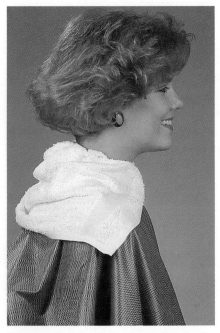

Fold towel over the cape.

Be sure cape is draped over back of chair.

Figure 5.8
Shampoo Drape

3. **Chemical drape.** Two towels are used for this method (Figure 5.9). One towel is placed around the client's neck and spread across his or her shoulders underneath a plastic cape. The

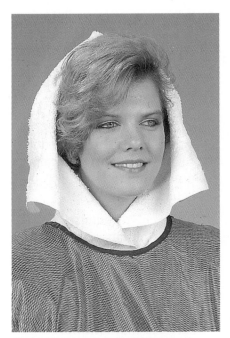

Place towel across shoulders and gather in front of neck. Place another towel on crown of head, and slide bottom corners of towel around in front of the neck.

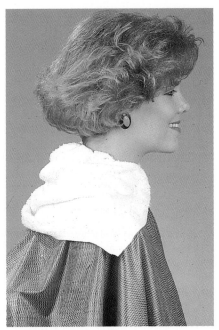

Figure 5.9
Chemical Drape

Fold towel over cape and across shoulders to catch any type of solution that may drip from chemicals processed on the hair.

other towel is placed around the client's neck and spread on top of the cape. This method is used for all chemical services.

Supplies

- client release form*
- laundered towel
- sanitized comb and brush
- neck strip
- shampoo cape
- shampoo
- neutralizing rinse, if necessary

Procedure

1. Greet the client and ask him or her to sign a release form. Take off any jewelry you are wearing. Politely ask the client to put any jewelry in a purse or pocket. If the client prefers, put the jewelry in a safe place, such as a drawer.

Rationale

1. Since services are performed by students, clients need to sign a release form. Removing jewelry protects it from chemicals and from getting lost. Always treat the client courteously.

*To avoid excessive repetition, the release form will not be listed for all procedures. It is included, however, in all chemical services and in a few others as a reminder of its importance. You must follow the policy of your school or salon.

2. Wash your hands with soap and water before beginning this and every other service.

3. Neatly fold down the client's collar. Place a neck strip or towel around the client's neck before securing the shampoo cape (Figure 5.10).

4. Observe the client's hairstyle before wetting the hair.

5. Ask the client what services are scheduled.

6. Determine step-by-step procedures to be followed.

2. **Preventing the spread of disease-causing bacteria is the responsibility of everyone.**

3. Since a cape is used on more than one person, a laundered towel or new strip is placed around the client's neck as a sanitary precaution before the cape is used.

4. If the client requests a similar hairstyle, you will have a clear mental picture of it.

5. Shampooing procedures vary according to the services that follow.

6. The hair usually **is not brushed before applying a lightener, permanent color retouch, permanent color for virgin hair, chemical relaxer, or permanent wave.** The hair is brushed before a shampoo and style

Figure 5.10
Placement of neck strip. (a) For wet services, fold the neck strip back against the collar of the shampoo cape. (b) Placement of neck strip for dry services.

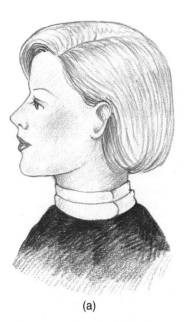

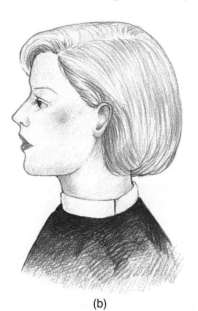

(a)   (b)

unless the scalp is irritated. It is brushed before a frosting, too. Some clients will also ask you to remove backcombing. If the client has an extraordinary accumulation of hair spray or soil, plan to shampoo twice or even three times.

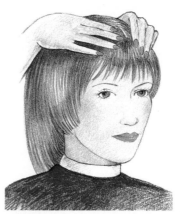

Figure 5.11
Examine the scalp.

◀ Safety Tip

7. Remove hairpins, bobby pins, and hair ornaments.

7. If the brush catches on something in the hair, the client will be uncomfortable.

8. Examine the scalp for cuts, scratches, abrasions, irritation, and other abnormal conditions or diseases (Figure 5.11). Consult your instructor or manager if abnormalities are visible.

8. **Examination is necessary because you must refuse service to anyone who has a contagious scalp disease.**

9. If the client has not scheduled a chemical service, begin brushing on the left front of the head using horizontal ½-inch to ¾-inch (1.25- to 1.88-centimeter) partings.

9. **This sectioning ensures** that all the scalp and hair will be brushed and **examined for scratches, abrasions, and diseases.**

10. Rotate the brush 180 degrees in your right hand while holding the section of hair in your left hand. (Figure 5.12).

10. Brushing increases the blood supply to the scalp and normalizes the activity of the sebaceous glands.

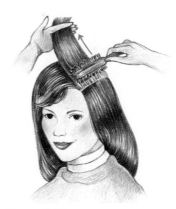

Figure 5.12
Scientific brushing

11. Be certain to rotate the brush on the scalp and then into the hair.

11. Brushing the scalp loosens soil and flaking skin so that the shampoo will clean more thoroughly.

12. Each section should be brushed thoroughly three times.

12. This ensures that the entire scalp and hair are brushed thoroughly.

13. Lay the first section over the right front area, then bring your hand down and

13. Brush from the top to the bottom of the left side of the section just brushed so

part off another ½- to ¾-inch (1.25- to 1.88-centimeter) horizontal section.

hair will not be in the way when you brush the next section down.

14. Repeat steps 10, 11, and 12 until all hair in that section has been brushed.

14. Again, immediately report any abnormal conditions to your instructor or manager.

15. Go on to the crown section on the left side of the head and begin brushing. Use ½-inch (1.25 centimeter) horizontal partings. Work from the top of the section until all scalp and hair have been brushed. Repeat step 12.

15. This procedure will save time because the brushing proceeds around the head—from the left side of the head to both the crown and nape sections and on to the right front section.

16. Using the information presented in this unit, analyze the condition of the client's scalp and hair and select the appropriate shampoo.

16. In performing the first seven shampoos on clients, consult your instructor or manager on the choice of shampoo. Depending on the condition of the scalp and hair, plain, nonstripping, medicated, or conditioning shampoos may be needed.

17. Check to make sure that the cape is secure but comfortable and that it drapes over the back of the chair.

17. **A loose or poorly secured cape can cause water damage to the client's clothing. Draping it over the chair will cause water to run onto the floor.**

Practical Objective 5
Shampoo the Hair

Safety Tip

(Remember that your instructor may show you the school method for shampooing the hair. In that case, the school method is the one you should learn.)

Procedure

1. Standing by the client's side, place your hand behind the **client's head**

Rationale

1. Shampoo bowls are made of porcelain-covered iron. If unassisted, **a client might**

and carefully lower it to the shampoo bowl. Make any necessary adjustments to ensure that the client is comfortable.

2. Pick up the nozzle of the spray hose and point it toward the drain. Then turn on cold water.

3. Hold the nozzle between your thumb and index and middle fingers. Slide the little finger of your right hand into the water's spray.

4. Any time that water is directed at the client's head, the little finger should be in the water's spray.

5. Gradually saturate the hair on the crown. **Use the back of your hand to shield the client's face from the water spray** (Figure 5.13). Cup your left hand around the client's left ear as you move the spray around the head.

6. Gently move the side of the client's right ear forward with your left hand as you saturate the hair on that part of the head.

lower his or her head too quickly and be injured.

2. If the water is turned on before the nozzle is pointed downward, someone may be sprayed. Always turn on cold water first, adding hot water as necessary.

3. In this position the little finger can monitor water temperature. A good, comfortable temperature for the average client is 90° to 110°F. (Water temperatures can be classified as follows: cool, 65°–70°F; tepid, 85°–90°F; warm, 95°–100°F; hot, 105°–110°F.)

4. **Water pressures and temperatures can change quickly. The little finger will detect changes so that water can be directed away from the client's head when necessary.**

◀ Safety Tip

5. This allows the client to react if water temperature is uncomfortable. Always protect the client from the spray.

6. Same as step 5.

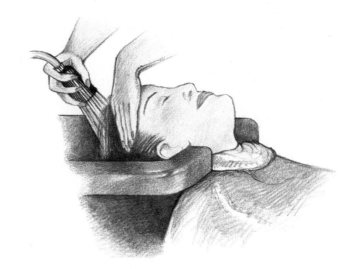

Figure 5.13
Use one hand to protect the client's eyes and face from the water.

7. Use your left hand to protect the client's nape area as you saturate it.

7. This will protect the client's clothing.

8. After all the hair is saturated, turn off the **hot water first,** then the cold. Check the shampoo you have selected.

8. If the cold water were turned off first, the client might be burned. Checking shampoo for correct viscosity, color, and fragrance is a good safety measure.

9. Apply shampoo sparingly about 2 inches (5 centimeters) from the hairline in small, even sections across the crown.

9. Since soiled hair doesn't lather well during the first application of shampoo, using a large amount is wasteful and unnecessary. If shampoo were applied at the hairline, some might drip onto the client's forehead and into the client's eyes. **If the shampoo does get in the client's eyes, use the corner of a clean towel saturated with cold water to blot the eyes immediately.** Consult your instructor or manager for help.

10. With one hand on each side of the client's head, manipulate your fingertips firmly in a zigzag pattern from the hairline toward the back of the head.

10. This lathers and evenly distributes the shampoo so that it can clean all the scalp and hair. Use the cushions of your fingertips to avoid scratching the scalp.

11. Repeat this procedure three times.

11. This ensures thorough cleansing.

12. Lift the client's head with your left hand while the client braces his or her neck against the shampoo bowl.

12. This procedure gives the client's head the proper support. The client braces his or her head against the bowl to keep shampoo from dripping onto his or her clothing.

13. Begin manipulations with your right hand behind the client's right ear and zigzag firmly across the back of the crown to the left ear.

13. This procedure cleanses the crown evenly.

14. Repeat the preceding step three times.

14. This ensures thorough cleansing.

15. Repeat these manipulations in the nape area, working across from the right ear to the left ear.

15. Same as step 14.

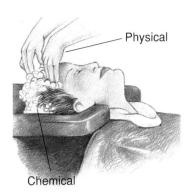

Figure 5.14
The cosmetic hairline is the place where makeup can collect around the client's face.

16. Use your thumbs to shampoo the **"cosmetic hairline"** (Figure 5.14).

16. The **cosmetic hairline** is the area where makeup has accumulated because the client has attempted to clean their face without disturbing the hairstyle.

17. Carefully lower the client's head into the neck of the shampoo bowl.

17. This protects the client.

18. **Rinse the hair thoroughly** by saturating it with water.

18. Rinsing removes soil, sprays, and other unwanted substances.

19. Repeat the steps for cleansing and rinsing the hair. No visible traces of

19. **Shampoo left in hair will interfere with other services.**

shampoo should remain in the hair, particularly in the **nape** area.

20. Raise the client upright and towel-dry the hair.

20. This removes excess moisture that could interfere with the next service.

21. Select and mix the creme rinse conditioner.

21. The rinse neutralizes the alkalinity of shampoo. Most creme rinses have a low pH so that they, too, can neutralize.

22. Lower the client's head to the shampoo bowl and apply the rinse according to the manufacturer's directions.

22. Products vary widely. Always read and follow directions.

23. Thoroughly rinse again if required.

23. A product left in the hair could interfere with the next service.

24. Raise the client to a sitting position and towel-dry the hair.

24. The client is more comfortable.

25. Sterilize the shampoo bowl. Give special attention to the neck rest after each client.

25. This protects other clients.

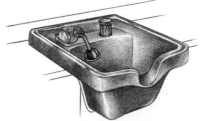

Figure 5.15
Leave the hose nozzle in the drain position.

26. Return the hose nozzle to the drain position (Figure 5.15).

26. Leaving the nozzle as shown in Figure 5.16 will allow any dripping water to drain into the sink, rather than onto the floor.

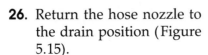

Glossary

Acetic acid A natural acid found in vinegar.
Acid A product that has a pH rating under 7.
Acid-balanced products Products that have the same pH rating as skin and hair (4.5–5.5).
Acne (AK-nee) An eruption of the skin caused by irritation of the sebaceous glands. It usually appears on the face, chest, and back.

Alkaline (AL-kah-lin) A product that has a pH rating over 7.

All purpose shampoos Shampoos that have a lower alkaline content than some specialty shampoos and will not strip color.

Asteatosis (as-tee-ah-TOH-siss) A condition caused by underactivity of the sebaceous glands; it results in dry, scaly skin and/or hair that lacks luster.

Blackheads See **Comedones.**

Chronic (KRON-ik) disease A long-term or recurring disorder (such as emphysema).

Citric acid A natural acid found in lemon juice.

Comedones (kahm-eh-DOH-neez) Raised, clogged pores caused by sebum hardening around a speck of dirt or dust; commonly called blackheads.

Conditioning shampoos Shampoos that have small amounts of animal, vegetable, or mineral additives that improve the tensile strength and porosity of the hair.

Congenital disease A disorder that has existed since birth (such as a heart condition).

Dandruff See **Pityriasis.**

Epidermis (ep-eh-DER-mis) The thinnest, outermost layer of the skin.

Herpes simplex (HEHR-peez SIM-pleks) An inflammation of the skin and mucous membranes, especially those of the face and lips, caused by a virus. Often called cold sores.

Imbrications (im-breh-KAY-shunz) Overlapping layers of cuticle scales of the hair.

Liquid-dry shampoo A solution that loosens soil so that it can be removed by towel-blotting the hair. The solution then evaporates. It is used mostly on wigs and hairpieces.

Medicated shampoos Shampoos that contain ingredients for treating scalp and hair problems.

Milia (MIL-ee-ah) Cysts that contain sebum trapped in a sebaceous duct; commonly called whiteheads.

Miliaria rubra (mil-ee-AR-ee-ah ROOB-rah) An acute, noncontagious inflammation of the sweat glands, usually occurring in hot weather; commonly called prickly heat.

Neutral point A point (7) on the pH scale where a product is neither acid nor alkaline.

Nonstripping shampoos Shampoos that cleanse without removing permanent hair coloring or toning colors used on prelightened hair.

Orrisroot An ingredient found in many fragrances that is known to cause an allergic reaction.

Pediculosis (pi-dik-yah-LOH-siss) A parasitic condition of the scalp caused by head lice that lay their eggs on the scalp and hair shaft.

pH (potential hydrogen) Indicates the concentration of hydrogen in a solution. This concentration determines whether a product is acid or alkaline.

Pityriasis (pit-i-RIGH-ah-siss) A skin disorder characterized by an excessive number of flat scales or flakes shed from the outermost layer of the skin of the scalp; it is commonly called dandruff. Two types are known: pityriasis capitis simplex (KAP-eh-tis SIM-pleks), characterized by dry, flaky, white scales; and pityriasis steatoides (stee-ah-TOI-deez), characterized by yellow, oily, or waxy scales close to the scalp.

Powder-dry shampoos Shampoos consisting of powder or granules that absorb soil and oil as they are brushed through the scalp and hair.

Psoriasis (sah-RIGH-eh-siss) Noncontagious skin disorder characterized by inflamed (red) patches and overlapping yellow or white scales on the skin; can be chronic or acute.

Scabies A parasitic condition of the scalp caused by itch mites that burrow into the scalp.

Sebaceous (see-BAY-shuhs) glands The glands that supply sebum (oil) to the hair.

Seborrhea (seb-ah-REE-ah) A disorder of the sebaceous glands that causes the scalp and hair to be excessively oily.

Steatoma (stee-ah-TOH-mah) A cyst beneath the skin occurring when the duct from the sebaceous gland to a hair follicle becomes clogged or blocked; commonly called a wen.

Tinea (TIN-ee-ah) A very contagious skin infection caused by a fungus, which appears as a circular inflamed areas of little blisters; commonly called ringworm.

Whiteheads See **Milia.**

Questions

1. What is a shampoo?
2. The letters pH are an abbreviation for what two words?
3. What range of numbers indicates that a product is acid-balanced?
4. Name at least six different classes of shampoos.
5. What is herpes simplex?
6. What is another name for whiteheads?
7. Does a shampoo have to lather heavily in order to clean the hair?
8. What type of shampoo would you recommend for lightened (bleached) hair?
9. Why would you refuse to allow a client to smoke a cigarette while you applied a liquid-dry shampoo?

10. What is the name given to small white flakes on the scalp?
11. What is the medical name for dandruff?
12. Would you serve a client with pediculosis?
13. Tinea of the scalp is another name for what condition?
14. Would you serve a client who has psoriasis?
15. What is the technical term for an oily scalp?
16. What is the cosmetic hairline?
17. After finishing with the shampoo bowl, where should you leave the nozzle of the hose?

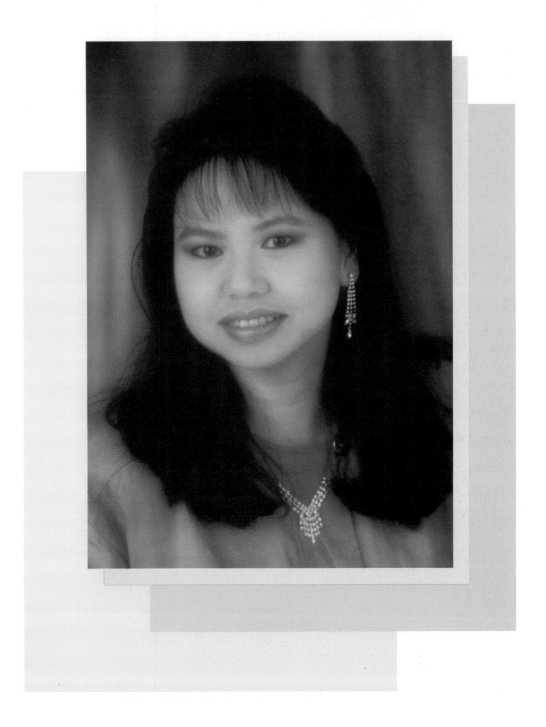

Conditioning

Learning Objective

Select a specific conditioner that will improve the condition of a client's damaged hair. Perform the learning objective according to the principles discussed in this chapter. Score 85 percent or better on a multiple-choice exam on the information in this chapter.

In order to achieve the above level of competence, you should master the following chapter objectives.

Theory Objectives

1. List the physical and chemical actions that damage hair, and define five terms that describe hair condition.
2. Describe how proteins are used in conditioning the hair.
3. Classify and describe the different types of conditioners.

Practical Objective

4. Assess hair damage and select and apply the appropriate conditioner.

You may already have seen some of the available products that have been designed to improve the condition of the hair. At this point, you may even feel that you have "seen them all," but in fact, you probably have only scratched the surface. When you become a practicing cosmetologist, you will be exposed to hundreds, if not thousands, of hair conditioners. How can you know which one to use? This chapter is designed to answer a few basic questions:

1. **Why** is the hair conditioned?
2. **What** is used to condition the hair?
3. **When** should the hair be conditioned?
4. **How much** conditioning should be done?
5. **How** should the conditioner be sold to the client?

So many different conditioners are available both professionally and over-the-counter that it would be impossible to discuss all types and their effects here. Nevertheless, hair conditioning is one of the most frequently requested services, so it is very important that you learn as much as possible about it. Therefore, this chapter will discuss the composition, use, and application of the **general types** of conditioners. As in all other cases, you should ask your **instructor or manager** which conditioner should be used to solve a specific hair-conditioning problem.

Theory Objective 1
Physical and Chemical Actions That Damage Hair and Five Terms That Describe Hair Condition

To use any conditioner effectively, you must understand why conditioners are needed at all! Conditioners are needed to correct physical or chemical damage to the hair.

Physical damage to the hair may be caused by natural forces such as sunlight (ultraviolet rays), drying winds, air oxidation, hard (high mineral content) water, or chlorinated water. Physical damage may also occur unnaturally from the following:

1. **Brush rollers** (used at home), which split and break the hair.
2. **Heated rollers,** which have points that can split and break the hair and damage the scalp.
3. **Thermal curling irons and hand dryers** (used at home), which burn and singe the hair.
4. **Incorrect teasing** (back-combing), which causes the hair to break.

5. **Incorrect brushing** using a nylon brush without rounded bristles. A natural boar-bristle brush or vent-brush is better for use at home. Sharp-pointed nylon-bristle brushes tend to cut the hair shaft and scrape the scalp.

The scalp and hair can be damaged chemically by the improper use of chemical relaxers, cold waves, hair lighteners (bleaches), tints, styling lotions, and conditioners.

Physical and chemical damage to the hair affects its porosity, elasticity, texture, appearance, and manageability:

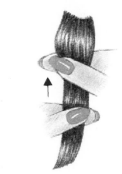

Figure 6.1
Porosity test

1. **Porosity** refers to the amount of liquid a strand of hair can absorb (Figure 6.1). Damaged hair is said to be overporous if the imbricated outer layers of the cuticle are in an open position.

2. **Elasticity** refers to the degree to which a hair can be stretched without breaking (Figure 6.2). The amount of "stretch" or elasticity hair has is related to its **tensile strength.** A hair can be stretched almost 50 percent when wet, but only 10 to 20 percent when dry. If the hair has been physically and/or chemically damaged, it may be very weak and may break **easily** when stretched. It also may not return to its original length when it is released after stretching.

3. **Texture** refers to the feel of the hair and diameter of the hair shaft. If the hair feels smooth, hard, and "glassy," the imbricated layers of the outer cuticle are lying flat against the hair shaft. When the imbrications are open, the hair feels rough. If the hair "feels" soft and fluffy and the hair shaft has a small diameter, the hair is called **fine hair.** When the hair shaft has a larger diameter, the hair is **coarse hair.** Hair in which the diameters are between these extremes is referred to as average or **medium hair.**

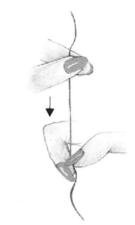

Figure 6.2
Elasticity test

4. **Appearance** refers to the luster, sheen, or shininess of the hair. Damaged hair is lackluster and does not shine. Its dull appearance is due to the lack of natural scalp oil or **sebum** that gives hair its beautiful shine.

5. **Manageability** refers to the ease or difficulty with which a comb passes through the hair, both when the hair is wet and when it is dry. For example, if it is very **difficult** to comb through the hair when it is wet, the hair is said to be "unmanageable," and it needs conditioning. Dry hair may also be unmanageable and difficult to comb. Dry, "flyaway" hair can be caused by static electricity created by low humidity. The humidity inside buildings, especially in colder climates, is often too low.

Manageability is affected by the overall condition of the hair, which takes into account porosity, elasticity, texture, and appearance. Therefore, whenever one of these natural hair qualities is lost or weakened, the hair is said to be "damaged."

Whenever you see a scalp that is red and irritated or has cuts and abrasions, you should advise the client to visit the family doctor or a dermatologist. Only a medical doctor can treat diseases or injuries of the skin. You **cannot** legally **treat** such conditions and must refuse service to clients who have them.

Theory Objective 2
Use of Proteins in
Conditioning Hair

As was explained earlier in the text, **keratin** (KER-eh-tin) is the basic protein that forms the structure of the hair shaft. All preparations that are labeled or called protein conditioners contain protein. The proteins used on the hair differ mainly in (1) the size of their molecules and (2) their origin:

1. The size of the molecules that form the protein helps determine how well a conditioner will work on the hair. To penetrate the cortex of the hair shaft effectively, protein hair conditioners must contain **substantive proteins.** These proteins have been manufactured or processed. Because their molecules are **very** small, substantive proteins work better than other conditioners.

   Conditioning the hair can be compared to repairing a crack in the plaster wall of a building. Cement cannot be used to repair the crack because it contains sand and stone particles that are much larger than the particles of plaster. A mixture of plaster, however, will fill the crack so that it will not be noticeable. In the same way, a hair conditioner must contain proteins **small** (substantive) enough to penetrate the hair's cuticle layer and adhere (stick) to the damaged part of the hair.

   Some people use milk, egg whites, beer, and other foods containing proteins to condition the hair. In their natural state, these items are not very effective conditioners because their protein molecules are **too large** to penetrate the hair. Using these substances to condition the hair is somewhat like trying to force a bowling ball into a grape—it is impossible! These proteins can benefit the outside of the hair, however.

2. The **origin of the conditioner's protein** is also important. Most protein conditioners are made from **animal** or vegetable materials, although a few come from minerals.

   Some conditioners contain bovine serum, an **animal protein.** It contains refined and sterilized cattle tissues, such as blood and bone marrow. Bovine serum is diluted with buffering agents and water since animal protein can be used safely only at about 10 percent strength. The **placenta** (plah-SEN-tah) of female cattle and sheep is also refined and used in some hair conditioners. **Collagen** (KAHL-eh-jen) is another animal protein used to condition the hair.

Some other conditioners contain vegetable proteins. **Vegetable** proteins are made from soybeans, balsam trees, tong beans, olives, wheat germ, and other high-protein plants. These ingredients are refined and formulated for conditioning the hair.

The process by which both animal and vegetable protein conditioners are made is very complex and uses many different combinations of chemicals. Only the **most basic** ingredients contained in these products have been mentioned here.

A conditioner is often used **prior** to a strong chemical service to prevent hair damage; this application is called **preconditioning.** Conditioners **added** to products to improve or buffer their action on the hair **during** a service provide **in-process conditioning.** After a service, conditioners may be used to **recondition** the hair.

It **is possible to overcondition** the hair so that the conditioner stops the action of another chemical product. If too many chemicals are applied, the hair can act like a saturated sponge. The hair can absorb just so many protein molecules; if its capacity is reached with the conditioner, it will have no room for cold-waving lotion (or other chemicals). Another example of overconditioning would be the use of a very acid conditioner that closes the cuticle imbrications tightly against the cortex, preventing a tint from penetrating the cuticle to color the cortex. It is also possible to put so much oil on dry hair that it becomes greasy and unmanageable—even after rinsing!

Always remember that conditioners are **not** magic! If the hair has been severely damaged or abused, a **series** of conditioning treatments may be necessary to return the hair to a normal state.

Cosmetologists are always being asked to buy this or that conditioner because it contains some new scientific discovery that will "miraculously" improve the hair. Although scientific product research continues to make valuable contributions, cosmetologists must judge products by studying the available facts and observing how well the products actually work. The following checklist will be useful in applying conditioners and assessing their effectiveness:

1. Did you carefully read and follow the label directions?

2. Did you consult your instructor or manager before you used the conditioner?

3. Was the condition (moisture, elasticity, porosity, texture, or appearance) of the hair improved?

If you chose the correct conditioner, used it according to the instructions on the label, and followed the advice of your instructor, the hair's condition **should be improved.** If it is not, a series of conditioning treatments may be necessary, or a different conditioner may be needed.

Theory Objective 3
The Different Types of
Conditioners

So many hair conditioners are available that you must know exactly what those used in your school or salon can and cannot do. Five general types of conditioners are available; they are discussed here and summarized in Table 6.1.

1. **Instant conditioners** usually have a vegetable oil (for example, balsam) base, which benefits the hair by **restoring** moisture and **oils.** This type of conditioner often has an **acid** pH. The instant conditioner coats the hair and usually does **not** penetrate into the cortex to replace keratin in the hair shaft. Instant conditioners may make fine hair too oily and limp and, thus, difficult to comb out.

   Instant conditioners are applied to shampooed hair that has been towel-dried. When you use an instant conditioner, let it stay on the hair for one or two minutes; then rinse off the excess conditioner that has not been absorbed by the hair.

2. **Instant conditioning and setting aids** are mainly strong setting lotions that also contain a little animal or vegetable protein. These conditioners are intended to increase the diameter of the hair shaft. Parts of the setting aid have an **affinity** (attraction) for the cuticle of the hair shaft. The pH of these conditioners can be either acid or alkaline. Instant conditioning and setting aids are often used between cold waves to make the hairstyle last longer. They contain an **antihumectant,** which creates an antihumidity **barrier between the hair shaft** and the **moisture in the air** to help preserve the hairstyle. Conditioners of this type are particularly good for fine hair. Most instant conditioning and setting aids are made in different **strengths** for fine, normal (not tinted or lightened), tinted, and bleached hair.

   When applying an instant conditioning and setting aid, you should follow several important steps. Apply the conditioner to the hair after you have shampooed and towel-dried it. **Always** apply the conditioner immediately before setting the hair. Do not rinse it away. After you have

Table 6.1

Types of Conditioners

Category	Procedure	Analysis	Description of Problem
Instant conditioner	Applied, timed, then rinsed from hair.	Porosity test: OK Elasticity test: OK	Hair appears dry, lacks some shine and sheen, but generally in good condition. Conditioner adds sheen and may also protect hair from too much heat from curling iron/blow dryer.
Instant conditioning and setting aid	Applied and left in hair.	Porosity test: OK Elasticity test: Fair	Hair appears dry and lacks elasticity and shine. May be of fine texture. Conditioner adds bounce and body to finished hairstyle by clinging to hair and increasing the diameter of the hair shaft.
Protein conditioner	Applied, timed, then rinsed from hair. (Sometimes left in hair; this is called a "leave-in" conditioner.)	Porosity test: Fair to good Elasticity test: Fair to good	Hair appears dry and lacks elasticity and shine. Cuticle layer is rough and lackluster. Read and follow manufacturer's directions carefully. May be left in the hair and used as a reconditioner prior to styling, permanent waving, hair coloring, or recurling.
Normalizing conditioner	Applied, timed, then rinsed from hair.	Porosity test: OK Elasticity test: OK	Used mainly after a chemical service to restore the natural pH range to the hair after a treatment using a product with an alkaline base, i.e., a permanent hair color.
Nucleic acid conditioner	Applied, timed, then either rinsed or left in the hair depending on directions.	Porosity test: Fair to poor Elasticity test: Fair to poor	Used when a deep, penetrating type of conditioner is needed, i.e., for reconditioning hair either before or immediately after a strong chemical treatment such as hair lightening, recurling, or a permanent wave.

Occasional conditioning of the hair is similar to applying a protective coating to something to prevent damage. While regular conditioning repairs minor hair damage from the wind and sun. Hair reconditioning replaces proteins lost from the hair shaft through the application of chemicals, such as a hair lightening product; or physical abuse from using a curling iron that was too hot.

applied the conditioner and combed it through the hair, spray water onto the hair and then comb it through. Water works as a carrying agent to assist the conditioner in penetrating the cuticle. If the hair dries out during the setting procedure, add more water, not setting lotion or conditioner. Some of these products make hair feel "crisp" before combing.

3. **Protein conditioners** are the products that actually go through the cuticle of the hair shaft into the cortex to replace keratin that has been physically or chemically removed. This internal replacement results in **equal porosity** within the hair shaft, **greater elasticity,** and improved texture.

   Because of the strength of substantive proteins, protein conditioners are usually applied to hair that has been shampooed and then towel-dried. After a period of time and/or the application of heat, **protein conditioners are rinsed from the hair before setting!** This is the best way to use them. *Carefully read the label and follow its directions and those of your instructor or manager.*

4. **Normalizing conditioners** are made specifically to neutralize the **alkaline** effects of trace chemicals **after** such services as tints, relaxers, cold waves, or lighteners. Thus, the normalizing conditioner has an **acid pH.** If the traces of alkali are not neutralized by these normalizing conditioners, the alkali may damage the hair or irritate the scalp. Two minutes after application, they are rinsed from the hair.

5. **Nucleic** (NEW-klee-ik) **acid** is the newest and, scientifically, the best professional hair **reconstructor** (rebuilder) available. As you know, hair is made of hard protein, and this protein is composed of a combination of some of the 20 known **amino acids.** Each of these amino acids has a set of chemical "fingerprints," which enable us to tell one amino acid from another, e.g., the set of fingerprints is the way we identify each amino acid. Scientists call this chemical identification system RNA (ribonucleic acid). The RNA system is now so refined that scientists can easily detect the difference between amino acids that make up hair protein and those that make heart muscle protein. Scientists refer to the system by which the known amino acids are coded or copied (duplicated) as DNA (deoxyribonucleic acid). This DNA duplicating system (called **protein synthesis**) enables scientists to make nucleic acid hair reconstructor, so that when it is applied to the hair, it replaces any needed amino acid(s) that may be missing in the hair shaft. Animal and vegetable cells are used in the protein synthesis process. **Micropolysaccharide** is the gluelike substance that holds the hair together (see Figure 4.12h on

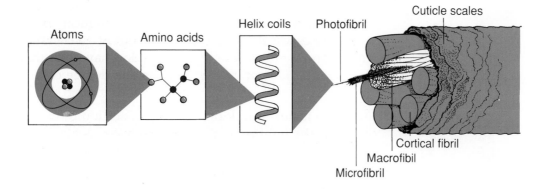

page 73). This cement resembles sap from a tree, only it is in your hair.

Figure 6.3
Breakdown of the hair shaft

Thus, nucleic acid conditioners rebuild damaged polypeptide (protein made of four or more amino acids) chains, hydrogen bonds, and sulfur bonds in the hair (Figure 6.3). These conditioners also protect hair from high-alkaline services, such as bleaching, tinting, cold waving, and so forth.

For these scientific reasons, nucleic acid is the best reconstructor for the hair because it (1) restores moisture; (2) rebuilds the helix of the polypeptide chain; (3) penetrates the cuticle and cortex; (4) strengthens the cuticle and the cortex without interfering (slowing down or diluting) with other chemical actions; (5) gives the hair greater elasticity and shine; (6) adds body to hair for easier styling; and (7) remains in the hair longer than other conditioners. In short, nucleic acid does more for hair reconstruction than any other conditioner.

The exact way in which nucleic acid conditioners work is not yet completely understood. Follow the advice of your instructor or manager so that you will be using this new product correctly.

Practical Objective 4
Damage Assessment and Application of an Appropriate Conditioner

Supplies

■ client release form
■ shampoo supplies
■ assortment of professional hair conditioners

Procedure

1. Drape the client and examine the scalp for scratches, abrasions, disorders and diseases, and general color.

Rationale

1. This is standard procedure.

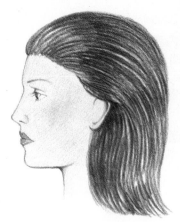

Figure 6.4
Note the luster or lack of luster of the hair.

2. If chemical services are not scheduled, brush the hair and then assess its condition.

3. Note the luster or lack of luster as the light reflects from the hair (Figure 6.4).

4. Feel the hair to determine if it is smooth or rough to the touch.

5. Analyze the porosity and elasticity of the hair.

6. Shampoo and analyze the hair, and explain the results of the analysis to your client.

7. Recommend two different conditioners at two different prices to the client, and explain how each will improve the condition of the hair. If you will have to spend a great deal of additional time to apply a conditioner, explain this as well.

8. **An example:** Ms. (Mrs., Mr.) Anderson, your hair needs conditioning. It seems to be dry and lacks natural oils. This may be due to overexposure to the sun and wind, or it may have been caused by chemical abuse. I would recommend either our Brand A or our Brand C conditioner to restore oils to your hair so that it will have a beautiful shine. Brand A

2. Due to widespread physical and chemical abuse, almost 9 out of 10 clients in the salon have hair that requires some degree of conditioning.

3. Luster indicates whether the sebaceous glands are functioning normally.

4. Dryness can be felt. To some extent, you also can feel the porosity of the hair if the cuticle imbrications stand away from the hair shaft.

5. This is standard procedure (explained in Chapter 4).

6. It is good practice to analyze the hair twice, once when wet and again when dry. Always explain the hair's condition to the client.

7. Giving the client two choices of price and conditioner is good sales practice. It puts the decision into an either/or instead of a yes/no category. The client has a right to know how the product will affect his or her hair and how long the application will take.

8. **Identify the problem** clearly for the client so that he or she understands the condition of the hair. Describe **what the hair** lacks. Explain **why the conditioner is needed.** Recommend **two** conditioners that will correct the hair damage so the client will have a **choice.** State the time required for each conditioner because the client may be operating on a

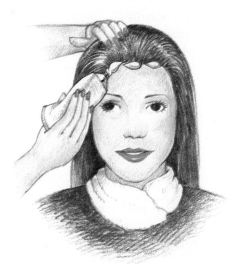

Figure 6.5
Apply the conditioner directly to the hair. Give the client the remainder of the tube or discard it. Do not reuse!

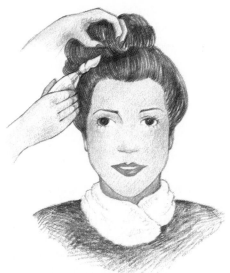

Figure 6.6
Work the conditioner thoroughly through the hair.

requires only 3 or 4 minutes and sells for $2. Brand C takes 10 to 12 minutes to apply and penetrates the cuticle of the hair shaft. It sells for $5.

9. Apply the conditioner and work it through the hair (Figures 6.5 and 6.6). Next place a protective plastic cap and then a heating cap over the client's head (Figure 6.7).

10. **An example:** Ms. (Mrs., Mr.) Anderson, I have assessed the condition of your hair, and it is in very

tight schedule. The price difference may also be important to a client who has forgotten his or her checkbook and may have only enough cash for the scheduled service. The steps outlined here should be standard procedure for recommending all salon services.

9. The heat helps the conditioner penetrate the hair.

10. **Never attempt to sell a client an unneeded service.** The best way to win your client's confidence is to

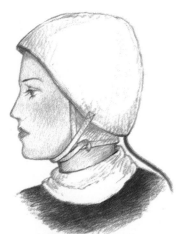

Figure 6.7
Place a protective plastic cap on the client's head and cover it with a heating cap.

good shape. Although you have asked for a conditioner today, I honestly do not think that your hair needs it now. If your hair needs conditioning in future visits to the salon, I will call it to your attention.

give honest, accurate, and professional advice. The reward for doing the right thing will be tenfold because it will enhance the client's trust in your technical competency.

Glossary

Affinity The attraction between chemicals or substances.

Animal proteins One kind of protein in hair conditioners.

Antihumectant A chemical that creates a barrier between the hair shaft and moisture in the air.

Appearance The luster, sheen, or shininess of the hair.

Collagen (KAHL-eh-jen) An animal protein used in some skin and hair cosmetics.

Elasticity The degree to which a hair can be stretched without breaking.

In-process conditioning Adding conditioners to products to improve or buffer their action during a service.

Instant conditioner A conditioner with a vegetable oil base and often an acid pH; it does not penetrate into the hair shaft.

Instant conditioning and setting aids Strong setting lotions that also have a little animal or vegetable protein; can be either acid or alkaline.

Keratin (KER-eh-tin) The basic protein that forms the structure of the hair shaft.

Manageability The ease or difficulty with which a comb passes through the hair, whether the hair is wet or dry.

Micropolysaccharide (migh-kroh-pah-lee-SAK-e-righde) A gluelike substance that is believed to cement the cortical fibers together.

Normalizing conditioners Conditioners with an acid pH that neutralize the alkaline effects of trace chemicals after such services such as tints, relaxers, cold waves, or lighteners.

Placenta (plah-SEN-tah) The nutrient-providing organ in female mammals—in this case, cattle or sheep—that is refined and used in some protein hair conditioners.

Porosity The amount of liquid a hair strand can absorb.

Preconditioning Using a conditioner before a strong chemical service to prevent hair damage.

Protein conditioners Products that penetrate the hair shaft to replace keratin that has been physically or chemically removed.

Reconditioning Using a conditioner after a service.
Substantive proteins Manufactured or processed proteins.
Tensile strength The amount of elasticity hair has.
Texture The feel and diameter of the hair shaft.
Vegetable proteins One source of protein in hair conditioners. The proteins come from high-protein plants, such as balsam trees.

Questions

1. Name the five characteristics that are used to describe the condition of the hair.
2. Using your own words, explain the difference between instant conditioners and protein conditioners.
3. What is keratin?
4. Briefly explain what hair texture is.
5. Do all clients need their hair conditioned?
6. When the hair is wet, what percentage of its length can it be stretched?
7. What term is used to describe the ability of the hair to absorb moisture?

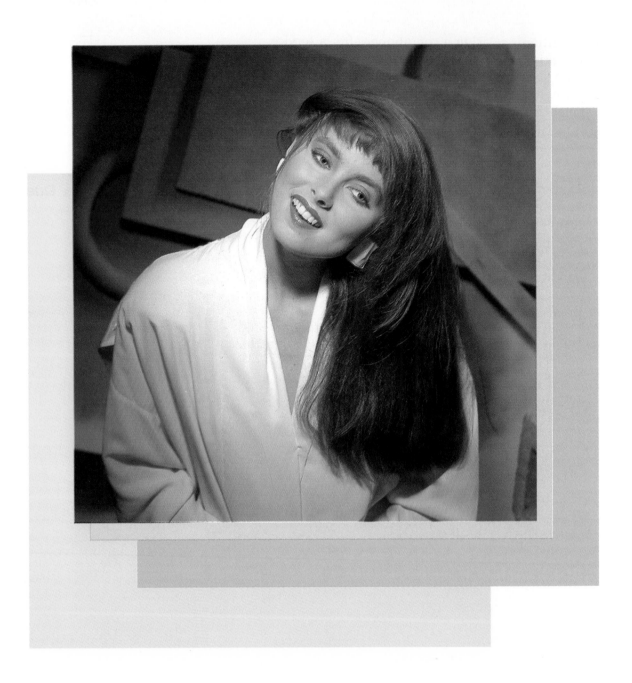

Scalp Treatments

Learning Objective

From the information in this chapter and practice under the supervision of your instructor, follow the proper steps to manipulate the scalp of the client after the shampooing service. Be able to manipulate the scalp in 30–40 minutes. Score 85 percent or better on a multiple-choice exam on the information in this chapter.

In order to achieve the above level of competence, you should master the following chapter objectives.

Theory Objectives

1. Describe the benefits of scalp manipulations.
2. List the basic safety precautions for a scalp treatment.

Practical Objective

3. Give a scalp treatment.

Introduction

Scalp manipulations are a separate service offered in schools and salons. They can be given after brushing the hair and shampooing to help maintain a healthy scalp. The purpose of these treatments is to increase the flow (circulation) of blood to the scalp. A clean, healthy scalp will also lead to healthy hair, although, as Chapter 4 explained, other factors are important, too. Nevertheless, improving the flow of blood to the papilla with a scalp treatment will certainly help preserve the health of a client's hair and scalp.

Theory Objective 1
Benefits of Scalp
Manipulations

Because a scalp treatment brings the blood supply closer to the surface of the skin, the treatment should **not** be given before a chemical service. For example, a client who is scheduled to receive a permanent wave (or chemical relaxer) should not be given a scalp treatment before the chemical service. Having a scalp treatment before the chemical service may cause the scalp to become red and inflamed. A skin allergy could also develop because the increased blood supply to the scalp could make the skin more sensitive to something that will cause the client to have an allergic reaction.

Scalp manipulations are very beneficial. They stimulate the nerves and glands in the scalp, and they soothe the muscles. They also increase the circulation of blood, which nourishes the scalp tissues, and they make the scalp more flexible.

Although there is no scientific evidence that scalp manipulations promote hair growth, you may observe that a client's scalp looks healthier after a scalp manipulation. Anything, including a scalp manipulation, that contributes to a healthy scalp is an appropriate service. Nevertheless, you must not promise a client that scalp manipulation will promote hair growth.

Theory Objective 2
Basic Safety
Precautions for a
Scalp Treatment

Scalp manipulations are given immediately after the shampoo service. They should not be given, however, if the hair is to be cold waved, permanently colored, chemically straightened, or lightened during the appointment. (Do not give a scalp treatment before any chemical service when the chemical will be applied directly to the scalp.)

Since some scalps are dry and others are oily, be sure to read the directions on the label before using the product. This will ensure that you use the correct product for the client's individual scalp condition.

In all scalp treatments, you should examine the scalp for disorders and diseases. If you are not sure about the condition of your client's scalp, consult your instructor. If a contagious disease is present, you may have to refuse the service and ask the client to visit a doctor.

You should also brush the client's hair and analyze its condition before giving the scalp treatment. After giving the manipulation, place your client under a steamer or heating cap. If you choose a heating cap, you will want to put a sanitized plastic undercap over the hair before placing the client under the dryer. If you choose the steamer, no undercap is needed because you want the moisture to seal the conditioner into the hair and scalp. In either case, the heat enables the scalp cream to penetrate better into the hair and scalp.

When working with any heating device, such as a steamer, be sure to check the temperature **before** you use the device on the client. If for any reason the client is severely burned (with an open wound), take him or her to a doctor. Do the same for any client who is **seriously burned with a curling iron** or any other cosmetology tool or chemical.

Practical Objective 3
A Scalp Treatment

Supplies

- laundered towel
- scalp conditioner
- sanitized or new plastic undercap
- electric steamer or
- heating cap

Figure 7.1 (pp. 130–132) illustrates the scalp manipulation procedure.

Sanitize your area as follows:

1. **Wash, wipe, and store bottles and supplies.**

2. **Discard used supplies.**

3. **Clean and sanitize the cape and apron.**

4. **Sanitize the work area; wash your hands.**

Figure 7.1   *Give a Scalp Treatment*

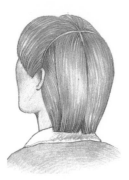

(a) Wash your hands after draping the client. Brush, shampoo, towel-dry, and section the hair into four quarters. This is standard procedure.

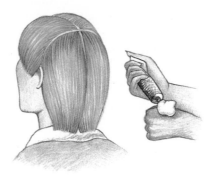

(b) Apply scalp conditioner to the back of your hand. This keeps the conditioner more sanitary.

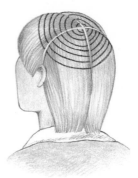

(c) Outline the four section partings; then divide the hair into ¼-inch (0.6-centimeter) subsections. Apply conditioner to all of the scalp partings until the entire scalp is covered.

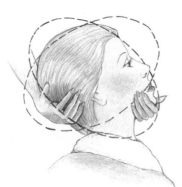

(d) Gently cup one hand underneath the client's chin, and place the other at the nape of the neck. Rotate the head carefully. Reverse the rotation. **Repeat each movement four times.** These movements will relax the client.

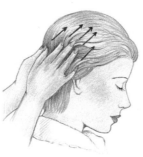

(e) At the base of the nape, slide your fingers through the hair to the scalp. Firmly slide and spread your fingers as you move upward toward the front hairline.

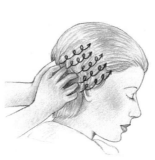

(f) Repeat the preceding step, but stop every inch and rotate the scalp with your fingertips.

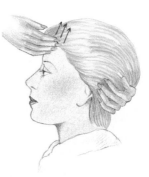

(g) Support the back of the head with one hand. Extend your thumb away from your index finger, and place your palm down on the client's forehead. Firmly slide your hand an inch or two into the hairline.

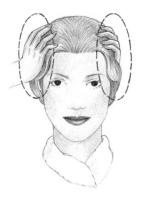
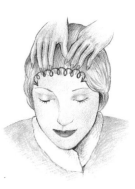
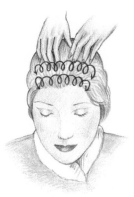
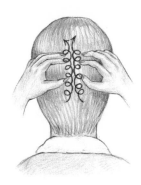

(h) Scalp rotation: Slide your fingertips through the hair above the ears; using the palms of your hands, apply even, circular pressure to each side of the head.

(i) Place your fingertips together along the front hairline. Use a lifting and rotating motion to work from the top-center to just below the temple area.

(j) Repeat the preceding step, but gradually slide back from the hairline 1 inch (2.5 centimeters).

(k) Slide your fingertips through the hair at the back of the head. Use the pads of your thumbs to rotate the scalp. Move thumbs up 1 inch (2.5 centimeters) and repeat the procedure upward to the top of the head.

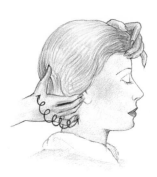
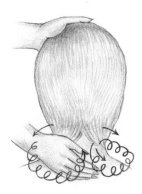
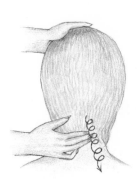
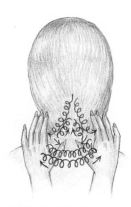

(l) Support the forehead with one hand. Slide your fingertips through the hair behind the ear on the nape. Rotate the palm of your hand in an upward direction. Work across the nape toward the other ear.

(m) Support the head with one hand, and use rotation movements along the base of the neck on one side; next move along the shoulder, then back across the shoulder to the spine. Repeat for the other side.

(n) Gently grasp the trapezius muscle at the base of the neck. Use circular movements with the fingers and palms. Work across the trapezius to the shoulder. Repeat.

(o) Next, rotate the middle and ring fingers from the occipital bone to the spine. This should be done using firm, slow, circular movements.

Figure 7.1   *Give a Scalp Treatment (cont.)*

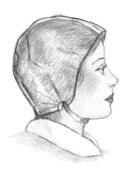

(p) Place a plastic
undercap over the hair.

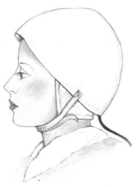

(q) Put on a heating cap.
Regulate and monitor
(check) temperature
carefully!

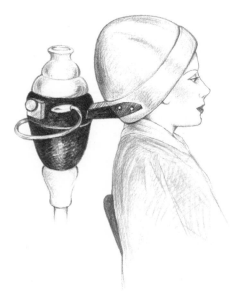

(r) Or you may seat the client under the
steamer. Regulate and monitor (check)
temperature carefully!

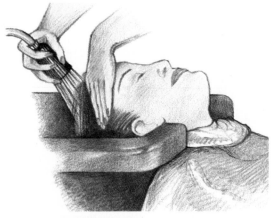

(s) Rinse conditioner from hair. (You may need to give the
hair a light shampoo to remove excess scalp conditioner.)
Proceed with the next service.

Anterior auricular (an-TIR-ee-ehr aw-RIK-yeh-lehr) arteries
Arteries located toward the front part of the ear (Figure 7.2).

Cervical vertebra (SEHR-vi-kehl VUHR-teh-brah) The part of the backbone located at the center base of the shoulders.

Mastoid (MAS-toyd) bones The bones behind the ears.

Occipital (ahk-SIP-eh-tehl) bone The bone located at the back of the skull.

Posterior auricular (pah-STIR-ee-ahr aw-RIK-yeh-lehr) arteries
The arteries located near the back of the ear.

Temporal (TEM-peh-rehl) arteries The arteries located at the temples.

Trapezius (tra-PEE-zee-us) muscle The muscle that raises and rotates the shoulders and draws the head back and to the side.

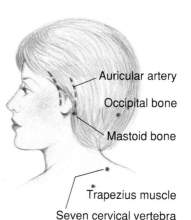

1. Locate and label the mastoid bone on the drawing.
2. Locate the seventh cervical vertebra on the drawing.
3. Identify the auricular artery on the drawing.
4. Label the occipital bone on the drawing.
5. Now label the approximate location of the temporal artery.
6. Should you give a scalp treatment before applying a hair lightener retouch?
7. How many sections should the hair be divided into for a scalp treatment?
8. Will a scalp treatment promote hair growth?
9. Using your own words, describe the benefits of a scalp treatment.
10. Where is the trapezius muscle located?
11. Before placing the client under the dryer, what should you place on the head first?

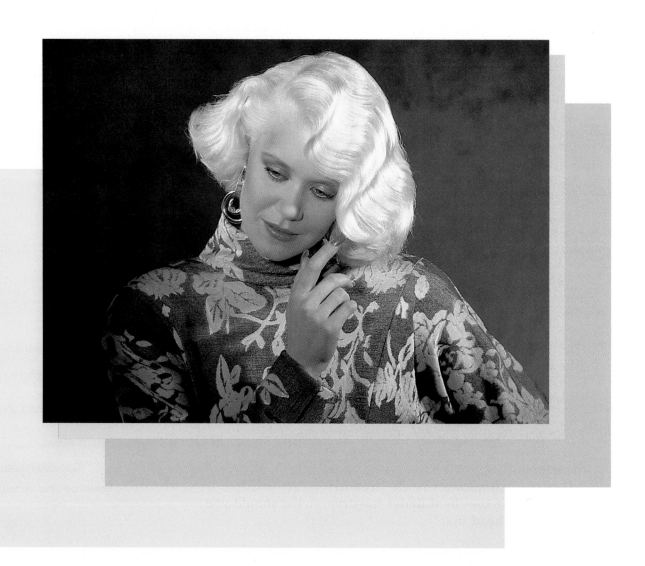

Finger Waving

Learning Objective

Comb, then brush, all of the client's hair in even, alternating rows of finger waves. Using a styling comb and the proper setting lotion, comb even and alternating waves with well-defined ridges that are parallel to each other. Design all the hair (length permitting) in finger waves in 30 minutes. Score 85 percent or better on a multiple-choice exam on the information in this chapter.

In order to achieve the above level of competence, you should master the following objectives.

Theory Objective

1. Describe the parts of a finger wave, and identify waves, shapings, sculpture curls, and base-directed hair.

Practical Objectives

2. Part off the five styling sections of the head.
3. Set and comb three alternating rows of horizontal finger waves in the crown section of the client's head.

Introduction

After you have shampooed the hair and, if necessary, conditioned it properly, you are ready to begin developing your hairstyling ability.

The first stage in this process is **finger waving,** or the art of combing the hair in alternating parallel arcs that have well-defined ridges. Cosmetologists call these ridges **waves.**

Practicing finger waves before going on to more complicated styles offers two advantages. First, it will give you experience in working on the curved surfaces of the head to create designs and patterns in the hair.

Second, it will give you the opportunity to create a hairstyle that has become popular in recent years. This basic, fairly simple, tight, curly hairstyle is a good way to get started on an important part of the cosmetologist's work. This style uses a basic pattern that will give you a foundation for your more imaginative and creative efforts.

By mastering effective finger-waving techniques, you will develop the dexterity, coordination, and strength that you will need to make the hair shapings, sculpture curls, and roller placements used for more advanced hairstyles.

Theory Objective 1
*Parts of a Finger Wave
and Waves, Shapings,
Sculpture Curls, and
Base-Directed Hair*

A finger wave is hair combed in alternating parallel semicircles. The hair between two parallel wave ridges is called the **wave trough** (Figure 8.1). A good finger wave must have the following characteristics:

1. A wave pattern, or "SS," must appear in the hair.

2. The hair in a given semicircle must be parallel to the hair on either side. If one pattern looks like an "S," the pattern before and after must be parallel to the first pattern—an "SSS."

3. The ridges must also be parallel to each other.

4. The wave troughs must have the same width.

Sculpture-wave patterns generally have wider or softer troughs between their ridges, and the ridges themselves are not as sharply defined as they are in finger waves. Otherwise, sculpture-wave patterns are almost the same as finger-wave patterns. Before sculpture curling, comb some of the hairs into a parallel, semicircular (half-circle) design. These designs are called **hair shapings** or moldings. These shapings make waves that can be combed in either a clockwise (c.w.) or counterclockwise (c.c.w.) direction (Figure 8.2).

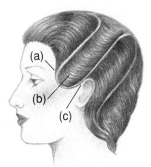

Figure 8.1
*Parts of a wave: (a) ridge,
(b) trough, and (c) ridge
parallel to (a).*

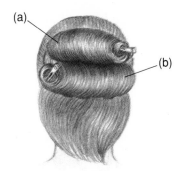

Figure 8.2
*Wave shapes:
(a) counterclockwise,
(b) clockwise.*

Hair direction usually refers to how a strand or section of hair is combed in terms of the overall hair strand or section from the scalp to the end of the hair shaft (see Figure 8.1).

The **base direction** of a hair strand is the movement of direction of the hair as it grows from the scalp. Base direction refers to the first inch or two of a hair strand as it leaves the follicles in the scalp. The **first** half of a semicircular shaping is the base direction.

*Practical Objective 2
Styling Sections of
the Head*

Supplies

- two styling combs
- mannequin
- mannequin clamp
- two laundered towels
- water applicator bottle
- duck-bill clips

Procedure

1. Fold a towel over the edge of the styling station and secure the clamp correctly. Place the mannequin on the clamp spindle.

2. Begin applying water in the nape section. Hold the applicator in your left hand, and spray the section. Comb the water through the hair with your right hand. Apply water in this manner until all hair is wet and easy to comb.

Rationale

1. This protects the laminated surface of the styling station. The mannequin is now in place.

2. The hair must be wet for any styling procedure because the water breaks the hydrogen cross-bonds in the hair, causing it to stretch. These bonds will re-form naturally, with the new design in the hair, as the hair dries.

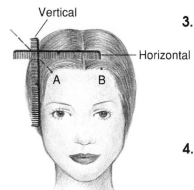

Vertical

Horizontal

A   B

Figure 8.3
Finding points to divide the top from the side sections

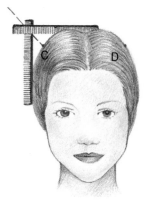

C   D

Figure 8.4
Finding more points to divide the side from the back (crown) sections

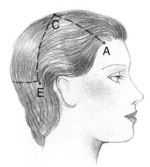

C

A

E

Figure 8.5
Lines AC, CE, and the hairline enclose the right side section.

3. Hold the bottom of one comb in a vertical position along the right cheekbone, and hold another comb horizontally just behind the hairline.

4. Imagine a straight line that divides the right angle formed by the two combs into two equal parts (Figure 8.3). The point where this line meets the hairline is A. Use this procedure to find corresponding point B on the left side.

5. Place a comb in a horizontal position along the side of the head and align the comb with point A (Figure 8.4). Hold another comb vertically at the back of the head. Divide the angle that the combs form as you did in step 4. The point where the line dividing the angle meets the surface of the head is C.

6. Repeat these steps on the left side of the client's head to find point D. Imagine a line connecting points A, C, D, and B.

7. Part the hair from point C to point E, which is 1 inch (2.5 centimeters) behind the right ear (Figure 8.5).

8. Part the hair on the left side in the same manner, working from point D to point F, which is 1 inch (2.5 centimeters) behind the left ear.

3. These combs will form a right angle. The vertical comb will be one side of the right angle, and the horizontal comb will be the other side of the right angle.

4. The top profile of the head forms an arc. If you divide the right angle placed on the arc, you will get the approximate middle of that arc. This exercise is not absolutely accurate, but it will help you estimate the lines that divide the top from the two side sections.

5. Same as steps 3 and 4.

6. The area enclosed by the lines that connect these points is the top section.

7. This completes the division of the side section. The area enclosed by lines AC, CE, and the hairline is the right side section.

8. This completes the division of the side section. The area enclosed by lines BD, DF, and the hairline is the left side section.

9. Part the hair in a slight arc from F to E through the occipital nerve point (at the top of the nape) (Figure 8.6).

9. This establishes the crown and nape sections. Lines connecting C, E, F, and D enclose the crown section. Line FE and the bottom hairline enclose the nape section.

10. You can use this exercise to find the five styling areas on any size head (Figure 8.7).

10. Considerable practice on a mannequin is helpful before working on a client.

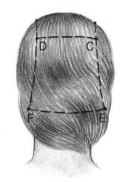

Figure 8.6
The crown section

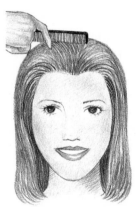

(a) Comb hair away from the hairline.

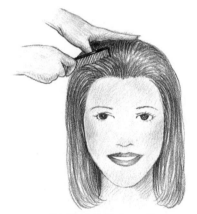

(b) Push hair from the crown forward.

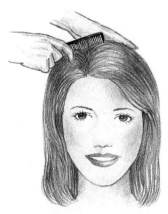

(c) Watch for the natural split of the hair.

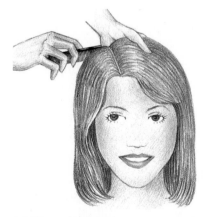

(d) The natural part

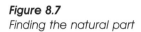

Figure 8.7
Finding the natural part

*Set and Comb Three
Alternating Rows of
Horizontal Finger Waves
in the Crown Section of
a Mannequin or Client*

Supplies

- finger-waving lotion
- finger-waving comb
- laundered or paper towels
- duck-bill clips
- mannequin and clamp
- hair-setting tape

Procedure

1. Assemble all supplies and implements in work area.

2. Beginning in the nape, carefully brush or comb tangles from the mannequin. Comb or brush from the ends of the hair and work toward the scalp.

3. Wet the hair on the mannequin or client. Ask your instructor about the wetting method and the application of creme rinse.

4. Towel-dry according to directions from your instructor or manager and the directions on the label of the creme rinse product you will be using.

5. Part the top and side sections and secure them with duck-bill clips.

Rationale

1. This practice will help you work more efficiently.

2. It is easier to remove tangles by beginning in the nape area. It is very difficult to remove tangles from wet hair. If you remove tangles and back-combing before wetting the hair, it will be much more manageable when you apply setting lotion.

3. The hair has to be wet for shaping. Water helps break hydrogen cross-bonds in the hair so that the strands will conform to the setting pattern. Mannequins may require only brushing and spraying with water, followed by a creme rinse, which increases manageability. A client may have to be shampooed and given a creme rinse or conditioner.

4. This is standard procedure.

5. In all finger-waving exercises and services, sections not to be waved should be clipped out of

6. Obtain finger-waving lotion from your instructor.

the way. In this case, this includes all sections except the crown. Duck-bill clips are used to hold large sections of hair.

6. A special semiliquid waving lotion is used for finger waving because its thick, or heavy, consistency (viscosity) makes it easier to form wave ridges.

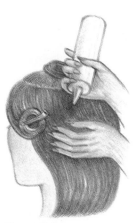

Figure 8.8
Apply finger-waving lotion.

7. Pour the lotion onto the crown hair with your right hand (Figure 8.8). Cup your left hand beneath the hair.

7. You must pour finger-waving lotion onto the hair because it is too thick to be sprayed on with a pump applicator. The cupped left hand catches dripping lotion, protecting the client's clothing and the floor. Water on the hair acts as a wetting agent to distribute the lotion onto the hair shaft.

8. Comb the hair straight back and flat against the head after evenly distributing lotion. Deposit excess lotion on a laundered or paper towel.

8. You should comb the lotion evenly through the hair so it will dry uniformly. Combing the hair straight back and flat against the head also softens and stretches the hydrogen bonds in the hair. These bonds make the waving pattern firm and enable it to last until the next shampoo. As the hair dries, it contracts, resulting in a bouncy setting pattern. The lotion gives body (surface substance) to the hair shaft.

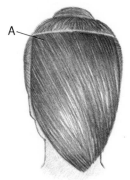

Figure 8.9
The hair is combed down and to the right to begin semicircular shaping.

9. Comb all crown hair downward and to the right side of the head (Figure 8.9).

9. These steps will give you the first half of the semicircular shaping that you will use to make a horizontal ridge pattern.

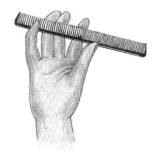

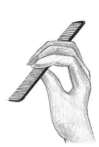

Figure 8.10
The correct way to hold the comb for finger waving

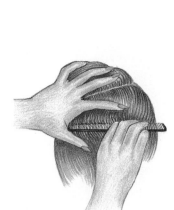

Figure 8.11
Move comb to the left to make the first ridge.

10. Hold the comb as shown in Figure 8.10.

11. Place the index finger of your left hand firmly across point A (see Figures 8.9 and 8.11). Hold your finger parallel to the floor.

12. Place the teeth of the comb just below your index finger and perpendicular to the head. Insert the comb into the hair at a 45-degree angle to your index finger.

13. To make the ridge, shift the comb along an imaginary line that is 1 inch (2.5 centimeters) to the left of your index finger (Figure 8.11). Do not remove comb. Flip the comb downward, but do not move it from its shifted position.

14. Move the middle finger of your left hand to the position held by the index finger of your left hand (Figure 8.12).

15. Rotate the teeth of the comb to a flat position on the hair and place the index finger of your left hand across the lower half of the comb toward the head (Figure 8.13).

16. Push firmly against the head with your index and

10. Holding the comb this way will make it easier to comb the ridges from the shaping.

11. Your index finger secures the base direction of the hair so that it will not move when you comb the first part of the ridge into the hair.

12. When the hair is shifted between the comb and index finger, the ridge begins to form. The teeth of the comb keep the strands closer together so that the hair will comb more smoothly.

13. If you remove the comb, the ridge will relax and settle close to the head. Placing the comb flat gives you room to move your middle finger to the position of your index finger, while your index finger secures the hair immediately above the comb.

14. This procedure secures the ridge before you reverse the direction of the comb.

15. Same as for step 12. Placing the comb flat allows room for the index finger. Your middle finger takes the position that was occupied by your index finger to help hold the hair and form the ridge.

16. If you do not hold the hair firmly, the ridge will be

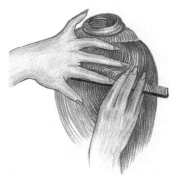

Figure 8.12
Shift finger position to secure the ridge of the wave.

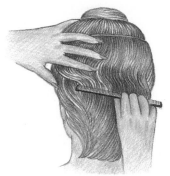

Figure 8.13
Rotate comb to smooth hair under index finger.

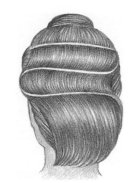

Figure 8.14
First wave shaping

middle fingers; then shift the comb to the right. Rotate the comb away from the head and through the ends of the strand.

17. Repeat this procedure in 1-inch (2.5-centimeter) strands across the top crown of the head to form the first wave ridge.

18. Carefully comb through the hair as needed until the ridge is well defined (Figure 8.14).

19. Beginning on the right side of the head, repeat this procedure to form the second ridge across the middle crown.

20. Start on the lower left side to comb the third ridge into the hair. Check the size of the wave troughs. Place hair-setting tape across the wave troughs and all loose hair (optional). Ask your instructor for an evaluation.

disturbed and will flatten out.

17. A 1-inch (2.5-centimeter) single-strand seems to be the easiest size for adding to the ridge.

18. The shaping and the ridge may have to be touched up a little to make all hairs in the shaping parallel to each other.

19. Be sure that the ridges are parallel and an equal distance from each other as you comb across from one side of the crown to the other.

20. Wave troughs should be about the same size from ridge to ridge (Figure 8.15). This first exercise must be correct if other waves are to be formed properly. The tape will not mark the hair (as clips will), but it is porous so the hair will dry

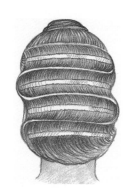

Figure 8.15
The hair is combed down and to the right to begin semicircular shaping.

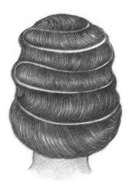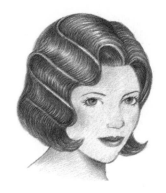

Figure 8.16
The completed finger wave

evenly. Also, the tape helps define the ridges by bringing the wave troughs closer to the head.

21. Dry the hair thoroughly according to your instructor's directions. Remove and discard the tape. Comb or brush through the wave pattern. Repeat these procedures for all the hair.

21. If mannequins are used, your instructor may give you special instructions. To maintain sanitation, do not reuse tape. Combing the hair will relax it. If the waves are too small, brush them to achieve more relaxation. The entire head should be finger waved (Figure 8.16).

Sanitize your area as follows:

1. Wash, wipe, and store bottles and supplies.

2. Discard used supplies.

3. Clean and sanitize the cape and apron.

4. Sanitize the work area; wash your hands.

Glossary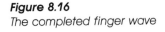

Base direction The movement of direction of the first inch or two of hair as it grows from the scalp.

Finger wave Hair combed in alternating parallel semicircles, or arcs, that have well-defined ridges.

Hair direction How a strand or section of hair is combed.

Hair shapings Combing some of the hairs into a parallel, semicircular design. These shaping designs make waves that can be combed in either a clockwise or a counterclockwise direction.

Wave trough The hair between two parallel ridges.

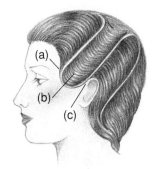

1. Label letter (a) on the drawing.
2. Label letter (b) on the drawing.
3. Label letter (c) on the drawing.
4. What kind of hair pattern results from combing the hair as shown in the drawing?
5. Write a definition for each part of the waves described in this chapter.
6. When hair is combed in alternating parallel arcs with a ridge in between, what is the formation called?
7. What are the designs called when hair is combed in a parallel pattern in a semicircular direction?
8. What is the term used to describe where the hair is combed as it leaves the scalp?

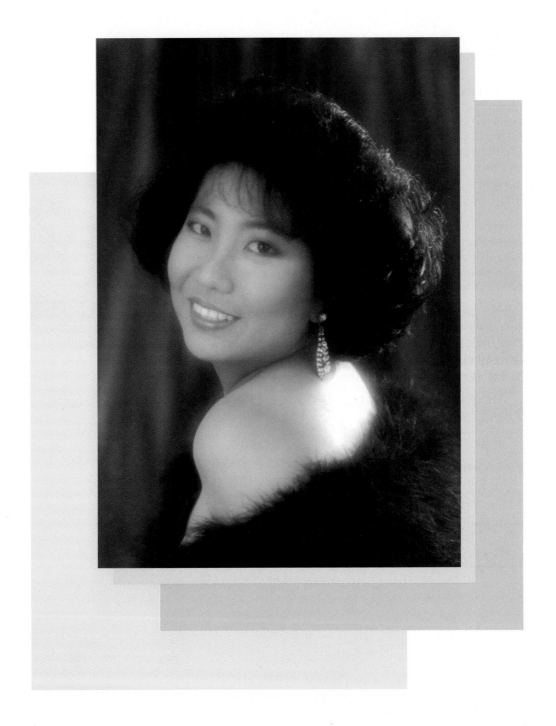

Sculpture Curls

Learning Objective

Using the proper implements, set all the client's or mannequin's hair in sculpture curls and comb it into place according to the proper styling principles. Set the hair in 30 minutes, dry as necessary, and comb into place in 20 minutes. Score 85 percent or better on a multiple-choice exam on the information in this chapter.

In order to achieve the above level of competence, you should master the following chapter objectives.

Theory Objectives

1. List the setting and combing implements used to style the hair.
2. Identify hairstyling terms and define the three parts of a sculpture curl.
3. Describe the basic types of sculpture curls and their variations and list the three strengths of sculpture curls.

Practical Objective

4. Set and comb sculpture curls: (a) in horizontal wave patterns in the crown and nape sections of the head; (b) in one large semicircular formation in both side sections; (c) in alternating diagonal-wave formations in both side sections; and (d) in the top section to form an outside movement away from the head.

Once you have mastered the basic techniques of finger waving, you can move on to learn advanced hairstyling techniques.

Your first two steps are basic, but very necessary. First, you will need to learn the basic hairstyling terms. Second, you will need to know and apply the basic principles used to create advanced hairstyles. There is a basic cause-and-effect relationship between the setting and combing patterns used for sculpture curls and the final style you wish to achieve. Thus, the results of using a specific set of principles for setting and combing are quite predictable. If you want a particular pattern of curls, you simply need to use a certain principle of setting. Because the results are predictable, you can apply basic hairstyling principles to unstyled hair and know that it will do what you want it to do.

In all cases, the key to good hairstyling is the mastery of the basic principles. High styling, or advanced styling, is simply a more advanced way of applying basic principles (with, of course, a little more imagination). When you master these principles, you will be able to create your own styles and give way to your imagination.

Theory Objective 1
Setting and Combing
Implements Used to
Style Hair

Like skilled workers in many fields, cosmetologists often are judged by the way they use and maintain their implements. Your skill as a cosmetologist is directly related to your implements. Always keep them sanitary and ready to use.

As a cosmetologist, you will use many different implements. You therefore need to know which implement is used to perform a particular task. For example, you will work with several different combs:

1. The **rat-tail comb** is often used for carving sculpture curls from their shapings or dividing the hair into sections for cold waving (Figure 9.1a). It can also be used for applying chemical relaxers.

2. The **rake comb** can be used to apply chemical relaxers (Figure 9.1b). It is also used to remove tangles by combing through the hair.

3. The **styling comb** is an all-purpose comb (Figure 9.1c). It is used for all services except applying chemical relaxers.

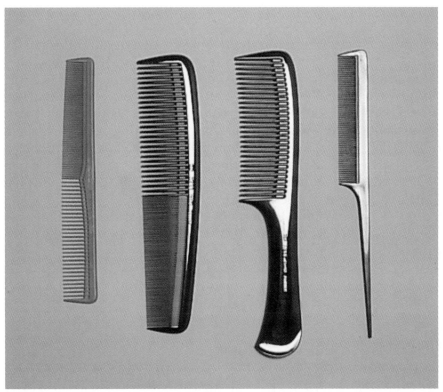

Figure 9.1
Combs

From left to right: barber comb, hairstyling/finger-waving comb, rake comb, and rat-tail comb.

The hair may be held in place by a variety of implements (Figure 9.2).

Hairpin   Bobbi pin   Single-prong clip

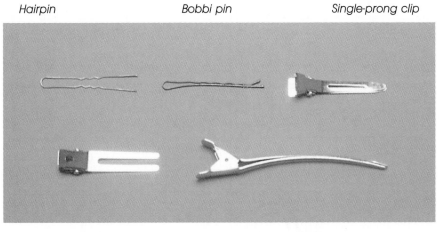

Figure 9.2
Implements to hold hair in place

Double-prong clip   Duck-bill clip

Theory Objective 2
Hairstyling Terms and Parts of a Sculpture Curl

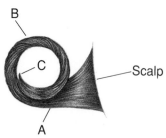

Figure 9.3
The base is from the scalp to A; the stem is from A to B; and the circle end is B to C.

Setting and combing procedures for all hairstyles and designs are based on **geometric forms.** In order to work quickly and accurately, you will need a working knowledge of these forms. The basic parts of a wave were described in Chapter 8, so you are familiar with them. However, the parts of a sculpture curl have their own particular names. Every sculpture curl has three main parts, as shown in Figure 9.3: the base (A), the stem (B), and the circle end (C).

The **base** (or **base direction**) of a hair was defined in Chapter 7. The base of a sculpture curl is the same. It is the direction the hair takes as it leaves the scalp to form a semicircle.

Chapter 7 used the term **hair direction** to describe the rest of the hair shaft. For sculpture curls, the hair direction consists of two parts: the stem and the circle end.

The **stem** (shown as arc AB in Figure 9.3) is the part of the curl that determines whether the **direction of the curl** will be **horizontal, vertical,** or **diagonal** (Figure 9.4).

Figure 9.4
Geometric forms

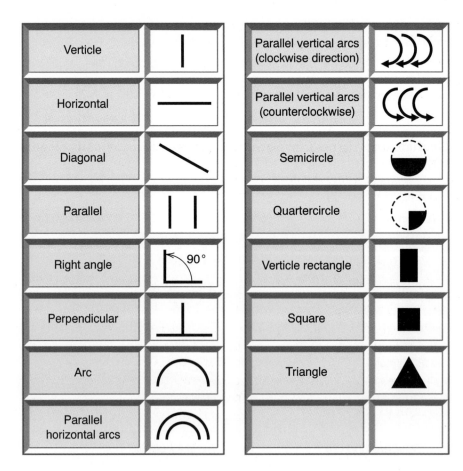

Verticle		Parallel vertical arcs (clockwise direction)	
Horizontal		Parallel vertical arcs (counterclockwise)	
Diagonal		Semicircle	
Parallel		Quartercircle	
Right angle	90°	Verticle rectangle	
Perpendicular		Square	
Arc		Triangle	
Parallel horizontal arcs			

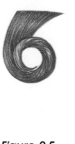 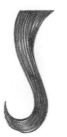 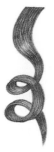 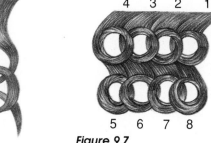

Figure 9.5
Wave

Figure 9.6
Curl

Figure 9.7
Alternating rows of sculpture curls to produce a wave

The **circle end** is the round formation (part) of a sculpture curl. The **size** of the **circle end** (sometimes called the circle) and the number of turns in it regulate the size and strength of the wave (Figure 9.5). The **tightness** of a curl depends on how large or small the circle is (Figure 9.6). Ordinarily, 1½ revolutions (turns) will result in a beautiful, uniform wave pattern (Figure 9.7).

If the ends are given more than 1½ turns, the wave pattern will be curly rather than wavy.

When making a sculpture curl, you should begin setting from the **open end** and let the circle end of the curl being made overlap the base of the **preceding** curl (the one before it). Note how the hair ends of curl 2 overlap the base of curl 1 in Figure 9.7.

As is true for all sculpture curls, the kind of shaping designed into the hair and set in curls will determine what the finished hairstyle looks like. All the semicircular **base** shapings must remain parallel to each other; otherwise, the base direction of the shaping will be **disturbed.** The hair has to pivot (turn) from a point at the bottom of the shaping to retain the parallel shapings for the curls (see point A in Figure 9.3).

Theory Objective 3
Basic Kinds of Sculpture Curls and Their Three Strengths

Sculpture curls get their name from the way they are combed into the hair. A design is combed into the hair, and the curls are then secured close to the head. This is similar to the way a sculptor makes a statue. The sculptor works the general pattern (or blueprint) of his or her creation into the marble and then chisels in the specific details. The design combed into the hair for sculpture curls is called a **shaping.** (Sculpture curls are sometimes called **pin curls,** although the old-fashioned pin curl was not carved from a shaping.) Shapings should be combed in either a clockwise (c.w.) or counterclockwise (c.c.w.) direction. Once you comb the shapings into the hair, you

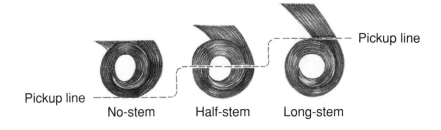

Figure 9.8
Types of sculpture curls

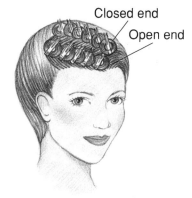

Figure 9.9
Set curls from the open end of the shaping and finish at the closed end.

can place single curls into it. However, you must not disturb the shaping after you have secured the curl with a clip. Secure curl according to directions from your instructor.

The curl is carefully carved (sliced) from the shaping in three different ways, which will determine how strong the curl will be when dried and combed into place. The point at which the curl is carved out of the shaping is called the **pickup line** or **pickup point.** The place in the shaping where the curl is picked up determines what **kind** and **strength** of sculpture curl it will be. The three types of sculpture curls are no-stem, half-stem, and long-stem (Figure 9.8).

The amount of **mobility** (movement) that a curl has depends on the type of stem that is used. The mobility indicates how tight, or firm, the curl will be. The **no-stem** curl produces the least mobility (tightest curl), and the **long-stem** (also called full-stem) curl produces the most mobility (loosest curl). The **half-stem** curl ranges between the other two.

A row of **secured** sculpture curls is correct only if all of the following are true:

1. The shaping was combed into the hair **before** the hair was set.

2. The parallel shapings next to the scalp are **not** disturbed or distorted.

3. The curls were set from the open end of the shaping and finished at the closed end (Figure 9.9).

4. The end of each curl has 1½ turns.

5. The end of each curl forms a perfect **circle.**

6. The extreme end of the hair used to make the curl is on the **inside** of the circle of hair.

7. The curl that has been secured is **overlapped** by the following curl.

While all three stems offer some flexibility and a certain range of design possibilities, the half-stem curl offers the widest range of patterns and combinations because it is between the two extremes of the no-stem and the long-stem.

The half-stem sculpture curl may be combed in either of **two** directions or in combinations of both. Depending on which combi-

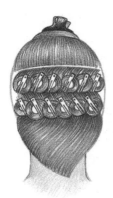
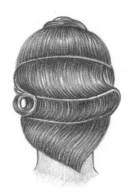

Figure 9.10
Alternating rows of sculpture curls to produce wave

nation you use, you will get curls that are tight (a small amount of movement) or loose (larger movement).

You can make a **wave pattern** by using **alternating** rows of c.w. and c.c.w. sculpture curls (Figure 9.10). These curls will have some movement, but it will be limited.

After you have secured a row of **c.w. sculpture curls,** it will be easy to figure out exactly where the **c.c.w. sculpture curls** should be placed. You can do this by carefully removing the clip from the last c.w. curl made and allowing it to unfold. The position of the hair **end** that forms the **last half** of the semicircle will determine exactly **where** the shaping should be made so that the c.w. curls will unfold into the c.c.w. curls (Figure 9.11).

Setting two rows of half-stem sculpture curls in the **same** direction results in a **larger** movement (Figures 9.12 and 9.13).

Skip-waving patterns are made by using alternating **combinations** of unset hair shapings and sculpture curls (Figure 9.14). Thus, if you make a row of sculpture curls, then a row of unset hair shapings, and so on, you will produce a skip wave (Figure 9.15).

Stand-away (stand-up) curls usually are made when the style calls for the hair to move **away** from the head to achieve height

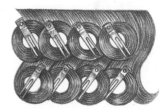

Figure 9.11
Determining where the c.c.w. sculpture curls should be placed

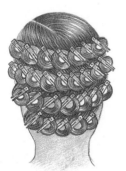

Figure 9.12
Soft wave setting pattern

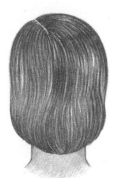

Figure 9.13
Soft wave comb-out

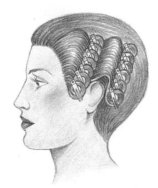

Figure 9.14
Skip wave

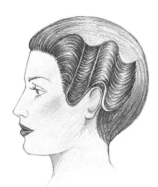

Figure 9.15
Diagonal wave

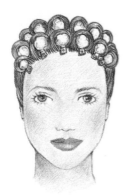

Figure 9.16
Stand-away curls

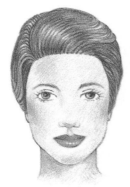

Figure 9.17
Stand-away curls comb-out

Figure 9.18
Stand-away curl

Figure 9.19
Barrel/cascade curls

or volume to silhouette or frame the head in a particular way (Figures 9.16 and 9.17).

Several steps are needed to make these curls. First, comb the hair **away** from the head. Next comb the hair **into** the required design. Then **carve (slice)** the curl from the shaping, and **secure** it in a **standing** position by using a **clip** (Figure 9.18). As with regular sculpture curls, you should pick the hair up from the **open end** of the shaping. The **base strand** for each of the these curls may be **square, rectangular,** or **triangular,** depending on the desired results. You can avoid splits around the front hairline by using curls with triangular bases. Small puffs of cotton may be inserted in the standing circles so that they will not be disturbed under the dryer.

When larger strands are used to make stand-away curls, they sometimes are referred to as **barrel curls** and **cascade curls** (Figure 9.19).

When selecting the strength or type (no-stem, half-stem, long-stem) of sculpture curl to be set, you should consider the following:

1. Hair movement desired

2. Location of the wave movement of the head

3. Texture and length of the client's hair

4. Setting lotion used to prepare the hair

Each of these points requires further explanation:

1. Large, soft, flowing waves are made by a combination of half-stem and long-stem sculpture curls carved from perfectly

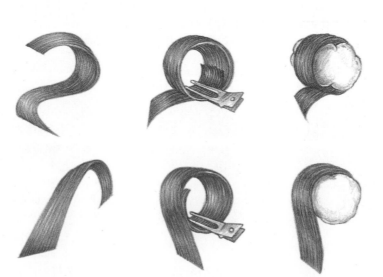

designed hair shapings. Circle ends are wound about 1½ turns so that the hair will not become too curly.

2. Larger movements of hair are ordinarily desirable in the top, upper crown, and sides of the head, depending on prevailing hair fashions and the wishes of the client.

3. Hair texture and length are important considerations. Coarse or medium hair textures may also have a little natural curl so **half-stem** and a **few long-stem** curls would be adequate for them. Fine hair may require the **exclusive use** of no-stem curls, and perhaps more of them, to preserve the hairstyle for even a short time. Long hair is usually set in rollers, which will be discussed in the next chapter.

4. Some setting lotions make the hair crisp or stiff and usually produce a more durable hairstyle. Others make the hair soft and pliable, which may decrease the durability of the set, depending on the style. When using stiff setting lotions, more **half-** and **long-stem** curls and fewer **no-stem** curls are needed because these lotions do not allow the hair to relax as easily as the softer preparations do. Softer setting lotions generally require more long-stem and half-stem sculpture curls because the long hair unfolds and relaxes more when combed.

Practical Objective 4
Set and Comb
Sculpture Curls in the
Crown and Nape of
the Head

Supplies

- combs (rat-tail and styling—Figure 9.20)
- brush
- setting lotion (Figure 9.21)
- creme rinse
- water in spray bottle
- mannequin
- laundered towels
- cotton coil
- end wraps
- mannequin clamp
- duck-bill and double-prong clips (Figure 9.22)

Preparation of Head

Procedure

1. Beginning in the **nape** section, carefully brush or comb tangles from mannequin. Comb or brush from the ends of the hair and work toward the scalp.

Rationale

1. If you remove tangles or back-combing before you wet the hair, the hair will be much more manageable when you apply the setting lotion. It is very difficult to remove tangles from wet hair.

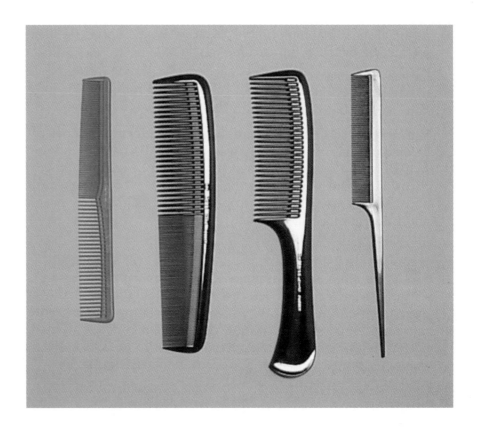

Figure 9.20
Combs

Figure 9.21
Supplies

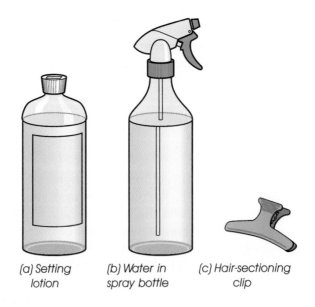

*(a) Setting
lotion*

*(b) Water in
spray bottle*

*(c) Hair-sectioning
clip*

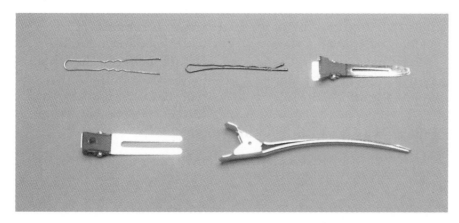

Figure 9.22
Pins and clips

2. Wet the hair in the shampoo bowl. Shampoo the hair if necessary.

3. Towel-dry the hair and apply the creme rinse or conditioner that your instructor recommended. Thoroughly rinse excess lotion from the hair according to the directions on the label.

4. Towel-dry the hair. Return to the styling area.

5. Comb all tangles from the hair. Begin in the nape area and comb toward the **front** of the head.

6. Part off both the **top** and **side** sections. Secure each section with a duck-bill clip or as advised by your instructor.

7. Spray the crown and nape with **setting** lotion. Evenly distribute the lotion through

2. Shapings for sculpture curls cannot be designed (combed) into the hair unless it is wet.

3. The application of the rinse should remove any tangles that you might have missed when you brushed the hair. If you did not apply the creme rinse, the hair could be difficult to comb. This would cause loss of hair.

4. This will keep water from dripping on tiled or carpeted floor.

5. Tangles remove easily when hair is combed from the bottom nape through the **top** and **side sections** of the hair.

6. The top side sections will not be set, so you can slip them out of the way to make it easier to set the hair in the crown and nape.

7. Thorough saturation and combing are needed to stretch the hair. As the hair

the hair. You can dilute the lotion by spraying **plain water** over the hair. Comb excess lotion and water onto a towel.

dries, it **contracts.** This gives a bouncy, durable setting pattern. The lotion adds body (surface substance) to the hair shaft.

Set the crown area with sculpture curls.

1. Determine whether a c.w. or c.c.w. horizontal shaping will be used in the crown. Ask your instructor for assistance.

1. This is standard procedure.

2. If you are going to shape the hair in a c.c.w. design, begin the **first half-base direction** of the semicircle by combing the hair to the left from the top parting (Figure 9.23). Hold the styling comb in your right hand.

2. A horizontal wave pattern requires a series of **parallel,** vertical arcs. They should look like this: (((. The first part of the arc moves to the left **before** you shift it to the right with the comb.

3. Start forming the horizontal **stem** direction by firmly placing the index finger of your left hand in a horizontal position at the **open end** of the shaping, just above the point where you want the hair to change direction.

3. The index finger is placed firmly (nail up) on the hair to prevent the first part of the arc from being **disturbed.** Shapings have to begin at the **open end.**

4. Place the comb **perpendicular** to the scalp and **slide** it along the index finger of your left hand. Shift the hair to complete the semicircular shaping (Figure 9.24).

4. By holding the comb perpendicular to the scalp and sliding it against your index finger, you can shift the hair easily and neatly to get the kind of wave pattern you want.

5. Move your index finger to the **left,** place the comb perpendicular to the scalp, and continue to shift the hair along your index finger. Hold the comb in

5. You should move your index finger to the left so that you shift the next strand of hair out of the way. Each shift has to be made at the same distance

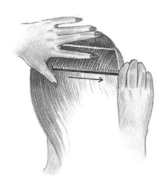

Figure 9.23
Place comb alongside finger. Shift hair against finger to create "(" shaping.

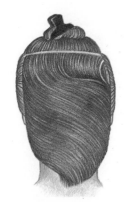

Figure 9.24
"(" shaping

your **right** hand. Continue until shaping is complete.

6. Place the index finger of your **left hand parallel** to the scalp at the **open end** and in the **center** of the shaping; carve out a half-stem curl in the direction you want the design to go.

7. Being careful not to disturb the shaping, lift the index finger and use the thumb, middle, and index fingers of both hands to manipulate the ends inside the completed circle. Secure with a single- or double-prong clip from the **right** side (Figure 9.25).

8. Put your index finger back on the shaping and carve the second curl. Lift your index finger (keep the circle end close to the head) and make the circle end **overlap** the first curl (from step 7). Secure this curl with single- or double-prong clip (Figure 9.26).

9. Fold an **end wrap** (paper) the long way into three equal panels (Figure 9.27). Carve out the curl as you have in the past; place the **circle end** in the center panel. Carefully fold the **right** and **left** panels **over**

from the top part, or the wave pattern will be uniform. This has to be repeated until **all strands** are shaped into parallel arcs that are the same size.

6. Always slice the curl in the **same direction** that the curl will be set.

7. After you have sliced the circle end of the curl from the shaping, you will need both hands to form the completed circle. Place the ends **inside** the circle to maintain curl form and strength. Be sure to secure the curl on the **right side.** If you secure it on the left side, the clip will be in the way of the next curl.

8. If the fingers used to form the circle end are not **close** to the head, the shaping will be disturbed. If the curls do not overlap (the second curl over the first, the third over the second), the shapings will not be parallel to each other.

9. **Paper curls** are used on hair that is very short, straight, coarse, or wiry. You can use them to help hold circular forms in place and achieve stronger curls on hair that is otherwise very difficult to set. Be

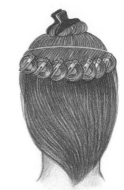

Figure 9.25
Row of c.c.w. sculpture curls. Note the base direction of the curls is undisturbed.

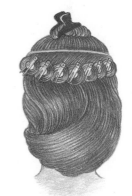

Figure 9.26
Row of c.c.w. sculpture curls. Note next section has been reshaped for carving.

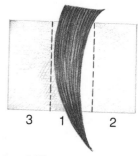

Figure 9.27
Paper curling technique for short hair

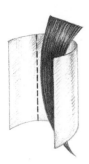

Figure 9.28
Folding the paper over the curl

the hair and complete the circle as usual (Figure 9.28). Secure with a clip.

10. Slice out the next sculpture curl. Spread a ¾-inch (1.88-centimeter) piece of cotton coil the long way. Place the **circle end** in the **center** of the cotton across the **top** of the end, then fold the second edge of the cotton **over** the first and complete the sculpture curl (Figure 9.29). Secure the curl with a clip.

11. Slice out the next sculpture curl. Hold the beginning of the stem between the thumb and index fingers of your left hand. Insert the comb in the stem in front of the fingers of your left hand (Figure 9.30). Rotate the comb ¼ of a turn and place the thumb of your **right** hand on the teeth of the comb. Slide the comb along the hair in a **circular** motion to complete the curl (Figure 9.31). Secure with a clip.

careful not to disturb or twist the circle end when folding the paper around the curl.

10. A **powder-puff** curl basically achieves the same thing as the paper curl technique. Use a piece of cotton instead of an end wrap (paper) to make one. This works very well on bleached (lightened) hair, which may be marked if it is held by a clip. Such a mark is sometimes called a **clip mark.** Ask your instructor for assistance.

11. This procedure is called **ribboning** the hair. Its effect is similar to drawing the edge of a scissors against a piece of wrapping ribbon. Ribboning causes the bonds in the hair to temporarily create a better circular form on the end of the curl. Ask your instructor for help.

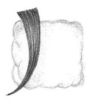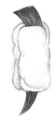

Figure 9.29
Powder-puff curl

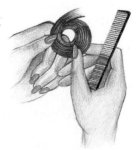

Figure 9.30
Ribboning the hair strand

Figure 9.31
Forming the curl

12. Checklist: (a) Curls should follow a **perfectly parallel semicircular arc.** (b) Starting with the second curl, all circle ends should **overlap** the **base** of the **preceding curl.** (c) The circle ends should be perfectly **round, not oval,** and they **should not be disturbed** by clips (Figure 9.32).

13. Remove the last clip and carefully unfold the sculpture curl.

14. After you have decided where the c.w. shaping will be, put the curl back in place and hold it with a clip. Set all the hair in this shaping in sculpture curls.

Set the nape section.

1. Comb all unset hair from the scalp to the right side of the lower crown. Then, set all remaining hair in c.w. sculpture curls (Figure 9.33).

2. Set the rest of the nape hair in **no-stem** c.c.w. curls. Turn them 1½ times if the hair is long enough to do so. Use end wraps or cotton if necessary. If the hair dries out while you are setting it, **spray with water only.**

12. The first row of horizontal c.c.w. sculpture curls should be checked.

13. This will help you see where the next shaping should be combed into the hair.

14. The curl has to be put back in place to complete the shaping.

1. The hair must be shaped again to set this row of sculpture curls.

2. Since so little hair is left at this point, you **should set** it in the **same** direction as the shaping above it. There is not enough space to change the direction of the hair completely. No-stem curls are used because the hair in the nape usually is subject to abuse from clothing collars and body heat. If the hair is quite short, cotton or end papers may be used. Water will reactivate the setting lotion that you have

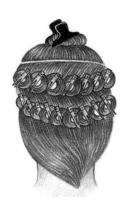

Figure 9.32
Check your work to this point.

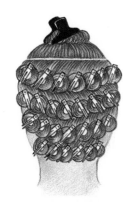

Figure 9.33
Setting the nape section

already applied. It is **not** necessary to apply more setting lotion. If you apply more lotion, **the hair may become sticky, stiff, or gummy.**

3. Check with your instructor to make sure you have set the hair correctly. If your instructor approves, then dry the set.

3. If the set is not correct, you should reset the areas that you did incorrectly. Because standard principles are applied to a set, you should be able to comb it out in a very predictable way.

4. Dry the set thoroughly by allowing the moisture to evaporate from the hair overnight, or use a hair dryer.

4. Mannequins are very expensive. They may be **damaged** if they are placed under a dryer. Consult your instructor.

5. Remove all clips from setting patterns and **make sure** that the hair is **dry.**

5. Any clips will interfere with brushing. If the hair is moist when you brush it, it will comb straight rather than wavy.

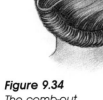

Figure 9.34
The comb-out

6. Comb through the curls with a clean, dry comb. This unfolds the setting pattern. Comb the hair in the same direction in which it was set (Figure 9.34).

6. Unfolding the hair with a comb causes the setting pattern to relax. If the set is too "tight," brushing may be needed to relax it.

7. Unless the set is too tight and is overly curly, you should not brush the hair straight down and flat against the head because it was not set that way. Brush it only in the direction in which it was set. Do not brush a long time because the hair may become too straight.

7. Brush the hair in the direction in which it was set. Begin at the open end of each wave and work toward the closed end.

8. Discuss the results of the combing with your instructor.

8. By checking with your instructor, you will be able to avoid repeating errors that you have made.

Set and comb sculpture curls in both side sections for a large semicircular formation.

Procedure

1. Prepare mannequin as described in the previous exercise.
2. Part off and secure the top section, then proceed to set the side sections according to the patterns in Figures 9.35 to 9.43.
3. Follow the usual procedure to dry the hair.
4. After you have removed the clips, comb through both side sections of the hair, following the design of the shapings.
5. Compare your combed-out design to the one in Figure 9.44.

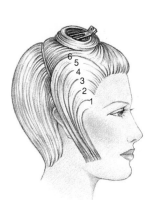

Figure 9.35
Part off the hair

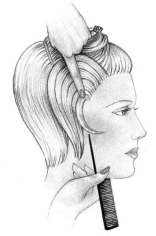

Figure 9.36
Begin setting at the open end.

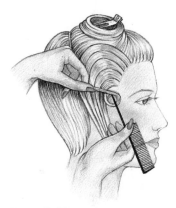

Figure 9.37
Set the first curl as a no-stem curl.

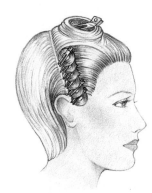

Figure 9.38
Complete curls.

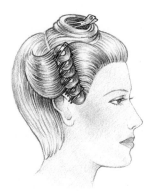

Figure 9.39
A diagonal column of c.c.w. curls

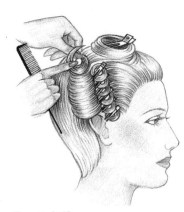

Figure 9.40
The end of each curl must be on the inside of the curl.

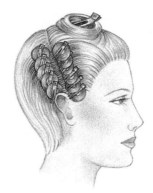

Figure 9.41
Completed rows of alternating c.c.w. and c.w. sculpture curls

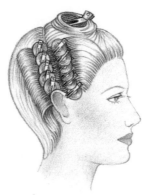

Figure 9.42
Always comb the shaping into the hair before setting the row of sculpture curls.

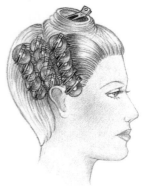

Figure 9.43
Completed pattern of diagonal sculpture curls

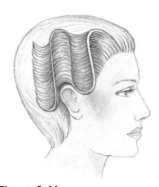

Figure 9.44
The comb-out

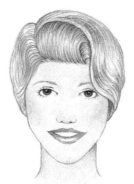

Figure 9.45
The shaping pattern is combed into the top front section before setting in sculpture curls.

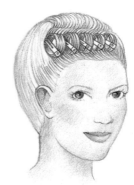

Figure 9.46
Setting pattern for first row of c.w. sculpture curls. Begin setting at point A.

Set the top sections in sculpture curls.

1. Follow the instructions in Figures 9.45 to 9.47.
2. Compare your combed-out design to the one in Figure 9.48.

Set the whole head in sculpture curls.

(At this point you should have mastered the techniques necessary for setting an entire head in sculpture curls. If you have any questions, look at the illustrations, review the previous objectives, and ask your instructor for help.)

■ Begin by making a part from the center of the eyebrow to the crown (Figure 9.49).

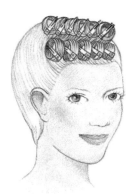

Figure 9.47
Alternating pattern of c.w. and c.c.w. sculpture curls

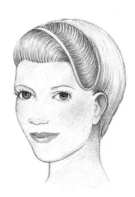

Figure 9.48
Finished wave pattern in top front section

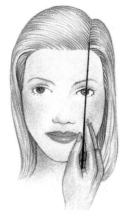

Figure 9.49
Make a part from the center of the eyebrow to the crown.

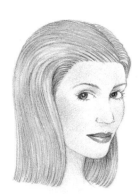

Figure 9.50
Comb hair away from part.

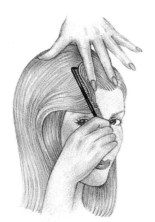

Figure 9.51
Shift comb forward to enable first shaping.

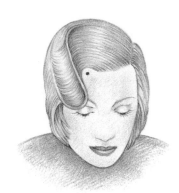

Figure 9.52
Start making curls at the bullet (●).

- Comb hair away from the part at a 45-degree angle (Figure 9.50). Shift hair to form a "(" shaping toward the face (Figure 9.51).
- Complete the shaping. The pickup point for forming half-stem curls is in the middle of the shaping. Start making curls at the open end of the shaping (the bullet [●] in Figure 9.52 shows where to start). Clip the curl across the base and finish making curls in this shaping (Figures 9.53 to 9.58).
- Comb the hair away from the face at a 45-degree angle (Figure 9.59). Begin your shaping by shifting the hair toward the face (Figure 9.60). Working from the left side of the head (Figure

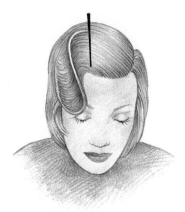

Figure 9.53
Slice curls one at a time from the imaginary line extending along the center of the "(" shaping.

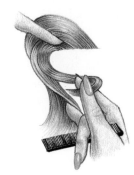

Figure 9.54
While making the curl, hold the base of the shaping in place with one finger.

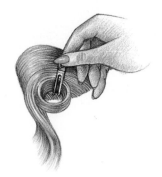

Figure 9.55
Secure with a clip.

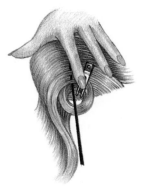

Figure 9.56
Make the second curl.

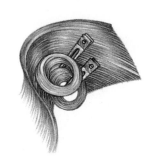

Figure 9.57
Clip may be inserted through the hair on one side of the curl.

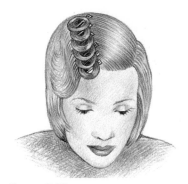

Figure 9.58
Completed row of sculpture curls.

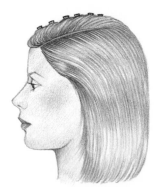

Figure 9.59
Continue shaping from left side, and across crown section to other side.

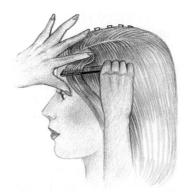

Figure 9.60
Angle, then shift comb forward to make next shaping.

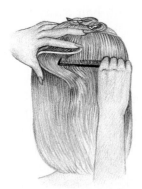

Figure 9.61
Completed shaping from left side.

9.61), continue your shaping all the way around the head (Figures 9.62 and 9.63).

■ Set the curls into the shaping around the head (Figures 9.64 to 9.67). Your last curl will be placed on the right side of the head.

■ Working from the right side of the head, comb your next shaping into the hair. The bottom of the shaping should be directed toward the face (Figure 9.68). The last two rows should be set in the same direction (Figures 9.69 to 9.73).

■ Thoroughly dry the hair, remove the clips, brush the hair straight back to relax it, and blend the curls from one section to the next. Comb out the hairstyle by following the pattern set with your curls (Figure 9.74).

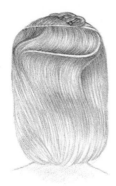

Figure 9.62
Continue shaping across crown of head.

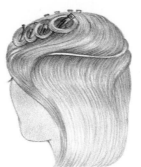

Figure 9.63
Complete shaping to front hairline. Remember to shift comb toward left.

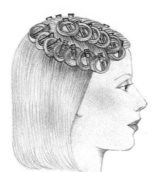

Figure 9.64
Set curls within shaping.

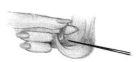

Figure 9.65
Catch end of curl with thumb and index fingers.

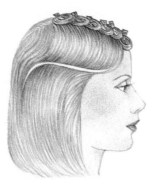

Figure 9.66
Work from left side toward right side of crown.

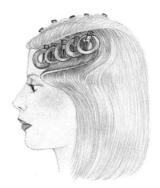

Figure 9.67
Rows of curls should be close together.

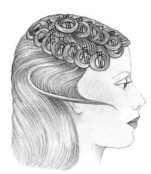

Figure 9.68
Now begin from right side section.

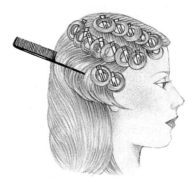

Figure 9.69
Finish this row at left side section.

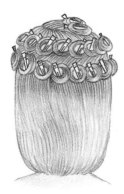

Figure 9.70
Continue setting curls across crown.

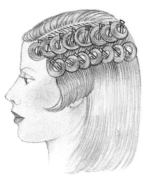

Figure 9.71
Completed curls.

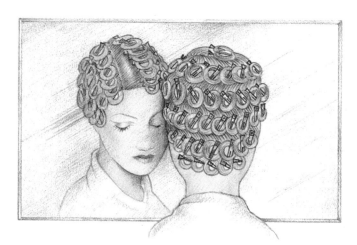

Figure 9.72
Completed set.

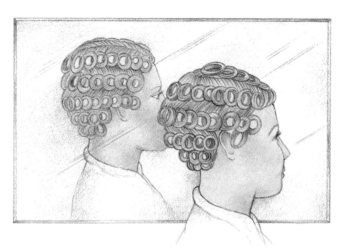

Figure 9.73
Dried set. Appearance after clips have been removed.

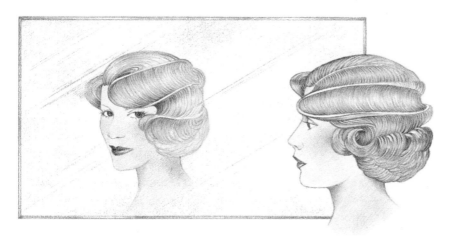

Figure 9.74
The comb-out

Set a skip (shadow) wave in the left side section of the head.

Comb a vertical shaping into the hair (Figure 9.75). Begin setting at the bullet (●) in Figure 9.75 and proceed as in Figures 9.76 to 9.78. Note the direction of the alternating wave formation in the comb-out in Figure 9.79.

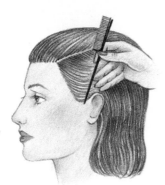

Figure 9.75
Comb hair away from the hairline as shown.

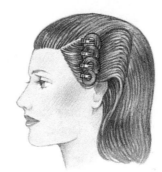

Figure 9.76
Start setting curls from open end (top) of shaping.

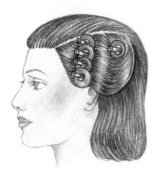

Figure 9.77
Note that the second wave shaping is not set.

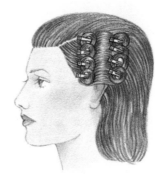

Figure 9.78
Set curls from top of third shaping.

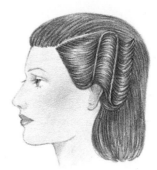

Figure 9.79
The comb-out

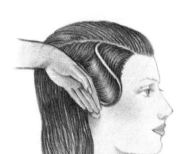

Figure 9.80
Comb a diagonal shaping into the hair.

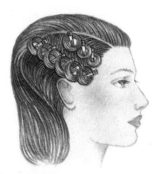

Figure 9.81
Set c.c.w. curls into the upper shaping first. Then set c.w. curls into the lower one.

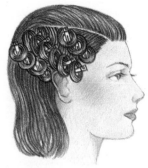

Figure 9.82
Finish with a third row of c.c.w. curls.

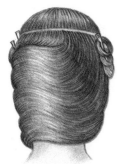

Figure 9.83
Comb the diagonal shaping.

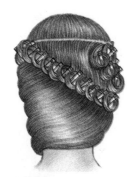

Figure 9.84
Begin setting c.w. curls from the top of the crown.

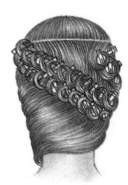

Figure 9.85
The second row is also c.w. curls.

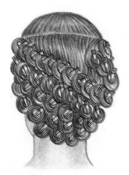

Figure 9.86
The remaining hair should be set in c.c.w. curls from your shaping.

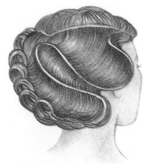

Figure 9.87
The comb-out for a diagonal side wave

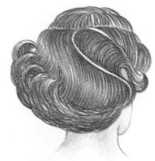

Figure 9.88
The comb-out for a diagonal back wave

Set a diagonal wave in the right side section of the head.

Follow the illustrations in Figures 9.80 to 9.82.

Set a diagonal wave in the back section of the head.

■ Comb the diagonal shaping from the crown to behind the right ear (Figure 9.83).

■ Begin setting at the (●) bullet in Figure 9.84. Proceed as in Figures 9.85 and 9.86.

■ Comb out the diagonal side wave and diagonal back brush wave (Figures 9.87 and 9.88).

Sanitize your area as follows:

1. Wash, wipe, and store bottles and supplies.
2. Discard used supplies.
3. Clean and sanitize the cape and apron.
4. Sanitize the work area; wash your hands.

Glossary

Barrel curls Large stand-away curls. See also **Cascade curls.**

Base direction The direction the hair takes when it leaves the scalp to form a semicircle.

Cascade curls Large stand-away curls. See also **Barrel curls.**

Circle end The round formation (part) of a sculpture circle that determines the curl's tightness; also called the circle.

Half-stem curl Halfway between a no-stem and a long-stem curl in mobility and tightness.

Long-stem (full-stem) curl The loosest kind of curl; it has the greatest mobility.

Mobility How tight or firm a curl will be.

No-stem curl The tightest kind of curl; it has the least mobility.

Pickup line Where the curl is carved out of the shaping.

Pin curl See **Shaping.**

Rake comb A comb used to apply chemical relaxers and to remove tangles from the hair.

Rat-tail comb A comb often used for carving sculpture curls, dividing hair into sections, and applying chemical relaxers.

Shaping The design combed into the hair for sculpture curls or pin curls.

Skip-waving pattern Alternating combinations of unset hair shapings and sculpture curls.

Stand-away curls Sculpture curls that are clipped in a standing position to form a movement away from the head.

Stand-up curls See **Stand-away curls.**

Stem The part of the curl that determines whether the direction of the curl will be horizontal, vertical, or diagonal.

Styling comb An all-purpose comb.

Wave pattern Alternating rows of clockwise and counterclockwise sculpture curls.

Questions

1. Name the three basic types of sculpture curls.
2. In your own words, write a definition for the open end of a shaping.
3. Using your own words, define the closed end of a shaping.
4. What is a "pickup point"?
5. What type of curl bases should be used around the front hairline to avoid splits?
6. What is the strongest type of sculpture curl?
7. What type of sculpture curl has the least strength?
8. If your sculpture curl set is too tight, how can you relax it?
9. If you try to brush the set and discover some wet sculpture curls, what will happen?
10. What will happen if too much setting lotion is used to set the hair?
11. During the setting process, where should the ends of each curl be set?

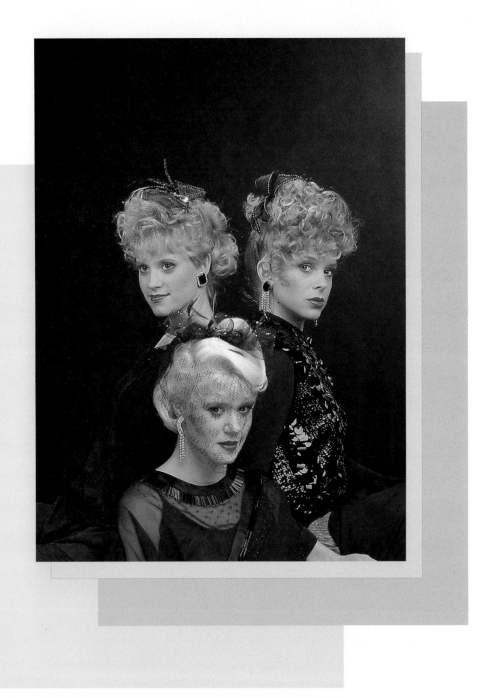

Setting the Hair with Rollers

Use the proper roller-placement principles to set all the mannequin's or client's hair in rollers and comb the style into place. Set the hair in rollers in 15 to 25 minutes and (after it is dried) comb it into place in 20 to 30 minutes. Score 85 percent or better on a multiple-choice exam on the material in this unit.

In order to achieve the above level of competence, you should master the following chapter objectives.

Theory Objectives

1. Explain the basic materials from which rollers are made and describe their shapes and sizes.
2. Describe the basic principles used to select the correct roller diameter for the hair's length and define inside and outside movements of hair.
3. Explain the purpose of no-stem, half-stem, and long-stem roller placements.

Practical Objectives

4. Set and comb roller curls in four different patterns in the top section of the head.
5. Set and comb roller curls in three different patterns in the top, sides, crown, and nape sections of the head.

Introduction

Do you have a hobby? Perhaps like many people, you enjoy working in your garden and may even have a "green thumb." But could you run a 2,000-acre farm? Managing a farm—for a living—is a long way from raising some tomatoes and beans in your backyard.

The difference is simple. You are an amateur, not a professional farmer. A professional knows and uses all the "tricks of the trade" to perform quickly, efficiently, and productively.

The same thing is true for cosmetologists. Many people could set hair if they had to (though not as many people as think they could—in recent years cosmetologists have seen more and more cases of hair damage caused by the improper use of home-care products). But they would have to work very slowly, and they would not know what to expect when they combed out the set.

As a professional you will learn to set hair efficiently (quickly but precisely), and you will be able to predict the outcome of your work. One important skill in reaching that goal is the mastery of rollers. Rollers are basic implements that all cosmetologists use to design hairstyles.

Mastering the setting and combing principles involved in using rollers is useful for two reasons. You will be able to save time by using one roller instead of having to set several individual stand-away curls. You will also be able to set a wide (almost limitless) variety of designs and styles.

You will be tested on the material in this unit, but the real test will be when a client (maybe an "amateur" hairstylist) sees the results of your work and realizes, "You can only get professional results from a professional."

Theory Objective 1
Basic Materials, Shapes,
and Sizes of Rollers

Over the years, beauty schools and salons have used many different kinds of rollers. Today, professionals generally use two basic kinds of rollers—**plastic** and **nylon.** Rollers made of these materials are especially popular because they are **magnetic.** Wet hair will cling to them. Both have small ventilating holes on their surfaces that help the hair dry more quickly.

Although plastic and nylon rollers are similar in some ways, the differences between them are greater than you might think. **Plastic rollers** are heavier than nylon ones and have a tendency to warp with continued exposure to dryer heat. If they warp, you must throw them away. **Nylon rollers,** on the other hand, are much lighter than plastic rollers, but temporary and semipermanent rinses will stain them.

Plastic and nylon rollers come in two shapes: **cylindrical** and **conoid** (cone-shaped). Most plastic and nylon rollers are also made in various lengths and diameters (Figure 10.1). Short rollers are called **filler** or **direction rollers.**

The wire mesh/brush roller is basically a wire cylinder covered with mesh netting with a circular brush inserted into the hollow part of the roller's frame. For many years, nearly all cosmetologists used brush rollers. Finally, it was realized that brush rollers quickly become unsanitary with salon use and need to be sanitized every day. Thoroughly sanitizing them daily is not practical, however. There also was evidence that the tips of brush bristles can puncture and damage the hair as the strand dries (contracts).

Back-combing and Back-brushing

Back-combing and **back-brushing** refer to the process of packing (pushing) the shorter (close to the scalp) hairs within the hair strand toward the scalp to give the hair volume.

After the hair has been dried and thoroughly brushed, a ¾-inch (1.88-centimeter) strand is sectioned off for back-combing. The hair is usually back-combed in the same order that it was set. Begin with the hair that was set first, and work your way toward the crown of the head. The hair strand should be held between the middle and index fingers; then the thumb is pressed against the index finger to prevent the strand from sliding through your fingers.

To avoid pulling the hair and causing the client discomfort, release the pressure from your thumb immediately after pushing the shorter hairs toward the scalp. Use a styling comb and back-comb the hair with the fine, closely spaced teeth of the comb. The hair is then surface cleaned using the wide teeth of the comb to smooth the hair-

Figure 10.1
Standard roller sizes

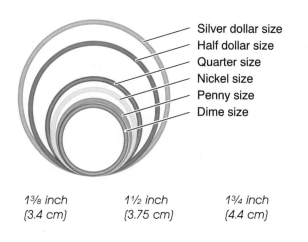

Silver dollar size
Half dollar size
Quarter size
Nickel size
Penny size
Dime size

1⅜ inch	1½ inch	1¾ inch
(3.4 cm)	(3.75 cm)	(4.4 cm)

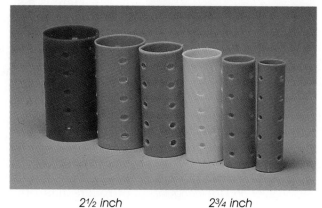

2½ inch	2¾ inch
(6.25 cm)	(6.9 cm)

style. Clients sometimes refer to **back-combing** as **ratting** or **matting,** but professionals prefer the terms **back-combing** or **French lacing.**

Back-combing can also be done using a brush; then it is called **back-brushing.** It is done the same way as back-combing except that the inside of the brush is used for **"ruffing"** the cuticle layer of the hair. Cushion-type, round brushes are the most popular for this technique.

Theory Objective 2

Basic Principles Used to Select Roller Diameters That Are Correct for the Hair's Length and Inside and Outside Movements of Hair

At this point you should have mastered the principles that apply to setting sculpture curls. Once you have learned those principles, you are well on your way to mastering the principles used for setting with rollers. These principles can be summarized as follows:

1. The hair must be **shaped.**

2. The shapings must be **parallel to each other,** and the hair must be combed and wound smoothly on the rollers.

3. Rollers are **set** into a shaping **from the open end** toward the closed end.

4. All the hair placed on a roller should form **all or part of a perfect circle.**

5. Rollers are set in **no-stem, half-stem,** and **long-stem** placements.

6. Probably the most important principle is that the hair should be wound 1½ to 2 turns around the roller (depending on the desired effect and hair texture).

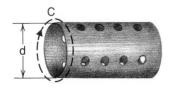

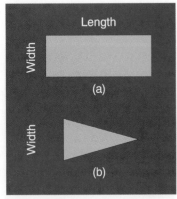

Figure 10.2

"C" indicates the roller circumference, and "d" indicates the diameter.

Figure 10.3

Subsections of a hair strand: (a) rectangular and (b) triangular.

This last principle deserves more explanation. The number of turns needed will tell you what diameter of roller to select (Figure 10.2). Roller diameters vary from about ½ to 1½ inches (1.25 to 3.75 centimeters).

Here is a simple problem to work out. If the hair strand is 6 inches (15 centimeters) long, what roller diameter should you use (Figure 10.3)?

You can use a combination of common sense and trial and error to arrive at the answer. You know that a large (1- to 1½-inch [2.5- to 3.75-centimeter] diameter) roller could **not** be used to set a strand of hair that is 1 inch (2.5 centimeters) long because the distance around the roller is 4½ inches (11.25 centimeters). A simple rule of thumb to remember is that the **shorter** the hair is, the **smaller** the roller diameter must be for the ideal wrapping of 1½ turns.

All of this figuring and choosing among types and sizes of rollers has one basic purpose: to make a wave in the client's

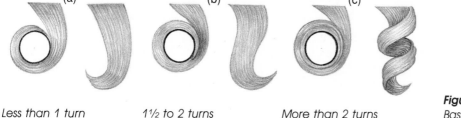

(a)	(b)	(c)
Less than 1 turn	1½ to 2 turns	More than 2 turns
Curved	Soft wave	Curly

Figure 10.4
Basic wave formations

hair. You will use rollers to produce three basic wave formations (Figure 10.4).

Although the number of styles and designs is almost limitless, all of them are made up of two basic kinds of roller movements. A pattern that gives height and volume, bringing hair away from the head, is called an **outside movement** (Figure 10.5a). A pattern that brings hair close to the head is called an **inside** or **indentation movement** (Figure 10.5b).

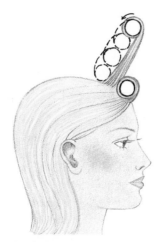

(a) Outside movement

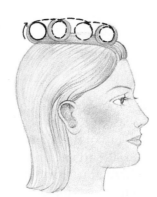

(b) Inside or indentation movement

Figure 10.5
Basic roller movements

Theory Objective 3
Purpose of No-Stem, Half-Stem, and Long-Stem Roller Placements

The **strength** of the curl produced by the roller depends on whether the roller is set in a **no-stem, half-stem,** or **long-stem** placement. You should remember these terms from the discussion of sculpture curls in Chapter 9. The direction that the hair strand is combed and held before the roller is placed decides where the base for the roller will be (Figure 10.6).

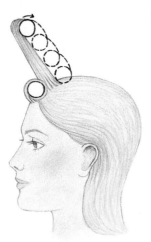

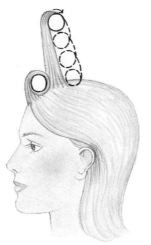

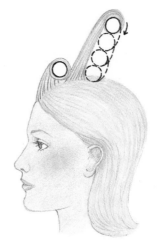

(a) No-stem; maximum height and fullness

(b) Half-stem; half as strong as no-stem

(c) Long-stem; the weakest stem

Figure 10.6
Basic roller placement

The three roller placements can be described as follows:

1. Directly on the base of the strand for a **no-stem** type (Figure 10.6a).
2. Half on and half off the base of the strand for a **half-stem** type (Figure 10.6b).
3. All the way off and usually below the base of the strand for a **long-stem** type (Figure 10.6c).

The size of the section of hair to be wound around a roller also affects the strength of the curl. The section of hair to be wound should **not** be wider than the diameter of the roller. The hair should not cover more than **80 percent** of the **length** of the roller (Figure 10.7).

When you want hair that is 6 inches (15 centimeters) or shorter to make an inside (indentation) movement, the width of the section should be larger than the diameter of the roller, and the strand should be located entirely above the subsection (Figure 10.8).

Figure 10.7
Roller length

Correct length of roller section

Incorrect length of roller section

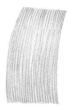

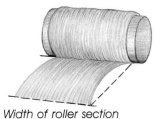

Diameter of subsection and roller

Width of roller section

Figure 10.8
Width of the hair section and diameter of the roller

The width of the subsection should be **50 percent** larger than the **diameter** of the roller.

Practical Objective 4
Roller Curls in Four Different Patterns in the Top Section of the Head

Supplies

- shampoo supplies
- roller rack (Figure 10.9)
- roller pins
- double-prong clips
- mannequin and clamp
- setting lotion
- spray applicator bottle for water
- rat-tail comb
- styling comb
- cushion brush
- neck strips
- protective comb-out cape
- hair spray

Top-setting Pattern 1: Half-bang

Procedure

1. Prepare mannequin for setting. Wet the hair. Apply setting lotion to hair and comb it through the hair.

2. Comb all hair straight back and flat against the head. Keep the hair wet at all times with water, not setting lotion.

3. Comb the hair at the hairline in the top

Rationale

1. Apply setting lotion (could be a gel or mousse) to wet hair because the water helps to distribute it onto the cuticle of the hair. Always spray or apply the lotion carefully.

2. This breaks the hydrogen cross-bonds in the hair. It also stretches the hair so it will be easier to set on magnetic rollers and will dry to a longer-lasting hairstyle.

3. Always follow any **natural wave** or **cowlick** (hair that

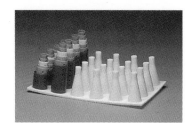

Figure 10.9
Roller rack

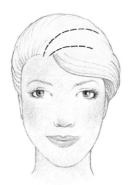

Figure 10.10
Diagonal "working" part

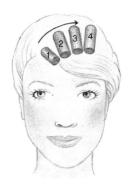

Figure 10.11
Placement of rollers 1 through 4

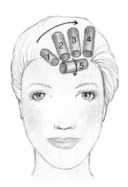

Figure 10.12
Placement of rollers 1 through 5 for the half-bang set

according to the natural growth. Comb the hair in a half-bang design.

4. Part off the hair that will be set first (Figure 10.10).

5. Set the first strand of hair on a filler (short) roller to produce a no-stem curl.

6. Rollers 2, 3, and 4* should be set in triangular sections of hair on long cylinder rollers (Figures 10.11 and 10.12).

7. Standing behind the head, part across each strand. Catch the strand between the middle and index fingers of your left hand. Recomb the hairs of the strand next to the scalp and through the ends until the strand is smooth. Keep the strand tense by holding it tightly with your left hand. Lay the strand **evenly** across the

stands upward, usually in a circular pattern) whenever possible. Doing so will make the hairstyle last much longer.

4. This is the best way to begin setting rollers. Parting the hair makes the panel of hair easier to set.

5. Since other rollers will be set toward the crown and right side of the head, a split in the style may occur if a long roller is placed right on the hairline. Most rollers (but not all, depending on the hairstyle) in the top section are set on their bases (no-stem) because this results in maximum height or volume (fullness) and durability when the hair is combed into place.

6. The panel of hair to be set is curved to conform to the contour of the head. To follow the curved part, you must use triangular sections of hair.

7. This is the easiest way to set the hair. You must comb the hair smooth to stretch the strand so that it is easy to place on the roller. Clip the strand where the roller meets the head to maintain the tension you placed on it as you wound it. As the hair dries and contracts, the hydrogen cross-bonds re-form around the roller.

***Roller** and **curl** will be used interchangeably in the context of **roller number** in the pattern.

roller and begin to turn the roller toward the head. Keep the strand tense until you have secured the hair. Place the clip where the roller meets the head (Figure 10.13).

The degree to which this takes place depends on the amount of tension you put on the strand of hair as you wind it around the roller toward the scalp. **The tension affects the degree of curliness.**

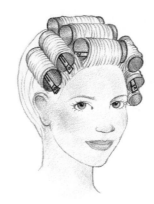

Figure 10.13
In any roller setting pattern, the clip is inserted where the roller touches the head. Generally, only one end of the roller needs to be clipped.

8. Place one double- or single-prong clip in the roller. (Figure 10.14).

8. Rollers may be clipped into place with single- or double-spring clips or roller clips or pins. Roller clips or pins are usually more expensive than single- or double-prong clips, but the use of any of these items is correct.

9. Pick up the roller with your right hand and place it beneath the middle finger of your left hand, which is holding the strand. Slide the strand between the middle and index fingers of your left hand while pushing the roller with your right hand. Spread the hair evenly across the roller. Hold the comb in the palm of your hand **at all times** (Figure 10.15). Use a rolling action to lay the hair across the roller. Using the thumb and fingertips of your hand, place the strand neatly on the roller.

9. This motion makes the hair cling to the magnetic rollers. The strand is spread across the roller so that it will dry evenly in a circular form. If you place the comb on the styling station, you will waste a lot of time reaching back and forth as you set the rollers. With practice, it becomes easy to set the hair while holding the comb throughout the procedure.

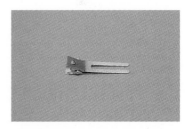

Figure 10.14
Roller clip and pin

Figure 10.15
Holding the comb

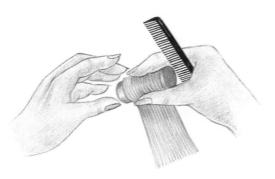

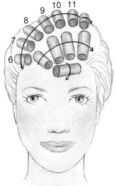

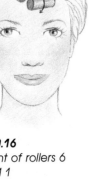

Figure 10.16
Placement of rollers 6
through 11

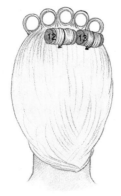

Figure 10.17
Placement of rollers 12 and 13

10. Set roller 5 half-stem or no-stem.

11. Shape the hair behind the first panel of hair from the left to the right (Figure 10.16). Set rollers 6 through 11 in triangular-shaped strands of hair and on the **next-to-largest-size** rollers. Use a filler roller for curl 6.

12. Set rollers 12 and 13 (Figure 10.17). Ask your instructor for an evaluation and drying instructions after you have set the rollers on the top of the head.

13. If you are working on a classmate or client, position

10. Since this hair will be combed down onto the forehead, you might want to use a half-stem roller. Do not use a long-stem placement because it may cause a split between the panel of hair on rollers 1 through 4 and the hair on roller 5.

11. Always comb the design into the hair before you set the rollers. This procedure will give a more defined, natural movement of hair. To give the hair dimension and form, the rollers in the top section that are **not** on the hairline are larger (by one size) than those used right on the hairline. This is done because the hair is longer toward the crown than around the hairline. You should seldom vary from this rule of thumb: as the hair becomes shorter, select the next smallest roller diameter. Do not vary the diameter of rollers more than two or three sizes from one section of the head to the next.

12. It is easier to see and correct setting errors **before** you have dried the hair. It is also easier to learn to relax, back-comb, back-brush (or tease), and control the style of the hair when only one section is used.

13. Since the same comb-out cape may be used by

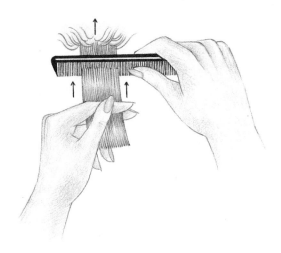

Figure 10.18
Back-combing the hair

the neck strip and comb-out cape.

14. Comb the hair through; then brush as needed to unfold and relax the setting pattern.

15. Back-comb the hair by panels in the same order they were set (Figure 10.18).

16. Repeat the back-combing until all panels are lightly packed.

17. Using your left hand, very carefully guide the hair into place. Hold the comb in your right hand. Clean up the back-combing with the wide teeth of the styling comb.

18. After your instructor has evaluated the comb-out of the top section, brush all back-combing from it.

everyone, a neck strip must be placed between the neck and the cape.

14. Combing and brushing relax and unfold the pattern. The more the hair is brushed, the more it relaxes.

15. This is the easiest place to begin. Back-combing supports the height of the style and also further relaxes the hair to blend roller sections.

16. This supports the hairstyle.

17. This procedure arranges the hair and removes visible back-combing from the surface of the hairstyle.

18. It is important to spot-check so that you can catch any errors as soon as possible.

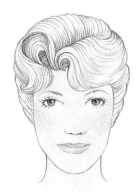

Figure 10.19
Half-bang comb-out

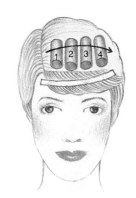

Figure 10.20
Full-bang set

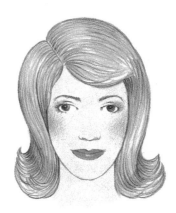

Figure 10.21
Comb-out for setting pattern 2

Top-setting Pattern 2

Procedure

1. Comb a few curls onto the forehead from the hairline. Use long cylinder rollers in half-stem placements in the front top section along the hairline. Use hair-setting tape on bang hairs (Figure 10.20).

2. Set the entire head if the hair is long enough for this style (Figure 10.21). Use long cylinder rollers in half-stem placements for curls 5 and 6 (Figure 10.22). Use a long cylinder roller in the no-stem position for curl 7.

3. Set rollers 8, 9, and 10 as in step 2.

4. Set curls 11 through 15 with long cylinder rollers in half-stem placements. Drape the center crown hair onto filler rollers that are turned upward. Use rollers that have progressively smaller diameters as you move down toward the nape hairline (Figure 10.23).

Rationale

1. Since very little back-combing will be needed because the hairstyle is not extremely bouffant (high) in the top section, long cylinder rollers set half-stem will produce the desired effect. Tape will keep bang hairs in place under the dryer.

2. Hair that is long enough for this set will be difficult to comb if only the top section is set. In this situation, it may be easier to set all the hair. Follow the directions of your instructor.

3. Same as step 2.

4. If the filler rollers are turned upward, the hair will flip upward. Draping the hair in the center crown brings the movement of the hair close to the head, which is the way you want the hair to move.

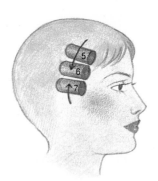

Figure 10.22
Set for flipping ends of hair

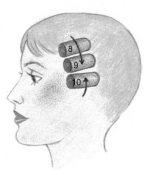

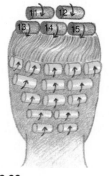

Figure 10.23
"Brick-laying pattern" to avoid splits

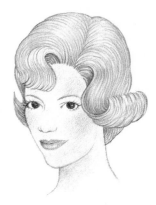 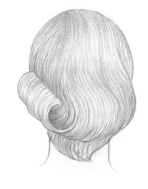

Figure 10.24
Comb-out for setting pattern 3

5. Comb through or brush the hair if necessary. The hair should be back-brushed slightly. If you have any problems, ask your instructor for help.

5. This unfolds and relaxes the pattern set into the hairstyle. Back-brushing will make the hair easier to control.

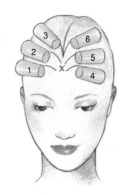

Top-setting Pattern 3

Procedure

1. Comb the design into the top section of the hair (Figure 10.24).

Rationale

1. This is standard procedure.

Figure 10.25
Pivotal half-bang set using conoid rollers

2. Note the pivot point marked ''X'' in Figure 10.25. Set long cylinder rollers or filler rollers as indicated in the figure. Use long-stem roller placements for rollers 1, 2, 3, 4, and 5. Set the rest of the top in half-stem roller placements (Figure 10.26).

2. The pivot point is a central point around which the hair movement flows. Long-stem roller placements are used because the hair will be combed close to, but **not** flat against, the head. Half-stem placements are used to complete the set in the top section because only medium, rather than maximum, height is desired.

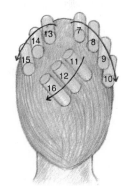

3. Set the crown, side, and nape sections if your instructor tell you to.

3. Your instructor may want you to set the entire head. If so, your instructor will give you additional directions.

Figure 10.26
Placement of rollers 7 through 16

4. Dry the hair after your instructor has evaluated the set.

4. It is easier to correct errors before the hair dries.

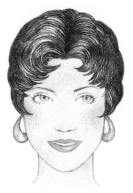

Figure 10.27
Classical Italian top comb-out

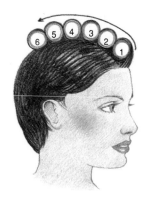

Figure 10.28
Italian top set

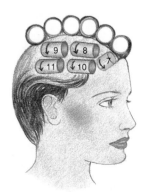

Figure 10.29
Italian top-setting pattern

5. Remove rollers and clips when the hair is thoroughly dry. Back-comb or back-brush as described in the setting pattern.

Top-setting Pattern 4

Procedure

1. Use rollers in no-stem placements for curls 1 through 6 (Figure 10.28).

2. Use a filler roller in a no-stem placement for curl 7. Set long cylinder rollers no-stem for curls 8 through 11 (Figure 10.29).

3. Use a filler-size roller to set roller 12 in a no-stem placement (Figure 10.30). Use long cylinder rollers to set curls 13 through 16 in

5. Back-combing and back-brushing techniques are the same, regardless of the top-setting pattern. The only thing that changes is the arrangement of the hair.

Rationale

1. Filler rollers in no-stem placements give maximum height and mobility to hair. It may be easier to comb the hair in different directions if you use filler (short) rollers rather than long rollers. In this set, it is easier to comb hair around either side of the forehead on the hairline.

2. A filler-size no-stem is used for roller 7 so there will not be a split between roller 1 and roller 7. Setting roller 7 (filler) at a slight angle, rather than using a long roller, will make it easier to comb the hair onto the forehead. Curls 8 through 11 are set no-stem with long cylinder rollers so there will not be a split in the style. The direction of the style changes between the rollers set away from the hairline (1–6) and the rollers set downward (8–11). If you did not use long cylinder rollers in a no-stem placement, the style could split.

3. Same as step 2. Do not count rollers because the head size of the mannequin and the length of the hair may change the actual

no-stem placements. (Do not count rollers exactly.)

number of rollers used. Just use roller numbers as a **guide.** The direction the hair will be combed and the stem direction of the rollers are important things you should remember.

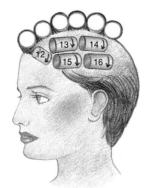

4. Unfold the setting pattern and comb or brush as necessary.

4. This is standard procedure.

5. Arrange the hair in the top section according to the style shown in Figure 10.27.

5. Unless the hair is extremely long or short, the top section should look like the illustration in Figure 10.27.

Figure 10.30
Side-wave setting pattern

Setting Pattern 1

Procedure

1. Set rollers 1 through 12 according to the pattern described in objective 4 (Figure 10.31).

2. Clip hair strands for rollers 14, 15, and 16 out of the way. These will be set on no-stem filler rollers; set curl 13 on a long cylinder roller in a no-stem placement. Use filler rollers with **larger** diameters when you set curls 14, 15, and 16 (Figure 10.32).

3. Repeat this procedure on the left side of the head.

4. Use long cylinder rollers at a slight angle in half-stem placements throughout the upper crown section.

Rationale

1. This is standard procedure (see Figure 10.31).

2. Roller 13 is set no-stem so that it will blend easily with the roller fillers above it. You should use rollers with larger diameters because hair lengths are longer toward the back of the head. Filler rollers are used for better hair control. The better the setting design is, the less back-combing or back-brushing will be needed.

3. By duplicating the set, the style will be **symmetrical** (the same on both sides).

4. Setting the hair this way creates the inside movement of the hair between rollers 10 and 11; the result will be

Practical Objective 5
Setting Three Different Patterns in the Top, Sides, Crown, and Nape Sections of the Head

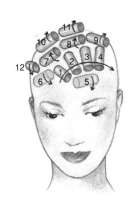

Figure 10.31
Placement of rollers 1 through 12

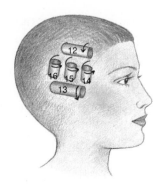
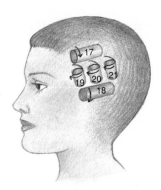

Figure 10.32
Side-wave setting pattern

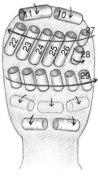

Figure 10.33
Placement of rollers 10 through 29.

a wave pattern. Hair from the top half of the roller will unfold in a c.w. direction, while hair from the lower half of the roller will unfold in a c.c.w. direction. The use of half-stem placements and the slight angle make the hair wave more easily.

5. Complete the set as shown in Figure 10.33. Dry your set, then comb out the hairstyle; it should look like the illustrations in Figures 10.34 and 10.35.

5. This is standard procedure.

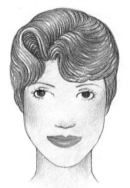

Figure 10.34
Comb-out for setting pattern 1 (front)

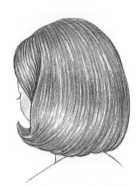

Figure 10.35
Comb-out for setting pattern 1 (back)

Setting Pattern 2

Follow the instructions in Figures 10.37 to 10.40. The finished hairstyle should look like the illustration in Figure 10.36.

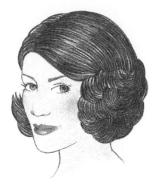

Figure 10.36
Comb-out for setting pattern 2

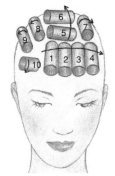

Figure 10.37
Set rollers in numerical order from 1 through 10

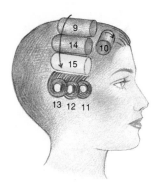

Figure 10.38
Clip hair to be set in rollers 14 and 15 to roller 9. Set c.c.w. sculpture curls 11 through 13. Place rollers 14 and 15.

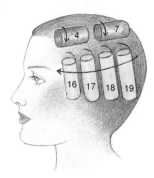

Figure 10.39
Complete setting pattern on the left side as shown.

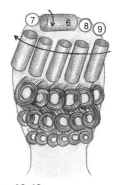

Figure 10.40
Beginning at the open end (tip of arrow) of the shaping, set c.w. rollers in the crown section. Complete the set with a row of c.c.w. sculpture curls; then finish nape section with two rows of c.w. curls.

Setting Pattern 3

Follow the instructions in Figures 10.42 to 10.44. The finished hairstyle should look like the illustration in Figure 10.41.

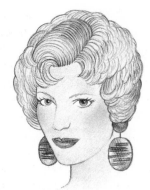

Figure 10.41
Comb-out for setting pattern 3

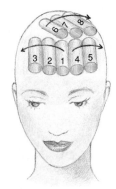

Figure 10.42
*Placement of rollers 1
through 8*

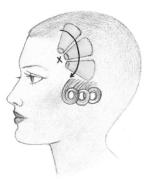

Figure 10.43
*Set conoid rollers and sculpture
curls as shown.*

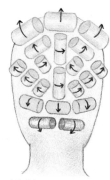

Figure 10.44
*Complete setting pattern on
the back as shown.*

Sanitize your area as follows:

1. Wash, wipe, and store bottles and supplies.
2. Discard used supplies.
3. Clean and sanitize the cape and apron.
4. Sanitize the work area; wash your hands.

Half-stem roller placement Placing the rollers half on and half off the base of the strand.

Inside movement (indentation) A hair pattern that brings hair close to the head.

Long-stem roller placement Placing the rollers all the way off and usually below the base of the hair strand.

Natural wave or cowlick Hair that stands upward, usually in a circular pattern.

No-stem roller placement Placing the rollers directly on the base of the hair strand.

Outside movement A hair pattern that gives height and volume, bringing hair away from the head.

1. What is a roller's circumference?
2. What is a roller's diameter?
3. How many turns must the hair be rolled to get soft waves?
4. To achieve a curly look, how many turns must the hair be rolled?
5. What determines the strength of the curl produced by the roller?
6. When setting with rollers, what determines the curliness of the hair?
7. Normally, the diameter of the subsection to be wound on a roller should be what size?
8. Where should the clip be placed to secure a roller?
9. Is tension on the hair important when winding the roller to the head?
10. Does back-combing give height to the hairstyle or bring the style close to the head?
11. Is an Italian top-setting pattern wound toward the face?

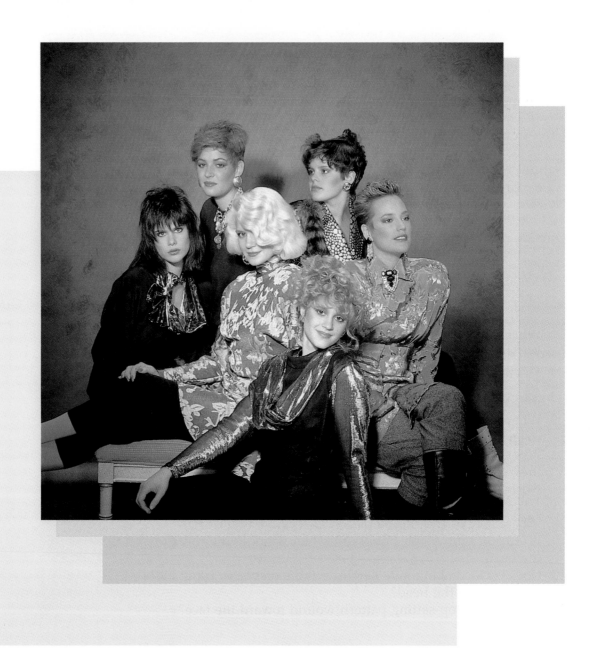

Selecting Hairstyles

Learning Objective

Correctly identify the facial shapes of six clients and recommend for each an appropriate hairstyle that demonstrates the principles presented in this unit. Using the information in this chapter, in addition to classroom instruction and practice, plan each hairstyle to create the illusion of an oval facial shape. Score 85 percent or better on a multiple-choice exam on the information in this chapter.

In order to achieve the above level of competence, you should master the following chapter objectives.

Theory Objectives

1. Identify the ideal facial and head features.
2. Describe the six facial shapes and identify ways an oval illusion can be created for them.
3. Describe the three common profiles.
4. Identify six other things to consider in hairstyling.
5. Give examples of hair braiding and corn rowing.

Introduction

Hairstyling involves arranging the hair to complement the features of a client's head, face, and body.

Have you ever bought something that you had to assemble yourself, but just when you had almost finished putting it together, you realized that a piece was missing? That missing piece was probably one little nut, or screw, or bolt—just one piece! But without that one little piece, your bicycle was just a jumble of metal parts, or your bookcase was little more than a pile of sticks. You had to have that piece.

Selecting a hairstyle is important in the same way. You may perform all of the necessary services perfectly. But when you stand back to look at the finished product, you realize that something is wrong: the style doesn't suit the client. If you know what to look for when selecting a style, it shouldn't take much time. Nevertheless, the selection process is very important because if your client does not like the hairstyle you choose, he or she probably will not have confidence in your ability and will not ask you to perform more expensive services.

In the past, cosmetologists did not learn these skills until they were on the job and already working in salons. Learning from experience may be the best way to improve your ability to select the proper hairstyle, but you can begin to develop these skills now.

Theory Objective 1
Ideal Facial and Head Features

It is easier to style the hair of a client who has an oval face. An oval face is considered the standard, and facial shapes that vary from the standard require more planning in the setting and combing stages.

First, a clear understanding of how to identify the standard oval is necessary. If you look at an oval face from the front, you will see that the three main divisions of the face are equal in size (Figure 11.1). In other words, the following three distances are the same:

1. Chin to the bottom of the nose.

2. Bottom of the nose to the top of the eyebrows.

3. Top of the eyebrows to the forehead (hairline).

A face that conforms to this description is easier to style because it does not have features that must be played down to improve the appearance of the client. A variety of hairstyles can be attractive on a client who has this type of face.

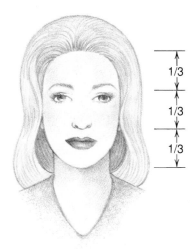

1/3

1/3

1/3

Figure 11.1
Proportions of the ideal facial type

In addition to facial shapes, you should be interested in the profile and silhouette of the hairstyle. The **profile** is the outline of the hair and head when viewed from the side. The **silhouette** (sil-eh-WET) is also an outline formed by the hair and head, but it may be viewed from any position, including the side.

When people look at someone's overall appearance, they will notice the hair first, then the eyes, and finally the clothes. A fashionable client will attempt to achieve a "total look."

1. Eyes are made up.

2. Hair is styled.

3. Clothes are coordinated.

Although the hairstyle is not everything, it is important. The most attractive and expensive clothes will not complement the client unless his or her hair has been styled attractively. (Eye makeup will be discussed later in the text.)

Theory Objective 2
Six Facial Shapes and Ways to Create the Oval Illusion for Them

There are six generally accepted facial shapes that differ from the ideal type: **diamond, heart, square, oblong, round,** and **pear.**

It is important to identify these problem facial shapes so that you will be able to create an optical illusion that will make the face appear oval (Figure 11.2). You must consider the facial shape in planning, setting, and arranging the final profile and silhouette.

■ **Problem 1** The **diamond-shaped face** is characterized by a narrow chin and forehead and wide cheekbones.

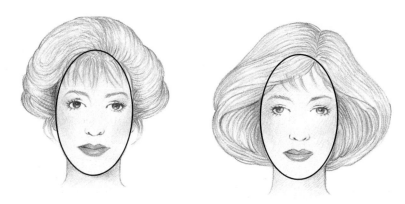

Figure 11.2
Oval-shaped face—the ideal

- **Solution** To achieve an attractive oval look, fullness or width is needed in the forehead hairline and the lower cheekbone areas of the face. Fullness is not needed in the area of the upper cheekbones. The hair should be styled close to the head in that area. The hair should be styled with a fringe or bang to disguise the narrow forehead and with fullness on the face around the jawbone to complete the oval illusion (Figure 11.3).

- **Problem 2** The **heart-shaped face** is characterized by a large, wide forehead (often with a widow's peak) and a narrow chin.

- **Solution** To remedy the heart shape, some hair is brought onto the forehead to reduce its width. A pageboy-type style is good for the lower sides of the face because the hair is close to the head at the eyes where narrowness is needed, but is slightly full around the jaw and below and in front of the earlobes where width is needed (Figure 11.4).

- **Problem 3** The **square-shaped face** is characterized by a wide hairline and jaw.

Figure 11.3
Diamond-shaped face

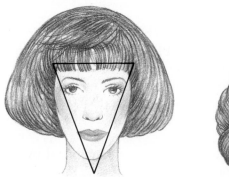
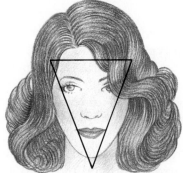

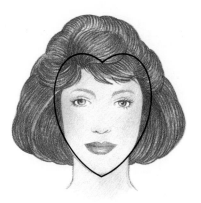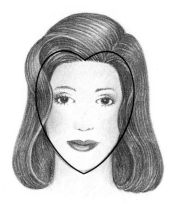

Figure 11.4
Heart-shaped face

■ **Solution**   An oval illusion can be created by bringing the hair forward and close to the face just below the cheekbones and by setting and combing the hair off the forehead (Figure 11.5). Combing the hair onto the sides of the face helps break the wide, straight lines of the square face, while combing the hair off the forehead adds the appearance of height.

■ **Problem 4   Oblong facial shapes** characteristically have a very long, narrow bone structure. A client who has an oblong face often also has a long, thin neck.

■ **Solution**   A fringe or half-bang across the forehead should be accompanied by soft waves or curls in the crown and nape areas (Figure 11.6). These curls flatter the face and neck by adding width and creating the oval illusion.

■ **Problem 5   Round facial shapes** are characterized by a wide hairline and fullness at and below the cheekbones. The contour moves from each cheekbone through the jawline and chin. The client may be overweight, and the neck may appear short.

Figure 11.5
Square-shaped face

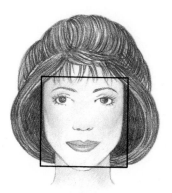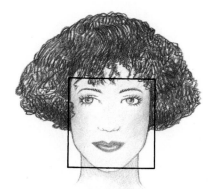

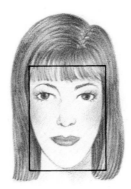
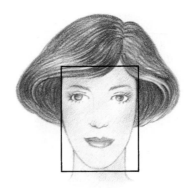

Figure 11.6
Oblong-shaped face

■ **Solution**   Setting and combing height in the top and crown sections tends to diminish some of the roundness (Figure 11.7). Setting and combing the hair close to the head on the side and nape sections also helps.

■ **Problem 6   Pear facial shapes** are characterized by a small or narrow forehead and a rather large pouchy-appearing jawline.

Figure 11.7
Round-shaped face

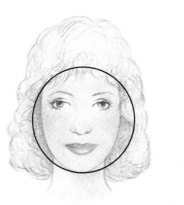
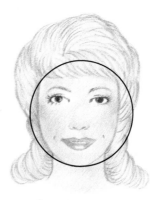

Figure 11.8
Pear-shaped face

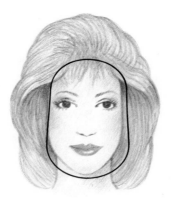
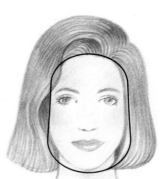

■ **Solution** Setting and combing the hair to add width from the eye level through the crown of the head is helpful (Figure 11.8). Hair in the side and nape sections should be set and combed close to the head.

There are three common profiles: **straight, concave,** and **convex.**

The straight profile is characteristic of the ideal facial shape — the oval. Viewed in profile, the nose is in proportion to the forehead and the area below the lower lip (Figure 11.9).

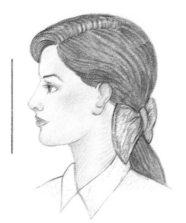

Figure 11.9
Straight profile

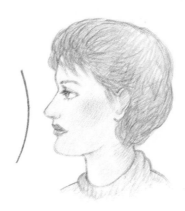

Figure 11.10
Concave profile

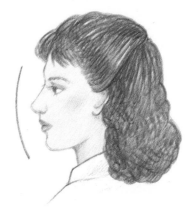

Figure 11.11
Convex profile

In the concave profile, the forehead and chin protrude, almost meeting a natural vertical line drawn perpendicular to the nose (Figure 11.10).

The convex profile is characterized by a prominent nose with the mouth and chin receding beyond the natural vertical line of the forehead (Figure 11.11).

Facial shapes and profiles are the most basic considerations you will take into account when you style the client's hair, but they are not the only things you should consider. Other factors are the client's distinctive physical characteristics, personal choices, and occupation; the occasion for which the hairstyle is requested; the client's personal eccentricities; and the color, texture, curliness, and shaping of the hair.

Physical imperfections, such as scars or large ears, may have to be camouflaged by arranging the hair to cover them.

Personal choices, such as the client's desire to have a half-bang on the right side of the forehead rather than the left, or no bang at all, must be considered.

The client's **occupation** often dictates the style chosen. Statistics indicate that more than 50 percent of all married women work outside the home. They usually consider weekly visits to the beauty school or salon a necessity rather than a luxury. The client's job also determines the type of hairstyle to some extent. Very long hair may be unacceptable in food service work. Hair, which is a collection point for germs, may fall into the food. Long hair may also create a hazard in a machine shop where it might get caught in a drill press or other equipment and cause an injury.

Professional hairstyling services are often requested for **special occasions,** such as weddings, anniversaries, graduations, birthdays, office parties, banquets, and holidays. A casual or formal style should be chosen according to the occasion.

Personal eccentricities (distinctive behaviors or ideas) of clients sometimes affect hairstyling. Occasionally, a client will insist on a hairstyle that you know is unbecoming. For example, the client may insist on a fringe or half-bang on the right side of the forehead when the natural growth direction indicates the half-bang should be on the left side. In such a case, once you have explained why the left side would be better, the bang should be set and combed on the right side! You should advise the client what is best, but then do as he or she requests.

The shaping, color, texture, and curliness of the hair also determine how it is styled. If the length is not correct for the style requested by the client, the hair should be shaped. If the hair is too short, the client should be advised to allow it to grow to the correct length. The hair shaping must also be correct for the desired hairstyle. If you are unsure of the relationship between the hairstyle and the hair shaping, ask your instructor for help.

Certain hairstyles also look better if in certain colors—in some cases lighter, in other cases darker.

Some hairstyles can be achieved on fine hair but not on coarser hair textures, and vice versa.

The curliness or straightness of the hair can also be important factors in selecting a hairstyle. Straight hairstyles are difficult to achieve on very curly hair unless it has been chemically relaxed. On the other hand, curly hairstyles are difficult to form on hair that has not been cold waved (chemically waved) or does not have natural curl.

Braided hairstyles are very popular, and you may be asked to create such styles. You can see an example of a three-strand braided hairstyle (Figure 11.12) and corn-rowing braiding technique (Figure 11.13). Some styles are especially suitable for black hair (Figure 11.14).

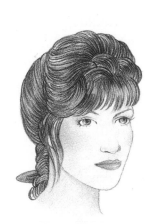

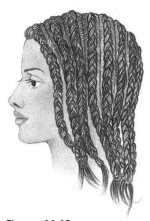

Figure 11.12
A three-strand braided hairstyle

Figure 11.13
A corn-rowing hairstyle

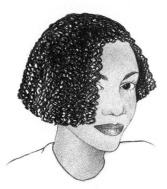

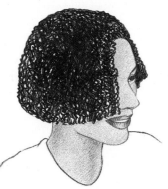

Figure 11.14
*An example of a hairstyle for
black women*

Glossary

Profile Outline of the head and hair as viewed from the side.
Silhouette (sil-eh-WET) Outline formed by the hair and head as viewed from any angle.

Questions

1. On a separate sheet of paper, sketch and label the six basic facial shapes. (Use a pencil.)
2. Write out the hairstyling solution for a diamond-shaped face.
3. Write out the hairstyling solution for a heart-shaped face.
4. Write out the hairstyling solution for an oblong face.
5. Is a heart-shaped face characterized by a large, wide forehead?
6. If the client has a heart-shaped face, should the hair be set and combed (styled) onto the forehead?
7. For a heart-shaped face, is it better to style some of the hair toward the face or away from the face?
8. Should the hair be styled away from a square-shaped face?
9. Does a concave profile protrude outward?
10. Does a convex profile slope inward?
11. Is one characteristic of a pear-shaped face a small, narrow forehead?
12. Does a person's occupation have anything to do with his or her hairstyle? If yes, write an explanation in your own words.

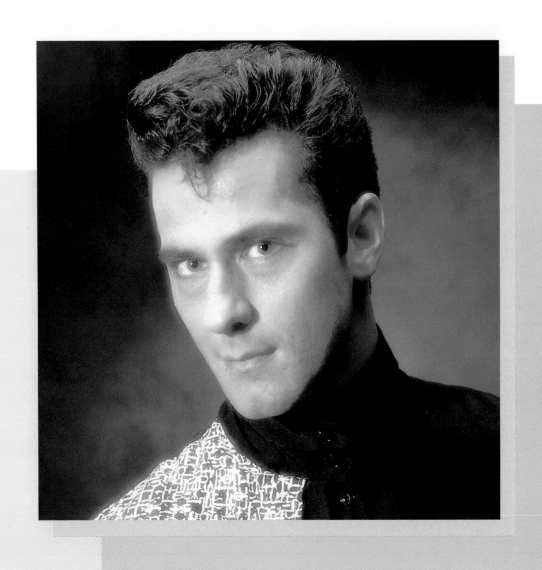

Hair Shaping

Learning Objective

Using hair-shaping implements and supplies, cut the client's hair for the hairstyle requested. Use the proper hair-shaping techniques and safety precautions to cut the client's hair in 15–25 minutes with a razor or 25–40 minutes with scissors (also called shears). You should also be able to perform some basic procedures with the electric clipper/trimmer/edger. Score 85 percent or better on a multiple-choice exam on the information in this chapter.

In order to achieve the above level of competence, you should master the following chapter objectives.

Theory Objectives

1. Describe hair-shaping implements and basic cutting movements.
2. Explain the differences between razor shaping, scissor shaping, and electric clipper shaping.
3. Locate the basic parting sections of the head.
4. Define the terms used in hair shaping and list the necessary safety precautions.

Practical Objectives

5. Give a basic scissor shaping for a female client.
6. Give a basic scissor shaping for a black female client.
7. Give a basic scissor shaping for a male client.
8. Give a basic clipper shaping for a female client.
9. Give a basic clipper shaping for a male client.
10. Give a basic razor shaping for a female client.
11. Trim a beard and a mustache.

Introduction

Hair shaping (hair cutting) is one of the most important services performed in the salon because it affects so many other services. For example, if the hair is not cut evenly from one subsection to the next, it will be very difficult to set on rollers. The same problem will occur when you try to wrap unevenly cut hair around permanent wave rods for chemical waving or curl reformation. Of course, you may have a real styling disaster if the hair has not been properly cut. In short, if the hair shaping is not done well none of your other hairstyling services will be successful.

Like other services a cosmetologist performs, hair shaping is a matter of doing many small tasks accurately rather than doing a few large tasks well. You must be able to shape the hair correctly to perform the other tasks within the program.

Since the whole family—mom, dad, and the children—comes into the salon now, it is important that you learn how to shape hair for men as well as women. The texture, condition, color, degree of curliness or straightness, and growth pattern of the hair will determine the overall appearance of your hair shaping.

Since most of the cutting implements you will be using have extremely **sharp edges** and almost **needlelike points, be careful not to cut, snip, or pierce the client's eyes or the skin around the ears, nose, or neck.** Public safety is an important part of your job. Be particularly cautious when giving a hair shaping to small children because they tend to move their heads without warning.

Theory Objective 1
Hair-Shaping
Implements and Basic
Cutting Movements

You should be able to identify and describe hair-cutting implements and their individual parts in much the same way an artist can explain why a certain brush is used for a particular purpose. The following are the basic implements you will use:

1. Probably the **double-edge scissors** is the implement most frequently used for shaping hair in the salon (Figure 12.1). Scissors come in a variety of sizes ranging from about 4 to 8 inches (10 to 20 centimeters) from the **finger tang** (a little finger brace) to the tip of the cutting edge (point). They are also made without a finger tang (Figure 12.2). The style of scissors you will use depends on the hair-cutting technique you will be performing.

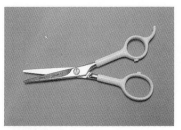

Figure 12.1
Double-edge scissors with finger tang

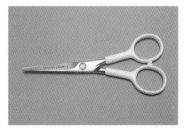

Figure 12.2
Double-edge scissors without finger tang

The two most popular sizes of double-edge scissors are the 5½-inch and 7½-inch (13.75- and 18.75-centimeter) models. The 5½-inch size is ordinarily used to cut wet hair straight across (blunt or club cut), while the 7½-inch scissors are used to cut dry hair. The 7½-inch scissors are generally used in a sliding (slithering or effilating) movement to shorten and thin hair. Double-edged scissors may be purchased in both left-hand and right-hand models.

2. **Double-notch scissors** are used to thin the hair (remove bulk), but not to remove length (Figure 12.3). They are also called **thinning scissors (shears).**

3. **Single-notch scissors** are also used to thin, or remove, bulk rather than length from the hair, but they remove or thin **more** hair than double-notch scissors do. Single-notch scissors are also called **thinning** scissors (Figure 12.4).

4. The **single-edge safety razor** is also called a hair **shaper** (Figure 12.5). This implement is used to shorten and thin the hair. It is always used on **wet** hair. If used on dry hair, the razor will "pull" the hair and cause discomfort to the client.

5. The **styling comb,** which is 7 inches (17.5 centimeters) long, has both fine and coarse teeth (Figure 12.6). It is used to control the hair during the shaping service.

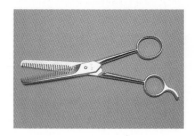

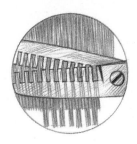

Figure 12.3
Double-notch scissors

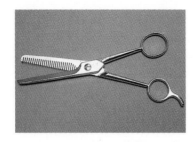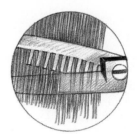

Figure 12.4
Single-notch scissors with finger tang

In addition to these basic implements, you will also use the **electric hair clipper.** Although this implement is discussed in greater detail in the next objective, Figures 12.7 and 12.8 show two clipper models. Figure 12.9 shows an assortment of clipper blades, and Figures 12.10 and 12.11 illustrate combs used with clippers and shears.

Figure 12.5
Safety razor

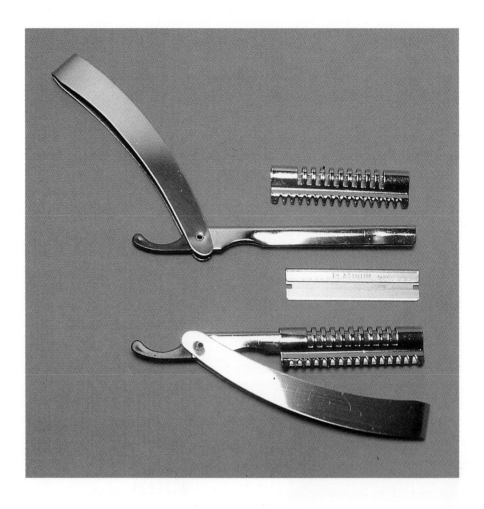

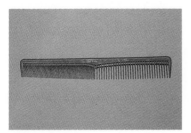

Figure 12.6
Styling comb (7 inches/17.5 centimeters)

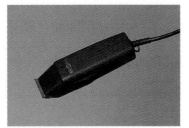

Figure 12.7
A small electric clipper

Cutting Movements

When you are shaping hair, either with a razor or scissors, you will need to make two basic kinds of motions with your cutting implement: **slither cutting (effilating)** and **blunt (club) cutting.**

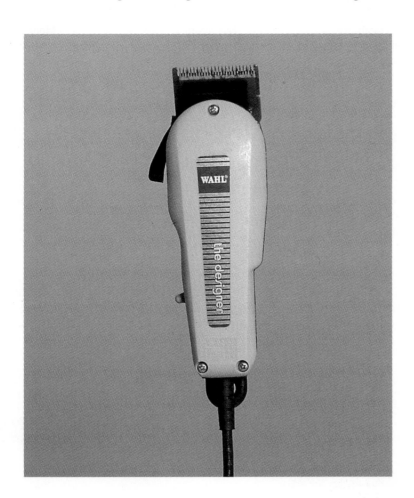

Figure 12.8
Electric clipper

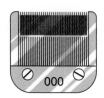

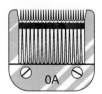

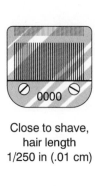

0000	**000**	**0A**
Close to shave, hair length 1/250 in (.01 cm)	Very close, hair length 1/100 in (.025 cm)	Close, hair length 5/64 in (.195 cm)

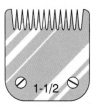

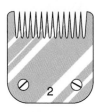

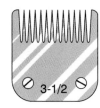

1	**18**	**1A**
Full tooth, hair length 1/8 in (.31 cm)	Skip tooth, hair length 1/8 in (.31 cm)	Medium, hair length 5/32 in (.39 cm)

1-1/2	**2**	**3-1/2**
Medium full, hair length 3/16 in (.47 cm)	Full, hair length 1/4 in (.625 cm)	Fullest, hair length 3/8 in (.94 cm)

Figure 12.9
Assortment of electric clipper blades

Slither cut the hair by sliding the cutting implement against the hair (Figure 12.12). If you are using scissors, close them **partially** as you slide them along the hair. This will give the hair a tapered, or

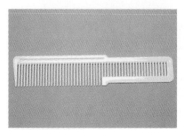

Figure 12.10
Clipper comb

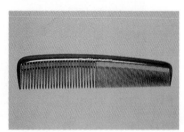

Figure 12.11
Barber comb

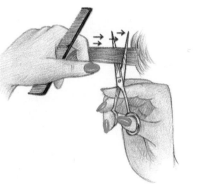

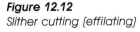

Figure 12.12
Slither cutting (effilating)

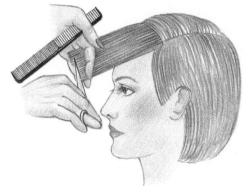

Figure 12.13
Blunt (club) cutting

"graduated" shape. **Do not** close the scissors completely. Slither cutting (effilating) is used to thin the hair, not to chop it off. If you close the scissors completely, you will cut the hair off completely. This will leave cutting **"marks" on the hair.**

Blunt, or **club, cutting** involves cutting the hair straight off the strand without slithering or thinning it (Figure 12.13). This movement will give the hair an even, well-defined ("blunt") edge or line. Blunt cutting may be done on dry or damp hair.

The hair-cutting task is more accurately called **hair shaping** because the professional cosmetologist does much more than simply "cut" lengths of hair from the client's head. **Hair shaping takes into account the natural growth patterns, texture,** and **condition of the hair; the facial features,** and **head structure of the client;** and the desired hairstyle. Although you may cut, and therefore shorten, hair in some areas of the head, you actually are shaping the hair to suit the hairdressing needs of a hairstylist client.

Although a skilled cosmetologist can use either scissors or a razor for most hairstyles—individual practitioners often have strong preferences for one or the other—it is more practical to use one implement instead of the other for some styles (Figures 12.14 and 12.15). This is because certain hairstyles can be cut or combed into place faster if you use a razor rather than scissors and vice versa. For example, if the client desires a bouffant, teased (back-combed) hairstyle that is very high in the top and crown areas and requires rollers with a few sculptured curls, the razor is probably the better choice. Of course, you could also use your blow comb and curling iron to style the hair. In this case, the hair could be slither cut with scissors and thinned with single- or double-notch scissors, but it would

Theory Objective 2
Differences between Razor Shaping, Scissor Shaping, and Electric Clipper Shaping

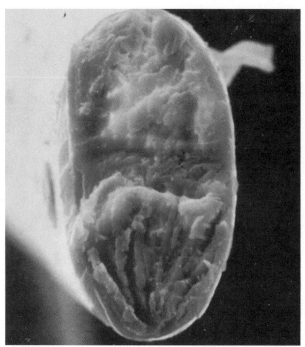

Figure 12.14
Scissor cut. Note how the action of the scissors squeezes the hair.

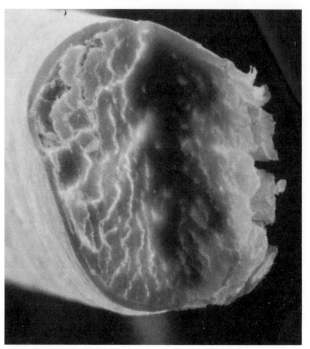

Figure 12.15
Razor cut. Note the edge of the outer cuticle.

probably be easier and faster to do it with a razor. On the other hand, some styles require blunt cutting, which is easier to do with scissors, even though a razor can produce similar results.

For some hairstyles, however, scissor cutting is a must. Hair that is to be air waved and/or curled with a curling iron to give fullness in the region of the eyes with a low top and crown should be shaped with scissors only. Therefore, your choice of scissors or a razor is determined partly by the styling principles that will be used after the hair shaping.

Some stylists do the entire haircut with the electric clipper because they feel it is faster (Figure 12.16). Your instructor will assist you in determining the best cutting implement for the clientele in your area.

Super-curly (black) hair is usually **cut dry.** Razor shaping is not recommended for this type of hair. It should be blunt cut or slither cut with scissors. Thinning shears are seldom, if ever, used on super-curly hair.

Precision or geometric haircuts are usually cut with a small scissors on wet hair. For example, 5- or 5½-inch (12.5- or 13.75-centimeter) scissors without a finger tang can be used (it is difficult to turn the wrist to hold the scissors at the correct cutting angles if

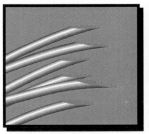 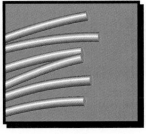 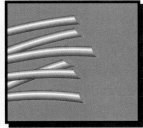

Hair cut with razor   Hair cut with scissors   Hair cut with electric clipper

Figure 12.16
Hair cut with different implements

it has a finger tang and longer blades). For this kind of style, the hair is always club or blunt cut, and the hair is not thinned very much, if at all.

The **electric hair clipper** is a cutting device made up of two closely spaced serrated (like the teeth of thinning scissors) blades. The cutting blade (called the **top blade**) is driven by a small electric or magnetic motor to vibrate back and forth against the nonmoving blade (**lower blade**). A portable, battery-operated clipper is also available. The hair caught in between the serrated blades is "sliced off" in much the same way as the hair is cut by the closing action of one scissors' blade against the other (Figure 12.17).

Hair clippers come in different sizes. Some have an adjustable lever on the side that allows blunt cutting, much like scissors, or varying degrees of tapering, somewhat like a razor. The **smaller clipper** model is sometimes called a **trimmer, outliner,** or **edger** because it is used mainly around the hairline to shorten the hair around the sideburns, ears, or neck (Figure 12.18). The trimmer/ outliner/edger is sometimes used to trim beards and mustaches. **Clipper shaping is generally done on dry hair to avoid the possibility of electric shock,** although many manufacturers offer a special

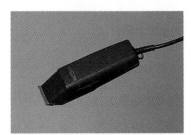

Figure 12.17
The cutting blade of an electric hair clipper

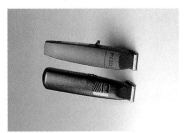

Figure 12.18
Examples of trimmers, outliners, or edgers used around the hairline and to outline beards and mustaches

model for cutting damp hair. **Remember,** if wet hair has not been towel-dried, water may drip into the clipper, causing a hazardous **electric shock** to the user or the client!

Theory Objective 3
Basic Parting Sections
of the Head

Since there are many good methods for parting and sectioning the hair for a hair shaping, you should ask your instructor which method you should use.

Because each person's head is a different size and slightly different shape, it is important to have a clear picture in your mind (a mental image of the design line) of how the head can be parted and sectioned. You probably already have some ideas about this from doing the exercise in objective 2 in Chapter 8 (Finger Waving the Hair).

To begin, the rectangle enclosed by points A, B, C, and D forms the **top section** (Figures 12.19 and 12.20). The area on the head enclosed by points A, C, and G is the **right side section** (Figure 12.21). Points B, D, and H enclose the **left side section.** The **crepe section** of the head is the area between the crown and nape sections. It is formed by points F, E, G, and H in Figure 12.22. The **nape section** is the area in the back of the head above the neck. It begins with the hairline and goes up to the occipital bone. It extends from ear to ear across the lower back of the head.

Sectioning is necessary because the hair is easier to "handle" in small sections, particularly if the client has long and/or very dense hair. Generally, the hair shaping is more accurate when the hair is sectioned first.

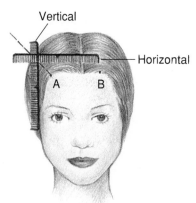

Figure 12.19
Finding points to divide the top from the crown section

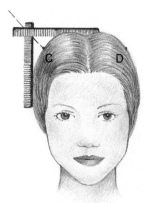

Figure 12.20
Finding points to divide the top from the side sections

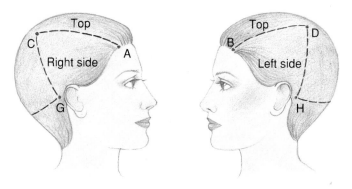

Figure 12.21
*Lines AC, CG, and the hairline
enclose the right side section.
Lines BD, DH, and the hairline
enclose the left side section.*

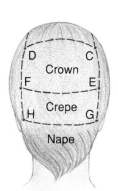

Figure 12.22
*Lines DC, CE, EF, and FD
enclose the crown section.
Lines FE, EG, GH, and HF
enclose the crepe section. The
nape extends from ear to ear
below line GH to the hairline.*

Theory Objective 4
*Terms Used in Hair
Shaping and Safety
Precautions*

Many of the words (terms) used in the hair-shaping service are not normally used in everyday conversations. You will need to learn these terms so that you can communicate with your instructors and other professional hairstylists. The following are the basic terms you will need to know: **guideline, hanging length, basic hair shaping, high elevation, low elevation, graduation, taper (layer), steps** or **marks, shingling, tailored neckline, feathering, angle, undercut, bi-level, fingerwork, scissors-over-comb,** and **clipper-over-comb.** An explanation of each term follows:

Guidelines   A guideline is one or more subsections (strands) of hair cut around the hairline or crown of the head. The purpose of the guideline is to give you a **measurement for cutting** the remaining hair (Figure 12.23). It is the yardstick by which you will cut the hair, a few strands at a time.

Hanging Length   The hanging length is the length of the hair when it is combed downward (Figure 12.24). The hanging

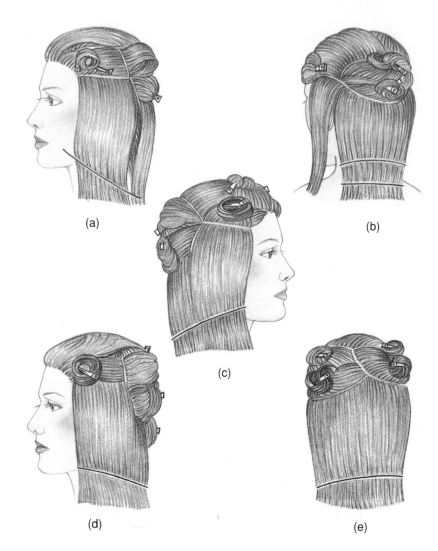

(a)

(b)

(c)

(d)

(e)

Figure 12.23
Once the guideline has been cut to indicate the length, many different shapes are possible. Here the black lines indicate shapes that can be cut using the guideline.

length is the longest hair around the bottom of the hairstyle.

Basic Hair Shaping Basic hair shaping is the general term used to describe a hair shaping that can be waved, blown, and styled in many different ways (Figure 12.25). Oftentimes, a basic hair shaping is a shorter hairstyle in the range of 3½ to 4½ inches (8.75 to 11.25 centimeters) in length (but may extend to as much as 6 inches/15 centimeters in length). This type of cut can be easily wrapped on cold-wave rods, set on rollers, set with an iron, blow combed, or set in sculpture curls. This versatile hair shaping is particularly useful in a school setting where it will allow you to practice many of the techniques you have learned.

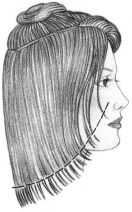

Figure 12.24
The dotted line shows the length of the hair after shaping—the hanging length.

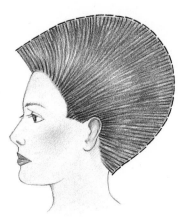

Figure 12.25
Proper distribution of hair lengths for a basic hair shaping

High Elevation   A high-elevation hair shaping is achieved by cutting subsections of hair held in an upward direction toward the crown or top of the head, rather than downward toward the nape of the head (Figures 12.26 and 12.27).

Low Elevation   A low-elevation hair shaping is achieved by cutting subsections of hair held in a downward direction toward the nape, rather than upward toward the crown or top of the head (Figures 12.28, 12.29, and 12.30).

Graduation and Taper   Graduation and taper mean about the same thing. Both terms refer to a shaping technique

Figure 12.26
A high-elevation hair shaping achieved by holding the hair at a 135° angle

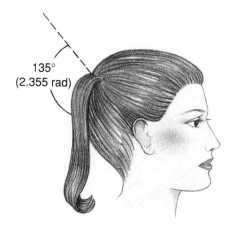

135°
(2.355 rad)

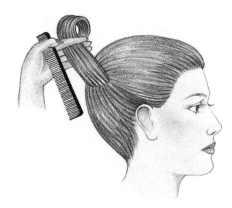

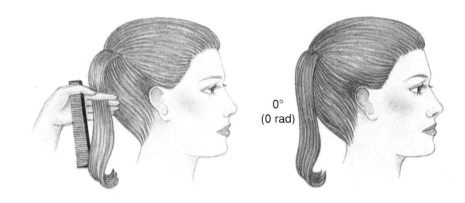

Figure 12.27
A high-elevation hair shaping achieved by holding the hair at a 180° angle

Figure 12.28
A low-elevation hair shaping achieved by cutting the hair at a 0° angle

(sometimes called layering) in which the hair is cut in layers that resemble the overlapping shingles on a roof except that the layers of hair are closer together (Figure 12.31).For example, if the guideline on the bottom nape is cut in one length, the layer of hair just above is graduated, or cut **slightly** shorter. Then the layer above that is cut **slightly** shorter than the one below it.

Steps or Marks   Steps or marks on the hair refer to a definite line(s) of demarcation between one layer of the hair and the layer just below it. Marks are the result of cutting the upper layer too short in relation to the layer directly underneath it. When the guideline is not followed, steps or marks can be easily seen, particularly on lighter hair colors or on hair that is naturally very straight or coarse. Remember not to cut the hair too short in the crown.

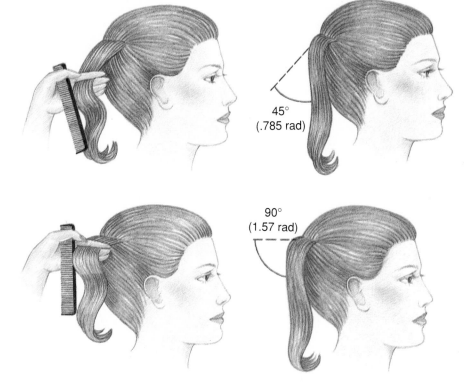

45°
(.785 rad)

Figure 12.29
A low-elevation hair shaping in which the hair is cut at a 45° angle

90°
(1.57 rad)

Figure 12.30
A low-elevation hair shaping in which the hair is cut at a 90° angle

Shingling and Tailored Neckline   These terms are used interchangeably: they usually refer to a hair shaping that is very short in the nape of the neck (Figure 12.32). If the hairline in the crown grows toward the center of the nape, the hair is graduated into a "V" shape in the nape area for women. However, men tend to have their nape shaped into a more squared-off design.

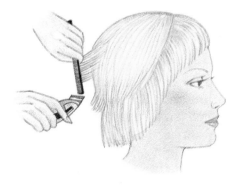

Figure 12.31
Graduating (layering) hair lengths with an electric clipper

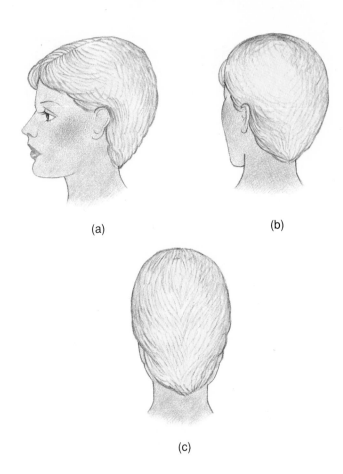

(a)

(b)

(c)

Figure 12.32
Shingling or tailored neckline shaping

Feathering Feathering and the term "feather edge" are sometimes confused. Feathering is a term clients use to refer to a shaping that is short and layered around the face (top and both side sections). The hair is about 3½ to 4½ inches (8.75 to 11.25 centimeters) long, and it is styled away from the face, so that the ends of the hair can be seen (Figure 12.33). Feather edge, on the other hand, generally refers to the nape area of a man's hair shaping in which the hair is gradually layered down the neck until it seems to disappear into the skin (Figure 12.34).

Angle The term angle is used in several different hair-shaping situations. For example, to cut an angle in the front section refers to parting the hair diagonally and parallel to the hairline to establish a cutting guideline (Figure 12.35). Angle may also refer to a design cut in the hanging length (Figure 12.36) or to how (the angle at which) the hair should be held when it is cut (Figure 12.37).

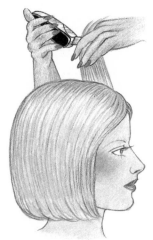

Figure 12.33
Feathering hair with an electric clipper

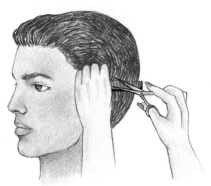

Figure 12.34
Example of cutting a "feather edge" for a male hair shaping. For safety, keep the comb between the client's head and the scissors.

Undercut   Undercut is a term used to describe longer hair lengths that are all one length on the bottom of the hairstyle (Figure 12.38). In this hair shaping, the nape guideline is cut, and then the client's head is tipped forward as far as is comfortably possible. The sections above the guideline are brought down one at a time and cut evenly on top of the skin along the bottom of the hanging length. The same principle can be used for an undercut for shoulder-length hair.

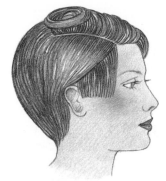

Figure 12.35
Hair parted and cut parallel on a diagonal angle

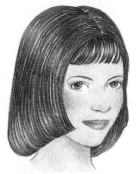

Figure 12.36
Note how the hanging length of the side sections is cut on an angle.

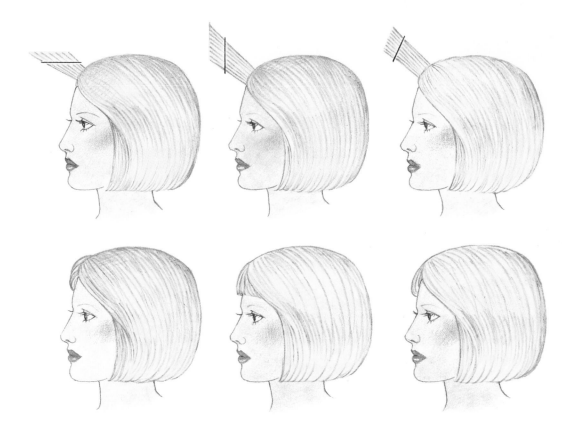

Figure 12.37
Holding the hair in different positions (angles) when it is cut produces different results.

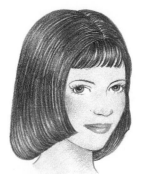

Figure 12.38
The hair flows under gracefully in the nape and side sections because it has been cut using the undercut technique.

Bi-level   A bi-level hair shaping is one in which the hair is cut in two different levels (Figure 12.39). It is quite short in the front hairline area and the front top section. The hanging length at the ear is usually short (about the middle of the ear or less). The top crown, crown, and back sections are left long (at about collar or shoulder length) and are usually all one length like an undercut.

Fingerwork   Fingerwork is a barber/cosmetology technique in which the comb and scissors are used to blend sections of hair from one area of the head to another (Figure 12.40). Fingerwork is used in very short hair shapings.

Scissors-over-Comb and Clipper-over-Comb   These terms are used to describe a barbering/cosmetology technique in which the hair is lifted away from the head with a comb and then cut with either the scissors or an electric clipper (Figures 12.41, 12.42 and 12.43).

You should also keep in mind that as hair fashions change, new terms and techniques will be used. Various regions of the country or provinces may also use terms that are different from those

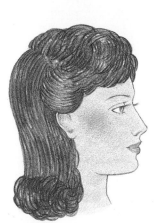

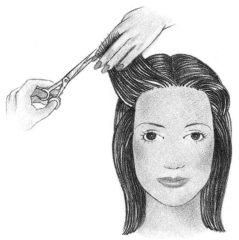

Figure 12.39
In a bi-level shaping, the hair is very short in the front side sections, but the hanging length is much longer.

Figure 12.40
Finger-work (finishing) blends subsections together for a "finished look." (See Figure 12.77 for an illustration.)

listed here. Your instructor will teach you the hair-shaping terms that are used in your particular area.

Safety Precautions

Be very careful not to cut yourself or your client during the hair-shaping procedure! Always follow the AIDS and HIV guidelines for your state. The following is a checklist of things to remember in order to work safely:

1. Always watch what you are doing. When not cutting, close your scissors; palm them when you comb through the hair (Figure 12.44). Hold the scissors as shown in Figure 12.45.

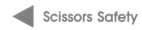 Scissors Safety

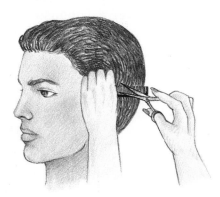

Figure 12.41
The scissors-over-comb technique is often used after the clipper to blend certain hair textures.

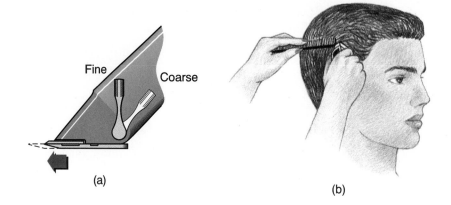

(a)

(b)

Figure 12.42
Using the clipper-over-comb technique to blend top and side sections. The clipper adjustment lever should be in the lower position as shown at the left.

2. Don't cut when you are talking to someone other than the client.

3. Never put scissors in your uniform pocket, or you may severely cut yourself when you reach for them. It is also an unsanitary practice.

4. Keep your scissors sanitized when not in use.

5. If you have a small hand, you may have to move along the hair strand by picking it up more than once.

6. **Use extra caution** when cutting hair in the area of the client's **eyes, ears, face, nose,** and **neck** (Figure 12.46).

7. **Be especially careful when shaping the hair of small children. A child may move his or her head quickly when you don't expect it. Try to anticipate dangerous situations and avoid them.**

8. **Sanitize your scissors with alcohol after each hair-shaping service.**

Razor Safety

1. **Don't attempt to change the blade of your shaper until you have asked your instructor for a demonstration** (Figure 12.47).

2. **Always use the guard on your razor.**

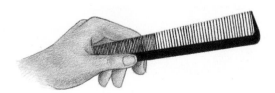

Figure 12.43
Holding the comb for the scissors-over-comb or clipper-over-comb cutting technique

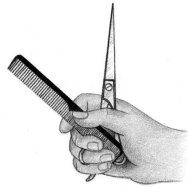
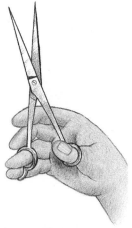

Figure 12.44
For safety, close scissors and rest them in your palm when combing through the hair. Hold your scissors at all times during shaping.

Figure 12.45
The correct way to hold scissors. Note the position of the thumb and ring finger.

3. **Never put your razor in your uniform pocket. Reaching for a razor in your pocket could put you in the hospital with a serious injury!** Pocketing razors is also unsanitary.

4. **Don't use a shaper with a rusty blade because it could cause an infection if a cut occurred. Always use a sharp blade to avoid painful "pulling" of the hair.**

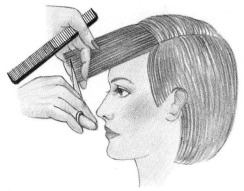
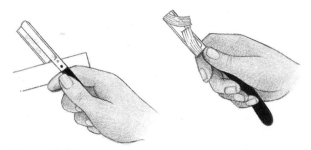

Figure 12.46
Note that fingers are placed between the scissors and face to protect the client's eyes and face.

Figure 12.47
Removing an old razor blade. Use the razor's guard to work the old blade out of the razor.

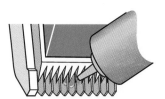

Figure 12.48
Oiling electric clipper blades

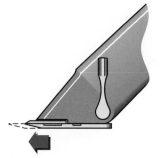

Figure 12.49
Taper adjustment lever

5. Use a razor only on wet hair.

6. Be careful not to "nick" facial or neck moles, scars, or other skin lesions of the client!

7. Don't remove the wrapper from a new razor blade until after it has been inserted into the razor.

8. Place tape over the old blade and dispose of it properly.

Clipper Safety ▶

1. Never use any electric (or battery-operated) clipper in the presence of water or other liquids. You or the client could get an electrical shock unless you have a special clipper with a waterproof case.

2. Use light clipper oil (one or two drops) daily to keep your blades working smoothly (Figure 12.48). Otherwise, the clipper may cause painful "pulling" of the hair.

3. Be careful not to "nick" facial or neck moles, scars, or other skin lesions of the client.

Figure 12.50
Removing blade for cleaning

4. Adjust your clipper as often as needed (Figure 12.49).

5. Remove blades, if necessary, for cleaning (Figure 12.50).

6. Never use a clipper that has a broken tooth in either blade. Keep a spare replacement set of blades.

7. Align replacement blades correctly. (Figure 12.51).

Figure 12.51
Check for correct alignment when changing electric clipper blades. The moving blade must not extend beyond the nonmoving blade, or the client will be cut.

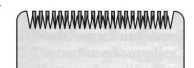

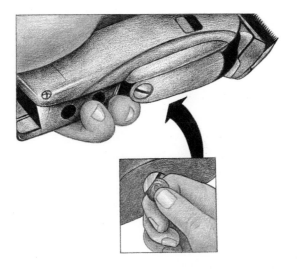

Figure 12.52
A coin may be used to turn the power adjustment screw.

8. **If you hear an irregular noise coming from your clipper, use a coin and turn the "power screw" counterclockwise to "tune" the clipper for quieter operation** (Figure 12.52). **(Not all clippers have this feature.)**

9. **Never use a clipper that has rusty blades. Never submerge your clipper in water! If you do, you will get an electrical shock!**

10. **Do not use a clipper if its case or power cord is cracked.**

11. **Never clean your clipper while the unit is turned on. Always store all hair-shaping implements safely away from the reach of small children!**

Practical Objective 5
Basic Scissor Shaping
for a Female Client

Supplies

- talcum powder
- shampoo cape or chair cloth
- neck strips
- spray applicator bottle for water

- styling comb
- duck-bill clips
- double-edge scissors

Preparation

Procedure

1. Drape the client with a shampoo cape and determine what services are to be performed.

Rationale

1. If the client will be having a chemical service, such as a tint or shampoo, a shampoo cape is necessary to protect his or her clothing from possible contact with chemicals or water. Also, the hair would be tinted before either shampooing or shaping. For a hair shaping when no chemical services including a shampoo are given, a chair cloth may be used for draping and will be more comfortable for the client because it is made of rayon or cotton or other woven fabric.

2. Shampoo the hair and part off the top section and secure.

2. It is easier to begin in this section, and it is much better to work on clean hair. Shampooing removes hair oils, loose hair, spray, dust, and the like.

3. Part off each side section, but leave enough hair to establish a guideline on each side (Figure 12.53).

3. The use of a guideline permits hair to be cut evenly from one subsection to the next.

4. Part off the crown, crepe, and nape sections, but leave a strip of hair in the nape to establish a guideline.

4. It is more convenient to cut the hair in small sections, rather than trying to control all the hair at once.

Figure 12.53
Part off sections of hair leaving a guideline at the bottom hairline.

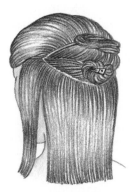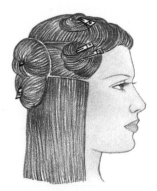

5. **Ask the client many questions** about the hairstyle desired. For example, how will the hair be styled—with a hot comb, hand dryer, or rollers? Or will it be air-dried or finger waved?

6. Position your comb at different places around the hairline and try to imagine where you will be cutting the hair for various hair lengths (Figure 12.54).

5. You should develop a mental image of exactly what the client has in mind before cutting the hair.

6. Placement of the comb is helpful to you, and it allows the client to visualize how long or short the hair will be after the shaping.

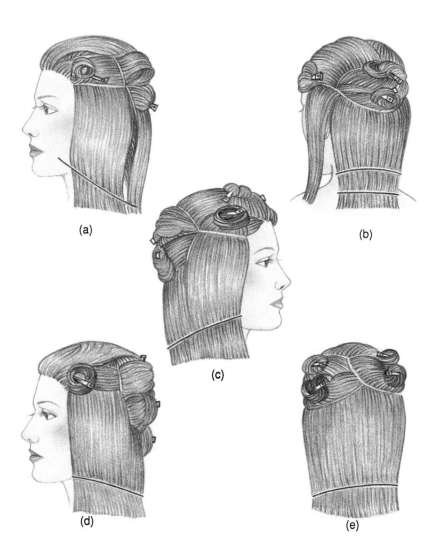

(a)

(b)

(c)

(d)

(e)

Figure 12.54
Possible imaginary guidelines for cutting. Consult with the client to determine the desired length.

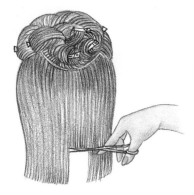

Figure 12.55
Begin cutting from the center nape and work forward to the next section.

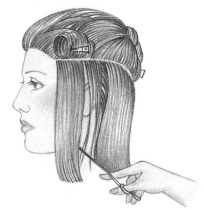

Figure 12.56
Continue cutting along the imaginary guideline. Carefully cut hair on the skin. Holding hair to be cut in the fingers causes it to become shorter.

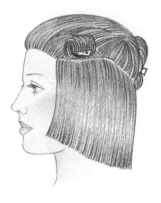

Figure 12.57
Hanging length of the first guideline

Shaping the Hair with Scissors

Procedure

1. Begin cutting the hair in the left nape section (Figure 12.55).

2. Work forward from the nape to the front of the left side section.

3. Repeat steps 1 and 2, cutting from the right nape section to the front of the right side section (Figure 12.56).

4. Release the crown and crepe sections and comb them smoothly into the guideline (Figure 12.57). Hold your comb in a vertical position and comb a strand of hair alongside the comb. Measure the hair to "half the comb" (3½

Rationale

1. This establishes a guideline in the nape section so that the subsections will be evenly cut from one section to the next.

2. Developing a system for working helps increase your accuracy and speed.

3. This is standard procedure.

4. After establishing the "hanging length" in the nape and side sections, it is necessary to establish the longest length in the crown section. **If the hair is cut shorter than 3½ inches/8.75 centimeters** (half the length of the styling comb), **you**

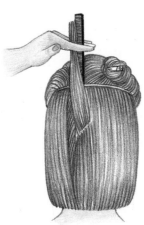

Figure 12.58
Hold the strand and comb straight up from the highest point on the head. Half of the comb will leave 3½ inches (8.75 centimeters) of hair for guidelines.

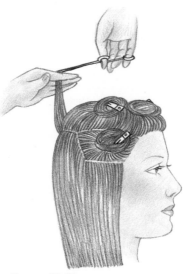

Figure 12.59
Cut a guideline. Allow more length if the client has a strong cowlick.

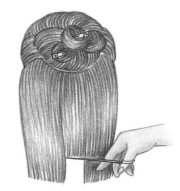

Figure 12.60
Cut the crown/crepe sections even with the hanging length.

inches/18.75 centimeters plus) as in Figure 12.58.

5. Starting in the center back of the crown, pick up a thin vertical subsection. Comb the subsection into the guideline from step 4 (Figure 12.59). Cut the hair that extends beyond the length of the guideline (Figures 12.60 and 12.61). Work from the center to the left ear until the crown has been cut. Repeat on the right side of the center of the crown.

6. Begin on the bottom of the crown section and part off a subsection of previously cut hair. Comb a thin,

will have difficulty wrapping the hair on cold-wave rods, setting it on rollers, and **using a curling iron.**

5. Using these thin subsections and the guideline will make your hair shaping more accurate (even) throughout the hair.

6. This will allow you to complete cutting the entire crepe section systematically.

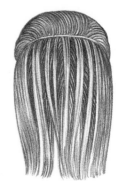

Figure 12.61
Use vertical partings to cut from the guideline.

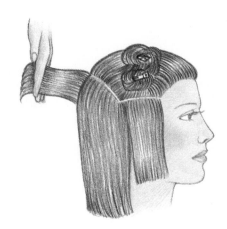

Figure 12.62
Note the guideline at the top of the hair strand.

vertical subsection from the crepe section into your fingers (Figure 12.62). Cut the hair that extends beyond the crown guideline and the nape guideline (Figure 12.63). Work from the center crepe to the left ear. Repeat by working from the center crepe to the right ear (Figure 12.64).

7. Go to the back of the right side section behind the ear.

7. This is standard procedure. Observing the hair closely

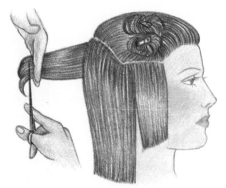

Figure 12.63
Use guidelines from the top and lower nape to cut the hair in between evenly.

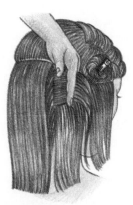

Figure 12.64
Cut from the center crown toward the right ear.

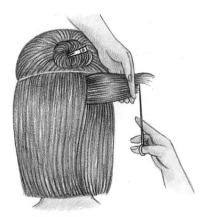

Figure 12.65
For each vertical subsection, hold the strand to be cut straight out from the head.

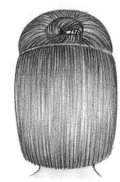

Figure 12.66
Keep the hanging length cut evenly to the guidelines.

Part off a thin, vertical subsection from the side section (Figure 12.65). Comb it into the last subsection cut in step 6, then observe the hair as you gradually comb both subsections forward (Figure 12.66). Cut off the hair that extends beyond the guideline (Figure 12.67). Repeat until all subsections have been cut.

8. Repeat step 7 on the left side section. Begin behind the left ear.

as you comb it will allow you to see the difference between the guideline and the hair that needs to be cut.

8. This is standard procedure for cutting the left side section.

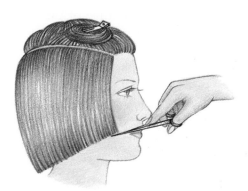

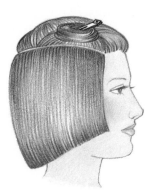

Figure 12.67
Carefully cut hair to the guideline. Be careful of eyes and skin. Watch what you are doing.

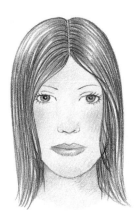

Figure 12.68
Release the top section, and part hair in the center.

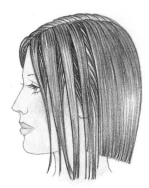

Figure 12.69
Use vertical partings to follow the guideline toward the front hairline.

9. Release the top section. Part in the center and comb into each side section (Figure 12.68). Make a vertical parting from the center part to the hairline behind the ear (Figure 12.69). Starting at the bottom of the part, "walk" a subsection of hair to a horizontal position on top of the head (Figure 12.70).

10. Hair that extends beyond the guideline when the hair is held in a horizontal position should be cut (Figure 12.71). Repeat for each subsection. Comb each subsection into the one previously cut, and then move your hand holding the hair forward before cutting (Figures 12.72, 12.73, and 12.74).

Keep raising your hand position to "walk" the strand to the top of the

9. This is standard procedure. You start combing behind the ear and comb the subsection to the top in order to "see" the guideline established in the hair that has already been cut.

10. It is important to use the guideline to measure each subsection **before** it is cut. Moving the hair forward takes into account the natural curvature of the head as it gradually slopes forward.

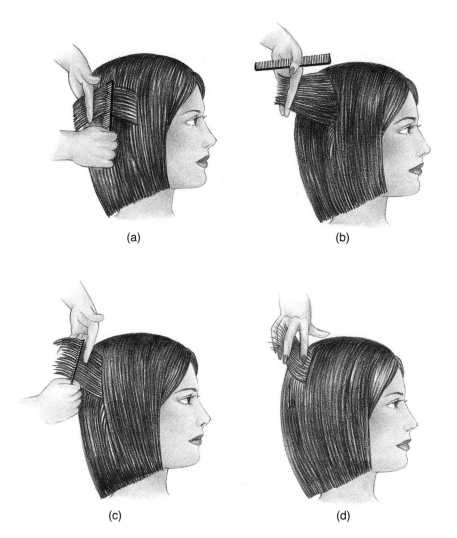

(a)

(b)

(c)

(d)

Figure 12.70
Keep raising your hand position to "walk" the strand to the top of the head.

head, but be careful not to cut the hair too short in the crown section.

11. Repeat step 10 on the left side of the top section. Begin parting behind the left ear and "walk" the subsection to the top of the head. Pick up a subsection of the hair cut on the right side of the top section, and use it as a guideline to begin cutting the left side

11. Since the right side of the top section is done, and you are reasonably sure it is correct, use a subsection from it as a guideline to cut the left side of the top section.

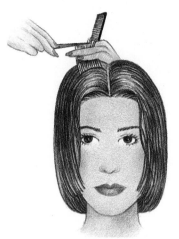

Figure 12.71
Cut hair that extends beyond the guideline.

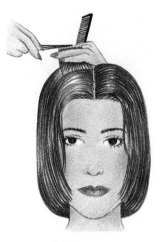

Figure 12.72
Comb through again to make sure no hairs have fallen from the strand you were cutting.

of the top section (Figure 12.75). Repeat until all subsections have been cut (Figure 12.76).

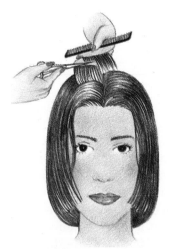

Figure 12.73
As you work toward the front hairline, move your hand slightly forward to allow for the natural curvature of the head.

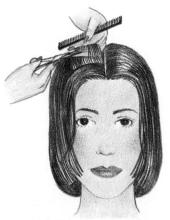

Figure 12.74
Continue cutting toward the front hairline.

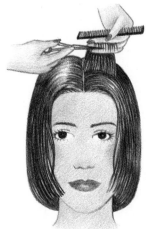

Figure 12.75
Cut the left side to match the right side. Use hair in the right section as a guideline.

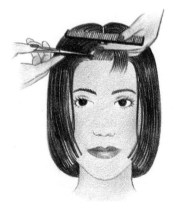

Figure 12.76
Remember to move your hand forward slightly to follow the shape of the client's head.

12. Check for hair that doesn't blend by systematically combing subsections between the top and side sections, and trim as needed for evenness (Figure 12.77). Double-check the hanging length for evenness and shape.

13. Using a small amount of talcum powder on a towel, thoroughly wipe hair clippings from the client's face, neck, and clothing. Sweep, comb, or vacuum all hair from the floor and work area. Dispose of hair clippings in a closed container. Continue with the next service. Sanitize and store cutting supplies and implements.

12. There will usually be a small "corner" of hair that doesn't fit into the hair cut between the top and side sections. Neck hair tends to "creep" up a little, so careful combing is needed to make sure it is even and shaped correctly.

13. The talcum powder allows the hair to slide freely off the client onto the cape or the floor. Many states have laws requiring the removal of hair from the floor and work area immediately after the shaping. Cutting implements must be sanitized after **each** use.

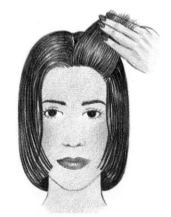

Figure 12.77
Checking hair lengths for "corners" between top and side sections

Practical Objective 6
Basic Scissor Shaping
for a Black Female
Client

Supplies

- talcum powder
- shampoo cape or chair cloth
- neck strips
- spray applicator bottle for pH-balanced wetting solution
- styling comb
- duck-bill clips
- double-edge scissors

NOTE: The same basic hair-shaping techniques are used for all clients: Nevertheless, in styling a black client's hair, you should give special consideration to curl control, texture, porosity, and the overall condition of the hair.

When working with hair that is excessively curly, wavy, wiry, or super-curly (kinky), it is usually better to cut the hair dry. Before cutting, the hair should be conditioned, thermally dried, and pressed so that even guidelines can be established.

The steps outlined here describe a basic wet shaping for a black female client. If the hair has been chemically relaxed or has received a soft perm (permanent wave for super-curly hair), it should be conditioned before shaping. When hair has been chemically relaxed, take care not to apply too much tension when you are combing and positioning the hair subsections during the shaping. Moisture balance is also very important because this type of hair is usually very porous (dry). An improper moisture balance leads to uneven porosity, which can result in an uneven hair shaping. The texture and density of the hair will also affect the resulting hairstyle.

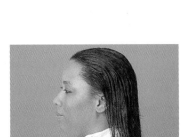

Figure 12.78
Chemically relax and condition the hair before shaping. Use a large-tooth comb to avoid breakage.

Preparation

Repeat steps 1 through 6 of objective 5.

Procedure	*Rationale*
1. Condition the hair, rinse, and comb smooth with a large-tooth comb. Take care not to allow the hair to dry or frizz (Figure 12.78).	**1.** Conditioning restores moisture balance to the hair. Combing with a large-tooth comb prevents breakage and frizziness.
2. Part off the hair into four or five sections (Figure 12.79).	**2.** Sectioning makes the hair easier to control.
3. Establish a cutting guideline (Figure 12.80).	**3.** The guideline should extend at least 1 inch (2.5 centimeters) into the perimeter of the hairline.

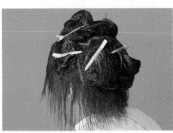

Figure 12.79
For control, comb and clip the hair into sections.

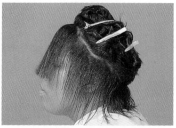

Figure 12.80
Part off a guideline around the hairline.

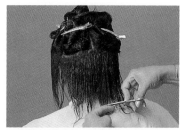

Figure 12.81
Blunt cut the hanging length for the hairstyle in the nape section.

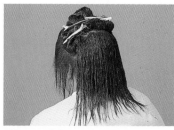

Figure 12.82
Parting the hair from ear-to-ear, use ¼-inch (.625-centimeter) horizontal subsections to work up the back of the head.

4. Comb the hair smoothly, then blunt cut a guideline in the nape section using zero-degree elevation to establish a hanging length for the hairstyle (Figure 12.81).

5. Starting at the middle of the ears on either side of the head, part off a ¼-inch (.625 centimeter) subsection. Bring down the subsection (using zero-degree elevation), and cut the hair along the established guideline. Apply more moisturizer as needed. Avoid placing too much tension on the hair (Figure 12.82).

6. Follow the guideline from the back to the left side section. Repeat this step on the right side section (Figure 12.83).

7. To achieve a layering effect, part the hair using ¼-inch (.625-centimeter) vertical subsections (Figure 12.84). Hold the hair at a 45° angle and cut along the guideline established in the nape section (Figure 12.85).

4. Be sure to keep the hair smooth and moist and avoid placing too much tension on the strands of hair.

5. Too much tension will create uneven lines. The hair will stretch very easily depending on the amount of natural curl remaining.

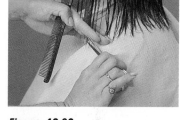

Figure 12.83
Comb hair from the back section into the side section to serve as a guideline.

6. This will create an even hanging length for your hairstyle.

7. The hair should be elevated to achieved a layered hairstyle.

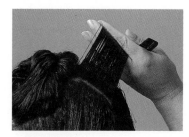

Figure 12.84
The partings should be clean and straight. Your fingers should be parallel to the partings.

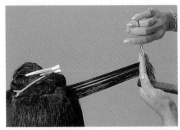

Figure 12.85
Before cutting, elevate the hair to a 45° angle.

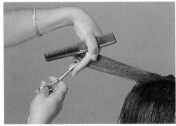

Figure 12.86
Comb the top, front part of the crown section forward. Use the guideline you established at the front hairline to cut the hair evenly.

8. Continue by parting above the temple area over the ear to the top crown section. Comb hair subsections forward, and cut at a 45° angle, using the established guideline. Using horizontal partings, continue parting upward to complete the top section (Figure 12.86).

9. Comb the back of the crown section downward at a 45° angle (Figure 12.87), using the established guideline to blend the hair with the occipital section.

10. Pick up a subsection at the top of the head and continue layering. Use vertical partings and cut the hair at a 45° angle to blend the top section with the back section. Create more layering in the top section by working a portion of each guideline into the section. Hold each strand at a 90° angle before cutting to blend (Figure 12.88).

8. This technique will result in the layering of the back sections of the hair.

9. This technique blends the hair from one section to the next.

10. Holding the hair at a 90° angle gives a greater amount of layering.

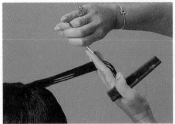

Figure 12.87
Comb the back of the crown section downward at a 45° angle to blend with the guide established in the crepe section.

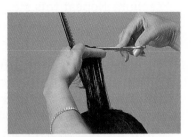

Figure 12.88
Hold the hair at a 90° angle to blend the top section with the back and side sections.

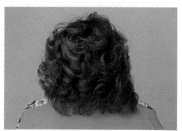

Figure 12.89
Note how blunt cutting in the nape section gives fullness in the finished hairstyle.

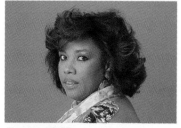

Figure 12.90
A front view of the finished hairstyle

11. Before calling your instructor to check your shaping, comb one section into the next. Finish the side section by establishing a length suitable for the client's facial features, wishes, and life-style. The hair may now be thermal styled, wet set, or wrapped to finish (Figures 12.89 and 12.90).

11. This will determine how all the hair blends from one section to the next.

*Practical Objective 7
Basic Scissor Shaping
for a Male Client*

Supplies

- talcum powder or hair vacuum
- shampoo cape or chair cloth
- neck strips
- spray applicator bottle for water
- styling comb
- duck-bill clips
- double-edge scissors
- barber comb (Figure 12.91)
- electric clipper/outliner

NOTE: The basic difference between a shaping for a man and a shaping for a woman is that the growth pattern is different around both the hairline in front and the nape hairline at the back of the head. The shaping on the man will be somewhat more square around the sideburns and the nape of the neck. A shaping on a woman tends to be cut around the hairline with a more oval shape. The sideburns are also angled more, almost to a point for the female client. For the male client, the cutting procedure after the guideline has been established is nearly the same as described in the previous objective. A man's hair shaping, however, is often

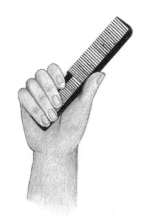

Figure 12.91
Holding a special flat-top comb

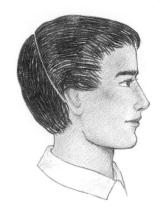 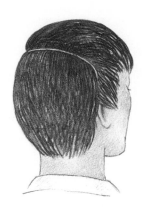

Figure 12.92
Section hair from the top of the crown section to behind each ear.

cut much shorter. If a permanent wave or curl reformation is not scheduled, the guideline for the male client is usually 2 to 3 inches (5 to 7.5 centimeters). The texture and density of the hair, along with the wishes of the client, will also influence the length of the guideline.

Rationales for the steps of this objective have been omitted because they are essentially the same as those for objective 5.

Preparation

Repeat steps 1 through 6 of objective 5.

Shaping the Hair

Follow the instructions in Figures 12.92 through 12.107.

Figure 12.93
If the hair isn't too short, clip the crown and crepe sections out of the way. Leave a strip of hair at the bottom of the nape for a cutting guideline.

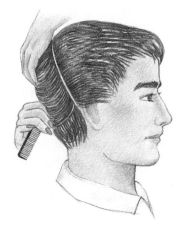

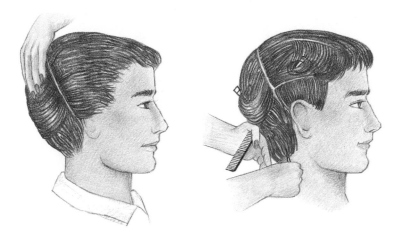

Figure 12.94 (far left)
Side sections may be combed out of the way or secured with a clippie or duck-bill clip.

Figure 12.95 (left)
Secure side sections if hair is not too short. Leave a strip of hair over the ears as a guideline.

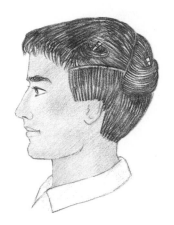
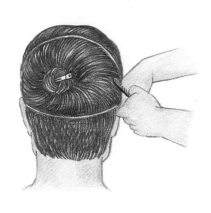

Figure 12.96 (far left)
Cut a guideline in the nape section.

Figure 12.97 (left)
Continue to cut the guideline from the ear to the nape along the hairline.

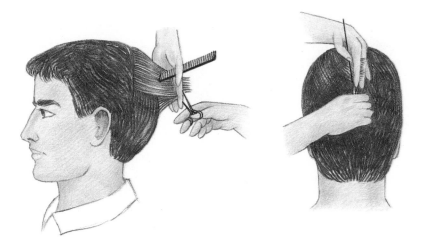

Figure 12.98 (far left)
Use vertical sections to work the nape guideline into the crepe section.

Figure 12.99 (left)
Continue to work into the upper crown section.

Figure 12.100
Cut the hair using vertical sections. Work from the center of the head to the left and right ears.

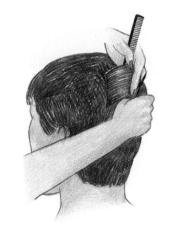
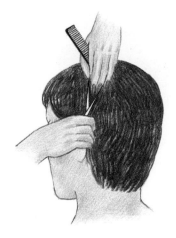

Figure 12.101 (right)
Part off hair at the top of the ear. Cut a guideline on either side of the ear.

Figure 12.102 (far right)
Consult the client to determine the desired length of hair over the ears. Repeat on the left side section.

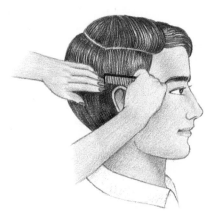
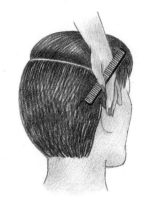

Figure 12.103
Use the bottom guideline to cut hair in the right and left side sections. Hold hair straight out from the head for cutting.

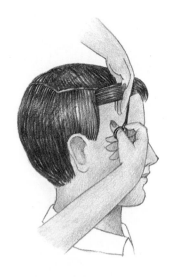
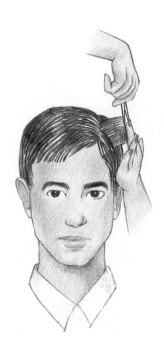

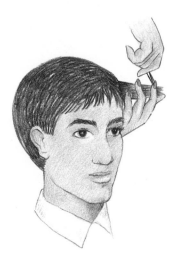

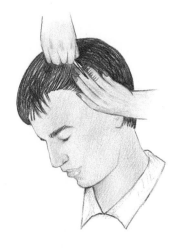

Figure 12.104
Move your hand slightly forward as you cut the hair to follow the curvature of the head.

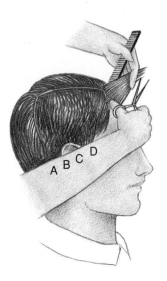

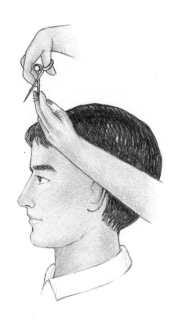

Figure 12.105 (far left)
Begin at section "A," and "walk" the hair to the top of the head. Use a guide from the side section for cutting the top section.

Figure 12.106 (left)
Repeat the steps in Figure 12.92 to cut the left top section to match.

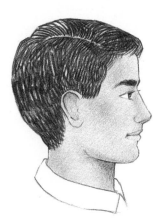

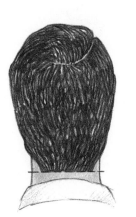

Figure 12.107
The finished shaping.

Practical Objective 8
Basic Clipper Shaping for a Female Client

Follow the instructions in Figures 12.108 through 12.120.

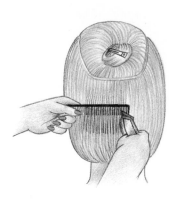

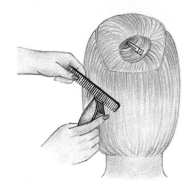

Figure 12.108 (right)
Section the hair and cut a guideline in the nape section.

Figure 12.109 (far right)
Work from the center of the nape toward the left ear.

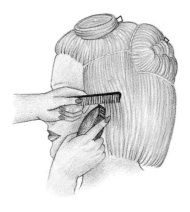

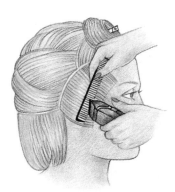

Figure 12.110 (right)
Cut the side section guideline.

Figure 12.111 (far right)
Work from the center nape to the right side section.

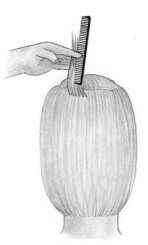

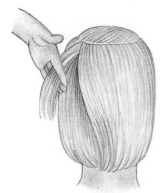

Figure 12.112 (right)
Establish the crown guideline and cut.

Figure 12.113 (far right)
Use clipper to blend hair between top and bottom guidelines.

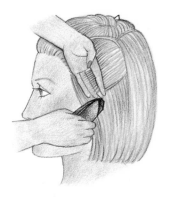
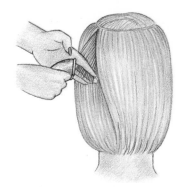
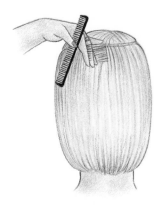

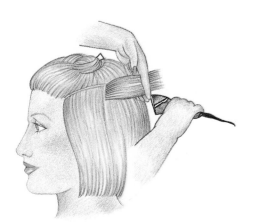
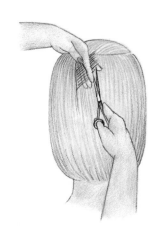

Figure 12.114 (top left)
Cut between the top and bottom guidelines using vertical partings.

Figure 12.115 (top middle)
Blend top and bottom sections.

Figure 12.116 (top right)
Work from the center of the crown toward the right side using the vertical subsections.

Figure 12.117 (far left)
Closely follow the guideline from the previously cut section.

Figure 12.118 (left)
Blend as needed using scissors.

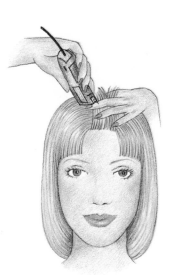
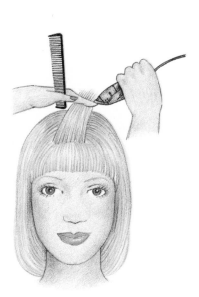

Figure 12.119 (far left)
Cut the guideline for the bang section.

Figure 12.120 (left)
Use the previously cut guideline to complete cutting of top section.

Practical Objective 9
Basic Clipper Shaping for a Male Client

Follow the instructions in Figures 12.121, 12.122, and 12.123.

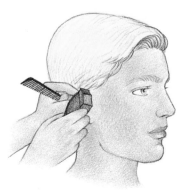

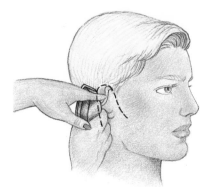

Figure 12.121
Give a basic haircut with the implement of your choice. Then establish a guideline at the side hairline.

Figure 12.122
Fold ear out of the work area to establish the shape of the hairline. Do not cut into the natural hairline. The dotted line indicates the shape of a short haircut for male clients.

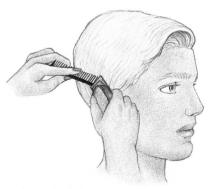

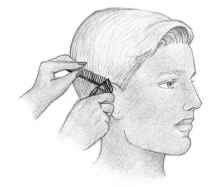

Figure 12.123
Use the clipper-over-comb technique to blend sides with hair above.

Follow the instructions in Figures 12.124 through 12.138.

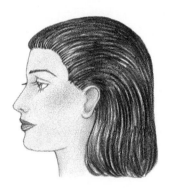

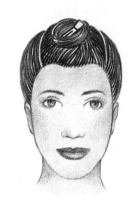

Figure 12.124 (far left)
Bulky, untapered hair.

Figure 12.125 (left)
Part off the top section.

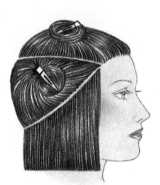

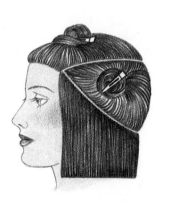

Figure 12.126
Part off the side sections.

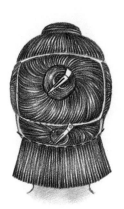

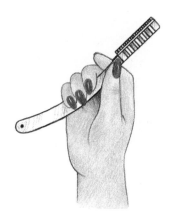

Figure 12.127 (far left)
*Part off the crown and crepe
sections, but leave a strip of
hair to cut the guideline at the
bottom.*

Figure 12.128 (left)
*Manner in which the razor
should be held*

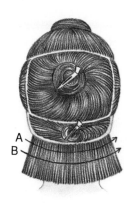
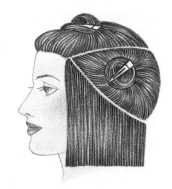

Figure 12.129
Decide the guideline for hanging length A or B. Decide the hanging length for both side sections.

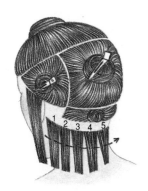
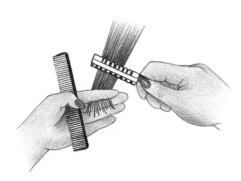

Figure 12.130 (right)
Begin cutting behind the left ear to make a guideline.

Figure 12.131 (far right)
Hold razor almost flat against the hair strand. The pressure of the razor against the hair will determine how much hair is removed.

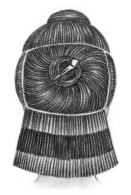
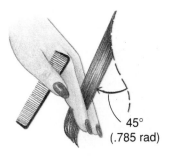

Figure 12.132 (right)
Bring down the crepe section. The dark area indicates the guideline.

Figure 12.133 (far right)
Hold hair at a 45° angle. Slide fingers down the strand until the guideline begins to fall. Then begin cutting.

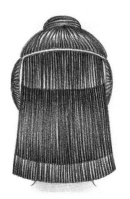

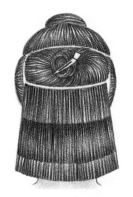

Figure 12.134 (far left)
Divide the crown section in half and bring down. Slide fingers down vertical strands until the crepe guideline falls. Then begin to cut.

Figure 12.135 (left)
Bring down the other half of the crown and blend with the lower half. Comb down both side sections, and repeat the procedure using the bottom guideline.

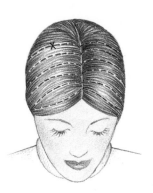

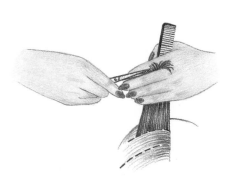

Figure 12.136 (far left)
Make a center part. Begin at point "X", and use vertical parts to "walk" the hair to the top of the head. Cut using your guide. Continue until all subsections are cut. Repeat procedure for other top section.

Figure 12.137 (left)
Check hair lengths to make sure they are even from one section to the next.

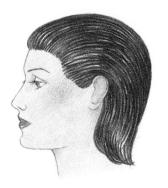

Figure 12.138
Properly tapered hair

Practical Objective 11
Beard and Mustache Trim

Follow the instructions in Figures 12.139 through 12.148.

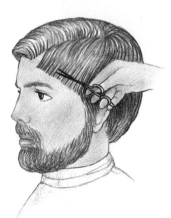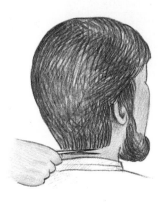

Figure 12.139
To begin, cut front and nape hanging length guidelines.

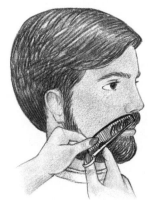

Figure 12.140
Use small, mustache comb for trimming mustache.

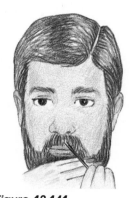

Figure 12.141
Use one hand to guide scissors. Be careful not to cut skin.

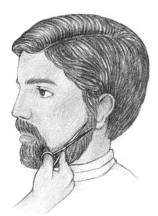

Figure 12.142
Trim outline of beard. Be careful of ear.

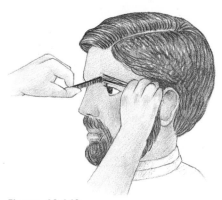

Figure 12.143
Use mustache comb to trim eyebrows.

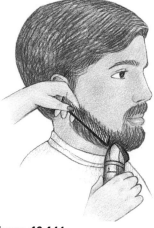

Figure 12.144
Use clipper-over-comb technique to remove fullness from beard.

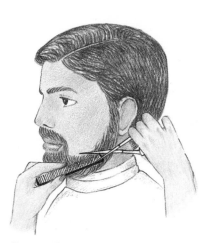

Figure 12.145
Overly curly hairs can be trimmed into form using scissors.

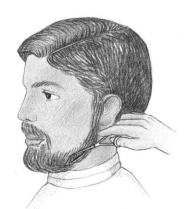

Figure 12.146
Use fingerwork to remove additional fullness from beard.

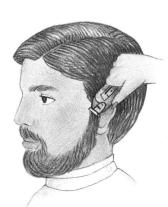

Figure 12.147
Use edger (trimmer) to define the border of the beard.

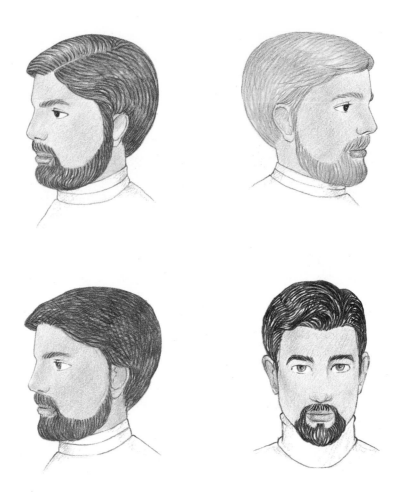

Figure 12.148
Finished beard shapings

Sanitize your area as follows:
1. Wash, wipe, and store bottles and supplies.
2. Discard used supplies.
3. Clean and sanitize the cape and apron.
4. Sanitize the work area; wash your hands.

Glossary

Angle A term that can be applied to different hair-shaping
situations in which the hair is cut on the bias.
Basic hair shaping A hair shaping that can be waved, blown, and
styled in many different ways.
Bi-level shaping A hair shaping in which the hair is cut in two
different levels.
Blunt cutting Cutting straight across the hair.
Clipper-over-comb The technique of lifting the hair away from
the head with a comb and then cutting it with a clipper.

Club cutting See **Blunt cutting.**

Crepe section The area of the head between the crown and nape sections.

Double-edge scissors An implement used frequently for hair shaping.

Double-notch scissors An implement used to thin the hair (remove bulk rather than length).

Edger See **Trimmer.**

Effilating Slither cutting.

Electric hair clipper A cutting device made up of two closely spaced serrated blades.

Feather edge The nape area of a man's hair shaping, in which the hair is gradually layered down the neck.

Feathering A shaping that is short and layered around the face.

Fingerwork The technique of using the comb and scissors to blend sections of hair from one area of the head to another.

Graduation A shaping technique in which the hair is cut in layers.

Guideline One or more strands of hair cut around the hairline or crown to provide a measurement for cutting the rest of the hair. Also, a narrow strip of hair used on both sides of the head and nape to establish the hanging length of a hairstyle.

Hair shaping Cutting the hair with scissors, razor, or electric clipper while taking natural growth patterns, facial features, the desired style, and other factors into account.

Hanging length The longest hair around the bottom of the hairstyle.

High-elevation shaping A hair shaping achieved by cutting subsections of hair held in an upward direction toward the crown or top of the head rather than downward toward the nape.

Low-elevation shaping A hair shaping achieved by cutting subsections of hair held in a downward direction toward the nape rather than upward toward the crown or top of the head.

Lower blade The blade of an electric clipper that does not move.

Marks The line of demarcation between one layer and the layer below it.

Nape section The area in the back of the head above the neck.

Outliner See **Trimmer.**

Scissors-over-comb The technique of lifting the hair away from the head with a comb and then cutting it with scissors.

Shaper An implement used to shorten and thin wet hair; also called a **single-edge razor.**

Shingling A hair shaping that is very short in the nape.

Single-edge razor An implement used to shorten and thin wet hair.

Single-notch scissors An implement used to thin the hair (remove bulk rather than length).

Slither cutting Cutting the hair by sliding the blade along the hair to give it a tapered shape; also called **effilating.**

Steps The line of demarcation between a layer and the layer below it.

Styling comb An implement used to control the hair during shaping.

Tailored neckline A hair shaping that is very short in the nape.

Taper A shaping technique in which the hair is cut in layers.

Thinning Removing bulk during a haircut.

Thinning scissors See **Double-notch** and **Single-notch scissors.**

Top blade The cutting blade of an electric clipper; it moves back and forth against the still blade.

Trimmer A small hair clipper that is mainly used around the hairline.

Undercut Hair subsections from the crepe and crown sections are cut so they are longer than the nape guideline.

Questions

1. Write a short paragraph explaining the importance of hair shaping.
2. What is effilating?
3. With what implement is super-curly hair generally cut?
4. On a separate sheet of paper, sketch the basic haircut taught in your school.
5. Write a paragraph comparing and contrasting low-elevation and high-elevation hair shapings.
6. Which hair-shaping implement is used to blunt cut and shape the hair around the sideburns of a male client?
7. Which cutting implement should only be used on hair that is wet?
8. On the electric clipper, is the top or the bottom blade the adjustable blade?
9. What is the name for the comb that is very tapered at one end and is used to cut short hair?
10. Which type of hair should not be cut with a razor?
11. Make a drawing, showing the sectioning divisions of the head.
12. Is the strand held upward for a high-elevation shaping?
13. What is the name for a shaping that is very short in the nape of the neck and is cut in a "V" shape?

14. Should you store your scissors or razor in your pocket when it is not in use?
15. Is a shampoo cape or a cloth cape more comfortable for the client when he or she is draped for a hair shaping?
16. Should you shape the hair the way you think it should be cut or consult the client?
17. True or false. Hair that is cut at 2½ inches (6.25 centimeters) can easily be wrapped on permanent wave rods.
18. If the hair is very thick, what size subsections should you use?
19. Is a guideline really necessary to achieve an even hair shaping?
20. If you don't have a blower or vacuum, what is the easiest way to remove hair from the client's skin after a hair shaping?
21. Should there be excessive tension on black clients' hair when cutting wet?

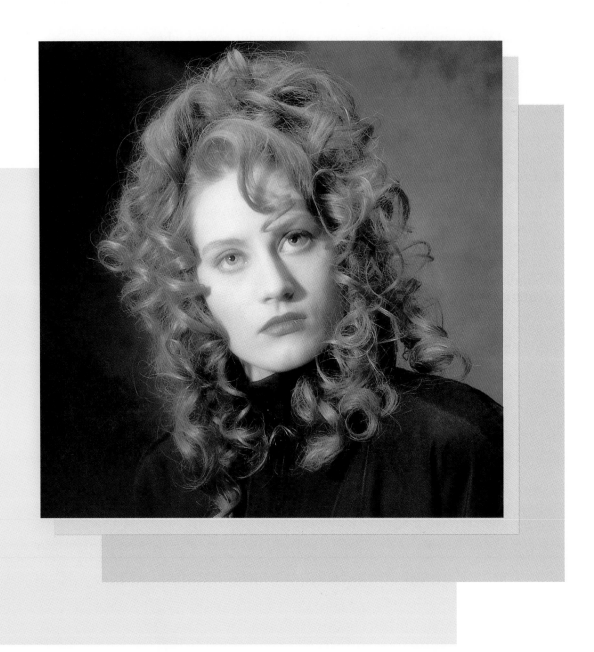

Air Waving and Blow-Drying (Waving)

Using a professional air waver or blow waver, dry the client's hair in a current hairstyle. The client's hair should be air waved (with air waver or blow waver) in 30–40 minutes. It should be thoroughly dried and arranged in a current hairstyle. Score 85 percent or better on a multiple-choice exam on the information in this chapter.

In order to achieve the above level of competence, you should master the following chapter objectives.

Theory Objective

1. Explain "quick-service" hairstyling and describe the implements used.

Practical Objectives

2. Blow wave the hair.
3. Air wave the hair.

Fashions, like the weather, are sure to change. Sometimes they seem to change almost as quickly as the weather; other times they change more slowly.

Hairstyles are an important part of fashion, and like fashion, they change as "looks" change. Air waving and blow waving are two examples of new styling techniques that have become quite popular. The use of a hand dryer to produce special effects is not completely new, but the hand dryers used for air waving and blow waving have new features and can be used in ways older hand dryers could not.

Special styles often require some kind of special treatment or care. This is true for air waving and blow waving. If you use these techniques, you must be sure to give the hair a very good scissor shaping. With practice, you will be able to master these skills.

Theory Objective 1
"Quick-Service"
Hairstyling and the
Implements Used

Air waving and blow waving are "quick-service" types of hairstyling (Figure 13.1). "Quick-service" hairstyling **saves time for the client.** After the hair is shampooed, it can be styled into place with an air waver or blow waver. Setting, drying, and combing the hair, which take quite a bit of time, are not necessary.

Air waving uses electrically heated air from an **air waver (blow comb)** and combing techniques to dry the hair into **wave patterns.**

Figure 13.1
Examples of "quick-service" hairstyles

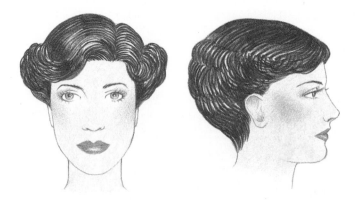

Blow waving uses electrically heated air from a **blow waver (hand dryer)** and combing and brushing techniques to dry the hair. Blow waving results in **larger wave patterns** than air waving does. As a result of these larger wave patterns, blow waving can give the hair more volume (height) than air waving and also produces a more casual hairstyle.

The appliances used for air waving and blow waving have several features with which you should be familiar:

1. The amount of **electrical power** needed to run air wavers and blow wavers and the degree to which they heat the air vary. The law requires that the amount of **electrical power** in **watts** (a unit of measurement) must be stamped somewhere on all these appliances. Their power ratings range from about **250 to 1350 watts.** The higher the rating, the **hotter** the appliance will heat the hair.

2. High-powered air wavers and blow wavers have from two to five heat settings (from hot to cold) that work best for particular hair types. Hotter settings are for normal and coarse hair that has **not been chemically treated.** The lower settings with cooler temperatures are for tinted, fine, and bleached hair.

3. In addition to the amount of heat, you should also be interested in the speed (force) of the air coming from the air waver or blow waver. The **speed** of the heated air leaving the appliance determines how fast the hair can be arranged and dried into a hairstyle. Most professional air wavers have more than one air speed setting.

4. Air wavers and blow wavers can be bought with a variety of attachments, but the most useful ones are the **fine-tooth** metal comb for the air waver and the **standard nozzle** (plastic or metal) **attachment** and **diffuser** for the blow waver (Figure 13.2). The **nozzle attachment** directs a narrow flow of air quickly through the barrel and out the end of the blow waver to rapidly dry the hair. The **diffuser** spreads the flow of air over a greater area so that it does not come out of the end of the dryer so fast. Thus, the drying process is slower with the diffuser.

To ensure that you and your client will be safe, all air wavers and blow wavers used in the beauty school or salon must be "U.L." **(Underwriters Laboratories) approved.** The "U.L." **seal means** that the dryer has been tested and **judged safe.** It should not overheat or cause accidental electric shocks.

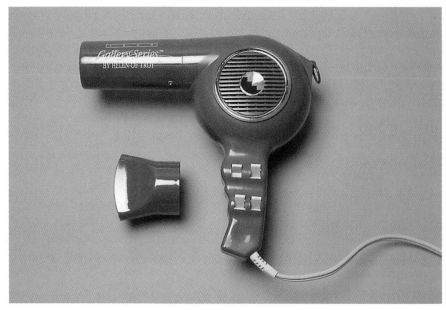

Figure 13.2
A blow waver with a nozzle attachment and a diffuser

Nozzle   Diffuser

Practical Objective 2
Blow Wave the Hair

Supplies

- shampoo supplies
- electric blow waver (hand dryer) with attachments including diffuser(s)
- brush selection: vent, Denman, round, cushion

- styling comb
- hair styling preparations: gel, mousse, lotion, spritz, hair spray, lacquer

Procedure

1. Shampoo, condition, and towel-dry the hair; thoroughly comb out tangles. Carefully apply styling preparation. Begin sectioning in the back nape of the head.

2. Select the brush you will be using (Figure 13.3).

Rationale

1. This is standard procedure. Long hair will be much easier to handle if the hair is sectioned.

2. For long hair or larger wave formations, use the brush with longer bristles or a larger circumference. For short hair, use a **Denman brush.** The **vent brush** is a good all-purpose brush. Use

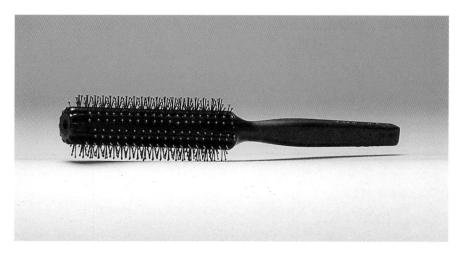

Figure 13.3
Round brush

the **round brush** when more curl is desired. **Be careful when drying long hair to make sure that it is not drawn into the air intake vent of the dryer.**

3. Turn the brush into the strand next to the scalp. As the hair dries, slide the strand through the brush. Direct the flow of warm air parallel to the scalp or at the hair as it lies across the brush (Figure 13.4). Never direct the hot air toward the scalp.

3. This gives the hair an outside movement away from the scalp. **Avoid directing the flow of hot air at the scalp, or you will burn the skin.**

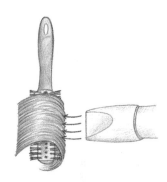

Figure 13.4
Directing the air flow at the hair as it lies across the brush

4. Thoroughly dry and shape the hair from the back of the head, in the nape, and then the crown, sides, front hairline, and side sections (Figure 13.5).

4. You must dry the hair thoroughly as it is styled to get a long-lasting style. On short hair, you may want to use the hot brush.

5. As the hair dries, rotate the brush to help shape all hair next to the scalp.

5. This procedure gives the hair curl as well as height and volume.

6. Rotate the brush in a vertical, horizontal, or diagonal position (Figures 13.6 and 13.7).

6. The way you hold the brush will depend on the section of the head you are styling and the style you are trying to create.

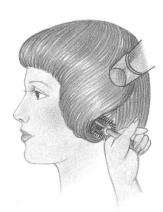

Figure 13.5
Curling the hair forward

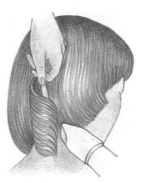

Figure 13.6
Rotating the brush in a vertical position

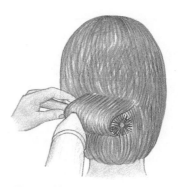

Figure 13.7
Rotating the brush in a horizontal position

7. Dry and shape the hair ends in the nape, top, and crown sections into place.

8. Arrange stray ends with the styling comb as needed to complete the coiffure (Figures 13.8 and 13.9). Spray with fixative of your choice. Screen the client's face with the edge of your hand when you spray.

7. This is standard procedure for finishing the hairstyle.

8. The ends may need arranging. The hair becomes sticky if too much spray is used. Apply the fixative from at least 12 inches (30 centimeters) away from the hair to avoid "wetting" the hair with droplets of spray, which will cause the hair to straighten. **Be careful** not to spray into the client's eyes or ears or on his or her clothing.

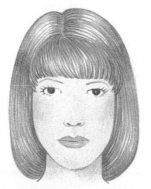

Figure 13.8
Hair styled forward, toward the face

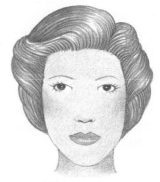

Figure 13.9
Hair "feathered" away from the face

Supplies

- shampoo supplies
- electric air waver (hot comb)
- 28-tooth comb attachment for air waver

- hard rubber air-waving (styling) comb
- air-waving lotion

Procedure

1. Shampoo and towel-dry the hair. Analyze and condition the hair if necessary. Apply air-waving lotion and comb it evenly through the hair.

2. Turn on the air waver to low temperature and fast air speed. Subdivide the hair into strands about the same size as those used for a roller setting.

3. Hold the end of the strand with your left hand and place the metal air comb close to, **but not on,** the scalp (Figure 13.10). Moving your right wrist in a circular pattern, turn the comb attachment against the hair (Figure 13.11). Fasten dried hair with a clip until it has cooled.

4. Use a regular styling comb (hard rubber) on very short strands.

5. Slide the air comb close to the scalp toward the face at an angle that matches the desired wave pattern.

Rationale

1. Special air-waving lotions are best for the hair and the air-waving implements; regular styling lotions may stick to the air comb and styling comb.

2. Starting at a lower temperature helps prevent accidentally burning the client's scalp or face. Smaller strands are easier to control and dry quickly. Roller-size sections afford the most durable hairstyle.

3. Rotating the air comb gives height and strength to the base of each hair strand. The hair will relax into a straighter position if it is not clipped into place and allowed to cool at room temperature.

4. Hard rubber combs stand up to heat better than plastic combs. The large hard rubber air-waving comb is easier to use except on very short hair.

5. This technique shapes the hair into the desired formation.

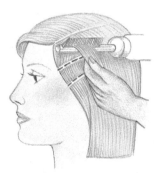

Figure 13.10
The air comb is next to the scalp, not on it.

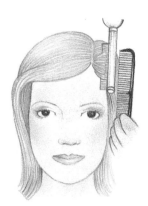

Figure 13.11
Turn the air comb against the hair.

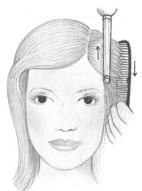

Figure 13.12
Slide the air comb to the right while moving the styling comb to the left.

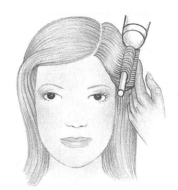

Figure 13.13
Direct the flow of air away from the scalp. Use your left hand to support the hair.

6. Insert the air comb into the hairline, shaping toward the crown. Insert the styling comb behind the air comb and the first ridge of the wave pattern (Figure 13.12). Slide the air comb upward toward the right while shifting the styling comb to the left.

7. Use your left hand to support the hair in the side section while flipping the ends there (Figure 13.13). Continue to dry the hair until a diagonal wave is formed in this section.

6. Gentle but correct use of the comb against the attachment gives the base and ridge of the wave their form. Be sure that the air does not blow on the client's face or scalp.

7. Using the fingers of either hand to assist the air-waving comb is often easier than using a styling comb (depending on the length of the hair).

Sanitize your area as follows:
1. Wash, wipe, and store bottles and supplies.
2. Discard used supplies.
3. Clean and sanitize the cape and apron.
4. Sanitize the work area; wash your hands.

Air waver (blow comb) An electrical appliance that blows heated air that is used in air waving the hair.

Air waving Using electrically heated air and combing techniques to dry shampooed hair into small wave patterns.

Blow comb See **Air waver.**

Blow waver (hand dryer) An electrical appliance that blows heated air that is used in blow waving the hair.

Blow waving Using electrically heated air and combing techniques to dry shampooed hair into large wave patterns.

Denman brush A brush that is good for blow waving short hair.

Diffuser A blow waver attachment that spreads the flow of air over a greater area so that it does not come out of the end of the waver so fast; it dries the hair more slowly.

Hand dryer See **Blow waver.**

Hot comb See **Air waver.**

Nozzle attachment A blow waver attachment that directs a narrow flow of air quickly through the barrel and out the end of the waver; it dries the hair more rapidly.

Round brush A brush that is good for blow waving when more curl is desired.

Vent brush A good all-purpose brush for blow waving.

Watt A measure of the amount of power needed to run hair-drying appliances.

1. Write a brief paragraph explaining the difference between air waving and blow waving.
2. What do the initials "U.L." stand for?
3. Why is it important to direct the flow of air in the same direction as the cuticle of the hair shaft?
4. In your own words, write at least two sentences explaining how a client could be injured with an air waver or blow waver.
5. What is the name for the blow-waving attachment that directs a narrow flow of air toward the hair?
6. What is the name for the blow-waving attachment that spreads out and reduces the flow of air toward the hair?
7. Explain what would happen if the hair fixative (spray, spritz, and so forth) is held too close to the hair when sprayed.
8. What can you use to shield the client's face from hair spray?

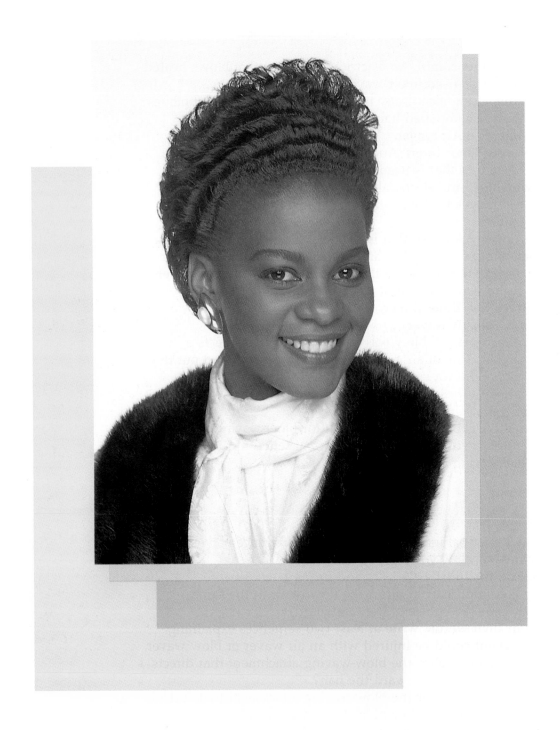

270

Iron Curls

Learning Objective

Using a professional curling iron and supplies, curl the hair with the curling iron and comb the curls into a hairstyle. Use the proper steps and safety precautions to curl the hair in 20–30 minutes; then comb in the hairstyle in 20–30 minutes. Score 85 percent or better on a multiple-choice exam on the information in this chapter.

In order to achieve the above level of competence, you should master the following chapter objectives.

Theory Objectives

1. List the types of electric curling irons and the different sizes of irons.
2. Identify the parts of a curling iron.
3. Describe basic types of curls made with the marcel iron.
4. Explain how curls are formed using the marcel iron.

Practical Objective

5. Give a basic hairstyle using the marcel iron.

Introduction

Previous chapters have been concerned with the curling of wet hair. This chapter presents a way to curl the hair when it is dry. You can give dry hair different degrees of curliness using a thermal (heat) process. Implements used in the thermal process are called thermal irons or curling irons. The process of curling the hair with an iron is called thermal waving or iron curling (the terms are used interchangeably). This can be done with several different thermal irons. Wigs and hairpieces made from human hair may also be curled by using the thermal process. In the salon, hairstyling with the curling iron will often follow blow waving or the drying services.

Theory Objective 1
Types of Electric Curling Irons and Iron Sizes

Thermal curling or waving of the hair was originally called **marceling.** It was named after Marcel Grateau, a Frenchman who perfected the curling iron and hair curling techniques in 1875. The original iron was called the marcel iron, and the service given with this iron was called **marcel waving.**

Three basic types of electric curling irons are in use today: the **spring-clamp iron,** the **marcel iron,** and the **crimping iron,** which is used for certain special effects. Of the first two, professionals tend to prefer the **marcel iron** because it is sturdier, the shell clamp of its barrel opens wider to accept more hair, and it heats faster and more evenly than the spring-clamp iron (Figures 14.1 and

Figure 14.1
Electric marcel iron

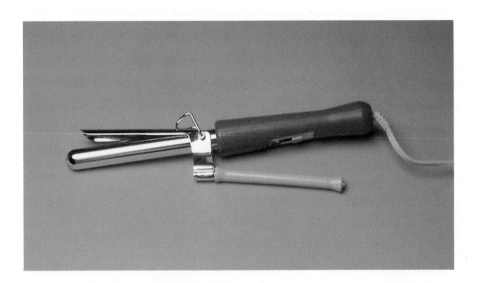

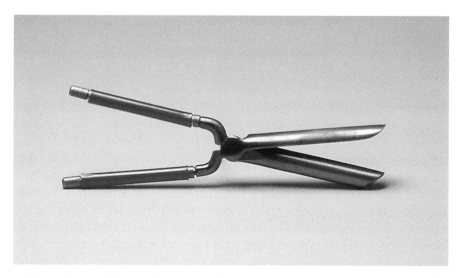

Figure 14.2
Marcel iron for use with heater

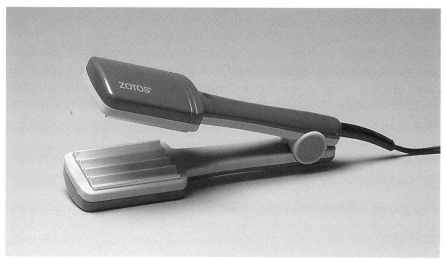

Figure 14.3
Crimping iron

14.2). The marcel iron is made of very fine-quality steel so that the barrel heats evenly. Years ago, a small gas burner was designed specifically for heating marcel irons. Gas burners are rarely used today, however.

The **crimping iron** comes with several sets of metal plates that form different curling or straightening patterns when used with **long hair** (Figure 14.3). These plates slide in and out of the basic electric heating mechanism that forms the handles. The crimping iron "presses" different degrees of curliness into long hair (strands of hair that are longer than 6 inches/15 centimeters) in much the same way that a waffle iron works in your kitchen. These curls create a "rippling" effect on the surface of the hair (Figure 14.4). Another set of plates can be used to straighten hair.

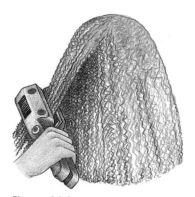

Figure 14.4
A rippling effect achieved with a crimping iron

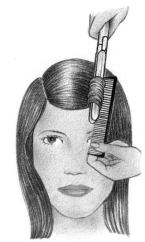

Figure 14.5
The comb protects the scalp.

Safety Tip ▶

Electric irons come in three sizes. The small **midget iron,** which is also called the **mini iron** (1/4 inch/.625 centimeters in diameter), is used to curl shorter hair (less than 3 inches/7.5 centimeters) or hair around the hairline; the medium (1/2 inch/1.25 centimeters in diameter) and large (3/4 inch/1.875 centimeters in diameter) irons are used to curl longer hair.

Modern electric curling irons heat more evenly than earlier irons, and the temperature of the iron is also easier to control. Nevertheless, curling irons become quite hot, and you should take several precautions when working with them. When winding the hair in the iron close to the scalp, the cosmetologist must put a comb between the iron and the scalp to **prevent the heat from burning the client's skin** (Figure 14.5). The styling comb used with the spring-clamp iron or the marcel curling iron should be hard, nonflammable rubber, new technology teflon, or some other heat-resistant material. Be careful when using inexpensive plastic combs because they may melt. You should also take care that your curling iron does not touch a **plastic cape because it also will melt.**

Remember, you and your client can be severely burned on the forehead, ears, neck, arms, and other parts of the body with your electric curling iron. You should practice on your mannequin until your instructor feels that you have developed enough control of the iron to use it on a client.

Theory Objective 2
Parts of the Curling Iron

The **barrel** (sometimes called **rod**) of the iron is the metal, nonmovable, hot part against which the hair is pressed to achieve curl (Figure 14.6). The curling iron has two moving parts that are used in the curling process: the shell/handle and the swivel base. The **shell clamp** is a C-shaped metal clamp that holds the hair against the barrel of the iron while you rotate the handle to form the curl. The other end of the clamp is the **shell handle,** which is held in your hand. The **swivel base,** which is located at the bottom of the iron, allows you to rotate the iron without twisting the power (electric) cord. When purchasing an iron, you should make sure that it has a swivel base. The swivel makes the iron safer in two respects. First, the swivel prevents the wires in the power cord from becoming twisted, which could cause an electrical fire. Secondly, since the wires won't become twisted, you are less likely to have a broken wire that would prevent your iron from heating properly. Some irons also have a **thermostat switch** that allows you to adjust the temperature of the iron.

Another moving part is the **safety rest (support clip),** which is used to rest your curling iron on your work station without burning the countertop.

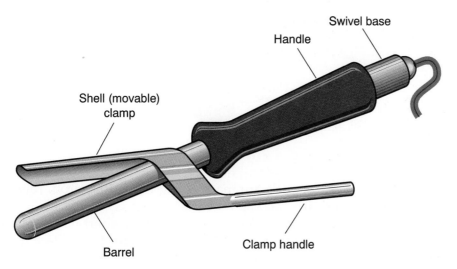

Figure 14.6
Parts of the curling iron

When curling the hair, you should consider the amount of volume you want in the finished hairstyle. The same principles that apply to rollers set in wet hair (see Chapter 10) apply to the thermal curling of dry hair.

No-stem iron curls placed on their bases will result in the maximum amount of **volume** (fullness and height) in your hairstyle. **Half-stem iron curls** (half on and half off base) will result in half as much volume as the no-stem curls. **Long-stem iron curls** placed off-base will give your hairstyle the least amount of lift and volume (Figure 14.7).

Figure 14.7
Types of curls made with a marcel iron

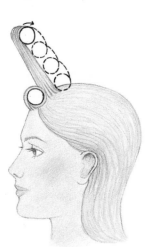
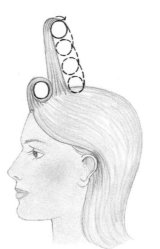
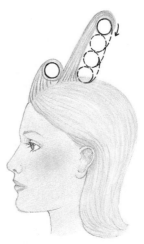

(a) No-stem: maximum height and fullness

(b) Half-stem: half as much volume as no-stem

(c) Long-stem: least amount of volume

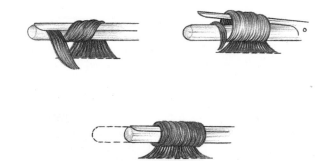

Figure 14.8
Forming a round curl

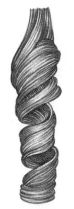

Figure 14.10
Candlestick curl

Three types of curls are made using the curling iron: roller curls, croquignole curls, and spiral curls.

The **roller curl** (round) involves winding a short hair strand from the end of the strand toward the scalp (Figure 14.8). Place the comb between the iron and the scalp for protection. When the heat penetrates the strand to the outside hair, hold the strand with the edge of your comb and slip the iron out of the side of the curl. Then (for a tighter curl) clip the curl into place and allow it to cool at room temperature.

For the **croquignole curl,** use your fingers to rotate the handle and turn your wrist to wind the strand in small or large sections from the scalp to the ends. If you release the tension on the hair strand often enough, you will be able to "feed" the hair entirely around the barrel of the iron. This technique will require a lot of practice.

The **spiral curl** (poker curling) is really a combination of the spiral and croquignole methods. Wind the strand from the scalp in a spiral fashion (Figure 14.9). The resulting curl looks like a spiral candle, and this technique is sometimes called candlestick curling. Then the curls are called **candlestick curls** (Figure 14.10).

Figure 14.9
Forming a spiral curl

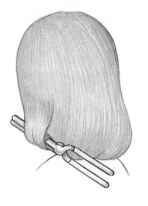
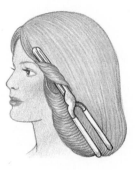
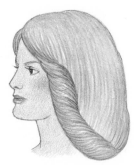

The electric curling iron should be used to make curls only on clean, dry hair. **If the hair is wet, steam will cause damage (scorching) to the hair**. Normal penetration of the heat rising from the barrel of the iron up through the hair strand causes the hair to curl. The amount of curl will be determined by the length of the hair and the diameter of the barrel of the iron used. For example, if you only want to curl the ends of medium-length hair, you would probably use a large-diameter iron on the ends of the hair strands. The temperature of the iron also determines the amount of time the process will take and the amount of curliness that will be achieved. The hotter the iron, the faster the hair will curl.

Always **pretest** the temperature of your iron before using it. This is important because some fine, lightened, or chemically treated hair will scorch very easily. One way to pretest the temperature of your iron is to clamp the barrel across a piece of white tissue paper or Sanek-type neck strip for 4–7 seconds. If the barrel scorches the paper, the iron is too hot. Turn the temperature control to a lower setting, and allow the iron to cool off. Another method is to **towel cool** your iron. Spray a towel with cool water and clamp your iron across the damp towel for a couple of seconds. Then clamp the iron across a dry towel to remove any traces of moisture.

Figure 14.11 reviews the parts of a curling iron, and Figures 14.12 through 14.19 explain the basic techniques involved in using the iron. Then Figures 14.20 through 14.23 show how curls are formed on short hair; Figures 14.24 through 14.28 show how to curl

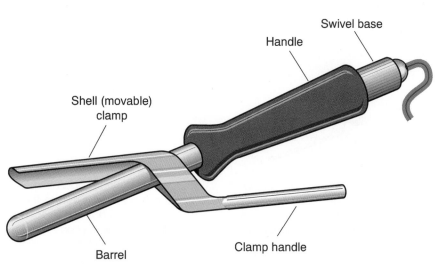

Figure 14.11
Parts of the curling iron

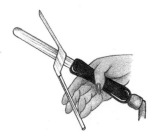

Figure 14.12
To open and close the shell clamp, use your little finger as shown.

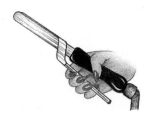

Figure 14.13
Use your ring, middle, and index fingers to close the clamp against the barrel.

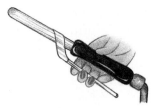

Figure 14.14
Note the position of the thumb has changed to help rotate the handle of the iron.

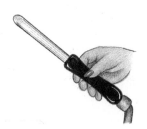

Figure 14.15
The iron has been rotated 1/4 turn in a counterclockwise direction away from your body.

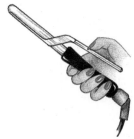

Figure 14.16
In rotating the iron 1/2 turn, note how the thumb opens the clamp to allow the iron to be rotated.

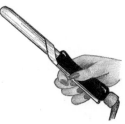

Figure 14.17
To achieve a 3/4 rotation, press the thumb against the clamp handle to continue the rotation of the iron.

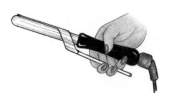

Figure 14.18
Practice turning your curling iron.

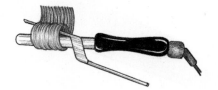

Figure 14.19
Practice the two basic curling manipulations—opening and closing the iron. The iron should be opened and closed using a quick, "clicking" action to release tension from the hair and avoid binding the hair strand. Rotate the iron as you practice the clicking manipulation.

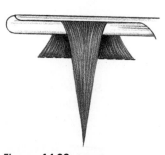

Figure 14.20
With the clamp open, apply the barrel of the iron to the base of the hair for 5 seconds (time will depend on the heat of the iron and the condition and texture of the hair).

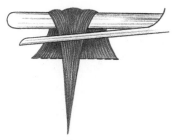

Figure 14.21
Using the medium tension, close the clamp, rotate the iron toward yourself as shown, and remember to place your comb between the hair and the scalp for the protection of the client.

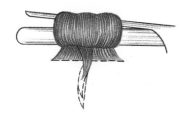

Figure 14.22
As you open and close the clamp, feed the hair strand into the curl.

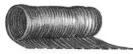

Figure 14.23
After the hair has been wound into the curl, allow the heat to penetrate the hair. Hold the curl in place with the edge (teeth) of your comb, and slide the barrel of the iron out of the curl.

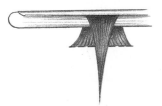

Figure 14.24
For medium hair lengths, form the base of the curl as shown in Figure 14.20 for short hair.

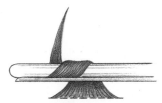

Figure 14.25
Click and rotate the clamp 1/2 turn downward, and hold the end of the strand with your other hand.

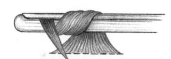

Figure 14.26
Continue rotating the iron and feed the end of the strand into the curl.

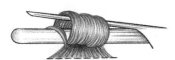

Figure 14.27
As you near the end of the strand, open the clamp a little, and slip the end of the strand between the clamp and the barrel of the iron. Close the iron.

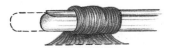

Figure 14.28
Slide the iron toward its cord to bring the end into the center of the curl. Rotate your iron to distribute the heat evenly across the curl. Open the clamp and slide the barrel out of the curl.

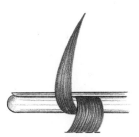

Figure 14.29
For long hair, form the base; wind the hair one revolution around the iron.

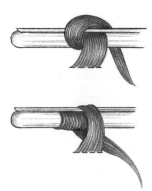

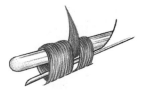

Figure 14.30
Wind the hair over the clamp, and let the end hang toward the cord of the iron. Use a 1/4 turn and clicking rotations; quickly feed the hair into the curl. Slide your iron so that the end of the strand falls toward the center of the curl.

Figure 14.31
Use a 3/4 turn, and clicking rotations to draw the hair into the curl formation.

medium-length hair; and Figures 14.29 through 14.31 illustrate how these techniques are applied to long hair.

Practical Objective 5
Basic Hairstyle Using the Marcel Iron

Supplies

- shampoo supplies, plus chair
- cloth and neck strip
- combs: hard rubber or heat resistant (rake, rat-tail, styling comb)
- hair spray
- temperature testing tissue
- electric outlet for iron
- duck-bill clips

Preparation for Curling

Procedure	Rationale
1. Drape the client in a heat-resistant cape. Shampoo and thoroughly dry the hair. Condition hair as needed. Apply styling preparation.	**1.** A plastic shampoo cape would melt from the heat of the curling iron. A cape made of cotton, rayon, and the like will not melt. It is also cooler and is therefore more comfortable for the client.

2. Preheat your iron(s).

2. This should be standard procedure. The temperature of your iron will be determined by the texture, length, and condition of the client's hair.

3. Select an iron with a small, medium, or large barrel.

3. The circumference of the iron is determined by the length and texture of the hair. The large barrel is best for medium to long hair. The large iron will not give a small enough curl on long hair, however, and the small (mini) iron will give a better curl on short hair. Short, fine hair (especially strands around the hairline) requires an iron with a smaller diameter (mini) than long, coarse hair does.

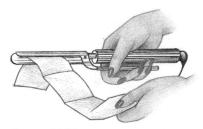

Figure 14.32
Pretest the temperature.

4. Pretest the temperature of the iron (Figure 14.32).

4. This helps you avoid applying too much heat to the hair and helps you control the heat of the iron. Use the ring and little fingertips of your hand to control the clamp handle (Figure 14.33). Be careful not to burn the client's skin, hair, or scalp!

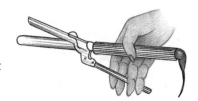

Figure 14.33
Control the clamp handle with the ring and little fingers.

Making Roller Curls

Procedure

1. Dry drape the client with a cloth or nylon cape. Begin curling the hair in the same sequence you used to set wet hair. Select the first strand to be curled.

Rationale

1. This is the easiest way to curl the hair if a roller-type hairstyle is desired. The size of the subsection will be determined by the texture and density of the hair. Fine, thin hair will normally require larger sections than coarse, dense hair. A plastic cape will **melt.**

2. Hold the hair strand and comb in one hand and hold the iron in your other hand. A metal comb is **not** recommended.

2. This is standard procedure. A metal comb may transfer heat to the scalp, causing a **burn.**

3. Practice holding the iron and clicking it (opening and closing the clamp) while rotating the comb. The barrel, not the clamp of the iron, curls the hair. The clamp merely holds the hair between movements.

3. Effective thermal waving takes practice. You can practice by using a cold iron on a mannequin.

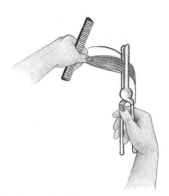

Figure 14.34
Wind the hair strand around the barrel of the iron.

4. Grab the hair near the scalp with the clamp on top of the barrel (Figure 14.34). Rotate the iron ½ turn downward; then, use your clicking technique to "feed" the hair onto the iron (Figure 14.35). Continue to rotate the iron using your thumb, middle, ring, and little fingers to manipulate your iron.

4. You will scorch the hair and damage it unless you keep the clamp moving as you are rotating the iron. Maintain control of the iron at all times. Long hair will require more rotations (turns of the iron) than short hair.

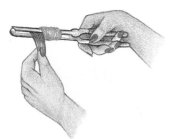

Figure 14.35
Slowly "feed" hair around the iron.

5. Hold the strand away from the scalp, and put the barrel of the iron against the hair next to the scalp. Push the iron against the scalp hair and bring the end of the strand toward you. Rock the iron against the base of the strand to form the base of the curl.

5. This directs the base of the hair strand to give it the same height and strength as a curl formed when setting wet hair.

6. Open the clamp and wind the strand between the barrel; then close the clamp to where it pivots next to the handle.

6. This is standard procedure.

7. Hold the end of the strand with your left hand. Curl this part of the strand (next

7. This procedure gives an even curl to each section of the strand.

to the head) by rocking the iron against the strand in a movement horizontal to the head. Spiral the strand between the clamp and the barrel next to the first part of the strand; repeat until the entire length of the strand has been curled.

8. **Place your comb between the iron and the scalp** (Figure 14.36). Carefully place your fingertips on the hair that is wound around the barrel.

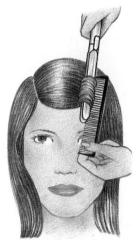

Figure 14.36
Protect the scalp with your comb.

8. You must place the comb carefully between the iron and the scalp. You can "feel" the heat as it radiates from the barrel through the hair.

9. Hold the curl in place with the edge of your comb. Slide the iron horizontally out the side of the curl and clip the curl to the scalp in the same way you would clip a roller curl. Do not allow the curl to unwind before clipping it into place. If you need assistance, consult your instructor.

9. The hair is quite warm when the iron is removed. A more durable curl is formed if the hair is allowed to cool in a clipped rather than an unclipped and unwound position.

10. Use the curling iron on all of the hair strands.

10. This is standard procedure.

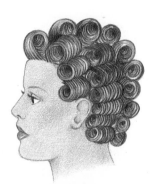

11. Clip the curls and let them cool. All curls should be allowed to cool before the clips are removed for styling.

11. This is standard procedure.

12. Remove the clips and arrange the hair into the desired hairstyle (Figure 14.37).

12. This is standard procedure.

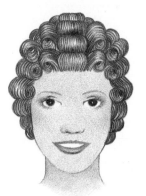

Figure 14.37
The completed curling pattern

Making a Wave Shaping

Procedure

1. To make a wave pattern, insert the iron diagonally in the hair to the outside

Rationale

1. This is how you should begin to form the wave ridge.

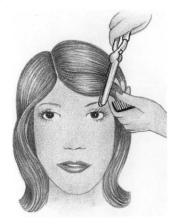

Figure 14.38
To make a soft wave, place the iron diagonal to the front hairline.

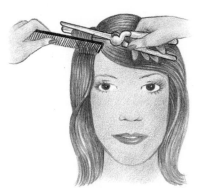

Figure 14.39
Shift hair beneath the iron to form a wave.

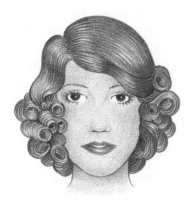

Figure 14.40
The finished thermal wave

corner of the left eyebrow (Figure 14.38).

2. Reverse the rotation of the iron, but return it to the original position.

3. Place the iron across the ridge, but do not close the clamp. Shift the hair beneath the iron with the comb to make the wave pattern (Figure 14.39).

4. Repeat steps 1, 2, and 3, until the hair on the bottom of the side hairline has been waved (Figure 14.40).

5. Wipe iron(s) with 70 percent alcohol.

2. This gives you an even ridge.

3. This is standard procedure.

4. This is standard procedure.

5. Keep your iron clean and sanitized using 70 percent alcohol. A towel with some ammonia on the corner will also dissolve residue from the barrel of your curling iron. Use steel wool too, if needed.

Sanitize your area as follows:
1. Wash, wipe, and store bottles and supplies.
2. Discard used supplies.
3. Clean and sanitize the cape and apron.
4. Sanitize the work area; wash your hands.

Barrel (of the iron) The metal, nonmovable, hot part of the iron that the hair is pressed against to achieve curl; sometimes called the rod.

Candlestick curls Curls made using a combination of the spiral and croquignole methods; also called poker curls.

Crimping iron An iron that creates a rippling effect on long hair.

Croquignole curl A curl formed by rotating the handle of the curling iron.

Half-stem iron curl A curl that is half on and half off base, resulting in half as much volume as a no-stem curl.

Iron curling The process of curling the hair with an iron; also called thermal waving.

Long-stem iron curl A curl that is placed off base, resulting in hairstyles with the least amount of lift and volume.

Marcel waving The service given by the original marcel iron.

Midget iron A small iron ¼ inch (.625 centimeters) in diameter; also called a mini iron.

Mini iron A small iron ¼ inch (.625 centimeters) in diameter; also called a midget iron.

No-stem iron curls Curls placed on their bases, resulting in maximum volume (fullness and height) in a hairstyle.

Pretest The process of checking the temperature of the iron on white tissue paper or a Sanek-type neck strip for 4–7 seconds before using it on a client.

Roller curl A curl made by winding a short hair strand from the end of the strand toward the scalp.

Safety rest The moving part that is used to rest the iron on the work station; also called the support clip.

Shell clamp The C-shaped metal clamp of the iron that holds the hair against the barrel.

Shell handle The end of the clamp of the iron that is held in the hand.

Spiral curl A combination of the spiral and croquignole methods; also called a poker curl.

Spring-clamp iron A type of curling iron with a spring attached to the clamp.

Support clip The moving part that is used to rest the iron on the work station; also called the safety rest.

Swivel base The part of the iron that allows it to be rotated without twisting the power cord.

Thermal irons Implements used to curl the hair with a thermal (heat) process; also called curling irons.

Thermal waving The process of curling the hair with an iron; also called iron curling.

Thermostat switch The switch that allows the user to control an iron's temperature.

Towel cooling The process of cooling the iron by clamping it across a damp towel for a few seconds.

Questions

1. What implements are used to curl the hair using heat?
2. What name is commonly used for the professional iron?
3. What are the differences between the spring-clamp iron and the marcel iron?
4. Explain the difference between the marcel iron and the crimping iron.
5. Which iron is used to achieve a special rippling effect on the hair?
6. Which iron would you recommend for curling very short hair?
7. During the marceling process, what should you do to avoid burning the scalp?
8. When iron curling the hair, what kind of cape should you use?
9. What material is the barrel of the curling iron made of?
10. What is another term for marceling or marcel waving?
11. Name the main chemical used to clean the thermal iron.
12. What part of some curling irons allows you to adjust the temperature?
13. Before using the marcel iron on the hair, what safety precaution should you take?
14. Write a short definition for the croquignole, spiral, and roller techniques, respectively.
15. Is it necessary to examine the scalp before curling the hair?
16. Is thermal curling given on wet or dry hair?
17. Should the hair be shampooed before the thermal service?
18. Should you use the same iron temperature on all types of hair?
19. How dry should the hair be before you use your curling iron?

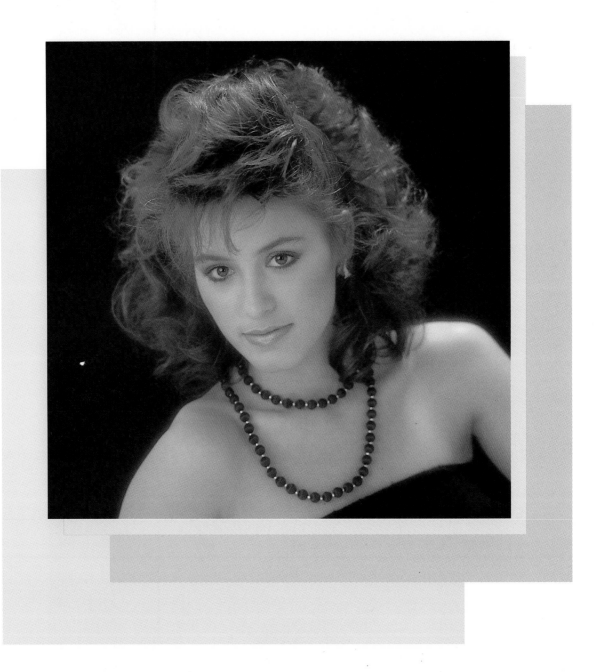

Temporary Hair Coloring

Learning Objective

Use the proper steps to apply temporary hair color(s) to the client's hair. Using the proper safety precautions and following label directions, apply a temporary hair color to the client's hair in 3 to 5 minutes. Score 85 percent or better on a multiple-choice exam on the information in this chapter.

In order to achieve the above level of competence, you should master the following chapter objectives.

Theory Objectives

1. Define temporary hair coloring and describe the early use and development of hair-coloring techniques.
2. Describe the advantages and disadvantages of different types of temporary hair colors.
3. Define the primary, secondary, and tertiary colors.

Practical Objective

4. Select and apply temporary rinses.

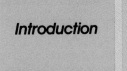

Introduction

Dyes, lighteners, frosts, tints, streaks, and tips—you may have heard some of these terms, and you may know a little about some of them. Or you may not know a thing about any of them. All of these products and many more besides have been used to make the color of the hair somehow different and better. For centuries, men and women have tried to give the hair more "exciting" or more "natural" looking color; sometimes they have done this by changing the hair color, sometimes by highlighting the natural color.

You will learn about these processes and products in this and the following chapters. Temporary hair-coloring services are one of the five most profitable services salons have to offer. By mastering the skills presented in this chapter, you will be able to improve your client's appearance and earn quite a bit of money.

Salons offer many different kinds of hair-coloring treatments. **This chapter shows** the techniques used for applying **temporary colors.** The chapters that follow will deal with other color treatments.

Theory Objective 1
Temporary Hair Coloring and Early Use and Development of Hair-Coloring Products

Any preparation that deposits color on or into the hair is called a **hair dye.** Dyes that color the hair from shampoo to shampoo are called **temporary rinses.** All hair colors should be applied immediately before the hair is styled. Temporary hair coloring is the process of changing the hair color by coating the clear cuticle of the hair with a color pigment. **Pigment** is the substance that gives color to something. The color of the hair is determined by the number and color of particles of **melanin** (MEL-eh-nehn), a kind of pigment, it contains.

For thousands of years, people have changed their hair color, using hair-coloring products made from a variety of substances. Vegetable dyes were among the earliest kinds of hair color used. Temporary colors were made from certain vegetables and herbs. About four thousand years ago, the Egyptians used vegetable dyes called **henna** (HEN-ah) and **camomile** (KAM-ah-mighl) (Figure 15.1). **Henna** colors the hair red (henna is made as a semipermanent hair color), and **camomile** colors the hair blonde. Both of them coat (cover) the cuticle (outside) of the hair shaft (Figures 15.2, 15.3, and 15.4). They are called **progressive dyes,** because with each application they build up on the hair and make the color darker and darker. This buildup is called a **color buildup.**

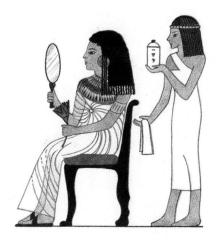

Figure 15.1
The ancient Egyptians used vegetable dyes such as henna.

Metallic salt dyes came into use later. They are combinations of copper, lead, silver, and other metals as well as **pyrogallol** (pigh-roh-GAL-ol), a weak acid.

Over the years, compound dyes were developed. They are combinations of vegetable dyes and metallic salt dyes.

All these dyes have serious disadvantages. Vegetable and herbal dyes coat the hair too much. The color tends to look unnatural, and it is difficult to remove. Metallic salt preparations can cause discoloration of the hair, and compound dyes can cause all these problems. The hair may feel brittle and have a dull appearance. Although some hair-coloring products for home use contain metallic salts and compound dyes, the salon products that you will use do not contain these substances.

Have you ever seen someone with orange, green, or purple hair? He or she certainly wasn't born with it! This person probably

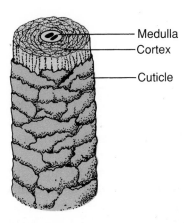

Medulla
Cortex

Cuticle

Figure 15.2
Imbricated cuticle layer of the hair shaft

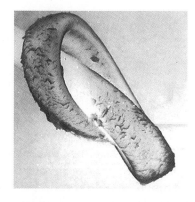

Figure 15.3
A knotted piece of hair. Note that as the hair is twisted, the cuticle layers stand away from the shaft.

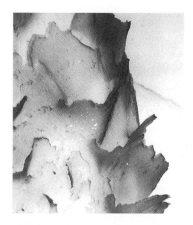

Figure 15.4
Cuticle layers of a hair as seen by a scanning electron microscope

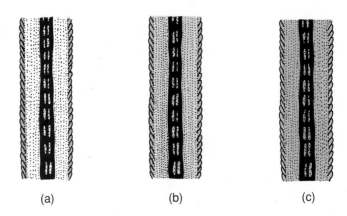

Figure 15.5
Action of hair-coloring products: (a) temporary color coats cuticle; (b) semipermanent color partially penetrates cortex; (c) permanent color completely penetrates hair shaft.

(a)   (b)   (c)

used a home-care product that did not react properly with a product that was already on the hair.

The same thing is true for professional products. **Never cold wave, lighten, or permanently color** hair that already has a metallic salt product on it. Salon products do **not** combine well with metallic salts and will result in unnatural hair colors.

Three types of hair-coloring products are used in the salon today: temporary, semipermanent, and permanent. Temporary coloring products only remain in the hair from one shampoo to the next. Semipermanent colors last through 4 to 6 shampoos. Permanent hair-coloring preparations remain in the hair until the dyed hair grows out and is cut off (Figure 15.5).

Each type of hair color has a different chemical makeup, different effects, and different uses. This chapter will focus on temporary coloring and present a few principles common to all three types. Semipermanent and permanent coloring will be discussed in the next two chapters.

Theory Objective 2
Advantages and Disadvantages of Different Types of Temporary Hair Colors

Temporary colors remain on the hair for a short time—only until the next shampoo. They thinly **coat** the hair cuticle but do not penetrate into the cortex because their molecules are too large. They are available as rinses, sprays, creams, powders, crayons, and shampoos. All, except powders, are in ready-to-use form.

Color rinses are the most commonly used form of temporary color. This is why temporary colors are often called **temporary rinses.** These rinses generally come in plastic applicator bottles (Figure 15.6). Many kinds of rinses are on the market. They can have different combinations of chemicals and colors, but they usually contain water, **azo** dyes (a group of synthetic dyes), and colors made

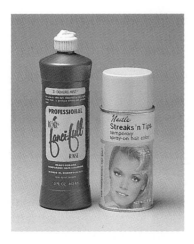

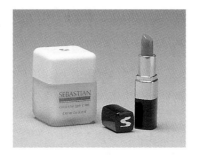

Figure 15.7
*Cream color and crayon hair
colors*

Figure 15.6
*Color rinses come in plastic
applicator bottles while spray
colors come in aerosol cans.*

from vegetables and herbs. These products are often acid-balanced. The cuticle layer of the hair shaft (the layer that protects the cortex) attracts rinses. The color settles into the scaly crevices of the cuticle and lightly coats it.

Spray colors come in aerosol cans (Figure 15.6). These aerosols contain water, color pigments, and a gas propellant called freon, which shoots the pigment from the can. They can be sprayed onto the hair after a shampoo or comb-out, depending on the kind used. They are used mainly to create unusual effects.

Cream colors come in small jars or tubes (Figure 15.7). They are used mostly by persons performing on stage, because they can be removed easily.

Powder colors need to be mixed with water before they are brushed through the hair. They are not ordinarily used in the salon.

Crayon hair colors, which look very much like tubes of lipstick, contain color pigments combined with a synthetic wax base (Figure 15.7). Crayons color the hair as they are rubbed against it. They are used to cover gray or to blend in new growth in permanently colored hair.

You probably have seen advertisements for "miracle" coloring products. Always keep one thing in mind: no product can work "miracles!" Instead of miracles, each product can offer only advantages and disadvantages. Be cautious and skeptical. By doing so, you will be doing yourself and your client a big favor.

Temporary color rinses offer several **advantages:**

1. The natural pH of the hair is not changed to any great extent, so the condition of the hair remains the same.

2. Clients can highlight or darken natural color, cover gray, and improve off-shades, all with the convenience of quick removal by shampoo.

3. Unless specified by the manufacturer, a predisposition (allergy) test is not required.

4. Since temporary colors usually do not need time to develop, they are quick and convenient to apply.

5. Many ready-to-use colors are available.

6. Temporary colors may be mixed to achieve different colors: However, only products manufactured by the same company may be mixed. Thus, a color of Brand X may be mixed with another color of Brand X, but not with Brand Y.

Temporary colors rinses also have several **disadvantages:**

1. Some temporary rinses rub off on clothing and pillowcases.

2. Excessive perspiration from the scalp may carry color from the hair onto clothing.

3. Temporary rinses **cannot lighten** natural hair color.

4. Temporary rinses may not color the hair evenly.

5. The color has to be applied after every shampoo.

6. Since it is a coating process, the color may not have the natural luster that semipermanent and permanent colors give the hair. For example, resistant hair may not accept very much color at all, and porous hair may accept too much color.

When deciding on a product, you must first ask, What is the client's purpose or need? For example, a client who is cautiously experimenting with hair coloring may see quick removal as an advantage. On the other hand, a client who is comfortable with coloring may see quick removal as a disadvantage.

Theory Objective 3
Primary, Secondary, and Tertiary Colors

To master hair-coloring techniques, you must first have a basic knowledge of color and color mixing.

Colors are divided into two types: chromatic and achromatic. Black, white, and gray are **achromatic** (ak-rah-MAT-ik) **colors.** All other colors are **chromatic** (kroh-MAT-ik). In addition to studying the mixing of chromatic colors, you must learn how to apply specific coloring principles to select or correct a client's hair color. The chart on pages 298–99 shows the principles of color mixing that you will use in selecting appropriate colors and correcting color problems.

Chromatic colors are divided into primary, secondary, and tertiary colors:

- The **primary** (PRIGH-mehr-ee) **colors** are red, yellow, and blue. All hair colors can be mixed from two or more of these three colors (Figure 15.8).

- **Secondary colors** (orange, violet, and green) are achieved by mixing equal amounts of two of the primary colors (Figure 15.9). Yellow and red are mixed in equal parts to make orange; red and blue make violet; blue and yellow make green.

- A **tertiary** (TER-shee-ehr-ee) (or intermediate) **color** is created by mixing a primary color with a secondary color (Figure 15.10). The six tertiary colors are made by the following combinations:

  - Yellow + orange = yellow-orange
  - Yellow + green = yellow-green
  - Red + orange = red-orange
  - Red + violet = red-violet
  - Blue + violet = blue-violet
  - Blue + green = blue-green

Complementary (kom-pleh-MEN-tah-ree) colors are directly opposite each other on the chart (Figure 15.11). These opposites (for example, yellow and violet) have a tendency to neutralize each other. Cosmetologists use these opposites to correct hair-coloring problems. For example, if a client has gray hair with unwanted yellow streaks, the cosmetologist would apply a violet-base color called a **bluing rinse. The violet neutralizes the yellow streaks,** and the client's hair appears consistently gray. Similarly, if the hair has a

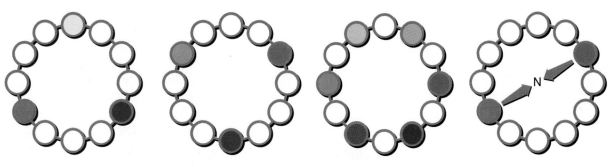

Figure 15.8
Primary colors

Figure 15.9
Secondary colors

Figure 15.10
Tertiary colors

Figure 15.11
Complementary colors

green cast, a red-base color would be used to neutralize the green.

These 12 pure colors form the basis for hair-coloring products used in the salon. If they were used as pure colors, however, they would be unattractive, so manufacturers darken and lighten them. Pure colors are darkened by the addition of black, resulting in a certain **shade of a color.** For example, if blue is darkened by black, the result is navy blue. White added to a pure color produces a **tint of the color.** For instance, pink is a tint of red. When a combination of black and white (in other words, gray) is mixed with a pure color, the result is a **tone of the color.** Rust is a tone of orange.

The federal **Food and Drug Administration (FDA)** labels as **certified** the pure colors used in professional temporary rinses. This means that the colors are safe for application on the scalp and do not require a predisposition (allergy) test.

Because color varies with each application on each client, **it is wise to make a strand test before applying hair coloring to the entire head.** This test of the color in a small area is especially important for semipermanent and permanent coloring, but it is also advisable for temporary rinses.

Practical Objective 4
Selecting and Applying
Temporary Rinses

Supplies

■ shampooing supplies
■ temporary color chart
■ temporary color rinse

■ gloves
■ protective apron

Procedure

1. Shampoo the hair twice and towel-dry.

2. Ask the client what services are desired. Use the color chart to help the client choose a color.

Rationale

1. This removes sebum, soil, sprays, and other residues. Water molecules adhere to cuticle layers, so you must be sure that the hair is fairly dry. Too much water will interfere with the application of color to the cuticle. Do not use an acid rinse before applying temporary color because it will close the cuticle imbrications so much that the color will not stick to the cuticle.

2. If the hair is to be shaped, this should be done before coloring. The client usually has a certain color effect in

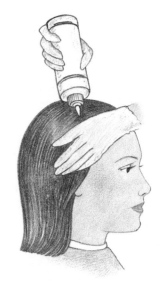

Figure 15.12
Evenly distribute the rinse through the hair. Wear gloves to protect your hands during the application.

3. Ask the client to show you the choice on the color chart. If you feel another selection would be better, explain to the client why you think so.

4. Select a color and read the label directions.

5. Apply the selected rinse (according to directions) around the entire front hairline and **comb it through the hair toward the back of the head.** (Figures 15.12 and 15.13). Towel-blot dripping color from the crown area of the head.

6. Apply a small amount of color across the nape area and comb it toward the bottom hairline.

7. Towel-blot dripping color and begin styling the hair.

mind, but it is your responsibility to discuss color selection with the client.

3. You must find out exactly what color effect the client has in mind. Not all clients know what a temporary color does to hair, so you may have to explain what the rinse can or cannot do.

4. Many temporary coloring products are available; they are applied differently, so you must read the label directions carefully. The label will indicate whether a predisposition test is required.

5. This evenly distributes color through the hair and prevents color from dripping into the client's eyes.

6. Applying small amounts makes it easier to distribute color evenly throughout the hair.

7. Not all temporary colors are set in the hair. **Some must be rinsed** before the hair is styled. Follow the directions on the label.

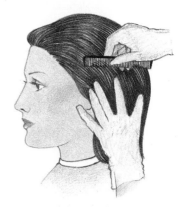

Figure 15.13
Apply the rinse in a chair or at the shampoo bowl.

Sanitize your area as follows:
1. **Wash, wipe, and store bottles and supplies.**
2. **Discard used supplies.**
3. **Clean and sanitize the cape and apron.**
4. **Sanitize the work area; wash your hands.**

ROUX fanci-tone® professional creme hair tint

Color Guide with Shade Level and Base Color Designations

		SHADE LEVELS Code Numbers Indicated on Bottle Label 10 - Lightest 1 - Darkest		Green **Gn** (Drab)	Blue **B** (Ash)
HIGH LIFT BLONDES	Can be used as toners on pre-bleached hair	10	High Lift Blondes	***10 Gn** 101 Lightest Ash Blonde	***10 B** 102 Lightest Smoky Ash Blonde
		9	Palest Blondes	***9 Gn** 19 Sweet Cream *Palest Ash Blonde*	***9 B** 51 Demure Mist *Palest Silvery Ash Blonde*
		8	Pale Blondes	**8 Gn** Whisper Blonde *Pale Ash Beige Blonde*	....
BLONDES AND LIGHT REDS		7	Light Blondes/ Light Red-Blondes	***7 Gn** 18 Spun Sand *Light Ash Blonde*	....
		6	Medium Blondes/ Strawberry Red-Blondes	***6 Gn** 17 Very Vanilla *Medium Ash Blonde*	***6 B** 74 Delicate Dawn *Medium Smoky Ash Blonde*
		5	Dark Blondes/ Bright Red-Blondes	***5 Gn** 16 Hidden Honey *Dark Ash Blonde*	....
REDS AND BROWNS		4	Light Browns/ Light Reds	***4 Gn** 15 Muted Maize *Light Ash Brown*	....
		3	Medium Browns/ Medium Reds	***3 Gn** 14 Pretty Beaver *Medium Ash Brown*	**3 B** 71 Subtle Slate *Medium Smoky Ash Brown*
		2	Dark Browns/ Dark Reds	***2 Gn** 13 Chocolate Kiss *Dark Ash Brown*	....
BLACKS		1	Blacks	***1 Gn** 12 Black Rage *Black*	***1 B** 11 Blue Jet *Blue Black*

Natural Haircolor Levels

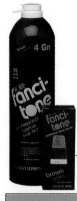

BASE COLOR CODES ON LABELS

R –	Red
G –	Gold (Yellow)
B –	Blue (Ash)
O –	Orange
V –	Violet
Gn –	Green
RGB –	Beige

45 BEAUTIFUL TINT COLORS

All colors are available in 1-application bottles.
*Starred colors also available in economical Professional Dispensers.

PREDOMINANT TINT BASE COLOR

Gold G		Red R		Beige RGB (Red/Gold/Blue)		Violet V	
*10 G 104 Lightest Golden Blonde		————		***10 RGB** 103 Lightest Beige Blonde		***10 BV** 49 ultra White Minx *Lightest White Blonde*	
9 G 27 Tempting Taffy *Palest Golden Blonde*		**9 RV** 54 Barely Pink *Palest Pink Blonde*		**9 RGB** 59 Gentle Doe *Palest Beige Blonde*		***9 BV** 52 White Minx *Palest White Blonde*	
8 G Misty Champagne *Pale Golden Beige Blonde*		————		***8 RGB** 56 Bashful Blonde *Pale Beige Blonde*		**8 BV** 43 Platinum Plus *Pale Platinum Blonde*	
*7 G 26 Golden Spell *Light Golden Blonde*		**7 RG** 35 Just Peachy *Light Red Blonde*		***7 RGB** 57 Saucy Beige *Light Smoky Beige Blonde*		**7 BV** 42 Silver Lining *Light Silver Blonde*	
6 G 25 Gilded Lily *Medium Golden Blonde*		***6 RG** 34 Strawberry Blush *Medium Red Blonde*		————		***6 BV** 41 True Steel (Drabber Only) *Medium Steel Gray*	
*5 G 24 Forbidden Gold *Dark Golden Blonde*		***5 R** 33 Wild Fire *Bright Red*		————		————	
*4 G 23 Frivolous Fawn *Light Golden Brown*		***4 RO** 32 Lucky Copper *Light Auburn*		***4 RGB** 63 Tantalizing Titian *Light Red Brown*		————	
4 GR Sugar & Spice *Light Warm Brown*							
3.5 G 22 Ardent Amber *Medium Golden Brown*							
3 GR Chocolate Royale *Medium Warm Brown*		***3 R** 31 Dark Blaze *Medium Auburn*		***3 RGB** 61 Sizzling Spice *Medium Red Brown*		**3 RV** 81 Russet Rose *Medium Mahogany*	
*3 G 21 Plush Brown *Deepest Medium Golden Brown*							
2 GR Brown Raisin *Dark Warm Brown*		————		————		————	
————		————		————		————	

See reverse side for additional information on Fanci-tone.

Glossary ▮▬▬▬▬▬▬▬▬▬▬▬▬▬▬▬▬▬▬▬▬▬▬▬▬▬▬▬▬

Achromatic (ak-rah-MAT-ik) colors Black, white, and gray.

Azo dyes Synthetic dyes used in hair-coloring products.

Bluing rinse A violet-based temporary color used to neutralize yellow streaks in gray hair.

Camomile (KAM-ah-mighl) A vegetable dye that colors the hair blonde.

Chromatic (kroh-MAT-ik) colors All colors that are not black, white, or gray.

Color buildup A darkening of the hair resulting from the use of progressive dyes that coat and recoat the hair with repeated applications.

Color rinses The most commonly used forms of temporary hair colors; they are applied with an applicator bottle.

Complementary (kom-pleh-MEN-tah-ree) colors Colors directly opposite each other on a color chart.

Crayon hair colors Temporary hair colors that contain pigments combined with a synthetic wax base. They come in a tube and are applied by rubbing against the hair.

Cream colors Temporary hair colors that come in small jars or tubes. They are most often used by persons performing on stage because they can be removed easily.

Hair dye Any preparation that deposits color on or into the hair.

Henna (HEN-ah) A temporary vegetable hair dye that colors the hair red.

Melanin (MEL-eh-nehn) A kind of pigment in the hair that gives it color.

Metallic salt dyes Hair dyes made from combinations of copper, lead, silver, and other metals as well as pyrogallol.

Pigment (PIG-mehnt) A substance that gives color to something, such as hair, skin, or paint.

Powder colors Temporary hair colors that are mixed with water and brushed through the hair; not ordinarily used in the salon.

Primary (PRIGH-mehr-ee) colors Red, yellow, and blue.

Progressive dyes Hair dyes that coat the cuticle of the hair and build up with repeated applications, making the hair darker each time.

Pyrogallol (pigh-roh-GAL-ol) A substance with weak acid properties found in metallic hair dyes.

Secondary colors Orange, violet, and green; these are obtained by mixing equal amounts of two primary colors.

Shade of a color The color obtained when a pure color is darkened by adding black.

Spray hair colors Temporary hair dyes that come in aerosol cans and are sprayed onto the hair after a shampoo or comb-out.

Temporary rinses Temporary hair colors applied with an applicator bottle. They coat only the cuticle of the hair.

Tertiary (TER-shee-ehr-ee) colors Colors obtained by mixing a primary color with a secondary color.

Tint of a color The color obtained when white is added to a pure color.

Tone of a color The color obtained when gray is added to a pure color.

_____ *Questions*

1. What are the three layers of the hair?
2. How long do temporary rinses stay in the hair?
3. Do temporary rinses completely cover gray hair?
4. What are progressive dyes?
5. Is the cuticle layer on the outer or inner part of the hair shaft?
6. What are chromatic colors?
7. What are complementary colors?
8. What name is given to a hair color that lasts only from one shampoo to the next?
9. What is a product or substance that gives color to something else called?
10. Identify the layer of the hair to which temporary colors cling.
11. Can a temporary rinse lighten natural hair color?
12. What name is given to the color used in a temporary rinse?
13. Does a temporary rinse change the natural pH of the hair?
14. Will a temporary rinse completely cover hair that is 70 percent gray?

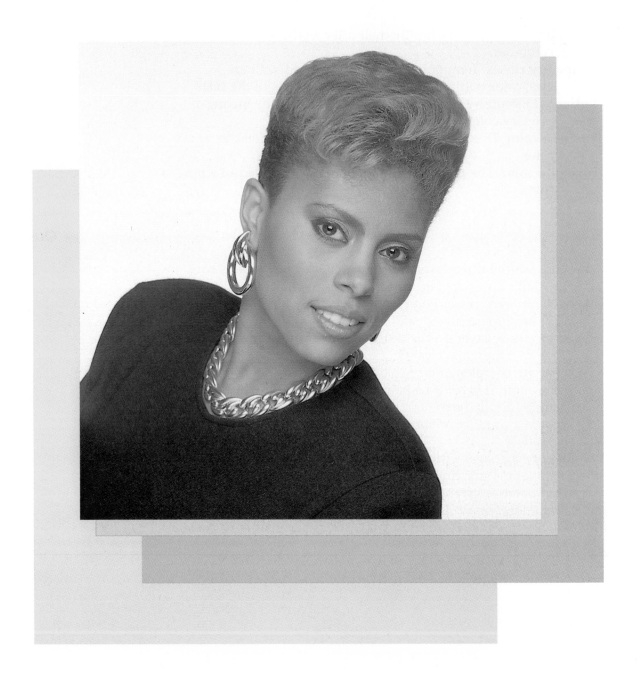

Semipermanent Hair Coloring

Learning Objective

Using an assortment of semipermanent hair colors and a hair-coloring chart, color the client's hair by following the proper steps. Using the proper safety precautions, evenly apply a semipermanent color to the client's hair in 5–10 minutes. Score 85 percent or better on a multiple-choice exam on the information in this chapter.

In order to achieve the above level of competence, you should master the following chapter objectives.

Theory Objectives

1. Define semipermanent hair color; compare it with temporary color; and list the advantages and disadvantages of semipermanent color.
2. Identify the client's hair color.

Practical Objective

3. Select and apply semipermanent hair colors.

Introduction

Many of your clients who have had their hair colored many times in the past will have a fairly good idea of what they want. While they may still ask you for advice, they probably will be fairly comfortable with the whole idea of hair coloring. They will want a semipermanent hair color because it will last up to 4 to 6 shampoos.

If you master the principles involved in applying semipermanent hair colors, you will be able to provide a service that is both fun and profitable.

Theory Objective 1
Semipermanent Hair Color: Definition, Comparison with Temporary Color, and Advantages and Disadvantages

Do you know what the prefix semi means? It means half or midway. **Semipermanent hair-color** rinses are about halfway between temporary and permanent hair colors. They partially penetrate the cortex and put some color inside the hair. But they do not completely penetrate the cortex, and they do not remain in the hair until the hair grows out. Because they usually last through 4 to 6 shampoos, semipermanent colors are called 6-week rinses.

Semipermanent coloring products last longer than temporary hair colors because of their ingredients. Like temporary coloring products, semipermanent hair colors contain water, certified vegetable dyes, and azo dye. But they also contain various combinations of **sulfur** and **ammonium thioglycolate** (ah-MOHN-ee-uhm thigh-oh-GLIGH-kah-layt), or **thio.** These substances enable the color to partially penetrate the cortex by raising the pH level to an alkaline range of 7 to 9. This alkalinity causes the cuticle to swell so that some of the color pigment can enter the cortex (Figure 16.1). The sulfur molecules contain the color pigment. These molecules attach themselves to the keratin (hard protein fiber) of the cuticle and to some of the salt bonds in the cortex. As a result, the cuticle is stained, and the cortex is also partially colored.

The physical and chemical actions of every shampoo cause semipermanent color to fade. Since the semipermanent color only partially penetrates the cortex of the hair, the color gradually tends to slip out of the cortex. Most of the color has faded by the fourth or sixth shampoo.

The U.S. Food, Drug, and Cosmetic Act requires a patch test before each application of all permanent colors and some semipermanent colors. This **patch test (predisposition (pree-dis-peh-ZISH-**

ehn) test) shows whether the client is allergic to any ingredient in the product. This test is very easy to give. Apply a small amount of the chosen color to the client's skin at least 24 hours before the coloring appointment. If the client does not have an allergic reaction, such as a skin irritation, nausea, or vomiting, during this period, you may use the product.

When a client does have an allergic reaction from the patch test (or later from the actual application of a coloring or cold-waving product), tell him or her to take the product box to a physician. The doctor can contact the local branch of the **Poison Control Center** for further details about the product. Most cosmetic firms furnish such information to these centers.

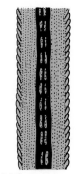

Figure 16.1
Cross section of the hair showing the cortex, cuticle, and medulla

Because an allergy may develop even after a product has been used with no reaction, **the test must be given before** every application of any product requiring it.

Semipermanent hair-coloring products offer several **advantages:**

1. The color lasts longer than one shampoo.

2. Many ready-to-use products are available.

3. The color will not easily rub off on the client's clothing.

4. Retouching is not necessary.

5. Semipermanent color covers gray hair better than temporary color does.

6. The colors may be used on decolorized (lightened) hair when frosting, streaking, or tipping.

7. Semipermanent colors manufactured by the same company may be mixed to achieve primary, secondary, or tertiary colors (in other words, Brand X with Brand X, but not Brand X with Brand Y).

Semipermanent colors also have several **disadvantages:**

1. The Food and Drug Administration requires a predisposition test (patch test) for most semipermanent colors 24 hours before the color application.

2. The colors need time to develop—perhaps 15 to 30 minutes (or more).

3. Semipermanent coloring is more expensive per application than temporary coloring.

4. After 4 to 6 shampoos, the color has usually faded so much that it must be applied again.

5. Semipermanent colors work best on hair that is 50 percent or less natural gray. In addition, semipermanent colors usually will not lift (lighten) the natural hair color.

NOTE: Read the manufacturer's instructions carefully before applying semipermanent hair color. Do not add hydrogen peroxide to a semipermanent hair color unless specifically directed to do so by the label instructions.

Theory Objective 2
Identifying the Client's Natural Hair Color

Because semipermanent color partially penetrates the hair, it is important for you to be able to identify different hair colors. You will also need to learn some new words so that you can refer to colors by their correct names. This will make it easier for you to communicate with other professional cosmetologists.

Identifying the client's hair color is a simple matter if you approach the problem systematically. If you think about it, only three hair colors are possible: **blonde, brown,** and **black.** Gray or white hair (canities) is not a color. Red hair is actually a color of brown. Differences within a particular color are called **levels.** In this system, each color has a number that indicates how much light the color reflects to the eye. Colors with low numbers are dark because they reflect only a small amount of light. Lighter colors have higher numbers because they reflect more light.

For example, if you look around your classroom, you will discover that some classmates have dark brown hair, some have medium brown hair, and others have light brown hair. All these variations of brown are **levels of color.** The following chart will help you identify other color levels:

1 Black
2 Dark brown
3 Medium brown

4 Light brown
5 Dark blonde
6 Medium blonde

7 Light blonde
8 Very light blonde
9 Pastel blonde

All hair colors should fall into one of these categories.

In addition to color levels, hair color also has a **"tone"** level, which indicates the differences from one tone to the next. The tone of the hair color is usually described in terms of its warmth or lack of warmth. **Warm tones** include red, orange, or gold tones. These tones reflect light and tend to highlight the hair. **Cool or drab tones** include **ash** or gray tones and have a blue, green, or violet base. These tones have no red or gold highlights. The following chart gives each tone a number:

> **Cool Tone Levels**
>
> 1 ash
> 2 mauve (purple)
>
> **Warm Tone Levels**
>
> 3 gold/yellow
> 4 copper (orange/red)
> 5 tobacco (red/gold)
> 6 auburn (red-red/brown)

Therefore, if your classmate has medium brown hair with a gold tone to it, you would describe the hair color as "medium golden brown." Another way to express this is to use two numbers from the color level/tone level charts, or 3/3. The first number 3 tells you the color is medium brown, and the second number 3 indicates the tone is gold.

In addition to helping you identify natural hair colors, this system should make it easier for you to compare the hair colors of one manufacturer to those of another manufacturer. Many of the companies that make hair-coloring products use the hair color names in these charts. Therefore, if you are using a semipermanent color in a medium ash blonde made by **Professional Company X** and run out of stock in that color, you could find the comparable color made by **Professional Company Y** by using the color level/tone level system. This same system is used for both semipermanent and permanent hair colors.

Practical Objective 3
Selecting and Applying Semipermanent Hair Colors

Supplies

- shampooing supplies
- gloves
- talcum powder
- timer
- color product
- color chart
- applicator bottle/brush
- stain remover
- protective apron

Steps for Selecting Color and Giving a Patch Test

Procedure	Rationale

1. Show the client the color chart and tell him or her whether a predisposition test is required (Figure 16.2).

1. Read the label directions. Most semipermanent colors require a skin test.

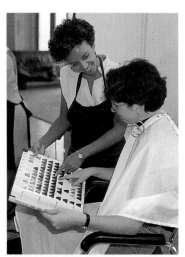

Figure 16.2
Help the client select a color from the color chart.

2. If the test is needed, pour $\frac{1}{4}$ ounce (1 capful or 7.7 milliliters) of the selected color into a small container and get a small, clean cotton swab from the dispensary. Explain to the client that the product to be used must be applied to the bend of one elbow or directly behind the ear (Figures 16.3 and 16.4).

2. This is standard procedure. A positive patch test that inflames the skin is called **dermatitis venenata** (VEN-en-ah-TAH).

3. Explain that the color must remain on the skin for 24 hours. Using a swab, apply a small amount of color to the bend of the elbow or behind the ear (Figure 16.5). Dispose of leftover supplies in a closed receptacle.

3. This is standard procedure.

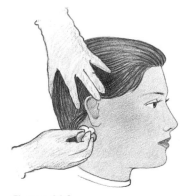

Figure 16.3
Cleanse the test area before applying the color.

4. Proceed to style the hair while explaining that the test site must be examined the next day. Inform the client what type of allergic reactions might occur.

4. Possible reactions to any chemical service performed in the school or salon might include redness and swelling of the skin, itching, headache, nausea, and vomiting. Although some reaction may occur before 24 hours have passed, the full time should be allowed for added protection.

5. **Advise the client to call the school or salon immediately if any discomfort occurs in the test area.**

5. Depending on the reactions the client describes, the school instructor or salon manager may ask the client to have the test site inspected by a doctor.

6. Record the location of the patch test, the product used,

6. Keeping accurate records is necessary to protect yourself

and the date on the client's service form.

7. Perform and complete the scheduled services.

8. Record the information for the client's appointment.

and the salon against any possible legal action.

7. This is standard procedure.

8. This helps you to follow up the results of the patch test. Even a client who regularly uses the same color must be tested before every application.

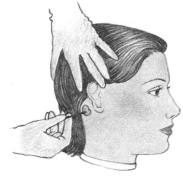

Figure 16.4
Apply the product to be used.

Steps for Applying Semipermanent Coloring

Procedure

1. Remove the client's service form from the file and inspect the patch test. Ask the client if there were any reactions.

2. Record the client's response on the service form. Drape the client for a chemical service.

3. After examining the scalp, carefully **read the label directions.**

Rationale

1. Checking the form will help you remember the client and the product to be used.

2. Cosmetologists perform so many services for different clients that it is almost impossible to remember all the important facts about them. You must use the same product and color that were used for the patch test.

3. Do not proceed if cuts, abrasions, or contagious diseases are present. Application procedures vary from one brand to another. **Some require shampooing** before a color application, while **others do not.**

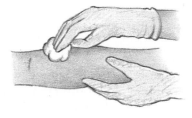 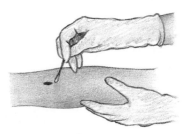

Figure 16.5
The predisposition test can also be applied to the bend of the elbow, but remember to cleanse the area first.

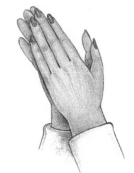

Figure 16.6
Wearing gloves protects your hands.

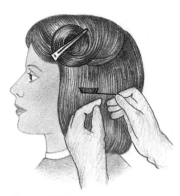

Figure 16.7
Strand test

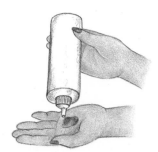

Figure 16.8
Apply the color according to the manufacturer's instructions.

4. Put gloves on both hands (Figure 16.6). **Follow the manufacturer's directions.**

5. **"Strand test"** the color on $\frac{1}{2}$ inch (1.25 centimeters) of hair in the lower crown (Figure 16.7). Apply color from the scalp all the way through the ends of the strand. Allow the color to remain on the test strand for approximately a third of the time specified for developing the whole head of hair. Blot with a clean, dry towel.

6. Apply color according to the directions on the label (Figure 16.8).

7. Set the timer for half the time the directions say should be allowed for developing.

8. Test one or more strands when the timer rings. If the color is not ready, set the timer for the rest of the developing time indicated on the label, and apply color to the hair that was used for the initial strand test.

9. When the timer rings at the end of the full developing time, remove the plastic

4. This will protect your hands and nails from direct contact with the coloring product. If a client can develop an allergy to the color, the cosmetologist can, too. The gloves also protect your fingernails from staining.

5. Always "strand test." This professional technique will enable you to see how a specific color will appear on a particular client's hair. If the strand test produces an unsatisfactory color, you will know that there may be a problem before you color the entire head. If necessary, a different color may be scheduled when the strand test indicates a problem.

6. Some colors are applied to shampooed hair that has been towel-dried. Other products that combine hair color and shampoo are applied to dry hair.

7. Porosity of hair varies from person to person, so the developing time will not be the same for all clients.

8. This is standard procedure.

9. Process the strand according to directions. If the color is not dark (or

cap (if the label said that one should be used) and strand test the color.

10. Thoroughly water rinse the hair until the water runs clear and the scalp is free of color. Semipermanent colors are usually **not** shampooed from the hair.

11. Apply an acid or normalizing rinse (Figure 16.9).

12. Style the hair. Note the color results on the client's service form and file it.

light) enough, you may want to rinse the color off and dry the hair. Then, reapply the color.

10. Semipermanent hair colors will not "set" into the hair unless they are rinsed first. The client's scalp around the hairline should be completely free of color stains.

11. This restores the natural pH of the hair by neutralizing the alkali of the coloring product.

12. The form will provide information for future decisions on coloring.

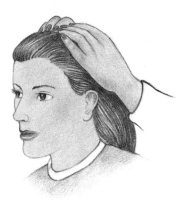

Figure 16.9
Applying the normalizing rinse

Sanitize your area as follows:
1. Wash, wipe, and store bottles and supplies.
2. Discard used supplies.
3. Clean and sanitize the cape and apron.
4. Sanitize the work area; wash your hands.

Glossary

Ammonium thioglycolate (ah-MOHN-ee-uhm thigh-oh-GLIGH-kay-layt) A chemical sometimes contained in semipermanent hair coloring that enables the dye to partially penetrate the cortex of the hair.

Cool (drab) tones Color variations that correspond to the cool secondary colors on the color chart. They include ash, silver platinum, smoke, and steel gray.

Dermatitis venenata A positive skin patch test that inflames the skin.

Drab tones See **Cool tones.**

Levels of color Variations within the three hair colors of blonde, brown, and black.

Patch test See **Predisposition test.**

Poison Control Center An agency that provides information about poisonous and potentially hazardous or allergy-producing products.

Predisposition test A test for allergy to hair coloring given by applying a small amount of color to the client's skin at least 24 hours before the product is used on the scalp.

Semipermanent hair coloring A hair dye that partially penetrates the cortex of the hair and lasts 4 to 6 shampoos.

Sulfur An element contained in semipermanent hair coloring that enables the coloring pigment to partially penetrate the cortex of the hair.

Tone level The variation from one tone to the next, such as drab tones, warm tones, and so forth.

Warm tones Color variations including red, orange, and gold.

Questions

1. What federal act requires a patch test for certain hair color products?
2. Using a dictionary, write a definition for the word "allergy."
3. Before applying a semipermanent color, what should you look for when you examine the scalp?
4. Where are the two points on the body where patch tests are given?
5. Does the application of a semipermanent hair color require a predisposition test?
6. What two chemicals are found in semipermanent hair colors?
7. Does a semipermanent color penetrate the hair shaft?
8. Is it necessary to give an allergy test before each application of a semipermanent color?
9. What are the three basic natural hair colors?
10. Is gray a hair color?
11. Is the color green a warm tone or a drab tone?
12. Is orange a warm tone or a drab tone?
13. Write a definition of dermatitis venenata.
14. Is it really necessary to keep a record of the color used on a client, or can you simply remember the client's formula?
15. Do you need to wear protective gloves when applying a semipermanent color?

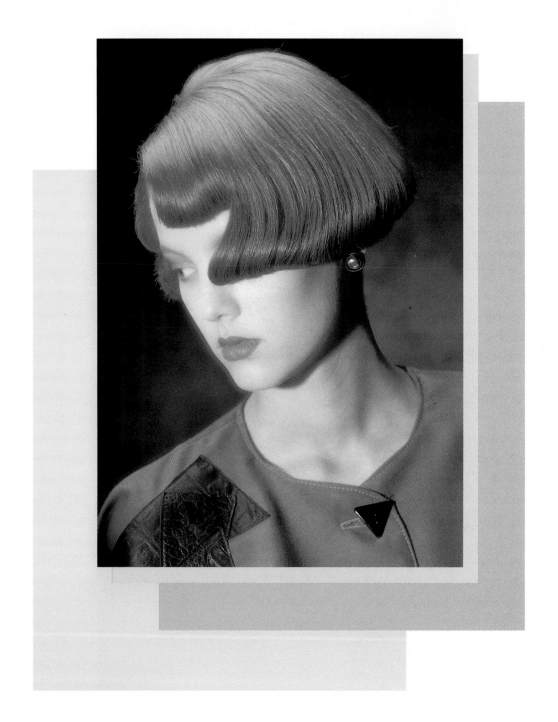

Permanent Hair Coloring

Use the proper steps to apply permanent hair color(s) to the client's hair. Provided with permanent hair-coloring products and supplies, permanently change the client's hair color. Using the proper safety precautions and following label directions, apply a permanent hair color to the client's hair in 10 to 15 minutes. Score 85 percent or better on a multiple-choice exam on the information in this chapter.

In order to achieve the above level of competence, you should master the following chapter objectives.

Theory Objectives

1. Define permanent hair-coloring services, terms, and chemicals.
2. Describe the advantages and disadvantages of permanent hair color and the safety measures required when using permanent hair-coloring products.

Practical Objectives

3. Test the hair for metallic salts.
4. Apply a virgin tint to lighten or darken hair.
5. Apply a tint retouch.

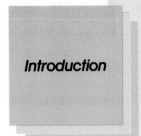

Introduction

The demand for permanent hair coloring has increased dramatically in recent years, and this demand will probably continue to grow. As requests for this service have increased, so have the number of professional permanent hair-coloring products. New procedures to achieve unusually beautiful hair-coloring effects have emerged and so, of course, have problems. This means that mastering permanent hair-coloring techniques will be a continuing challenge and source of satisfaction for you.

Since permanent hair coloring is probably the second or third most profitable service in schools and salons, mastering basic scientific coloring principles will also be important to your financial success.

Theory Objective 1
Permanent
Hair-Coloring Services,
Terms, and Chemicals

Hair colors that permanently penetrate the cuticle of the hair and deposit color in the cortex of the shaft are called **penetrating tints** (Figure 17.1). Because of their chemical action within the hair shaft, they are also called **oxidizing permanent hair colors** or **oxidation tints.** When these products are given in one application, the process is called a **single-application** coloring service.

Another method of permanently coloring the hair is called **double-application** hair coloring. **Lightening** (bleaching) and **toning** are double-application methods of coloring because two different products are applied separately to the hair (for these and other terms, see Table 17.1). First, the hair is lightened (decolorized), and then a toner is applied to achieve the desired color. Lightening and toning will be discussed in Chapter 18.

Hair that has not been overexposed to the sun or treated by tints, chemical straighteners, cold-waving solutions, or other chemical services is called **virgin hair.** The process used to color virgin hair is called a **virgin tint.**

As the tinted hair grows, the new growth of hair has to be colored. This is called a **retouch tint,** or a **tint retouch.** The purpose of a retouch is to color the hair that has grown from the scalp so that it matches the permanent color previously applied to the rest of the hair. A retouch is normally done every 3 to 5 weeks, depending on how fast the hair grows.

Occasionally, a client will request that the hair's natural color be permanently highlighted rather than drastically changed. This service, called a **soap cap,** combines permanent hair color with shampoo and hydrogen peroxide to **slightly change,** or **highlight,** the natural color. The soap cap is applied like a shampoo to dry hair. It is left in for 10 to 15 minutes (or as directed) before the hair is rinsed thoroughly.

The main chemical compound in the bases of most permanent color is **para-phenylene-diamine** (PA-rah-FEN-a-leen-DIGH-eh-meen), a synthetic (artificial) organic dye compound that scientists developed around 1900. It is an **aniline** (AN-ehl-ehn) **derivative** that comes from **coal tar.** Products containing this compound are called **tints.**

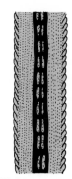

Figure 17.1
Cross section of the hair showing the cortex, cuticle, and medulla

Tinting products work by **oxidation,** which is the process of combining hydrogen peroxide with a color base so that the peroxide gives up some of its oxygen. The peroxide that supplies (or gives up) the oxygen is called the **oxidizer** (oxidizing agent). The color base that receives the oxygen is said to have been oxidized. The standard strength **hydrogen peroxide** is **20 volume (6 percent),** but higher and lower volumes are also available.*

Hydrogen peroxide is the oxidizer or developer in most modern tinting products. Its chemical symbol is H_2O_2 (hydrogen and oxygen). The tinting process produces color within the cortex of the hair. The para-phenylene-diamine dye bases (para dyes) have small molecules that easily pass through the imbrications of the cuticle into the cortex. After they have entered the cortex, the colored molecules of the dye base combine with oxygen from the hydrogen peroxide to make large molecules of dye. These newly formed molecules of dye are too large to pass back through the imbrications so they are permanently held within the cortex. The cross-bonds that develop between color molecules and keratin also hold the color in place. Hydrogen peroxide and the base (dye) must be kept in separate containers. The reaction (oxidation between the dye and hydrogen peroxide) takes 20 to 45 minutes. It begins when they are mixed, so you must keep them separated until you are ready to use them.

Hydrogen peroxide is an **acid.** It has a **pH of between 3.5 and 4.**

In most tinting products, ammonia is part of the dye base. This ammonia compound (an alkali) is the activator; that is, it helps start the tinting process in the following ways:

1. As an alkali, it makes the cuticle swell so that the molecules of the tint base can easily pass into the cortex.

---

*Volume strength indicates the amount of oxygen gas released from a certain amount of hydrogen peroxide; 20-volume peroxide is equal to a 6 percent solution of peroxide in water.

Table 17.1
Hair-Coloring Terms

Accelerator Peroxide in powder form that is added to peroxide lightener mixtures to increase the lightening effect. Also called "activator" or "booster."

Bleaching/Lightening Removal of some or all of the hair color, whether the color is natural or a previously applied artificial color. Also called "lifting."

Bleach Lotion or Oil See **Lightener Lotion.**

Conditioners Ingredients in color lotions, or applied independently to the hair, that improve its sheen, softness, and manageability.

Cream Colors An oxidation hair dye product that forms a thick creamy lotion when mixed with developer. It is applied by "parting and sectioning" and may then be combed through the hair tips. This product is usually purchased for home use.

Creme Rinses A rinse sometimes applied after coloring and shampooing to restore the initial condition of the hair, i.e., its normal acidity, softness, and manageability.

Developer Hydrogen peroxide (usually 20 volume, which equals 6 percent strength) supplied as a clear liquid or cream lotion and used either to lighten the hair or to develop the color of an oxidation dye.

Double Process A two-step process by which the hair is first lightened, usually drastically, and then recolored with a toner.

Frosting Lightening and toning the entire length of random strands of hair over the entire head.

Gentle Lightener A mild peroxide formula that provides only a slight lightening effect when added to another product.

Lightener Lotion The vehicle to which developer (peroxide) and accelerator are added to produce an effective lightening mixture. It is usually an ammoniacal (alkaline) soap solution and is often called "oil bleach."

Metallic Dye A hair dye product that contains metallic salts, usually lead acetate, as the active ingredient.

Oxidation Hair Dye A dye containing para-phenylene-diamine and other hair dye intermediates that must be mixed with a peroxide developer just before application to the hair in order to develop the color.

Para Dye A hair dye product containing para-phenylene-diamine as the primary hair dye intermediate. See **Oxidation Hair Dye.**

Patch Test A test on the forearm, bend of the elbow, or behind the ear to detect allergic sensitivity; federal law requires that a warning to perform such a test before each application of a hair color appear on the product label (unless the product contains only color approved by the Food and Drug Administration for cosmetic use).

Permanent Color See **Oxidation Hair Dye.**

Prelightening Lightening the hair before application of a hair color or toner.

Progressive Dye A dye that colors the hair gradually over repeated applications; a metallic dye.

Restorer (Hair Color Restorer) Euphemism for a metallic dye. This product is normally purchased for home use.

Retouching The process of lightening or dyeing the new growth (roots) with a permanent dye. First, the hair must be parted and sectioned; then, the applied lightener or dye is worked through the entire hair.

Rinse (Color Rinse) A temporary hair color of low strength in the form of a rinse. It is removed by the first shampoo.

Semipermanent Color Color that lasts through several shampoos. Usually, a nonoxidation hair dye product.

Table 17.1, Continued

Shampoo-in Hair Color Permanent dyes of the oxidation type that are applied like a shampoo. Also called color shampoo.

Single Process Lightening and recoloring the hair in one step, as in the oxidation hair-dyeing process.

Streaking The application of lightener to predetermined or random sections of hair.

Stripping The total removal of all natural and artificial color from hair using a soapy peroxide solution.

Temporary Color Color that is removed by the first shampoo.

Tipping Lightening of predetermined or random tip ends of the hair.

Toner A light (pastel) hair color applied to prelightened hair. Sometimes an oxidation dye, but semipermanent colors are also used.

Vegetable Dye A color formed by applying only natural plant products, usually from the henna plant.

2. It creates the alkaline conditions needed to develop the color.

3. It causes the hydrogen peroxide (H_2O_2) to give up oxygen for oxidation of the para dyes.

The addition of the ammonia makes the ready-to-use coloring product alkaline. Most products have a pH of about 9.5 to 10.5.

Manufacturers have made great improvements in professional tints. Tints can **lighten** or **darken** the hair in a single application. Hair can be lightened by softening the cuticle. Different products have different strengths, so the amount of lightening will vary with the product you use. Natural hair color is also an important factor. For instance, light brown hair can be lightened much more easily than dark brown or black hair because the lighter hair contains less color pigment.

Theory Objective 2
Advantages and Disadvantages of Permanent Hair-Coloring Products and Safety Measures Needed When Using Them

As you know, you must protect your client and yourself when you are using products that might be harmful. Tints containing para-phenylene-diamine may be harmful to the client, so you must give the client a **predisposition** or **patch test.** This test should indicate whether the client is **hypersensitive** (high-per-SEN-seh-tiv)— allergic—to the product to be used. Details on the patch test can be reviewed in Chapter 16. The best way to protect yourself from allergies is to wear an apron and protective gloves whenever you mix or apply permanent hair colors.

All professional products used in the school or salon are required by the Federal Food, Drug, and Cosmetic Act to have directions on the label or inside the package. Professional hair tints are made to color **only hair on the head.** To use a tint in any other way may be very dangerous (for example, using a tint to color eyebrows or eyelashes **may cause blindness**). Never tint eyebrows or eyelashes with any product unless the label directions state that the product was made for that purpose!

Tints usually are packaged in amber-colored bottles, small boxes, or tubes because light alters their chemical makeup. If they are exposed to light, heat, or air, they may become ineffective (and turn dark in color)—they should not be used. Always mix permanent hair coloring in a plastic or glass container. Do not use a metal mixing container for any oxidizing-type service. Peroxide reacts adversely with metal and may change the color.

Also, remember that permanent waves and chemical relaxers should be used **before** a hair color because their chemicals tend to remove artificial color from the hair.

Permanent hair coloring offers several advantages for the client:

1. Permanent color products (tints) are more effective at covering resistant gray hair than temporary or semipermanent colors are. Usually, tints completely **cover gray** hair.

2. Many persons experiment at home with cold-waving and coloring products, which frequently discolor the hair. As a result, many of them seek professional services to restore their natural hair color.

3. Cosmetologists are becoming extremely creative in using new methods of producing decorative and accenting effects. These new coloring effects (and methods) are so much in demand that many salons are starting to specialize in them. These services include framing, painting, frosting, streaking, and tipping, to name just a few. They will be discussed in Chapter 19.

4. An America's youth-conscious society, many persons want to avoid gray hair—a sign of aging. Although cosmetology offers services to enhance the natural beauty of gray hair, many persons choose to cover it. For those who want to appear younger, permanent hair coloring is a valuable service.

5. Clients have discovered that if their natural hair color does not flatter their eye color or skin tones, they can use penetrating tints to do what nature did not. Generally, clients with blue or hazel eyes and fair or creamy complexions should use warm, light hair colors. Light or dark colors without red accents or overtones generally flatter persons with green eyes and florid

and pinkish complexions. Brown-eyed clients with olive or yellowish complexions should use darker and ash colors.

You will quickly realize that permanent hair colors also offer cosmetologists several advantages:

1. Satisfaction of the client because gray hair can be completely covered.
2. The possibility of a permanent return to the client's natural hair color, which requires professional services.
3. Recognition and satisfaction for the cosmetologist because the appearance of the client has been improved.
4. An increase in money because permanent coloring is a more expensive service than temporary and semipermanent coloring and requires regular retouches.

Don't be misled, however. Permanent hair coloring does have some disadvantages for the client:

1. A **patch test** is absolutely required before **each** tint. Although this test takes only a few minutes, it is slightly inconvenient for the client.
2. Once the hair has been tinted, a **regular appointment** should be made for retouching the new growth to keep the color even. Thus, the client must spend more time in the school or salon than is required by temporary or semipermanent coloring services.
3. Tinting requires **extra time** not only in terms of additional appointments for retouches but also in respect to the time spent in the individual coloring sessions. The developing time (period in which the peroxide oxidizes the tint) is 20 to 45 minutes. Counting application and full processing, tinting adds 30 to 45 minutes to the time needed for a shampoo and styling. Temporary and semipermanent colors can be applied more quickly than permanent hair colors.
4. Since tints give color that cannot be shampooed out of the cortex, the **client cannot** quickly and **easily change** the hair color. It can be changed only by cutting or applying another tint.
5. The tinting service requires more supplies at a **greater cost** than do temporary or semipermanent coloring services; therefore, the client must pay more for permanent coloring.

Permanent hair colors also have some **disadvantages** for the cosmetologist:

1. Since color selection is very important, you may spend a considerable amount of time advising the client on it. Time is money, so you must use it as efficiently and profitably as possible. Although color selection requires a lot of time in the initial service, repeat color services may make the investment of time very profitable in the long run.

2. Patch testing for possible allergies can be time-consuming. You must figure the proportion of peroxide for the very small amount of color needed for the test, and you must also keep accurate records for each hair-coloring service. The date of the patch, the results, the formula proportions, and the brand of the product must be recorded **before each** tint.

3. Hair coloring is a complicated process that requires skill and judgment. Every product you use will react somewhat differently on each client. An endless variety of colors can be mixed, but skill is required to formulate just the right color for a particular client. Even experienced cosmetologists soon realize they can always learn something new about hair coloring.

4. The school or salon and the individual cosmetologist must be careful in using aniline or oxidizing products because the risk of legal action increases with these services. A client who has an allergic reaction to a color service can sue the cosmetologist. Much time and money can be spent in legal processes. The best way to protect yourself is by taking the following precautions:

   - Follow label directions **exactly.**
   - Give a predisposition test before **each** application of permanent color.
   - Keep current, accurate, legible hair-coloring records.

5. Tinting is a service requiring a number of supplies, such as shampooing items, many bottles or canisters of the complete range of hair colors, hydrogen peroxide, stain removers, cotton swabs, color applicator bottles, and protective gloves. Since you do not know exactly what colors your clients will select, **all** of the colors usually are stocked in the dispensary. **Fixed costs,** such as large inventories of a particular item, are always "built into" the cost of the service.

Supplies

- plastic or glass dish
- 20-volume peroxide
- 28 percent ammonia water

Procedure

1. Analyze hair texture and condition (Figure 17.2).

2. Ask the client if any home hair-coloring products have been used in the last 12 months. If the client answers "yes" or if the hair feels harsh or coated, test for a metallic salt color.

3. Cut a small strand of hair from the bottom of the crown area of the client's head (Figure 17.3). Wind hair-setting tape around one end of the hair.

4. Mix 1 ounce (30 milliliters) of clear 20-volume peroxide with 20 drops of 28 percent ammonia water in a plastic or glass—not metal—dish (Figure 17.4).

5. Submerge the strand in the prepared solution for 30 minutes. Watch for a chemical reaction.

Rationale

1. Always check to make sure that the client's hair is in good condition before you give any chemical process.

2. Metallic salt color coatings discolor the hair when combined with professional products.

3. A strand missing from this area will be less noticeable.

4. This solution will detect the presence of metallic salts on the strand. Mixing peroxide and a chemical in a metal bowl can cause the peroxide to react badly.

5. If metal is present, the strand will show a reaction in 30 to 40 minutes. The presence of lead will cause

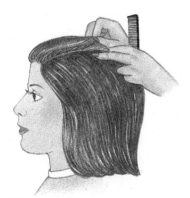

Figure 17.2
Examine the scalp.

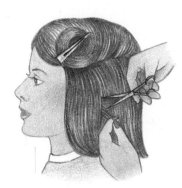

Figure 17.3
Cutting the test strand

Figure 17.4
Use only a plastic or glass mixing bowl.

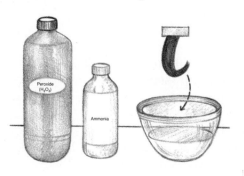

the hair to change color almost immediately. If copper is on the hair, the solution will boil, the strand will feel hot to the touch, and the hair will easily fall apart. Also test the hair for elasticity and breakage.

6. Explain to the client why the tint cannot be given.

6. Explain that it is for the client's protection.

Practical Objective 4
Applying a Virgin Tint to Lighten or Darken Hair

Supplies

- client hair-coloring record form
- client release form
- color-safe shampoo
- shampoo supplies plus two laundered towels
- sanitized plastic tint applicator bottle and top
- one pair of rubber or surgical gloves

- protective apron
- talcum powder
- 20-volume peroxide
- tint
- color chart
- comparison chart
- brush applicator
- plastic mixing bowl

Procedure

1. Double drape the client for a chemical service. If necessary, shampoo lightly and use a lukewarm dryer to remove moisture. Shampoo the hair only if it is very soiled.

2. Analyze the condition of the hair and scalp (see Chapter 7) and make conditioning recommendations as needed; ask the client what home or professional coloring products have

Rationale

1. Try not to stimulate circulation of blood to the scalp because this increases the likelihood that the client will react to the tinting material. Normally, the hair is **not shampooed** before a tinting service. The hair must be dry before tint is applied.

2. Hair that is very porous needs conditioning so that the tint will remain in it. If the hair is extremely porous or chemically damaged, a conditioning filler may be needed. Fillers equalize the porosity of the

been used in the last 12 months.

hair shaft so that color will penetrate evenly (Figure 17.5). The filler also acts as a primer coat on porous or damaged hair. Most fillers are ready to use and should be applied like a shampoo. Fillers usually are left in the hair, but follow label directions. It is important to know if other dyes are on the hair because they may interact unfavorably with the tint.

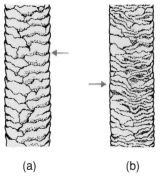

(a)   (b)

Figure 17.5
Conditioning filler used to equalize hair porosity

3. Explain the cost, process, and upkeep of the tinting; answer the client's questions.

3. Some clients do not realize that permanent color does not shampoo out of the hair. They also may not realize the tint has to be retouched.

4. Use the color chart to help the client decide on a color.

4. This helps you and your client visualize the best color. Consider color of the client's eyes and skin tones. (Recall the discussion of the color choice earlier in the chapter.) If the hair was not shampooed and dried, it will appear slightly darker.

5. Lift a small amount of hair on top of the client's head; look through the strand of hair. Examine the scalp for scratches, open cuts, or abrasions.

5. Lifting the hair makes it easier for you to feel its texture—fine, coarse, porous, or resilient—and helps you see if the hair has red or gold overtones, which should be considered in color selection.

6. Select the chart color that is closest to the client's natural color.

6. It is best to use the natural color as a guide.

7. When a client who does **not have gray hair wishes to lighten** the natural color,

7. Tinting products vary in strength. It is always better to have a color lighter than the one

select a tint that is one color lighter than the client desires.

desired rather than darker. If a color is too light, it is easy to go one or two shades darker. It is very difficult to lighten a tint that is too dark (whether you do it right away or at a later appointment). If the color is too dark, the client may be very unhappy. The same probably will not be true if the color is a little too light.

8. When a client who has **gray hair wants a lighter** color, again select a color that is lighter than the client's choice.

8. Remember that tints lighten and deposit color in the hair. The lighter colors have more lightening action than the darker ones. If the color selected by the client is very light, prelightening and toning may be necessary. (This double application—lightening and toning—will be discussed in the next chapter.)

9. If a client who does not have gray hair wants a darker color, use the color that the client picks.

9. This produces the best results. As a preliminary safeguard, always strand test a color before applying a virgin tint to the entire head.

10. If a client who has gray hair wants a darker color, use a color one shade darker than the client's selection.

10. Some gray hair is resistant to color. Such hair has a resilient, "glassy" feel because the cuticle layers are closed tightly around the cortex. After some coloring experience, you will develop a fingertip touch that identifies resistant gray hair. Because of this resistance, normally use a shade one color darker than the one desired

11. Tell the client that a predisposition (patch) test is needed and explain how it will be applied.

to be sure that the gray is covered.

11. Inform the client that a patch test is required by law. Describe the symptoms of a positive reaction. Advise the client to phone the school or salon if these symptoms occur.

12. Give the patch test with the same tint color that will be used.

12. Be sure that the client wants the color you are testing. Only the color you test can be used in the tinting service.

13. Record the location of the patch test and the product used on the client release form. Date and initial the entry.

13. Accurate records protect you and your client. They also save you the trouble of remembering all the mixing formulas for clients.

14. If needed, study the color comparison chart.

14. The color comparison chart is a table that lists and compares the professional colors of most manufacturers. The chart shows tints that are approximately the same.

15. Schedule the tinting service for at least 24 hours after the patch test began. Record the service in the appointment book and give this information to the client.

15. The results of the test must be negative. If the results are positive, do **not** give the tint.

16. Record the results of the patch test on the client release form.

16. This protects the school, the salon, and you!

Sanitize your area as follows:
1. **Wash, wipe, and store bottles and supplies.**
2. **Discard used supplies.**
3. **Clean and sanitize the cape and apron.**
4. **Sanitize the work area; wash your hands.**

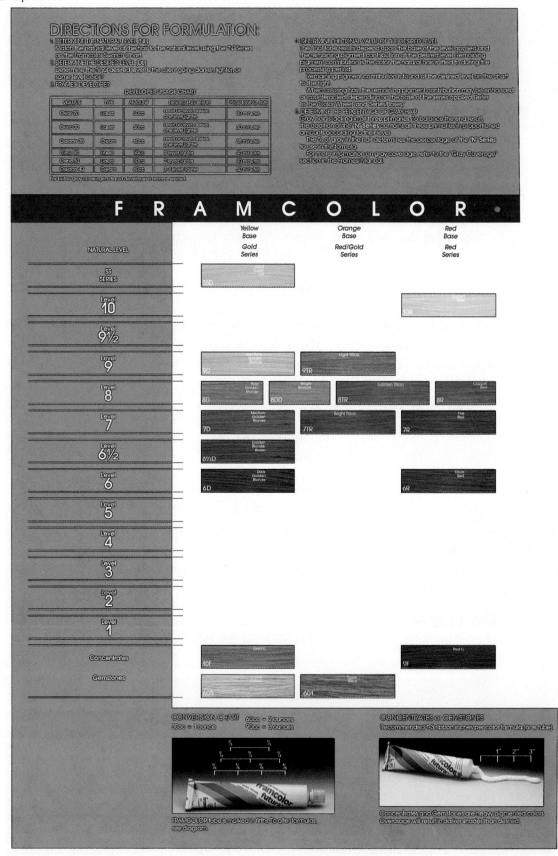

DIRECTIONS FOR FORMULATION:

1. DETERMINE THE NATURAL LEVEL (NL)
   Match the natural level of the hair to the natural level using the "N" Series on the Framcolor Swatch Chart.
2. DETERMINE THE DESIRED LEVEL (DL)
   Determine the final desired level. Is the client going darker, lighter, or same level color?
3. FRAMESI DEVELOPER

DEVELOPER USAGE CHART

VOLUME	TYPE	AMOUNT	DESIRED END RESULT	PROCESSING TIME
Clear 20	Liquid	50cc	Level on level, darker, one level lighter	30 minutes
Oxina 20	Liquid	50cc	Level on level, darker, one level lighter	30 minutes
Oxidon 25	Cream	60cc	Level on level, darker, one level lighter	35 minutes
Clear 30	Liquid	60cc	2 level lighter	40 minutes
Oxina 30	Liquid	60cc	2 level lighter	40 minutes
Oxidon 40	Cream	60cc	3-4 level lighter	50 minutes

For better gray coverage, a liquid developer is recommended.

4. DETERMINE THE TONAL VALUE OF THE DESIRED LEVEL
   The final tone results depend upon the base of the level applied and the remaining pigment contribution of the desired level. Remaining pigment contribution is the color the natural hair is lifted to during the processing period.
   Remaining pigment contribution is found at the desired level on the chart to the right.
   When coloring hair, the remaining pigment contribution may be enhanced or counteracted, depending on the base of the series applied. Refer to the "Color Wheel" and "Series Bases".
5. DETERMINE THE PERCENTAGE OF GRAY HAIR
   Gray hair is lacking in all three primaries. To balance the end result, the addition of the "N" Series contains all three primaries in proportioned amounts according to their level.
   The % of gray in the hair determines the percentage of the "N" Series to use in the formula.
   For more information on gray coverage, refer to the "Gray Coverage" section in the Framesi Manual.

F R A M C O L O R

	Yellow Base	Orange Base	Red Base
NATURAL LEVEL	Gold Series	Red/Gold Series	Red Series

- SS SERIES — SSD
- Level 10 — 10R
- Level 9½
- Level 9 — 9D, 9TR
- Level 8 — 8D, 8DD, 8TR, 8R
- Level 7 — 7D, 7TR, 7R
- Level 6½ — 6½D
- Level 6 — 6D, 6R
- Level 5
- Level 4
- Level 3
- Level 2
- Level 1
- Concentrates — 10F, 9F
- Gemstones — 605, 601

CONVERSION CHART
60cc = 2 ounces
30cc = 1 ounce
90cc = 3 ounces

FRAMCOLOR tube is marked in fifths. To alter formulas, see diagram.

CONCENTRATES or GEMSTONES
Recommended 1-3 ribbon inches per color formula (one tube).

Concentrates and Gemstones are heavy pigmented colors. Overusage will result in darker shades than desired.

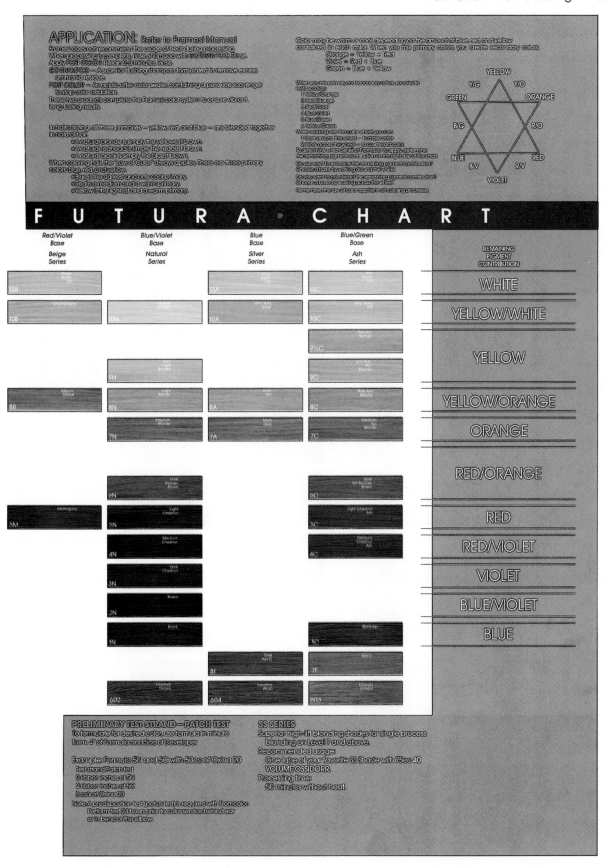

FUTURA · CHART

THE COMPLETE SOCOLOR® COLLECTION

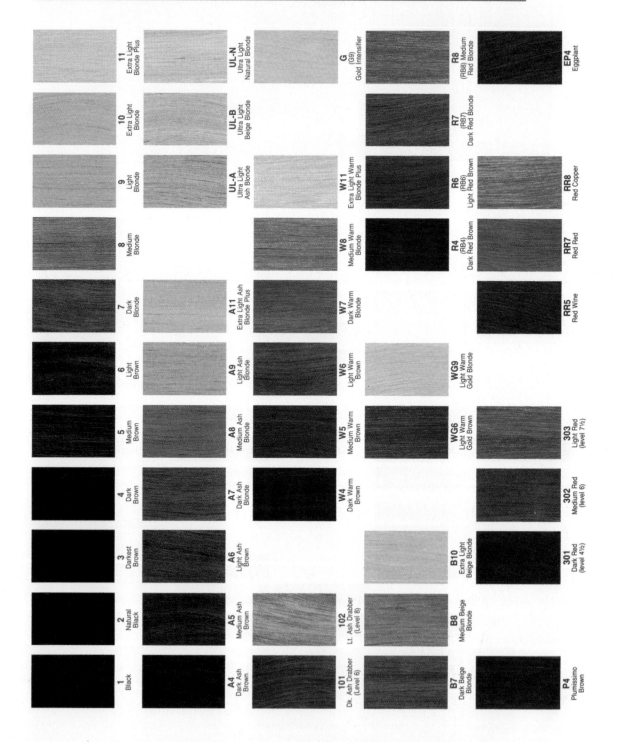

CONVERTING TO SOCOLOR®

Matrix — HAIR AND SKIN CARE

SOCOLOR	Miss Clairol	Wella Color Charm	L'Oreal Preference	Koleston 2000	Redken Amino Color	Redken Deco Color	Wella Color Perfect	Majirel Majiblond	Framesi	Goldwell	Clairol Logics
UL-N Ultra Light Natural Blonde								900	SS/C		
UL-B Ultra Light Beige Blonde								902	SS/B		
UL-A Ultra Light Ash Blonde								901	SS/A		
11 Extra Light Blonde Plus	20	1290		1200N				M10			
A11 Extra Light Ash Blonde Plus	30	1120	9.1Ba	1030A	12S	10N	12N	M10.1	5F	10N	12A
W11 Extra Light Warm Blonde Plus	12	1070	9BB	1190G	12G		11G		4F	10B	11G
10 Extra Light Blonde			9	900N				M9		10GB	12N
B10 Extra Light Beige Blonde	12B1	1030	9.2	1070G		10D	10B	M9.13	9D	10A	
9 Light Blonde				800N	10G		9N	M9.01		10P	
A9 Light Ash Blonde			9.1	740A	7N			M9.1	9N	11A	11A
WG9 Light Warm Gold Blonde			9.3		8G			M9.04	9C	8G	8G
8 Medium Blonde	26/28	740	8	700N		7C	8N	M8	8N		
A8 Medium Ash Blonde		1060	8.1	542A	6N			M8.1	8C	8P	
B8 Medium Beige Blonde			8.3					M8.13	8D		
W8 Medium Warm Blonde	41	841	8.4				8G	M8.3	8R	8G	
R8 (RB8) Medium Red Blonde	43	643		5440R			7RG	M8.34	8TR	8R	6R0
RR8 Red Copper	660R0		43					M7.43			
7 Dark Blonde	42	542	7	600N				M7	7N	7N	6V
A7 Dark Ash Blonde	32	632	7.1					M7.1	7C	7A	
B7 Dark Beige Blonde	25	544				8C		M7.13	6E		
W7 Dark Warm Blonde			7.3	725G	5G			M7.3	7D	7B	
R7 (RB7) Dark Red Blonde	33	633		347R				M7.4	7R	6K	
303 Light Red				7290R	6F/A		6RG	M7.40	9F	6R	4R0
RR7 Red Red	670R								7TR		
6 Light Brown		246	6	500N		8	6N	M6	6N	6G	6G
A6 Light Ash Brown	36	336	6.1	336A	4N	6C	6A	M6.1	6C	5A	5V
W6 Light Warm Brown	39	435		643G			6G	M6.23	75D	7G	
WG6 Light Warm Gold Brown			6.3								
R6 (RB6) Light Red Brown								M6.6			
302 Medium Red	64					7RU	5RV				
5 Medium Brown	44	257	5	400N	2G		4N	M5	5N	6B	4G
A5 Medium Ash Brown	57	237	5.1		2N	7C	4A	M5.1	5C	4B	
W5 Medium Warm Brown	39		5.3			6D	4G	M5.3			
RR5 Red Wine								M5.62			
4 Dark Brown	48	148	4	300N	1N	6	3N	M4	4N	3N	4V
A4 Dark Ash Brown			4.1								
W4 Dark Warm Brown					1G				4C		
R4 (RB4) Dark Red Brown				3560R	2A						
P4 Plumissimo Brown								M4.26			
301 Dark Red	68		41		2FA	5RU	3RV	M4.45	4R	4R	
EP4 Eggplant	680RV							M5.20			2RV
3 Darkest Brown	51	051	3	200N		4	2N	M3	2N	2N	
2 Natural Black											
1 Black	52	052	1	100N		2		M1	1N	2A	1V
G (G9) Gold Intensifier					Tr.Bl.Cor.		G		9/0		
102 Light Ash Drabber		050	Light Drabber		6S	91	V		7F	P	
101 Dark Ash Drabber		049	Dark Drabber						8F	A	

Matrix SoColor is based on pigmented hair. The above comparisons are guidelines only. We recommend a strand test to determine exact color results.

©1991 Matrix Essentials, Inc. Solon, Ohio 44139 USA Printed in USA FP60M2/91-LX02702

PLEASE RECYCLE

Mixing and Applying Tint

Procedure	*Rationale*

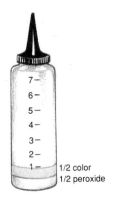

Figure 17.6
Mix 1 ounce (30 milliliters) of coloring material for the strand test.

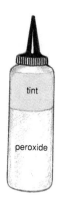

Figure 17.7
Double peroxide

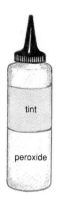

Figure 17.8
Equal peroxide

Procedure

1. Read the label directions that accompany the tint.

2. Prepare a strand test. Using the proportions in the label directions, mix a small amount of color with a small amount of hydrogen peroxide in a glass or plastic container or applicator bottle. **Remember: do not mix peroxide in a metal container.** Usually, 1 ounce (30 milliliters) total material (color and hydrogen peroxide) is enough (Figures 17.6, 17.7, and 17.8).

Rationale

1. Tints are always mixed with peroxide, but the proportion of color to peroxide varies from one product to another.

2. Follow the label directions to proportionately mix 1 ounce (30 milliliters) of tinting material. Tint bottles usually contain either 1½ or 2 ounces (45 or 60 milliliters) of coloring material. The directions usually require "double peroxide" or "equal peroxide." **Double peroxide** means twice as much peroxide as color should be used. **Equal peroxide** means that the same amount of peroxide and color should be used. For convenience in mixing a very small amount of coloring material for the strand or predisposition test, you can use milliliters (1 ounce equals 29.573 milliliters, which for this purpose can be rounded to 30). To mix approximately 1 ounce of coloring material, use 15 milliliters of color and 15 milliliters of peroxide if the directions call for equal peroxide; use 10 milliliters of color and 20 milliliters of peroxide if the directions require double peroxide. All tints must be mixed in glass or plastic containers. The chemicals could react with a metal container, releasing metal particles into the tint mixture. A **hydrometer** (high-DROHM-eh-tehr) may be used to test the strength of the peroxide.

3. Explain to the client the reasons for strand testing. Since cold waving and chemical relaxing can strip the color, explain that they should be done one week before tinting.

3. Make a strand test before applying peroxide to the entire head. Watch for discoloration resulting from previous chemical services, uneven coloring caused by overly porous hair, and unwanted red or brassy highlights.

4. Lightly powder the insides of the gloves and slip your hands into them.

4. Wear gloves to protect your hands.

5. Select a strand of hair in the lower crown area. Using the applicator bottle or brush, apply the color mixture along the entire strand (Figure 17.9).

5. Use the lower crown area because any discoloration that might occur will be covered by the hair above it.

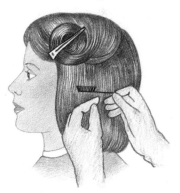

Figure 17.9
Strand test

6. Set the timer for 15 minutes and dispose of any remaining tint. Wash any color residue from the inside of the bottle.

6. Color usually takes 20 to 45 minutes to oxidize completely, but after the first test, you should check the strand at 10-minute intervals. Except when you must obtain supplies, **never** leave the client unattended during a chemical service. Accurate measurements for the next mixture cannot be made when color residue is clinging to the inside of the bottle.

7. When the timer rings, check the test strand for discoloration.

7. Consult the instructor or manager for assistance. Usually, the color will not be fully developed after only 15 minutes. If the hair has had a prior application

8. Reset the timer to allow the color to oxidize completely according to the label directions.

8. Clockwatching is a bother when you are concentrating on doing things in the correct order. It is much easier to depend on a timer to indicate the proper amount of time.

9. When the timer rings, saturate the corner of a towel with water and then shampoo to remove coloring material from the strand. Thoroughly towel-dry the strand.

9. The ideal way to see exactly when color has developed is to remove the coloring material and thoroughly dry the hair. Wet hair will always appear darker than it really is. Removing the tint and drying the hair will enable you to determine how long the color should be allowed to develop (remain) on the hair. After testing, reapply tint to the hair strand.

10. Discuss the color with the client and agree on the color to be applied.

10. If the color is all right except for too much red highlight, adjust it by adding a small amount of drabber. A **drabber** is concentrated color with a blue or violet base that neutralizes red or gold overtones in the hair.

of metallic color or is in need of conditioning, uneven or unnatural color will result.

11. Using the comb, part the hair in four equal sections (Figure 17.10).

11. This step is a standard way to begin a virgin permanent hair color for darkening the hair.

12. Following the label directions, pour clear 20-volume peroxide into a clean applicator bottle. (Cream developers also are used.)

12. Never mix a tint unless you are ready to apply it immediately. It is much easier to measure the correct proportions if you add the peroxide first!

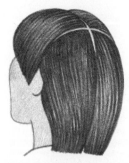

Figure 17.10
Part the hair in four quadrants (sections).

When the color is poured first, it stains the inside of the bottle and makes it difficult to see how many ounces (milliliters) of either liquid are in it.

13. Pour the correct amount of tint into the bottle. Check the total ounces (milliliters) of material in the bottle against the directions.

13. If the directions for 1½ ounces (45 milliliters) of color call for double peroxide (3 ounces/90 milliliters), the applicator bottle should have 4½ ounces (135 milliliters) of ready-to-use material after the color and peroxide are mixed. Always recheck measurements of coloring materials!

14. Secure the nozzle firmly on the applicator bottle and shake (gently or vigorously according to the directions).

14. Some manufacturers advise shaking the bottle gently because more vigorous shaking causes the combination to thicken too much. On the other hand, some color and peroxide combinations are applied in a gel form, which requires vigorous shaking for 10 to 15 seconds.

Sanitize your area as follows:
1. Wash, wipe, and store bottles and supplies.
2. Discard used supplies.
3. Clean and sanitize the cape and apron.
4. Sanitize the work area; wash your hands.

Applying a Virgin Tint to Lighten the Natural Hair Color

Procedures

Rationale

1. If the color selected is several shades lighter than the client's natural color, begin to apply it 1 inch (2.5 centimeters) away from the scalp area.

1. When you are coloring lighter, body heat causes the color to develop faster at the scalp than toward the middle of the hairshaft. Color also develops

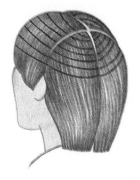

Figure 17.11
Part off horizontal ¼-inch (.625-centimeter) subsections.

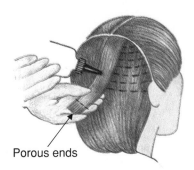

Porous ends

Figure 17.12
Apply tint only up to porous ends.

2. Use the nozzle of the applicator to part off horizontal ¼-inch (.625-centimeter) strands of hair in the right crown area (Figure 17.11).

3. Begin applying the color ½–1 inch (1.25–2.5 centimeters) away from the scalp to the top and bottom of the hair strand and work up to the ends of the hair (Figure 17.12). Work from the crown through the nape, using ¼-inch (.625-centimeter) partings.

4. After you have finished the right crown, go to the top left crown. Repeat application from the top crown through the nape.

5. Use the applicator nozzle to part off ¼-inch (.625-centimeter) strands on the left front top. Apply the color ½–1 inch (1.25–2.5 centimeters) from the scalp through to ½–1 inch (1.25–2.5 centimeters) from the ends of each strand. Work from the top to the bottom of the section.

6. Apply the color according to directions to the top right front section.

faster at the ends. If you apply color on the scalp first, the color will be uneven—lighter at the scalp and ends and slightly darker toward the middle of the hair shaft.

2. These partings ensure that all hair in the strand will be completely saturated.

3. Apply the color in the crown first. Hair around the front hairline is usually fine textured and less resistant than hair in the crown and nape.

4. **Do not allow coloring material to run into the client's eyes or onto his or her clothing.**

5. Since you have just completed the left nape, it is convenient to continue on to the left front top.

6. This will complete the application of color to all the hair except the scalp hair.

7. Set the timer for 15 minutes.

7. This allows the middle and ends of the hair shaft to start developing before you apply the color to the scalp hair. Body heat will cause this hair to oxidize the color faster.

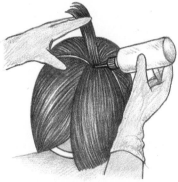

Figure 17.13
Apply color to scalp hair.

8. When the timer rings, make a strand test.

8. The strand tested should be lightened half as much as the desired final color.

9. Beginning in the right crown, apply color to the scalp hair and ends in ¼-inch (.625-centimeter) horizontal partings (Figure 17.13).

9. These partings help you color all of the hair.

10. Proceed to the left crown. Apply color in ¼-inch (.625-centimeter) horizontal partings. Work from the crown through the nape to color hair (Figure 17.14).

10. This is a good systematic way to apply the color.

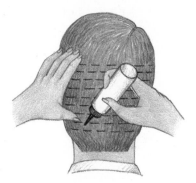

Figure 17.14
Working from the crown to the nape on a male client

11. Go to the left top front and continue to apply color to all of the scalp hair (Figure 17.15).

11. This is standard procedure.

12. Apply the color to the right top front section in ¼-inch (.625-centimeter) partings (Figure 17.16).

12. This is standard procedure.

13. Set the timer for 10 minutes; strand test when the timer rings and carefully check to be certain that all of the hair has color.

13. When the color on the ends of the hair matches the color on the hair next to the scalp, the color is even. It is easy to miss a small piece of hair, so check and apply color as needed.

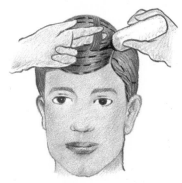

Figure 17.15
Application of tint to a male client. Note the horizontal partings.

14. Lightly spray lukewarm water around the hairline. Use your thumbs to work

14. This will begin the process of removing stain from the hairline.

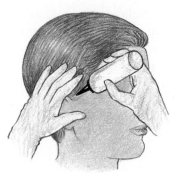

Figure 17.16
Applying tint to the right front section on a male client

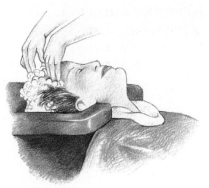

Figure 17.17
Shampoo gently, as the scalp may be sensitive.

the water into the color around the hairline.

15. Use circular thumb movements to work water and color into a lather. (Add shampoo as necessary.) Remove all color stains from the hairline.

16. Rinse the remaining color from the hairline, and shampoo the hair at least twice with a color-safe product.

17. Apply normalizing conditioner and discuss the results with the client.

18. Record the formula and results on the client's permanent hair-coloring card.

15. Warm water and the tint form a lather that removes stains along the hairline. This is the best way to remove stains. Quickly rinsing or shampooing color from the hair without lathering will not remove hairline stains. Lukewarm water is used because the scalp may be sensitive (Figure 17.17).

16. All coloring material should be removed from the scalp and hair. Dark colors may require more than two shampoos.

17. Since tints have a pH of between 9.5 and 10.5, it is necessary to neutralize traces of alkali.

18. Be sure to record the date, formula, result, and remarks.

Sanitize your area as follows:
1. Wash, wipe, and store bottles and supplies.
2. Discard used supplies.
3. Clean and sanitize the cape and apron.
4. Sanitize the work area; wash your hands.

Applying a Virgin Tint to Darken the Natural Hair Color

The steps and safety procedures for darkening the hair are basically the same as for previous services. The basic difference is that the tint is applied to the entire strand.

Practical Objective 5
Applying a Tint Retouch

Procedure

1. Prepare the client for a basic tinting service. Use the same procedures for applying a tint to new growth.

2. Apply the tint to outline partings, which divide the hair into four equal sections (Figure 17.18). Apply tint only to the new growth of hair (Figure 17.19). Stay ¹⁄₁₆ inch (.156 centimeter) from the previously tinted hair.

3. If hair is more than 50 percent gray, start applying the tint on the front top right section; then go to the front top left. Cover the crown section in ¼-inch (.625-centimeter) horizontal partings.

Rationale

1. Procedures and safety precautions are the same as for previously described services.

2. Do not overlap tint onto hair that has already been tinted. A **line of demarcation** will result from overlapping. If color is applied on tinted hair next to new growth, the color will build up on this part and cause a line of darker (or lighter) color. (It will look like marked hair caused by improper cutting.)

3. When hair is more than 50 percent gray, it is more resistant to coloring, so many cosmetologists begin applying color along the front rather than the crown. This gives better coverage of gray. If the hair is less than 50 percent gray, most cosmetologists begin applying in the right crown and work in ¼-inch (.625-centimeter) horizontal partings toward the nape.

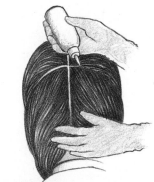

Figure 17.18
Always wear protective gloves. To begin, apply tint to the section outlines.

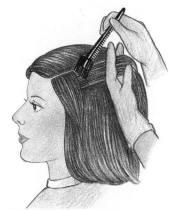

Figure 17.19
Apply tint to new growth.

4. After you have retouched all new growth, carefully inspect the areas in which you have applied the tint. Apply in any area missed. Gently lift the ends of the hair away from the head.

5. Develop color as usual. Shampoo and set the hair.

4. The tint oxidizes better if air is allowed to circulate through the hair. Do not mat the hair ends close to the head.

5. This procedure is the same as for the previously described services.

Sanitize your area as follows:
1. **Wash, wipe, and store bottles and supplies.**
2. **Discard used supplies.**
3. **Clean and sanitize the cape and apron.**
4. **Sanitize the work area; wash your hands.**

Glossary

Aniline (AN-ehl-ehn) derivative A substance used in tints. It comes from coal tar.

Coal tar An organic substance used to make synthetic hair dyes.

Developer A chemical that provides the oxygen to fix the color during a permanent hair-coloring process. Most modern products use 20-volume (6 percent) hydrogen peroxide for the developer.

Double peroxide Mixing twice as much peroxide as color in the permanent hair-coloring service.

Drabber Concentrated color with a blue or violet base that neutralizes red or gold overtones in the hair.

Equal peroxide Mixing equal amounts of peroxide and color in the permanent hair-coloring service.

Hydrogen peroxide An acid used to provide oxygen in chemical hair coloring. In this process, it is called the developer.

Hydrometer (high-DROHM-eh-tehr) An instrument used to determine the strength of the peroxide or other chemical in a mixture.

Hypersensitive (high-per-SEN-seh-tiv) Allergic

Lightening and toning A double-application method of coloring hair by using two different products, one to take color from the hair and another to add the new color.

Line of demarcation A line of darker or lighter color in the hair caused by overlapping the application of a tint onto hair that has already been tinted.

Oxidation The process of combining oxygen with other substances.

Oxidation tint A permanent hair color that deposits the color into the hair shaft through a chemical process. Also called a penetrating tint.

Oxidizer Any substance that gives up oxygen during the process of oxidation.

Para-phenylene-diamine (PA-rah-FEN-a-leen-DIGH-eh-meen) A synthetic organic compound that is derived from coal tar and used to give color to hair dye.

Patch test See **Predisposition test.**

Penetrating tint Hair coloring that permanently penetrates the cuticle and deposits color in the cortex of the hair shaft. Also called oxidation tint.

Peroxide See **Hydrogen peroxide.**

Predisposition (pree-dis-peh-ZISH-ehn) test The process of applying a small amount of hair color to the client's skin at least 24 hours before the service to determine if the client is allergic to the product. Also known as a patch test.

Retouch tint Coloring the new growth of hair that has already been permanently colored.

Single-application coloring service Hair coloring that is done in one application, such as darkening the hair.

Soap cap A service that highlights or slightly changes hair color by combining permanent hair color with shampoo and applying it like shampoo to dry hair.

Virgin hair Hair that has not been overexposed to the sun or treated by tints, chemical straighteners, cold-waving solutions, or other chemical services.

Virgin tint The process of using a permanent hair color on virgin hair.

Questions

1. What is virgin hair?
2. What are the three main parts of a soap cap?
3. What is the chemical abbreviation for hydrogen peroxide?
4. Write a definition for "double process."
5. Can hair tint be used to color eyelashes or eyebrows?
6. In your own words, write a paragraph(s) explaining the reasons a client might want a tint.
7. Does permanent color penetrate the hair shaft?
8. What layer(s) of the hair is (are) penetrated with a permanent hair color?
9. What is another name for an oxidation tint?

10. What is the name for hair that has not been previously treated with chemicals, such as cold-waving solutions or lighteners?
11. When the client's tinted hair grows out, what service will he or she need?
12. What is the activating chemical that makes an oxidizing tint work?
13. What is the name for the developer used in a tint?
14. What is the main ingredient in an aniline tint?
15. What is the pH range of hydrogen peroxide?
16. What name is given to an aniline derivative color that permanently colors the hair?
17. Can a single-process tint be used to lighten the hair?
18. Does an aniline tint completely cover gray hair?
19. If the client wants to change his or her hair color, will the tint shampoo out of the hair?
20. Is it necessary to wear protective gloves when tinting the hair?
21. Is it all right to mix tint in a metal bowl?
22. How can you determine beforehand how a color will turn out on a particular natural hair color?
23. In order to dilute the volume of the peroxide 50 percent, how much water would you add to the following formula: 2 ounces (60 milliliters) tint and 2 ounces (60 milliliters) peroxide?
24. When applying a virgin tint, should you begin by applying the color at the porous ends?
25. If you were doing a tint retouch, would you apply the tint to the new growth first?
26. Will the scalp be sensitive following a tint?
27. Should you keep a record of all tint clients, their formulas, and predisposition tests?
28. When applying a tint retouch, how far away from the previously tinted hair should the application be?
29. What device is used to measure the volume of peroxide?

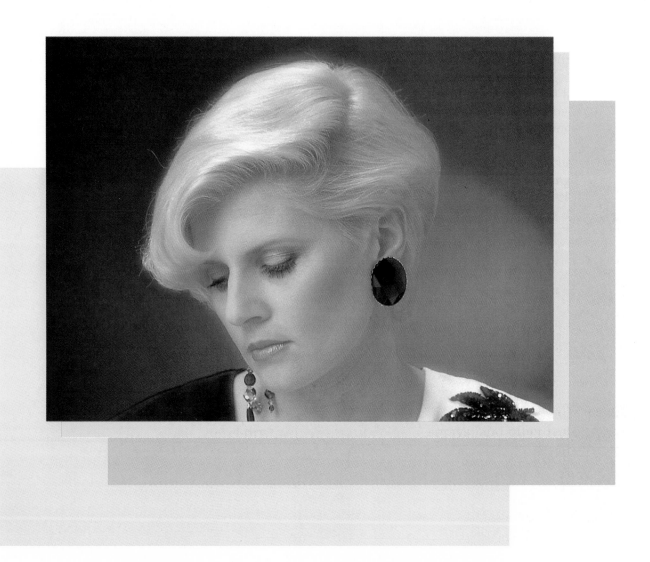

Lightening and Toning

Learning Objective

Provided with lightening and toning supplies, follow the proper steps to lighten and tone the client's hair. Using the proper safety precautions and following label directions, apply a virgin lightener and retouch lightener in 30–45 minutes for each. Score 85 percent or better on a multiple-choice exam on the information in this chapter.

In order to achieve the above level of competence, you should master the following chapter objectives.

Theory Objectives

1. Define hair lightening and toning; describe their chemical effects on the hair; and identify the seven stages of lightening hair.
2. Identify types of lighteners and services for lightening and toning and identify the toning colors.

Practical Objectives

3. Apply a virgin lightener.
4. Apply a lightener retouch.

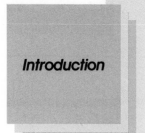

Introduction

You may remember from Chapter 17 that the second way to color the hair permanently is by lightening and toning it. This process, called a **double-application** service, involves some of the same basic steps that you used to tint the hair. The double application will be explained in detail in this chapter.

Theory Objective 1
Hair Lightening and Toning, Their Chemical Effects on Hair, and the Seven Stages of Lightening Hair

As Chapter 17 pointed out, a double-application service involves two separate services that use different products. When you lighten the hair, you apply a **lightening agent.** After the hair is lightened, the lightening agent is shampooed from the hair.

Toning the hair involves applying a special pastel coloring product to hair that has been lightened. These pastel colors, called **toners,** contain molecules of color that are so large that they can only penetrate the cuticle of lightened hair. Some toners are aniline derivatives. Hydrogen peroxide must be used with them. Other toners are semipermanent colors that do not need peroxide.

Lighteners have complicated chemical formulas. Like most products, they vary from one brand to the next, but they generally contain ammonium, potassium, and sodium persulfates, plus water, fatty acid soaps, alcohols, and a small amount of color (usually blue or white). Although you probably are most interested in the effects these chemicals have on the hair, for safety's sake, you should keep their general chemical makeup in mind.

Before these lightening chemicals are applied to the hair, they are mixed with 20-volume peroxide, which is the **catalyst** (KAT-el-est) (an agent that starts a chemical reaction). This mixture has a pH of about 8 to 9.5. It takes the brown, red, and yellow color out (decolorizes) of the cortex of the hair by oxidizing (adding oxygen to) the coloring pigment. The pigment actually vaporizes (evaporates) in the natural hair color. If you had a very powerful microscope, you could see that after a hair has been lightened, the melanin is no longer in the cortex (Figure 18.1). You would see spots in the hair shaft where the molecules of melanin, or pigment, once were. The toner fills these spots with new molecules of color. Many toners in a wide variety of strengths are available. The one you choose will, of course, depend on how light a color you want. Very light toners can be used only when the natural color has been completely lightened or "lifted."

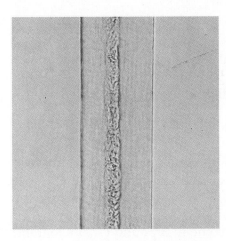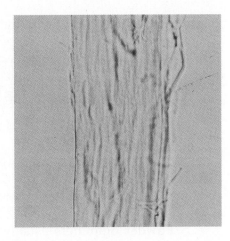

Figure 18.1
Two lightened hairs as seen under a light microscope. Note the absence of pigment in the cortex of each hair. The hair on the right has been overlightened.

Lightening is an oxidizing process that brings hair color to different stages of lightness. Counting black hair as the starting point, there are seven stages of lightening: **black, brown, red, red-gold, gold, yellow, and pale yellow**.

Hair must be porous enough as well as light enough to accept a toner; even hair that is naturally very light is not porous enough. All hair needs to be lightened before a toner can be applied.

Occasionally, you will be lightening a client's hair and planning to apply a toner. Suddenly, the client will look up and say, "That's it! That's the color I want." You can simply shampoo the lightener from the hair—you have saved your client some money and saved yourself some time.

The lightener may be shampooed from the hair at any time during the lightening process. Lightener can be applied to the hair to prepare it for a toner, or it may sometimes be used to lighten the hair to a desirable color without applying a toner.

Theory Objective 2
Types of Lighteners and Lightening and Toning Services

Lighteners are made in three basic forms: cream, powder, and oil.

In selecting a lightener, you should consider how and where you are going to use it. For example, a virgin lightener and a lightener retouch require direct contact between the scalp and the lightener, so a cream lightener, which is milder than the other forms, would be the best choice.

Packages of **cream lightener** usually contain one 2-ounce (60-milliliter) bottle of lightener and two packets of activators, also called protinators/activators or energizers. Half of the lightener base and one activator packet are used per application, so a package should be good for two applications. When you mix the lightener, put peroxide in the bottle first. Then add the activator and shake the bottle. Finally, add the cream lightener base and mix by shaking. Now the lightener is ready to apply.

The cream base contains a very small amount of white or blue color that slightly neutralizes unwanted red or brassy gold tones that are brought out during lightening. Cream lighteners also contain buffering, or conditioning agents, which keep the hair and scalp in better condition during the lightening process than powder lighteners do.

When cream lighteners are mixed, they have a creamy consistency, like a gel, that makes them easy to apply. The lightener remains where it is applied; it does not dry out, drip, or run onto the forehead and neck.

Powder lighteners usually come in 3-pound (1.35-kilogram) cans and need only to be mixed with hydrogen peroxide. Because they contain few buffers or conditioners, powder lighteners may irritate the scalp and are therefore used for off-scalp lightening. They are used primarily for creative techniques, such as streaking, framing, frosting, and painting (tipping), because the bleach does not come in direct contact with the scalp in these services. Hair is **streaked** by using foil to lighten large sections around the face. In **framing,** a continuous lighter band is made around the hairline. Although a separate application of lightener is not required, the tints that are used contain lightener, so the process is covered in this unit. Hair is **frosted** by using a cap or foil to lighten or darken small strands of hair throughout the head. Once the hair has been frosted with light strands of hair, it may be given a **reverse frosting.** This process darkens strands of hair when too many strands have been lightened. Hair is **painted** by **tipping** small strands toward the front of the head. These strands can be either lightened or darkened. Powder lighteners are faster and stronger than cream or oil lighteners, but they have a tendency to dry out when they are being used. Always remember **not** to use powder lighteners on the scalp.

Oil lighteners decolorize the natural pigment and also add a slight amount of certified color to the hair during the process. They come in the following colors: neutral, which sometimes is added in small amounts to regular tints to make the tint lighter; silver, which neutralizes red or brassy gold tones; gold, which adds golden highlights to otherwise drab hair; and red, which adds reddish highlights to the hair. Remember that all oil lighteners deposit a small amount of color and lighten the hair so a toner may not be needed.

Cream, powder, and oil lighteners do not require a patch test, but the test must be given if you are going to apply a toner after the lightener.

Many manufacturers use one of the following terms to identify the color that their toner will leave on lightened hair: gold, yellow-gold-orange, red, platinum, silver, or ash.

Yellow, gold, orange, red, and brown are **warm hair colors.** Ash, silver, platinum, smoke, and steel gray are **cool** (drab) hair colors. Recognizing the manufacturer's terms for toning colors will help you use the color chart to select a toning color for the client. For example, after you have studied the toning chart, you will know that a silver tone has a blue base, which would be used to naturalize lightened hair that is a little too yellow.

Practical Objective 3
Applying a Virgin Lightener

Supplies

- client release form
- client permanent record form
- 20-volume peroxide
- cream lightener
- timer

- shampoo supplied, including non-color-stripping shampoo
- clean plastic lightener applicator bottle
- protective gloves
- protective apron

Procedure	Rationale
1. Record the results of the patch test. Double drape the client for a chemical service.	**1.** You must give a patch test if an aniline toner will be used.
2. Do **not** shampoo or brush hair.	**2.** Lightener can produce small or large red blisters on the scalp if the hair is vigorously brushed or shampooed before it is lightened.
3. Thoroughly examine the scalp and the texture and condition of the client's hair.	**3.** If cuts, scratches, or abrasions are present, do not apply lightener. Condition hair that is very porous, fragile, or chemically damaged before you lighten it. If the hair is badly damaged, do not lighten. No other coloring products should be on the hair. If there are any other products, do not lighten.

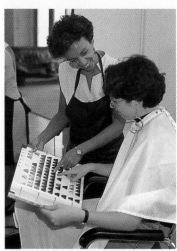

Figure 18.2
*Helping the client select a
toner from the color chart*

4. If a toner is going to be applied, use the color chart to help the client make a selection (Figure 18.2). See the chart for footnotes on lightening stages.

5. Part the hair into sections; then mix lightener according to label directions.

4. You will not be able to get light, delicate toning colors if the natural (virgin) hair color is very red. Do not tell a client who has dark red hair that the color selected will be the one he or she will get. Consult your instructor or manager for assistance. The bottom of the color chart describes the stages to which the hair must be lightened for a particular toner to give a certain color. Compare the stage needed to the condition of the client's hair. If the toner requires lightening to pale yellow and the client's hair is fine in texture and naturally black, the hair would probably break before it reached the pale yellow (seventh) stage. Ask your instructor for help and advise the client accordingly.

5. Cream lighteners usually have to be mixed in the following sequence. Put 4 ounces (120 milliliters) of clear 20-volume hydrogen peroxide in a bottle; add two activators (the protinators or energizers); cover and shake well. (Activators are really alkalizers. They speed up the lightening process by increasing the alkalinity of the product.) Then add 2 ounces (60 milliliters) of lightener base; cover and shake thoroughly. Mixing cream lighteners any other

6. Lightly powder the insides of surgical gloves and put them on.

7. Apply lightener in the same way that you would apply a virgin tint to **lighten** the hair—**away** from the scalp first (Figure 18.3).

8. Begin applying the lightener in the right crown section. Apply the lightener ½–1 inch (1.25–2.5 centimeters) away from the scalp and ends. Use ⅛-inch (.31-centimeter) horizontal partings. Apply the lightener in a bead across the strand. Following the proper steps, apply lightener carefully and quickly to all the hair.

9. Carefully examine the hair where the lightener has been applied.

10. Check the lightener application for dripping or running. Be sure that lightener has not dripped onto the hair next to the scalp.

11. Take a strand test after 30 minutes have passed (Figure 18.4).

way causes them to be "sandy" and unusable.

6. Always wear gloves to protect your hands during lightening or toning.

7. The principles for lightening are the same as for tinting, but lightener lightens the hair more. This is standard procedure.

8. These partings are needed to ensure that all hair will have enough lightener for even lightening. Apply the lightener generously so that it rests on and through the hair. Keep all lightener on hair strands moist. Allow air to circulate through the hair to oxidize the lightener. Apply lightener quickly so it will lighten the hair evenly.

9. There must be a generous amount of moist lightener on and through each strand.

10. Use the corner of a towel saturated with cold water to remove any lightener that is running down the hair shaft to the scalp. Lightener should not reach the hair next to the scalp because body heat will cause that hair to lighten faster, making it lighter than the area farther down the shaft.

11. When the hair is about half as light as you want it, you should apply the lightener

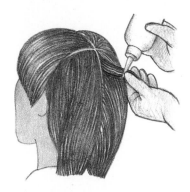

Figure 18.3
Virgin lightener application. Apply lightener away from the scalp first.

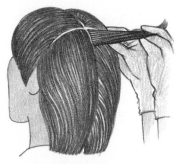

Figure 18.4
Strand testing hair

to the hair next to the scalp. Use horizontal partings ⅛ inch (.31 centimeters) apart. If the hair is not ready, reapply lightener to the strand used for the test. Strand test frequently as desired.

12. Carefully apply lightener to the hair next to the scalp, so that it meets the lightener that has already been applied to the hair. Apply the lightener in the same order you applied lightener to the middle and ends of the hair strands. Remove lightener by rinsing and shampooing when the hair has lightened to the correct stage.

12. Apply the lightener generously across the hair strands. Do not spread the lightener thinly across the strand. If it is spread too thinly, the hair will not be evenly lightened.

13. Use a towel or dryer to dry the hair according to the label directions of the toner; mix the toner and peroxide as directed. Apply according to directions.

13. Carefully read label directions because they vary from product to product. Wear protective gloves when applying toner.

14. Apply normalizing creme or conditioner.

14. Use a conditioner or normalizing creme to neutralize the alkalinity of the toner.

Sanitize your area as follows:
1. **Wash, wipe, and store bottles and supplies.**
2. **Discard used supplies.**
3. **Clean and sanitize the cape and apron.**
4. **Sanitize the work area; wash your hands.**

Supplies

- client release form
- client permanent record form
- 20-volume peroxide
- cream lightener
- protective gloves
- protective apron
- shampoo supplies, including non-color-stripping shampoo
- timer
- clean plastic lightener applicator bottle

Use the same steps that you used for a tint retouch. As you probably remember, tinting is a single-application process, whereas lightening is a double-application process. Therefore you have one additional step. After you have removed the lightener and shampooed the hair, apply a toner to the hair. If the lightener overlaps onto previously lightened hair, breakage may result.

Glossary

Catalyst (KAT-el-est) An agent that starts a chemical reaction.

Cool (drab) hair colors Hair color products that correspond to the cool secondary colors on the color chart. These are ash, silver, platinum, smoke, and steel gray.

Cream lightener A hair-lightening product with a gel-like consistency that makes it easy to apply.

Drab hair colors See **Cool hair colors.**

Framing Making a continuous lighter band of hair around the hairline.

Frosting Lightening or darkening small strands of hair throughout the head by using a cap or foil.

Painting Lightening or darkening small strands of hair toward the face. Also called **tipping.**

Powder lighteners Hair-lightening products that come in powder form and are mixed with peroxide for use. Because they contain few buffers or conditioners, they can irritate the scalp and are used primarily for applications where they will not come in contact with the scalp.

Streaking Lightening large sections of hair around the face by using foil.

Tipping Lightening or darkening small strands of hair toward the front of the head. Also called **painting.**

Toners Pastel colors used to color lightened hair.

Toning Applying a special pastel coloring product to hair that has been lightened.

Warm hair colors Hair color products with bases that correspond to the warm colors on the color chart. These are yellow, gold, orange, red, and brown.

Questions

1. Using a dictionary, write a definition for the term catalyst.
2. Give an example of a catalyst used in lightening the hair.
3. Generally, what kind of lightener is used to streak the hair?
4. Which colors are classified as "warm hair colors"?
5. What general term is used to describe the process of lightening and toning the hair?
6. What is the pH range of a lightener mixture?
7. Does lightener remove color pigment from the hair?
8. From which layer of the hair does lightener remove pigment?
9. Is lightening an oxidizing process?
10. Using your own words, write a description of the process for reverse frosting the hair.
11. What are the three basic forms of lightener used in the salon?
12. Write definitions for frosting, streaking, and tipping; then compare them to the textbook.
13. Is it necessary to give a patch test before applying a lightener?
14. Should you shampoo the hair before applying a lightener?
15. Should you give a patch test before applying an aniline toner?
16. How far from the scalp should a virgin lightener be applied?
17. What size horizontal subsections should be used?
18. Is strand testing ever done before lightening the hair?
19. Is it necessary to wear gloves when applying lightener?
20. What is "overlapping"?
21. Can overlapping cause breakage?

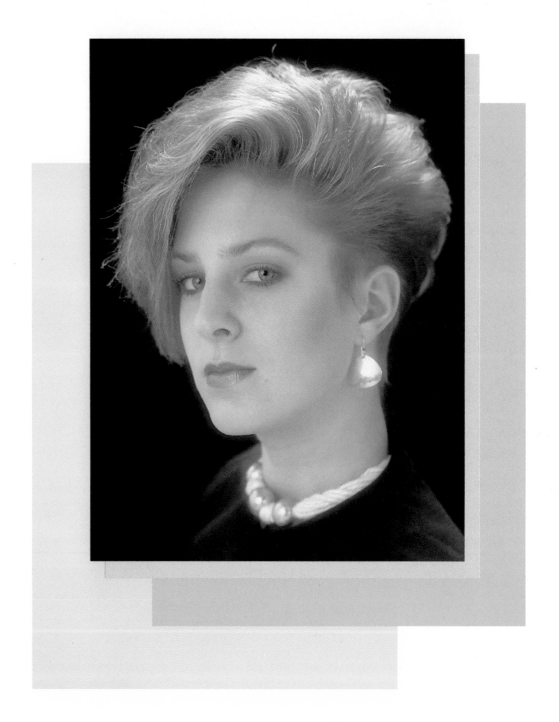

19

Creative Lightening and Toning Techniques

Learning Objective

Provided with the necessary supplies, follow the proper steps to achieve special lightening and toning effects—streaking, framing, frosting, and painting the hair and tinting it back to its original color. Score 85 percent or better on a multiple-choice exam on the information in this chapter.

In order to achieve the above level of competence, you should master the following chapter objectives.

Practical Objectives

1. Foil frost the hair.
2. Frame the hair.
3. Frost the hair.
4. Paint (freehand lighten) the hair.
5. Tint the hair back to its original color, lighter or darker.

Introduction

Chapter 18 introduced the basic principles of lightening and toning. This chapter will explain how to apply those principles to achieve special effect. Your instructor will also have methods and techniques which will be different from those presented in this chapter, and you will enjoy learning those techniques and products too. Remember that hair coloring is so vast that even your experienced teachers learn something new each day. So, don't be disappointed if it seems like there is almost too much to learn. Once you have picked-up on the basics, you will develop use of products and methods which you will feel comfortable using on your clients after graduating, becoming licensed, and working in the salon.

Practical Objective 1
Foil Frosting the Hair

Supplies

- client release form
- client permanent hair-coloring form
- shampoo supplies
- protective gloves
- 4–8 clips
- aluminum foil
- powder lightener
- 20-volume hydrogen peroxide
- color chart
- protective apron

Procedure

1. Review the client's permanent hair-coloring form and ask the client if any other products have been used.

2. Brush the hair according to its style.

3. Cut pieces of foil; place them at the base of the strands which have been separated using the weaving technique; and clip them into place.

4. Mix powder lightener with peroxide in a plastic or glass container according to the label directions.

Rationale

1. Always find out what other services or chemicals have been applied to the hair.

2. This helps you locate the streak(s).

3. Fit the foil to the hair's length. The longer the hair, the larger the pieces of foil should be. This helps you apply the lightener to the strand and immediately fold the foil around it.

4. Peroxide, ammonia, and other sulfonated lightening chemicals should not be mixed in metal containers.

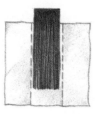
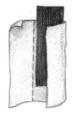
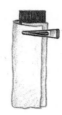
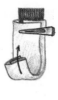

Figure 19.1
Carefully wrap foil around each strand of hair with lightener.

5. Apply the lightener to one strand and fold and clip the strand (Figure 19.1).

6. Apply lightener to the rest of the strands from the scalp through the ends of the hair (Figure 19.2). Then wrap the foil around them again and clip the foil. Leave the lightener on the hair until it is as light as you want it to be (Figure 19.3).

7. Remove all foil when the hair has lightened. Thoroughly rinse the lightener from the hair and shampoo it twice with colorsafe (nonstripping) shampoo. Apply normalizing cream if necessary.

8. Towel-dry the hair and apply temporary, semipermanent, or toning color, if necessary, to achieve the desired color.

5. Enough lightener should be used to lighten the strand thoroughly. Do not allow lightener to seep outside the foil or onto the scalp.

6. Since foil is used on each strand, the hair will decolorize evenly.

7. A nonstripping shampoo is milder for lightened hair. Lightener should be neutralized.

8. Temporary colors are often applied to streaks to neutralize unnatural gold or brassy tones.

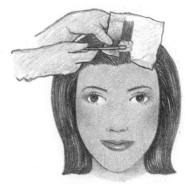

Figure 19.2
Lightener must be kept moist in order to lighten hair.

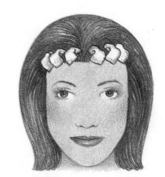

Figure 19.3
Leave the lightener on until the hair has lifted to the desired degree of lightness.

Sanitize your area as follows:

1. Wash, wipe, and store bottles and supplies.
2. Discard used supplies.
3. Clean and sanitize the cape and apron.
4. Sanitize the work area; wash your hands.

Practical Objective 2
Framing the Hair

Supplies

- client permanent hair-coloring form
- protective skin cream
- aluminum foil
- permanent hair colors
- 20-volume hydrogen peroxide
- applicator bottle with nozzle
- protective gloves
- talcum powder
- shampoo supplies
- color chart
- protective apron
- dispensary scissors

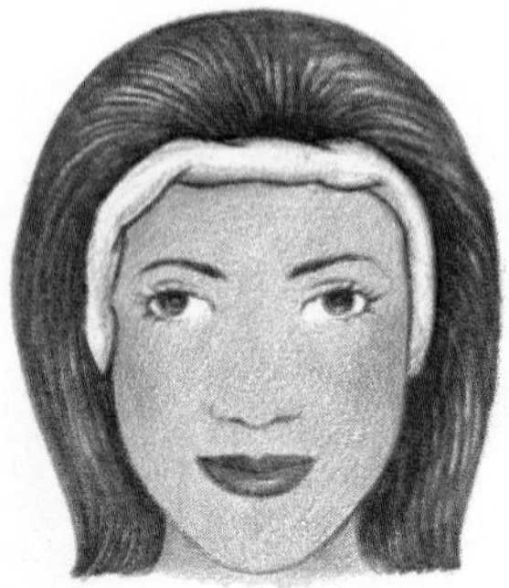

Figure 19.4
Apply protective cream around hairline.

Procedure	*Rationale*
1. Apply protective skin cream around the entire front hairline (Figure 19.4).	**1.** The protective skin cream acts like an adhesive or paste to keep the aluminum foil in position at all times.
2. Put enough aluminum foil around the hairline to extend from the left sideburn through the top center forehead and down to the right sideburn.	**2.** The foil protects the client's face (eyes, nose, mouth).
3. Use the tail comb to weave a 1/2-inch (1.25-centimeter) section of hair around the entire foil line (Figures 19.5 and 19.6). Clip the hair if necessary.	**3.** This is the first section that will be tinted. The lightest tint color will be applied around the hairline. Then progressively darker colors will be used.
4. Mix enough of the lightest tint to cover the hair you have sectioned (Figure 19.7).	**4.** Mix just enough color to cover this section.

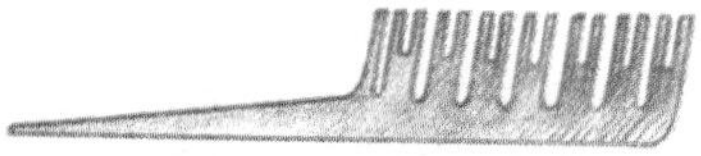

Figure 19.5
Hair weaving comb.

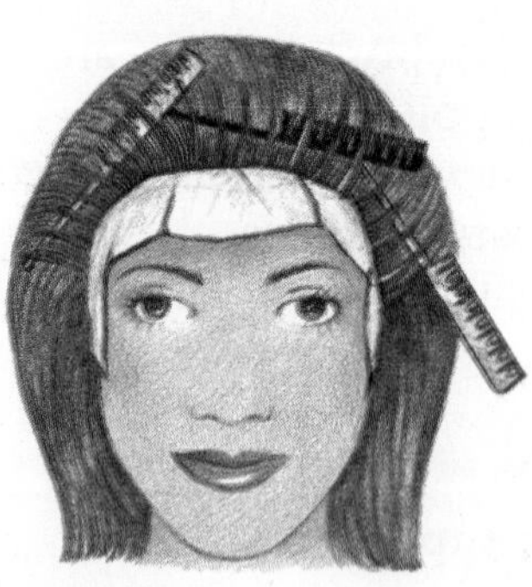

Figure 19.6
Weave comb through the hair.

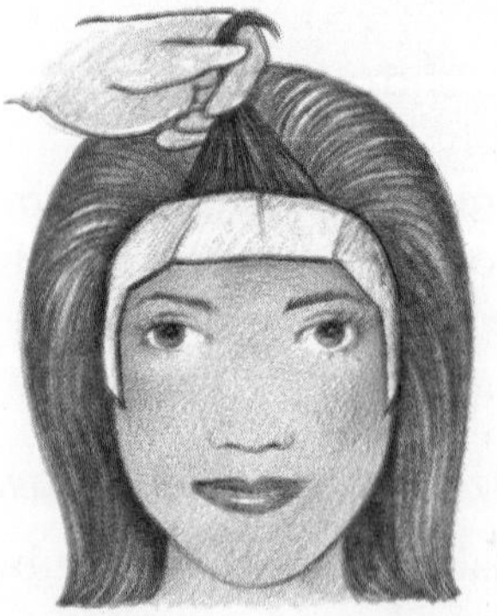

Figure 19.7
Start with the lightest tint.

5. Lay the tinted section on top of the foil (Figure 19.8) and put another length of foil on top.

6. Weave another 1/2-inch to 1-inch (1.25- to 2.5-centimeter) section of hair around the front of the hairline. Mix another tint preparation slightly darker than the first.

7. Apply tint to the strand; place the tinted strand along the new foil toward the face.

8. Apply foil and tint to the desired color.

5. The tinted strand is placed forward toward the face on the foil so that it will be out of the next strand to be tinted.

6. The change from one tint to another must be gradual.

7. The foil separates the individually tinted strands so that the tints do not come in contact with each other or with hair not to be colored.

8. The darkest tint should not be darker than the client's natural hair color.

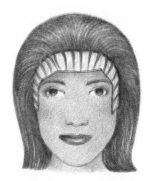

Figure 19.8
Lay the tinted section on top of the foil or cellophane.

Sanitize your area as follows:

1. **Wash, wipe, and store bottles and supplies.**
2. **Discard used supplies.**
3. **Clean and sanitize the cape and apron.**
4. **Sanitize the work area; wash your hands.**

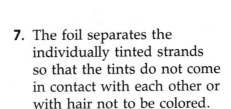

Practical Objective 3
Frosting the Hair

Supplies

- powder lightener
- plastic undercap
- frosting cap
- plastic overcap
- lightener applicator bottle with nozzle
- 20-volume hydrogen peroxide
- crochet hook

- toner color chart
- talcum powder
- protective gloves
- shampoo supplies
- client release form
- client permanent hair-coloring form
- protective apron

Procedure

1. Remove tangles from the hair, and comb the hair straight back and close to

Rationale

1. Preconditioning may be necessary. Frosting is not recommended for hair

the head. Precondition if necessary.

2. Place the undercap and frosting cap on the client's head. If the hair is quite long, lightly apply creme rinse before putting on the undercap.

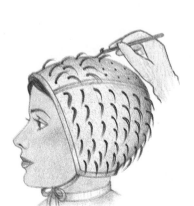

Figure 19.9
Pull hair through the frosting cap with a crochet hook.

3. Using a fine crochet hook, begin pulling strands of hair through the holes in the top section (Figure 19.9).

4. Begin just behind the front hairline. Pull 8 to 12 strands through the holes in the top of the cap. Pull 4 to 8 strands through the holes on each side of the cap, but avoid pulling strands that are on the hairline.

5. Pull 4 to 8 strands through the holes in the crown of the cap.

6. Finish by pulling 8 to 14 strands in the nape section.

7. If the client complains of too much frosting, reverse frost the hair.

8. Mix the powder lightener with hydrogen peroxide according to label directions and apply it generously from the cap through the ends of the hair (Figure 19.10).

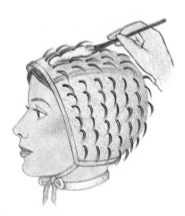

Figure 19.10
Apply lightener generously.

having a very dark tint because brassy streaks will result.

2. The undercap will prevent lightener from seeping (referred to as bleeding) through the frosting cap, which may have holes that are too large. A creme rinse makes long hair easier to pull through the frosting cap.

3. A fine crochet hook is the best implement to use. Do not pierce the scalp with the tip of the hook. Pull the hair slowly.

4. Begin behind the front hairline. Otherwise, an outgrowth of new hair will be visible in 4 to 6 weeks. The number of strands will vary with the amount of frosting desired.

5. Same as step 4.

6. This procedure completes the process of an even, attractive frosting.

7. Contact your instructor.

8. Powder lighteners, which are stronger than cream lighteners, can be used in frosting because the frosting cap protects the scalp from the lightener. Each strand must have enough lightener to remove the color pigment evenly.

9. Put the overcap on over the frosting cap (Figure 19.11).

10. Optional step: seat the client under a warm dryer for 15 minutes or until the hair is lightened enough.

11. After the hair is lightened and porous enough, rinse the lightener from the hair and shampoo once. Do not remove the undercap.

12. Dry hair under the dryer. Mix and apply toner. Allow toner to develop. Then rinse it out, remove the undercap, and shampoo the hair.

9. Natural body heat captured by the overcap accelerates the lightening action.

10. Some schools and salons use heat from the dryer to speed up the lightening action; others do not.

11. Lightener must be removed from the cap as well as from the hair, or the toner will not color the hair. Two shampoos may be necessary. If the undercap is removed, you will not be able to apply the toner.

12. Toners are usually applied to dry or towel-dried hair. This is standard procedure.

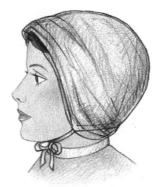

Figure 19.11
Cover with plastic cap.

Sanitize your area as follows:

1. **Wash, wipe, and store bottles and supplies.**
2. **Discard used supplies.**
3. **Clean and sanitize the cape and apron.**
4. **Sanitize the work area; wash your hands.**

Practical Objective 4
Painting (Freehand Lightening) the Hair

Supplies

- powder lightener and applicator bottle
- orangewood stick
- cotton
- shampoo supplies
- 20-volume peroxide
- cellophane
- hair-setting tape
- protective cream
- 4 clips
- protective apron
- protective gloves

Procedure

1. Carefully part off the top section of the hairstyle and

Rationale

1. Painting will be more difficult if you disturb the

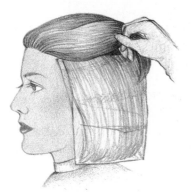

Figure 19.12
Protect the hair underneath the area you will be highlighting.

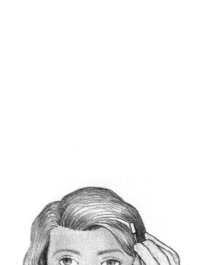

Figure 19.13
Apply lightener smoothly to the surface of the hair.

apply protective cream to the hair just below the top section. Apply sparingly from the hairline across the upper crown to the opposite side of the head.

2. Place the cellophane over the cream application and fasten it in place on the forehead with hair-setting tape (Figure 19.12).

3. Bring the top section into its regular styling position and spray lightly with a protein conditioner.

4. Wet the top of an orangewood stick with water; roll a bit of cotton around the point of the stick with about 1/2 inch (1.25 centimeters) of cotton on the stick.

5. Mix a frosting or powder lightener according to label directions, except add 1/2 to 1 ounce (15 to 30 milliliters) **more** peroxide.

6. Apply the lightener on the right or left side to accent the natural movement of the hairstyle.

7. When applying lightener along the top hairline for a half-bang, paint **very thinly** on very few strands (Figure 19.13).

8. If the top section is styled to one side of the head, begin painting a fine line of lightener; then branch off from one line into several others (Figures 19.14 and 19.15).

hairstyling lines. The cream will keep the cellophane in place.

2. Be very careful. If the cellophane falls from the head, it will be very difficult to paint the hair.

3. This is the section that will be painted. The conditioner will help keep the hair from moving while you paint it.

4. The orangewood stick tipped with cotton makes an excellent inexpensive applicator.

5. Using more hydrogen peroxide will make the lightener thinner and easier to apply (paint) to the hair.

6. The hairstyle will determine where you will begin painting.

7. If large strands are painted, the outgrowth of new hair will be obvious and unattractive.

8. Branching accents the hairstyle better than many individually painted streaks.

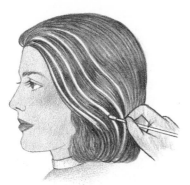

Figure 19.14
Apply lightener in the designed pattern.

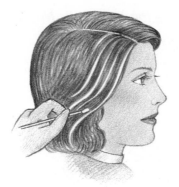

Figure 19.15
Begin applying lightener to side sections.

9. When you have finished, remove the hair-setting tape and cellophane.

10. Rinse the lightener from the hair. Shampoo twice. Condition the hair as needed and apply normalizing cream or acid rinse.

11. Air wave or set the hair.

9. When you stop depends on your judgment and artistic sense.

10. The lightening material must be removed. Some hair needs conditioning after lightening. Alkalinity from the lightener should be neutralized by normalizing cream or acid rinse.

11. This is standard procedure.

Sanitize your area as follows:

1. Wash, wipe, and store bottles and supplies.
2. Discard used supplies.
3. Clean and sanitize the cape and apron.
4. Sanitize the work area; wash your hands.

Practical Objective 5
Tinting the Hair

Supplies

- client permanent hair-color form
- color fillers
- dye solvent
- filler color chart
- 20-volume peroxide

- permanent hair-color chart
- color applicator bottle
- protective gloves
- protective apron
- shampoo supplies
- tint

Lightening the Hair to Its Natural Color

Procedure	*Rationale*
1. Analyze the hair's texture, elasticity, and porosity.	**1.** The hair should always be in good condition before any chemical service. This service is also called a **tint-back.**
2. Use a **dye solvent** to lighten the tinted color.	**2.** A dye solvent removes artificial and natural color. Neutral oil bleaches also remove both artificial and natural colors from the hair. Dye solvents are milder for hair, but they take longer to remove color. Dye solvents may require more than one application. Do not begin the tint until at least 24 hours after you have used the dye solvent.
3. Following the label directions, mix the dye solvent in a glass or plastic container.	**3.** For best results, dye solvents must be mixed and applied precisely according to label directions.
4. Apply the dye solvent along 3/4 of the strand (all except the ends).	**4.** Because the ends are more porous, the solvent removes color faster there than from the rest of the hair shaft.
5. Strand test for desired color.	**5.** Always strand test.
6. If dark streaks appear, rinse, shampoo lightly, and dry with a dryer.	**6.** Dark streaks can be removed on dry hair by **spot lightening.**
7. Apply the solvent to the dark spots (streaks) and leave only until desired lightening results.	**7.** Apply solvent or lightener only to dark spots. Removing a dark tint from hair by using a shampoo, dye solvent, lightener, or tint is called **stripping** the hair.

8. Rinse and dry when the desired color is achieved. Analyze the hair to determine if a **color filler** is needed, and apply if necessary.

8. A color filler is often needed before hair is tinted to equalize hair porosity, even out the color, or intensify the tint to be applied.

9. Apply the selected tint to the center of the strand.

9. Leave the scalp and ends until later. Color will develop more quickly at the scalp because of body heat and on the ends because of greater porosity. Start these areas later so color will be even.

10. Strand test until half the desired color is achieved; then apply tint to the hair next to the scalp.

10. Finish applying tint to the remainder of the hair.

11. Work the tint through the ends with your hands.

11. This spreads the color more evenly than combing does and does not irritate the scalp as much as combing.

12. Strand test until the color is even.

12. This is standard procedure.

13. Dilute tint slightly with warm water and remove hairline stains.

13. This is the best way to remove hairline stains from the scalp.

14. Thoroughly rinse the tint from the scalp and hair. Shampoo twice.

14. The hair will be gummy and sticky if you do not remove all tint from the scalp and hair.

15. Apply normalizing cream or conditioner. Record the coloring results on the client's form.

15. The alkalinity from the tint must be neutralized.

Sanitize your area as follows:

1. **Wash, wipe, and store bottles and supplies.**
2. **Discard used supplies.**
3. **Clean and sanitize the cape and apron.**
4. **Sanitize the work area; wash your hands.**

Darkening the Hair to Its Natural Color

Procedure	Rationale
1. Analyze the condition of the client's scalp and review the hair-coloring form.	**1.** The hair must be in good condition. This is a different procedure.
2. Explain the need for a filler, and use the color chart to select the proper color. Select and apply a gold or red filler according to label directions.	**2.** Fillers equalize porosity. They are available in ready-to-use form. The tint usually is applied over the filler. Thus, fillers are usually not rinsed before a tint. Select filler color according to desired color result.
3. Towel-dry the hair, or do as otherwise directed by the label or instructor.	**3.** Filler applications vary, so apply according to label directions.
4. Strand test with the selected tint.	**4.** When dark tint is applied to the hair, the tint has a tendency to "grab," resulting in a color that is too dark. Always strand test a tint before applying it all over the hair. Select a lighter color if the test strand indicates that the color is too dark.
5. Apply the tint, following the procedure for a retouch; blend immediately through the entire hair shaft.	**5.** Since the hair is being colored darker, the tint may be applied to the scalp hair first.
6. Allow the color to develop for 20 to 40 minutes.	**6.** Hair porosity will determine developing time. Strand test frequently.
7. Lightly rinse and remove stains from the client's hairline.	**7.** Darker colors have a tendency to stain the scalp more than light ones do.
8. Thoroughly rinse the tint from the hair. Shampoo twice.	**8.** Remove all traces of color and cleanse the scalp.

9. Record results and product formulas on the client's permanent hair-coloring form.

9. This is standard procedure.

10. Recondition if necessary.

10. This is standard procedure.

Sanitize your area as follows:
1. Wash, wipe, and store bottles and supplies.
2. Discard used supplies.
3. Clean and sanitize the cape and apron.
4. Sanitize the work area; wash your hands.

Glossary

Color filler A product used to equalize hair porosity, even the color, or intensify the tint to be applied.

Dye solvent A product that removes artificial and natural color from the hair.

Spot lightening Removing dark streaks from dry hair by applying a dye solvent or lightener.

Stripping Applying dye solvent or lightener only to dark spots to remove them from the hair.

Tint-back Lightening or darkening the hair to its natural color.

Questions

1. Using the information in Chapters 18 and 19, write a definition for each of the following terms: (a) streak; (b) painting; and (c) stripping.
2. Explain the basic steps that might be done during a tint-back.
3. During a tint-back, at what stage would you use a color filler?
4. Should a filler be shampooed from the hair before tinting?
5. Would you recommend mixing lightener in a metal mixing bowl?
6. Is it important to keep lightener moist when it is lightening the hair?
7. Should a protective cream be applied around the hairline to protect the skin?
8. If a client with medium brown hair complains that the frosting has lightened the hair too much, what would you advise?
9. True or false. Lightener should be applied as sparingly as possible.
10. Is heat from a hair dryer ever used to speed up a frosting lightener?

11. When painting the hair, should you apply the lightener in thin strips or in heavy strips?

12. What is the service called when a client with lightened hair wants to return the hair to its natural color?

13. When coloring lightened hair, what product is used to equalize the porosity of the hair?

14. What is the process in which you lighten random dark spots of hair after lifting the hair close to the client's natural hair color?

15. What is the name of the product that removes artificial color from the hair?

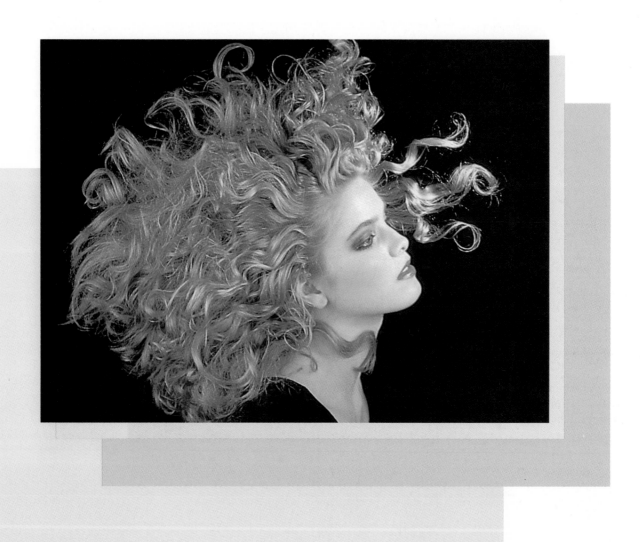

Permanent Wave

Learning Objective

Using professional permanent-waving chemicals and implements, permanently curl the client's hair to make it more manageable and durable from one styling to the next. Using safety precautions and following label directions, use the proper steps to curl the hair. Use water to wrap the client's hair on permanent wave rods in 25–45 minutes. Score 85 percent or better on a multiple-choice exam on the information in this chapter.

In order to achieve the above level of competence, you should master the following chapter objectives.

Theory Objectives

1. Describe three historical permanent-waving methods and list the advantages of the permanent cold-waving services.
2. Explain the difference between acid waves and neutral waves.
3. Describe the effects of cold waving, identify the basic cold-waving chemicals, and compare the pH, cost, and methods of giving an acid wave and the regular thio wave.
4. List other services included in cold waving.

Practical Objectives

5. Analyze the hair and select the proper cold-wave lotion and rods.
6. Section (block) and wrap the hair on permanent wave rods.
7. Process and neutralize the cold wave.
8. Give a perm on long hair using a ponytail wrap.
9. Relax an overly curly perm or naturally wavy hair.

Introduction

Are you one of those fortunate few whose hair falls exactly into place and has just the right amount of curl, not too much, not too little? No one has hair that is "just right" for every style. Many people have hair that is too straight. It needs a little—or maybe a lot—more curl. Others have hair that has too much curl.

Putting permanent curl into the hair is called **permanent waving** or a "perm." The process is also called a cold wave, acid wave, or neutral wave. (Permanent waving is also sometimes used to rearrange very curly hair into a different pattern.) Taking curl out of the hair is called chemical relaxing.

These services are very popular and financially rewarding. All of them are described in this chapter.

Theory Objective 1
Three Historical Permanent-Waving Methods and the Advantages of Permanent Cold-Waving Services

People have been attempting to put a permanent curl into their hair since the time of the ancient Egyptians and Romans, but these early attempts were not very successful. It was not until this century that cosmetology acquired a new art and science as three professional permanent-waving methods were introduced within about a 30-year period beginning in 1905. Since then **cold waving** has almost become a specialty service because of the technical knowledge and practice it demands.

The **machine permanent** method, invented in 1905, used electricity to heat large metal clamps that were placed over the client's hair (Figure 20.1). The hair was wound on rods from the ends to the scalp. Long flexible wires were attached directly to the clamps, which were then clipped over the rods on which the client's hair was wound. This version was called **croquignole** (KROH-kehn-ohl) wrapping (waving). The croquignole wrap was used mainly to wave **short** hair. When a **spiral** wrap was used, the hair was wound from the scalp to the ends. The machine permanent was not a very efficient way to curl hair because it required so much equipment: the machine, rubber scalp pads, small clamps, wool wave crepe, rods, and large clamps.

The **preheat permanent** wave, which was developed in 1931, was a "spin-off" from the machine permanent. The preheat permanent was an improvement over the machine permanent because it eliminated the long electrical wires between the machine and the client. The large clamps were heated on a machine before they were

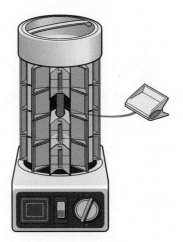

Figure 20.1
Permanent wave machine. If you are using a modern machine, it may be necessary to put cotton between the clamp and the scalp to prevent the heat from burning the client.

placed on the rods on which the hair was wound. Therefore electricity did not come close to the client's head.

With the **machineless permanent** wave, electricity was removed from the waving process altogether. The machineless wave used chemical pads that heated when they were moistened with water. After a pad was moistened, it was placed over a rod and held in place by a large clamp. This method produced a curl pattern that was "pressed into the hair" by steam heat from the chemical pads. Like the other methods, the machineless permanent used protective rubber pads, small clamps, rods, and large clamps; thus, the equipment and the process were essentially the same, except for the absence of electricity.

All three methods relied on two **physical** principles to curl the hair: winding the hair around a rod and applying extreme heat. All three also had certain disadvantages:

1. A large amount of equipment was required.
2. The expense for the client was considerable.
3. The client experienced discomfort.
4. The procedures were time-consuming for the client and cosmetologist.
5. Frequently, the hair and scalp were damaged.

The **cold wave** was accepted for professional use in 1940. It was called "cold" because it did not require heat. The croquignole wrapping system was still used, but chemicals, instead of heat, were used to curl the hair. This is the method used today; it is also known as chemical waving.

Cold waving uses a waving solution with a pH of 7.9–9.5, a neutralizer, rods, and end wraps. The physical effects of wrapping the hair on rods and the chemical changes produced by the waving solution and neutralizer give the hair its curl.

The liquid that causes the hair shaft to soften and swell (expand) is called the **waving lotion.** An **end wrap** or end paper is placed on the end of each hair strand to protect and control it as it is wound around the **cold-wave rod.** After all the hair strands have been wrapped and the waving lotion has been applied or reapplied, the hair begins to **process.** When the hair has softened enough to make a curl the same size as the rod being used, the hair must be **fixed** in this form. This is done by the **neutralizer** (stabilizer or fixative), which **hardens** and **shrinks** the hair shaft and **stops** the action of the waving lotion.

The cold wave has several advantages over other permanent wave methods:

1. It is less expensive for both the client and cosmetologist.

2. Less equipment and fewer supplies are required.

3. The wrapping takes less time.

4. The service as a whole requires less time.

5. Cold waving is more comfortable for the client.

Theory Objective 2
Difference between
Acid Waves and
Neutral Waves

Safety Tip ▶

Recently, several manufacturers have introduced neutral and acid permanent waves. The **acid wave** has been the more popular of the two. **Acid waves** generally have a pH in the range of 5.8–6.8 (some are a little higher—7.9). Although they are milder for the hair than neutral waves, sometimes they can be harsher on the skin. For this reason, special care must be taken when applying the wave solution. It must be applied only to the hair and should not be allowed to drip onto a towel and/or cotton; the towel or cotton could be left on the skin, which would cause a chemical burn.

Neutral waves have a pH in the range of 4.5–5.7, and many of them have not been very successful. All **neutral waves and acid waves need heat** in order to curl the hair that is wound around the permanent wave rods. The heat tends to be of two types: **heat from a hair dryer** and **chemical heat.** In order for the hair shaft to be "opened" so that the waving solution can penetrate the hair, a plastic cap is placed over the permanent wave rods; then, the client is placed under a hot dryer. The processing time is determined by the manufacturer, but "test curls" may be taken as advised by your instructor.

Neutral waves and acid waves make up a large part of the permanent waving done today. Together, the pHs of these products range from 4.5 on the low side to 7.9 on the high side. Remember that some form of heat is necessary for them to curl the hair effectively. It is also necessary to wrap the hair with even, moderate to firm tension, which breaks down the hydrogen bonds of the hair and gives the final curl the strength and firmness needed to hold the hairstyle in place.

Your instructor will help you select the correct permanent wave from the products used at your school.

Theory Objective 3
Effects of Cold Waving,
Basic Cold-Waving
Chemicals, and a
Comparison of pH,
Cost, and Procedures
of the Acid Wave and
the Regular Thio Cold
Wave

Cold waving involves three steps that produce physical and chemical effects on the hair:

1. **Wrapping** or winding strands on cold-waving rods (physical effects).
2. **Processing** with waving lotion (chemical effects).
3. **Neutralizing** with a separate solution (chemical effects).

Wrapping the hair on the rods **physically breaks** the hydrogen cross-bonds that help give the hair its form or shape (Figure 20.2).

In **processing,** the waving lotion softens and swells (expands) the hair. It also breaks the cystine (SIS-teen) disulfide (sulfur) bonds that help to maintain the shape of the hair (Figure 20.3). These bonds are re-formed around the rod (Figure 20.4). This means that the strand takes the shape, or circumference, of the rod. Thus, the hair becomes curly. As the cystine disulfide bonds are broken down and re-formed, the amino acid cystine is changed to a slightly different amino acid, cysteine.

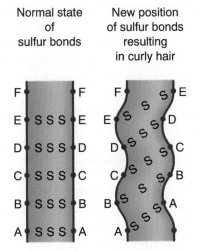

Figure 20.2
Amino acids form proteins and peptide linkages strengthened by cross-bonds.

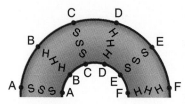

Figure 20.3
Cross-bonds are broken when the hair is wrapped on the rods.

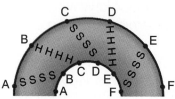

Figure 20.4
The bonds are re-formed as the hair dries on the rods.

After the hair has processed, it is rinsed with water; then neutralizer is applied to stop the action of the waving lotion and to change the cysteine back to cystine. The neutralizer **oxidizes** as well as neutralizes. It hardens the disulfide bonds in their new curly formation and shrinks the hair shaft. The hydrogen and salt bonds are also changed, but the effect on the cystine disulfide bonds is more important.

Cold waves are available in two types: thio and acid. Both have complex formulas that include chemicals to hide unpleasant odors, buffer harsh ingredients, and add protein to the lotion.

The most important chemical in the thio waving lotion is **thioglycolic acid (thio).** Ammonia is added to the acid to help the lotion penetrate, soften, and swell the hair shaft. With the addition of ammonia, the compound **ammonium thioglycolate (thio)** is formed. The ammonia makes the lotion **alkaline,** with a pH range of 8.5 to 9.5.

Acid waves are made from the same thioglycolate base as thio waves, but acid waves fall in a lower pH range of 5.8 to 6.8. They are called acid waves because they have a pH closer to acid than regular thio waves do. You may want to try a few acid waves to see their advantages and disadvantages for yourself.

Unlike the thio wave, which is basically a cold wave (although a little body heat is necessary for processing), the acid wave must have heat in a reliable form. The heated clamps used in one method of acid waving are reminiscent of the preheat permanent wave of the 1930s. Products using this acid-clamp waving method have one outstanding advantage: they cannot be sold over the counter and used at home (see Figure 20.1)!

At the proper time, the action of the waving lotion is stopped by the **neutralizer,** or **fixative.** The basic chemical in most neutralizers is either sodium bromate or 2 percent hydrogen peroxide; peroxide seems to be preferred by many cosmetologists and manufacturers. Peroxide neutralizers contain water and animal, vegetable, or mineral proteins with the peroxide in 2 percent strength. This preparation oxidizes the waving lotion. **Sodium bromate** is also used as a neutralizer, but its fumes can be combustible. The combustion can occur when soiled neutralizer towels are stored with soiled tint towels. The ammonia fumes from the tint combine with the sodium bromate fumes to make bromine gas, which can cause a fire.

Theory Objective 4
Other Services Included
in Cold Waving

For many years, the terms cold-waving **process** and cold-waving **service** have led to confusion. The process is included in the service. The price quoted for the service usually **includes** the following: (1) shampoo service, (2) cold-wave wrap, (3) cold-wave process, (4) cold-wave neutralizer, and (5) hairstyling service (setting and combing or air waving, and so forth).

Changes generally are made for conditioning or shaping (cutting). Thus, the cost of the code wave does **not** include hair cutting or conditioning, but it does include services other than the cold-wave **process.** Some state laws prohibit advertising a cold-wave price that includes hair shaping. It must be a separate charge; for example, if the cold wave costs $50 and the client requests shaping, which costs another $8, the total charge would have to be $58. Your instructor will tell you what to charge in your particular school.

Another consideration when determining the price of the service and what is included is the wrapping method. A basic wrapping method, which will be presented in the next objective, is normally used on short hair. **Short hair** is defined as hair that is less than 6 inches (15 centimeters) long. Depending on the rod size, you will use an average of 40–65 permanent wave rods on short hair.

Long hair, which is defined as hair longer than 6 inches (15 centimeters), may require a **stack, ponytail, spiral** or other wrapping method. These methods differ in the degree of curliness they produce. The **stack wrap** curls the hair on the ends so that the curl is farther from the scalp. The **ponytail** method gives the hair a medium degree of curliness, with the curl closer to the scalp than with the stack wrap.

The **spiral wrap** results in the curliest effect. Very small subsections of hair are used, and many more rods are needed for this method. Normally, 80 to 150 rods (depending on the hair density of the client) would be used when giving a spiral wrap.

Therefore, when determining what is included in the cost of the cold-waving service, you will want to consider the extra wrapping time needed and the permanent wave and other supplies required when permanent waving long hair.

Practical Objective 5
Analyzing the Hair and Selecting Proper Cold-Wave Lotion and Rods

Supplies

- client release form
- client permanent service form
- shampoo supplies
- shampoo cape
- protein conditioner
- styling comb
- 2 laundered towels

- protective apron
- cold-waving rods
- neutralizing bib
- cold-waving lotion and neutralizer
- hair-cutting implements
- protective garment for client

Procedure

1. Review the client's permanent-waving form,

Rationale

1. Always review the client's form so that you will know

◀ **Safety Tip**

noting chemical services that have been received in the past. **Do not brush,** but lightly **shampoo the hair** after you have analyzed it.

if the hair has been tinted or frosted or when the last cold wave was given. Brushing or **excessive** shampooing may irritate the client's scalp and may cause a cold-wave (chemical) burn.

Safety Tip

2. Analyze the porosity and elasticity of the client's hair.

2. This is standard procedure.

3. Carefully **inspect** the condition of the client's **scalp.** Ask the client what home and professional chemical services he or she has used in the past 12 months.

3. Cold waving is not permitted if **cuts, abrasions,** or **red irritation** appear on the scalp. Consult your instructor if necessary. Discoloration and breakage can result if a professional cold wave is given to hair dyed with home products containing a metallic salt tint. Some discoloration (color removal) will occur even if professional products were used in tinting.

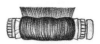

Figure 20.5
A thin rod used on short hair

4. Consider the texture and color of the client's hair. Determine if the hair is fine, medium, or coarse. Natural red and coarse gray hair will be more difficult to wave than other types and colors. Naturally curly hair is the easiest to wave.

4. Fine hair is fragile and may require a milder strength lotion than medium or coarse hair. If the hair has been tinted or frosted, use a lotion that is milder than one for medium or coarse hair, although coarse hair may also be very porous.

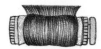

Figure 20.6
A medium rod used on medium-length hair

5. Assess the density and length of the client's hair (Figures 20.5, 20.6, and 20.7).

5. If the hair per square inch (centimeter) is very dense, smaller partings and larger rods seem to wave best. Very sparse (thin) hair waves best when small partings and small rods are used. If the hair is quite long (over 6 inches/15 centimeters), you may wish

6. Comb through the hair to determine whether it was cut with a razor or scissors. Ask the client if you are uncertain.

7. Ask the client the amount of curl desired—body, soft, or firm curl. Request picture(s) of the desired hairstyle and consider the length of the style shown.

8. Ask the client how often he or she gets a professional cold wave.

to use the procedure for cold waving long hair.

6. Razor cuts may have removed too much bulk from the ends of the hair strand. Slithering the hair with scissors may also remove too much bulk. In this case, the end has less resistance to cold-waving lotion and becomes frizzy or fuzzy. To avoid this, blunt cut the hair (with scissors) before waving (Figures 20.8 and 20.9).

7. The **diameter** of the cold-wave rods and the **number** of rods used will determine the degree to which the hair will wave or curl (Figure 20.10). Large, straight rods or concave rods can be used for a body wave. As noted in Chapter 9 on sculpture curling, the hair must rotate 1½ to 2½ turns to wave. A soft-to-medium curl will result from 2 ½ to 3½ turns. A firm cold-wave formation will be produced by 3¾ or more turns. For hair that is **not** very porous, add one additional turn (rotation) to these numbers. The size of the parting (blocking) also determines the size of the curl pattern.

8. The client who schedules a cold wave **once** *or* **twice** a year probably is accustomed to a **firm** curl. On the other hand, someone who has a cold

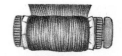

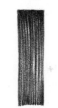

Figure 20.7
A thick rod used on long hair

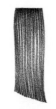

Figure 20.8
Tapered cut

Figure 20.9
Blunt cut

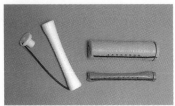

Figure 20.10
The size of the rod determines the degree of curliness

9. Recommend a particular wave to the client, stating the reason for the choice. If you make more than one recommendation, explain the differences.

10. Lightly shampoo the hair with a mild acid-balanced product.

11. Observe whether the hair absorbs water easily.

12. Shape (cut) the hair if necessary.

Safety Tip

13. Condition the hair if necessary.

wave three or four times a year may need only a soft or body wave.

9. Always explain the reason(s) for your recommendation. If different waves may be used, explain the different effects they have on the hair. Similarly, if perms at three prices are discussed, explain the advantages of each.

10. Cleanse the hair and scalp, but do not manipulate the scalp to the extent that scalp circulation is increased. Mild, **effective** cleaning, acid-balanced shampoos are preferred, unless an acid wave is to be used. If an acid wave is to be used, an alkaline shampoo gives better results.

11. This will help you determine the porosity of the hair.

12. The client's hair may need blunt scissor cutting to eliminate the possibility of fuzzy ends.

13. Preconditioning may be necessary to equalize the hair's porosity. **If the hair is conditioned too much, the hair shaft may not have room for the waving solution.** Thus, the waving solution may not penetrate the hair shaft. Be guided by your instructor when selecting a conditioner to be used **before** cold waving.

14. Dry the hair according to the manufacturer's directions.

14. Label directions vary from brand to brand, so it is necessary to read the instructions carefully.

15. If you must leave the client to get supplies, let the client know where you are going.

15. Once a chemical process has actually been started, **never** leave a client unattended without letting him or her know where you are going!

16. Select a waving lotion, neutralizer, and additives.

16. Waving lotions come in different strength for hair that is:
- overporous (lightened), use the mildest lotion.
- a little overporous (tinted), use a mild lotion.
- slightly overporous (fine or medium), use a mild lotion.
- not very porous (normal), use a medium lotion.
slightly porous or resistant
- (coarse), use a strong lotion.

Most cosmetologists who are concerned that a solution may be too strong for the client's hair use the next milder lotion. For example, if the client has frosted hair, the strength for tinted or lightened hair is used. If that strength does not produce a curl, the hair is towel-blotted, and the next strongest solution is used. Certain systems for cold waving the hair require protein to be added to the waving lotion and vitamins to the neutralizer, and so forth. Follow the advice of your instructor.

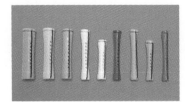

Figure 20.11
Rods come in a variety of sizes.

17. Select cold-wave rods that are appropriate for the length, condition, and texture of the client's hair and the amount of curl desired (Figure 20.11).

17. Cold-wave rods are concave, round, spiral, or oval. They are made of wood, plastic, or nylon. They are long, short, or very short (midget). The hair must be wound around the rod two complete turns in order to achieve a wave pattern.

Practical Objective 6
Sectioning (Blocking) and Wrapping the Hair on Permanent Wave Rods

Supplies

- timer
- end wraps
- rat-tail comb or styling comb
- 12 double-prong clips
- surgical or rubber gloves

- cold-wave processing overcap
- protective cream
- cotton coil
- plastic applicator bottle

Procedure

1. Test curl two or three subsections of hair in the lower crown. Using the length of the rods selected, section (block) off the hair and secure with double-prong clips (Figure 20.12).

Rationale

1. Whenever in doubt, use test curls to determine the curlability of the hair. Use waving lotion and neutralize according to directions. The length of each section (strand of hair) can be measured by the length of the rods selected. Although five sectioning (blocking) patterns are generally accepted, the choice of one pattern over another will not make much difference in the finished hairstyle. The size of the client's head seems to determine which pattern should be selected and the outcome of the hairstyle. Figures 20.13 through 20.17 show the five commonly used patterns.

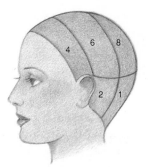
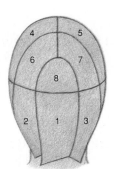

Figure 20.12
Wrapping order

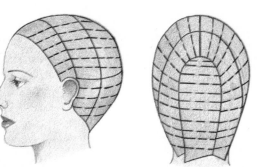

Figure 20.13
Double horseshoe (halo) wrapping pattern for
larger head sizes

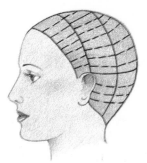

Figure 20.14
Single horseshoe (halo) wrapping pattern for
small-to-average head sizes

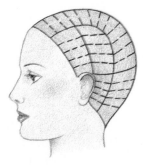
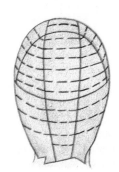

Figure 20.15
Straight-away (back) wrapping pattern for
off-the-face hairstyles

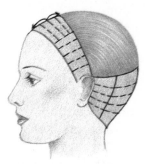
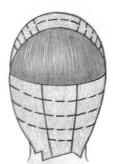

Figure 20.16
Modified straight-away wrapping pattern for
6- to 8-inch (15- to 20-centimeters) hair, where
the hair in the crown will be combed flat or
close to the head. This is also called a
dropped-crown wrapping pattern.

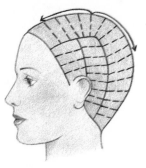
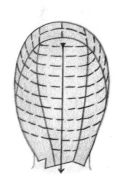

Figure 20.17
Forward wrap for larger-than-average head
sizes. Consult your instructor for assistance as
needed.

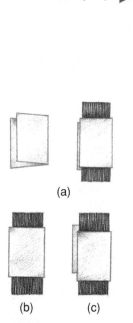

(a)

(b)   (c)

Figure 20.18
(a) Book-end fold; (b) single-end straight; (c) double-end straight.

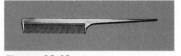

Figure 20.19
Rat-tail comb

2. **Put on surgical gloves or apply protective cream to your hands.** Select appropriate wrapping methods for end papers and begin wrapping the middle nape section (Figure 20.18). If you are wrapping the hair with water, gloves are not needed.

3. Use a rat-tail comb (or styling comb) to part the strand and wind it horizontally on the rod (Figure 20.19). The size of the rod will determine the size of the subsection (Figure 20.20).

4. Check the waving-lotion label and the cap's seal. Pour 1 ounce (30 milliliters) of lotion into the applicator bottle. Cap the lotion and screw the applicator nozzle on the bottle after adjusting the lotion.

5. Apply waving lotion ½ to 1 inch (1.25 to 2.5 centimeters) from the scalp before wrapping **each** strand (Figures 20.21, 20.22, and 20.23). Another method is to apply waving

2. Waving lotion may irritate your hands. End papers serve to protect porous ends of the hair, thus minimizing the possibility of "fishhook" ends. End papers also protect the hair against possible breakage. Papers also allows you to smooth the hair evenly across the rod, which makes the hair more controllable. Three basic wrapping methods are used:
   - Book-end fold
   - Single-end straight
   - Double-end straight

3. Either comb may be used, depending on advice from your instructor. The rectangular subsections should be slightly **less** than the **length** of the rod but should have the **same** diameter.

4. Check the seal to be sure that the lotion is active. The **seal should not** be broken. Tell your instructor if the seal is broken. Always double-check the label to make sure that the lotion, not the neutralizer, is used to wrap the hair. Your instructor may adjust the formula of the lotion to improve its performance.

5. A small amount of waving lotion will run along the strand toward the scalp, and natural body heat will process the scalp hair quickly when the lotion is reapplied after the entire

solution or water to the entire section to be wrapped, then reapply only if the hair becomes too dry to wrap. The hair may also be wrapped in water. Secure each rod by inserting the button attached to the elastic in the opposite end of the rod (Figure 20.24). The elastic should not be twisted or "bind" the hair next to the scalp.

6. Using horizontal partings, finish wrapping in the center nape section (Figures 20.25 and 20.26).

head has been wound. When practicing wrapping on a mannequin, or just beginning in a clinical experience center, you may be advised to wrap by moistening (not saturating) the hair with water. **Binding scalp hair with the elastic band will cause the hair to break.**

6. Because the nape hair is thought to be more resistant and therefore to require more processing

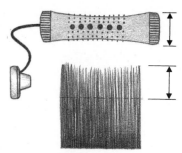

Figure 20.20
The subsection should have the same diameter as the rod but should not be quite as wide.

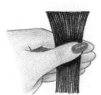

Figure 20.21
Apply waving lotion ½ to 1 inch (1.25 to 2.5 centimeters) from the scalp.

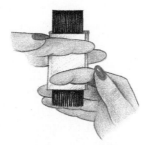

Figure 20.22
Slide paper toward end of each strand.

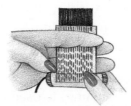

Figure 20.23
Use moderate, even tension.

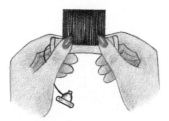

Figure 20.24
Insert the button attached to the elastic into the opposite end of the rod.

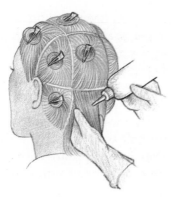

Figure 20.25
You may be instructed to begin in the nape section. Remember not to apply waving lotion too close to the scalp.

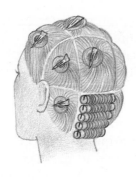

Figure 20.26
Completed nape section

time, schools usually advocate beginning in this section, although advanced students may use other methods. Moistening the hair only with water will soften the hydrogen bonds. They are further softened when the hair is wound around the rod.

7. Wrap the other sections, following the numbered sequence (see Figure 20.13) you used to wrap the nape sections. Carefully consider the length of the hair in each section before you wrap. **Do not apply excessive tension to the hair.** Apply moderate, even tension.

7. Wrapping the hair in sections that are too large will prevent the lotion from penetrating completely. As the hair length **increases,** a larger (diameter) rod must be used because a small rod will require too many rotations for long hair. Hair should be wrapped using moderate tension applied evenly across the rod. (Do not forget, though, that the **chemical** action of the thio causes the hair to curl.) If too much tension (stretching) is used on the hair, it will break. A combination of

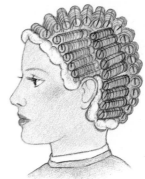

Figure 20.27
Completed wrapping

overstretching and overprocessing can also cause the hair to appear curly when wet and frizzy when dry. This is called **overprocessing.**

8. Wrap one top and side section and then the other. Follow the wrapping sequence of the pattern you have selected. Wrap each rod so that when it is fastened, it is just below the horizontal bottom parting.

8. Wrapping the hair this way will give maximum curl.

9. Wrap the crown sections smoothly and without too much tension to complete the wrapping procedure (Figure 20.27).

9. The hair is saturated more thoroughly when it is not wound too tightly. The hair must have room to **swell** when the lotion is applied. If it is wound too tightly, the hair cannot swell and may **break.**

◀ Safety Tip

Wrapping Check List

10. Check the width of **each** subsection and compare it to the diameter of the rod that you are using.

10. To achieve uniform curl, wrap the hair according to the rod's length and diameter. Consult the instructor for an evaluation.

11. Check the length of each subsection and compare it to the rod used.

11. Same as step 11.

12. Check the elastic band of each rod to ensure that none is binding the scalp hair. Adjust the bands if necessary. Unwind two or three rods immediately to test the curl.

12. If you used waving lotion to wrap the hair, the hair will be fragile because of the softening effect of thio. Improperly placed elastic bands can therefore cause the hair to break. Whether you use water or lotion for wrapping, always test the curl immediately.

13. Apply a piece of cotton coil around the hairline.

13. Cotton prevents the lotion from running into the client's eyes or ears or onto the face.

Applying Waving Solution

Procedure

1. Prepare waving solution according to the manufacturer's directions.

Rationale

1. Since some solutions are activated by adding two or more chemicals together, it is necessary to read the directions of each manufacturer.

2. Check to make sure the waving solution you are about to use is waving solution.

2. If you are not careful, you may apply the neutralizer in place of the waving solution!

3. Hand the client a clean, dry towel.

3. Should any waving solution drip into the client's eye(s), ear(s), face, and so on, advise the client to **blot, not rub,** the solution. Should waving solution drip into the client's eye(s), **flush the area with cool water, then dampen a clean towel with cool water and blot the affected area.** If irritation persists, consult your instructor. You may have to take the client to a physician.

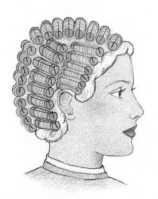

Figure 20.28
Begin applying waving solution in the nape section.

4. Beginning in the bottom of the nape section, apply a **very small amount** of waving solution to all rods in this section (Figure 20.28). Repeat until all rods in each section have been lightly saturated. Be careful to avoid dragging the nozzle of the applicator bottle across the hair on the rods.

4. Since the hair has probably dried out, it will not readily absorb the waving solution, and the solution may drip onto the client's face, eyes, ears, or neck. Minerals in the client's hair may cause the purple discoloration. The client has probably been shampooing his or her hair with "hard water." This

If the **solution drips purple** from the hair, continue the procedure.

5. Wait 60 seconds. Reapply waving solution to each rod. Apply only the amount of solution that the hair will accept (absorb).

6. Blot any excess waving solution that may be on the scalp between the rods. **Check the neck towel for dampness. If the towel is wet, replace it with a clean dry towel.**

usually will not affect the permanent wave.

5. The 60-second wait will allow the hair to become slightly wet. The **capillary action** set up by applying a small amount of solution in the previous step will allow the hair to neatly "suck up" the additional solution you are applying now. Slightly wet hair will absorb any solution much more readily than dry hair. This procedure will almost eliminate the need for cotton and an excessive number of towels.

6. If waving solution is allowed to collect between the rods or on the towel that is next to the client's neck, a **chemical burn will result!**

◀ Safety Tip

Practical Objective 7
Processing and Neutralizing the Cold Wave

Supplies

- timer
- end wraps
- rat-tail comb or styling comb
- 12 double-prong clips
- surgical or rubber gloves

- cold-wave processing overcap
- protective cream
- cotton coil
- plastic applicator bottle

Procedure

1. Remove the saturated cotton protective strip and neck towel. Replace the towel.

Rationale

1. The cotton and the neck towel can cause a chemical burn if they are left on after they have become saturated.

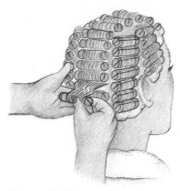

Figure 20.29
Definite "S" pattern. Unwrap rod a maximum of two turns.

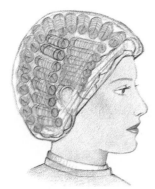

Figure 20.30
A plastic overcap will help retain body heat.

2. Immediately test the curl on one rod in the nape, crown, and front side. Unwind the rod 1¾ to 2 turns.

3. Look for a well-defined "S" formation in a depth equal to the rod diameter (Figure 20.29).

4. If very little wave appears in the test curls, touch the client's hand to see if his or her body temperature is normal or cool.

5. Using a timer, test the curl on **different** rods in each section of the head every 2 to 3 minutes.

6. Test the curl on a rod in each section of the head.

2. Hair may be adequately curled immediately or within 12 minutes. The temperature of the client's body, the room, and the waving lotion affect the processing time of the wave.

3. When a strong "S" pattern is observed in each section and back-to-back "S" formations appear, the hair has processed to its maximum.

4. The client may be cold from the air conditioning in the building. You can place a plastic overcap on his or her head to keep what body heat there is around the waving lotion (Figure 20.30). If the hair is waving properly in one section but not in another, use the cap; then place your hand on the cap where curls are processing slowly. The heat from your hand will accelerate the chemical action of the lotion in this part of the head.

5. The hair may curl very quickly, so frequent checking is necessary to avoid overprocessing. Since hair is very fragile after waving lotion has been applied, do **not** check the same rod twice.

6. If there is no apparent curling after 10 minutes, gently blot the rods with a towel saturated with warm-hot water. Apply the next strongest waving lotion. The first lotion may have been too weak. If the waving lotion is stored in a very cool part of the building, warm it by placing the bottle in tepid water. Natural body heat and room temperature (72°F) are needed for proper processing. Ask your instructor to help you select the right method of processing the cold wave.

7. Hand the client a towel saturated with cold water and advise him or her to blot any solution that may drip onto the forehead or around the hairline. **If a plastic cap is used to cover the rods, do not fasten it too tightly, as breakage may occur around the hairline** (Figure 20.31).

7. Cold water helps neutralize the alkalinity of the waving lotion. Tell the client to **blot,** not rub, because **rubbing may irritate the skin and cause a chemical burn.**

◀ **Safety Tip**

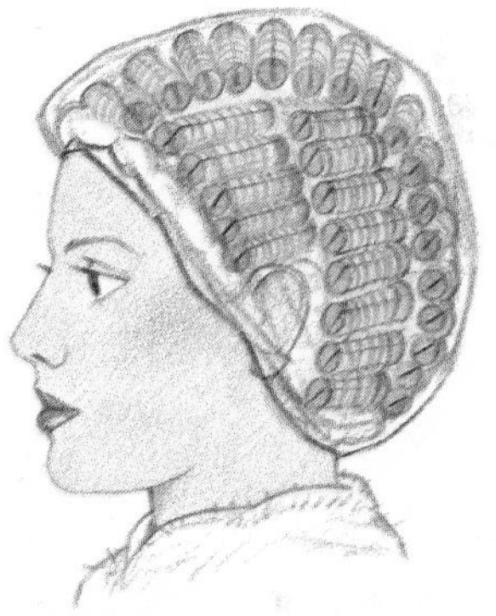

Figure 20.31
The plastic cap must be loose enough so fine or weak hair doesn't break! Check neck towel for wetness, and change if it is wet. A second coil of cotton must replace the coil used for initial saturation of the hair, or a chemical burn will result.

8. Test curl to the maximum processing time. Escort the client to the shampoo area to neutralize the hair.

8. Consult your instructor immediately before rinsing waving lotion.

9. Using tepid to warm water, thoroughly rinse the waving lotion from the hair for 3–5 minutes. Ask the client if the water temperature is too warm. Adjust temperature accordingly.

9. Warm water not only rinses the waving lotion from the hair, but it also provides oxygen that begins to partially oxidize and neutralize the waving lotion. Rinse the hair for at least 3 minutes.

10. Read the directions that are packaged with the neutralizer.

10. Manufacturer's directions generally work best, but two other methods may be used. Altogether, there are three methods:
    - **Instant.** Usually 5 to 10 minutes.
    - **Splash.** A small sponge or piece of cotton is used to "splash" the neutralizer

over the rods and through the hair. The neutralizer is caught in a bowl placed below the rods at the bottom of the basin; then it is poured and repoured over the rods for 10 minutes. The splash method is not used much now.

■ **Self-neutralizing.** The hair is blotted, not rinsed, with a damp towel and then is allowed to air dry naturally. Then, the rods are removed, and the hair is rinsed thoroughly. Style as usual. In this case, the oxygen in the air and water oxidizes and neutralizes the hair. This method works well, but it takes a long time.

11. Obtain dispensary scissors to cut off the top of the neutralizer bottle.

11. Use utility scissors to cut off the top of the neutralizer bottle. Neutralizer will corrode styling scissors, so usually a pair of dispensary shears is used just for this purpose.

12. Mix the neutralizer and additives as needed.

12. Many schools and salons believe that since the cuticle of the hair shaft is in the open position, conditioners will penetrate better if they are mixed with the neutralizer. This allows maximum conditioning to occur when the hair is rehardened and shrunk by the neutralizer. Follow the advice of your instructor for the best results.

Safety Tip ▶

13. Gently towel-blot each rod thoroughly. Paper towels

13. Since the hair is soft and swollen, it is very fragile; it

will remove the most water.

14. Attach the neutralizing bib along the client's hairline and secure it at the center of the forehead.

15. Apply neutralizer across the top and bottom of each rod; begin in the nape section and work forward (Figure 20.32). Ask the client to assume a sitting position, rather than lying back, during neutralization.

16. After 5–10 minutes, rinse thoroughly with tepid, then cool water. Gently towel-blot the hair and ask your instructor if additional reconditioning is necessary.

17. Remove the rods and end papers, carefully unwinding them without pulling or stretching the hair.

18. Consult your instructor to evaluate the results of the

can break if you manipulate the towel too firmly.

14. The bib protects the client's ears and clothing from the neutralizer. It also has a pocket at the bottom to catch the neutralizer so that it can be reapplied if desired. Neutralizing bibs have elastic around their perimeters, which may bind and possibly break the hair. Be careful! Bibs usually fasten with a **metal** eye hook near the center of the forehead. Cotton should be placed beneath the hook to prevent skin irritation.

15. Applying neutralizer to the top and bottom of the rod ensures thorough penetration across the hair. Neutralizer causes the **cysteine** in the hair to change **back to cystine** (see objective 3). The curl is "locked in." The weight of the client's head against the neck of the shampoo bowl could break the hair.

16. This removes excess neutralizer not absorbed by the hair.

17. The hair is still somewhat fragile, so you must be careful not to break the hair by stretching or pulling.

18. Your work should be continually evaluated by

◀ Safety Tip

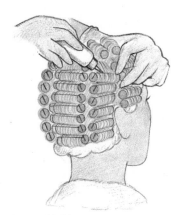

Figure 20.32
Apply neutralizer to top and bottom of each rod.

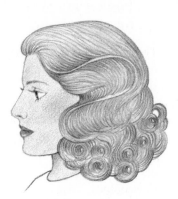

Figure 20.33
*A completed cold wave for a
female client*

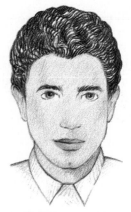

Figure 20.34
*A completed cold wave for a
male client*

cold wave (Figures 20.33 and 20.34). Record the results on the cold-wave card.

your instructor. **Make notes on the client's cold-wave record regarding products used, rod sizes, and time recommendations for future cold-waving services.** Cold-wave cards provide other useful information as well.

19. Discuss an appointment for the client one week from the date of the cold wave. The hair should **not** be shampooed or otherwise treated for a period of 48 hours.

19. Always recommend that the client schedule an appointment one week from the date of the cold wave. This is an opportunity to determine if the service was satisfactory and to correct any errors. If any areas on the head are not curly enough, pickup curls may be used (only) for those spots.

Sanitize your area as follows:

1. Wash, wipe, and store bottles and supplies.
2. Discard used supplies.
3. Clean and sanitize the cape and apron.
4. Sanitize the work area; wash your hands.

Practical Objective 8
*Giving a Perm on Long
Hair with a Ponytail
Wrap*

Supplies

- client release form
- client permanent service form
- shampoo supplies
- shampoo cape
- protein conditioner
- styling comb
- 2 extra laundered towels

- protective apron
- cold-waving rods
- cold-waving lotion and neutralizer
- hair-cutting implements
- protective garment for client
- rubber binders (bands)
- scissors

Procedure

1. Prepare client as for any cold-waving service. Discuss the advantages of the ponytail cold-waving methods with the client. Also discuss the cost.

2. After you have analyzed the condition of the hair, use a brush (or comb) to subsection it (Figures 20.35 and 20.36). Secure each

Rationale

1. The client should understand what service will be given. The advantage of the ponytail cold wave is that only the ends are curled; long hair does not need curl at the scalp. Placing a binder in subsections of the hair and using rods only in the hair ends makes sense. The client should agree to the cost of the services.

2. A brush gives better control of long hair than a comb does. The rubber binders secure the hair next to the scalp so that only the

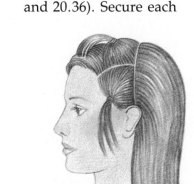

Figure 20.35
Larger subsections result in less curl.

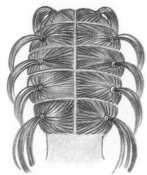

Figure 20.36
Smaller subsections result in more curl.

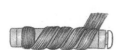

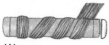

Figure 20.37
Spiral wrapping technique used for ponytail wrap

subsection with a rubber binder.

3. Secure the hair in rectangular subsections until all of it is held by rubber bands in columns (or rows) of ponytails.

4. Select rods according to desire curl. Spiral wrap each strand around the rod (Figure 20.37).

5. Begin wrapping at the bottom subsection of the right side, using 5 or 7 rods in each ponytail (Figures 20.38, 20.39, and 20.40). If you use a lotion, apply it 1 inch (2.5 centimeters) from the elastic binder. Following the instructions in Figures 20.41 through 20.48, continue until you have wrapped all sections of hair.

6. Test the curl immediately. (If spiral rods are used, take the test curl from the top of a rod by unwinding the strand 1½ turns to check for an "S" pattern.)

extreme ends are curled.

3. This allows you to work in uniform, well-defined sections and makes the wrapping procedure easier. The hair is curled more evenly, too.

4. Using the guides previously discussed in this unit, select the appropriate rod sizes.

5. Since the wound rods hang down, they would be in the way if wrapping started on the top of each subsection. If lotion is applied too close to rubber (elastic) binders, hair breakage will result from the tension of the binder.

6. Always test the curl even if the hair is wrapped with water. Water breaks the hydrogen bonds; if a sharp wave pattern appears, the hair will curl (process)

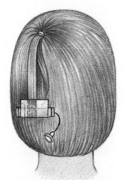

Figure 20.38
Begin wrapping at the bottom of each subsection.

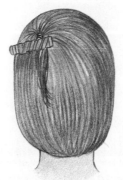

Figure 20.39
A wound rod

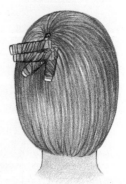

Figure 20.40
A completed subsection

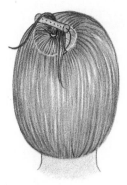

Figure 20.41
The ponytail piggy-back wrap gives an even curl to long hair. When actually wrapping, begin in the nape section; then work to the upper sections.

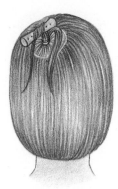

Figure 20.42
Spiral hair around rod using even tension. An end wrap is not needed for this step.

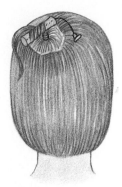

Figure 20.43
Wrap until hair covers most of the permanent wave rod.

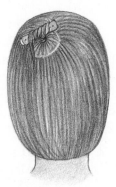

Figure 20.44
Fasten at bottom of wound rod.

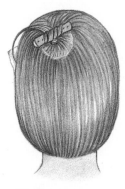

Figure 20.45
Put end wrap on the ends of the hair strand.

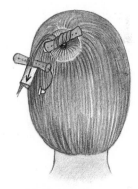

Figure 20.46
Slide end wrap down the strand, so the end wrap extends beyond hair ends. Use spiral wrap and finish wrapping the other rods.

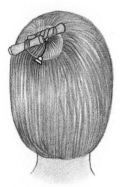

Figure 20.47
After wrapping short ends, secure the fastener at the bottom of the rod.

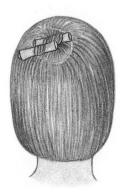

Figure 20.48
The number of sections, the number of subsections, and rod size will be determined by the length and texture of the hair and the degree of curl desired by the client.

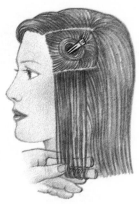

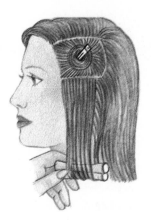

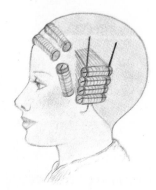

Figure 20.50
Hair wound on rods in a twin wrap

Figure 20.49
Twin wrap for longer hair

quickly when waving lotion is applied.

7. When you think the hair has the proper curl, test the curl again in the presence of your instructor before you neutralize the hair.

7. If the hair is neutralized before it is curly enough, the curl will be underprocessed. To make sure the curl is accurate, consult your instructor before rinsing or neutralizing the hair.

8. Use scissors to cut the elastic bands from each subsection.

8. It is faster, easier, and safer to cut the elastic bands.

9. Set or air wave the hair.

9. This is standard procedure.

A twin wrap may be used for longer hair (Figures 20.49 and 20.50), while a stack wrap gives greater curl at the nape (Figures 20.51 through 20.61).

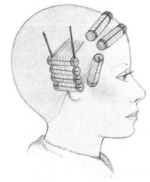

Figure 20.51
Remember to begin wrapping at bottom of each section.

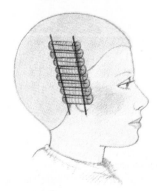

Figure 20.52
Stack rods on top of each other.

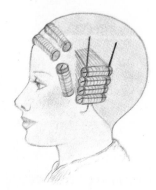

Figure 20.53
Begin wrapping on left-front section

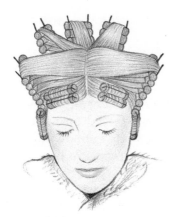

Figure 20.54
Continue wrapping until all sections are done.

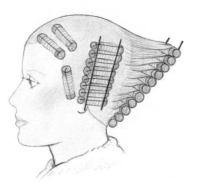

Figure 20.55
Note smoothness of crown, and rod placement on the ends.

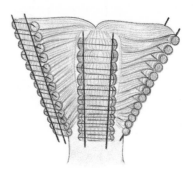

Figure 20.56
Completed wrap.

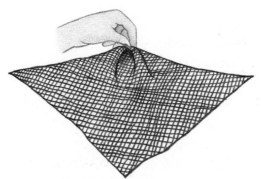

Figure 20.57
Pick up hair net in center.

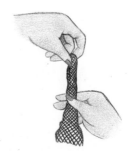

Figure 20.58
Gather net between fingers.

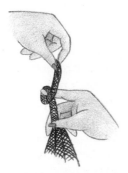

Figure 20.59
Wind around index finger.

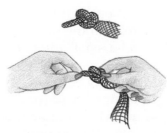

Figure 20.60
Tie knot.

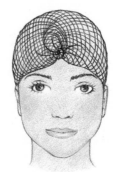

Figure 20.61
Place knot in center of forehead. Secure at nape. (Rods not shown)

Practical Objective 9
Relaxing an Overly
Curly Perm or Naturally
Wavy Hair

No matter how careful you are when permanent waving the client's hair, occasionally the client will complain that the permanent wave is too tight. Should this occur, you will find that the steps in this objective are very helpful in relaxing the client's hair to the desired degree of curliness. This procedure may also be used on naturally curly hair—provided the hair is not super-curly. The following procedure will allow the hair to be relaxed without excessive hair damage, and the steps are relatively simple to follow. Your instructor may have a better procedure or may require you to use a particular type of cholesterol.

Supplies

- towels
- comb
- shampoo cape
- one tube (approximately 2 ounces/56 grams) of cholesterol (check with instructor for specific brand)

- cold-waving solution
- plastic or glass mixing bowl
- cold-wave neutralizer
- mixing brush (and/or electric or manual mixer)

Preparation

Procedure

1. Drape the client for a chemical service. Analyze the condition of the client's hair and scalp, then select the waving solution. Prepare normal-strength waving solution according to label directions. Do not shampoo hair.

Safety Tip ▶ **2.** Squeeze an entire tube of cholesterol into the mixing bowl. Add a small amount of waving solution and blend with the cholesterol using a mixing brush (or electric mixer). Continue to add waving solution until your 3- to 4-ounce (90- to 120-milliliter) bottle is smoothly blended into a creamy mixture.

Rationale

1. Hair should not be dry, frizzy or brittle, or breakage may occur. **Don't use this procedure** on hair that has been tinted or lightened as the hair will be damaged. Some waving solutions require mixing.

2. The cholesterol waters down the strength of the waving solution and protects the hair from becoming dry. **Unless the waving solution is added slowly, it won't mix with the cholesterol—it will separate and will not blend correctly.**

3. Escort client to shampoo chair.

3. Since dripping can become a problem, this service should be performed in the shampoo bowl area.

Applying Curl-Relaxing Solution

Procedure

1. Begin application in the curliest section of the head first. If the hair is curly all over, begin application in the nape section of the head first. Then work your way toward the top of the head. Excess solution should be allowed to drip into the shampoo bowl.

2. Continue applying solution with the applicator bottle or applicator brush until all sections of the hair have been saturated with relaxing solution.

3. Carefully comb the solution through the hair using the **coarse** (wide) teeth of the comb. Change the neck towel if it becomes saturated with relaxing solution. **Do not allow any solution to drip into the client's eyes or ears or onto the client's face or clothing.**

Rationale

1. Curliest hair will take longer to relax, so it is wise to begin applying relaxer solution in that area first. By systematically beginning in the nape section, you will be applying the relaxing solution evenly to all of the hair.

2. If all sections of hair are to be relaxed, it is important to apply solution evenly.

3. Combing the hair with the fine teeth of the comb, or combing the hair firmly, flat against the head may cause breakage. If solution should contact the client's skin, **flush the area with tepid water.** Cool water may not rinse the cholesterol from the skin.

◄ Safety Tip

Processing the Curl Relaxer

Procedure

1. Continue to comb the hair slowly for about 5 minutes. Allow hair to process to the desired degree of straightness. If the hair is very resistant, you may want to place a plastic cap

Rationale

1. Combing the hair into a straighter position allows the curl to relax more evenly and quickly. Placing the client under the dryer to straighten resistant hair speeds up the straightening

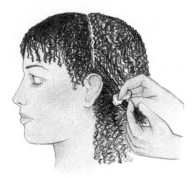

Figure 20.62
Strand test every 3 to 5 minutes.

over the processing hair. A hot dryer may also be used for 10 minutes if the hair fails to relax in 15 minutes.

2. Strand test every 3–5 minutes to check straightening action (Figure 20.62). When the hair appears shiny, feels silky, and looks straight, it probably has processed sufficiently.

process by enabling the relaxing solution to better penetrate resistant hair.

2. Check hair to ensure that it is processing properly, but not overprocessing. If the hair is resistant, put the client under a dryer for 10–15 minutes to achieve better penetration of the hair shaft.

Neutralizing the Curl Relaxer

Procedure

Safety Tip ▶

1. Thoroughly rinse hair with comfortably warm water, then towel-blot as much moisture as possible from hair (Figure 20.63).

Rationale

1. Rinsing stops the straightening action and begins the neutralizing process. **The scalp may be sensitive,** but the water must be warm enough to rinse the solution from the hair.

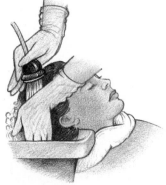

Figure 20.63
Rinse solution from the hair to stop the straightening action.

2. Using the coarse teeth of your comb, begin combing through the nape section. Carefully comb the hair downward to a straight position. Air dry for 5 minutes. **Apply neutralizer** according to the manufacturer's directions.

2. Use the coarse teeth of the comb and begin in the nape to avoid overstretching the hair. Air assists the hair in the neutralizing process. Since almost all manufacturers "buffer" their neutralizers, there is no need to worry about lightening the hair—even with a peroxide neutralizer.

3. Condition as needed and style the hair.

3. This is standard procedure.

Sanitize your area as follows:

1. Wash, wipe, and store bottles and supplies.
2. Discard used supplies.
3. Clean and sanitize the cape and apron.
4. Sanitize the work area; wash your hands.

Acid wave A type of permanent wave that has a pH of 5.8–7.9; it is milder than the thio wave.

Capillary action The method by which the hair "sucks up" the second application of waving solution after the first small application of solution.

Chemical heat Heat generated by adding an activator chemical to the waving solution.

Cold waving A hair-curling method that uses chemicals to wave the hair.

Croquignole (KROH-kehn-ohl) A method of wrapping hair from the ends to the scalp.

Cross-bonds Structures that help hold the hair's internal structure together.

Cysteine (SIS-teen) disulfide cross-bonds Bonds that help give hair its shape.

End paper See End wrap.

End wrap Paper placed at the end of a hair strand to protect and control it as it is wound around the cold-waving rod.

Fixative See Neutralizer.

Long hair Hair that is longer than 6 inches (15 centimeters).

Machineless permanent A hair-curling method that used chemical pads that heated up when moistened with water.

Machine permanent A hair-curling method in which electrically heated clamps were placed over the client's hair.

Neutralizer A solution that stops (fixes) the action of the waving lotion by hardening and shrinking the hair shaft.

Neutralizing Stopping the activity of the waving lotion.

Ponytail wrap A permanent wave wrapping method for long hair; it gives a medium degree of curliness.

Preheat permanent A hair-curling method that used large heated clamps to curl hair. Unlike earlier methods, it did not bring electricity close to the client's head.

Processing The action of the waving lotion on the hair.

Self-timing permanent wave A type of permanent wave for which the manufacturer does not recommend test curls.

Short hair Hair that is less than 6 inches (15 centimeters) long.

Spiral wrap A permanent wave wrapping method using very small subsections of hair and producing the curliest effect.

Stack wrap A permanent wave wrapping method that curls hair on the ends.

Thio See Thioglycolic acid.

Thioglycolic (thigh-oh-gligh-KOL-ik) acid The most important chemical in cold-waving lotion. It causes the hair to soften and swell.

Waving lotion A liquid that causes the hair shaft to soften and
swell.

Wrapping Winding hair on rollers or cold-wave rods.

Questions

1. During cold waving, how are the physical and chemical hair bonds broken?
2. How does waving lotion affect the hair shaft?
3. In what two ways does the neutralizer affect the hair shaft?
4. What determines the degree to which the hair is curled?
5. After applying the waving lotion, why should you remove the cotton from around the hairline?
6. Does cold-waving solution soften or swell the hair?
7. Can the neutralizer swell the hair?
8. True or false. Neutralizer shrinks the hair.
9. Are sulfur bonds and cystine disulfide bonds the same?
10. Can the neutralizer oxidize the hair?
11. What is the basic chemical in a cold-waving solution?
12. What is the pH range of a cold-waving solution containing ammonium thioglycolate?
13. Is hydrogen peroxide ever used as the active chemical in cold-waving neutralizer?
14. Some cold-waving neutralizers contain sodium _____ .
15. Is cold-waving neutralizer also called a fixative?
16. What determines the degree of curliness when giving a permanent wave?
17. In order to achieve a wave pattern, how many turns must the hair be wound around the rod?
18. If the client is allergic to the neutralizer, how should you neutralize the hair?

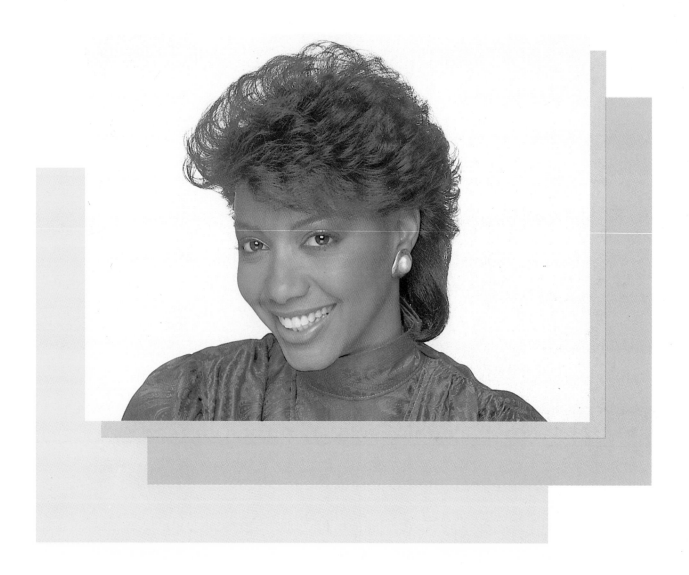

Chemical Hair Relaxing

Learning Objectives

Using professional hair-relaxing products, relax the client's hair to permit setting with sculpture curls or rollers in a less curly hairstyle. Following the proper safety precautions, label directions, and proper steps, straighten the hair. If you use a **no-base** relaxer, apply the relaxing cream in 15 minutes. If a base relaxer is used, apply both the base and relaxing cream in 30 minutes. Score 85 percent or better on a multiple-choice exam on the information in this chapter.

In order to achieve the above level of competence, you should master the following chapter objectives.

Theory Objectives

1. Describe chemical relaxing and straightening.
2. Explain the difference between a base and a no-base relaxer.
3. Identify safety precautions used in chemical relaxing and straightening.

Practical Objectives

4. Apply a base chemical relaxer to virgin hair; apply a retouch relaxer.
5. Give a chemical blowout relaxer.

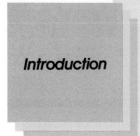

Introduction

The previous chapter described the cold-waving methods used to give hair the right amount of curl. Many people don't have to worry about putting curl in their hair. They have the opposite problem: they have more curl than they want.

Until 20 or 30 years ago, if you had very curly or super-curly hair and wanted it less curly, you had a real problem. The kinds of hairstyles you could wear were rather limited. Many people, both then and now, have liked curly hairstyles. But today people who have very curly or super-curly hair have an advantage. They can change easily to a style with less curl because the products used to relax hair have been improved greatly in recent years.

Today hair that is very curly or super-curly can be relaxed and styled with sculpture curls or rollers without much difficulty, although it must be relaxed quite a bit before it can be set with rollers. If used carefully, hair-relaxing products will relax the hair very nicely. The strength of the relaxer used and the application and processing time will determine the overall result. For example, fine hair will require a milder relaxer than coarse hair. This is also true of the fine hair around the hairline, which will require a shorter processing time than the hair in the crown of the head.

Some of your clients who have shorter hair and want to wear it in a slightly relaxed version of a basic Afro-American hairstyle may prefer a **blowout.** In this procedure, a milder chemical relaxer is applied to the hair, which is then processed, rinsed, neutralized, and conditioned. The hair is then shaped (trimmed with clippers or scissors) and **picked out** (lifted away from the head with a hair **pick,** working from the scalp toward the ends) during drying and styling. The pick-out eliminates the need for setting the hair with rollers, drying, and then brushing into a final hairstyle. Blowouts are very popular because they enable the clients to have a shampoo and pick-out and then go about their business.

A curling iron may be used for styling dry chemically relaxed hair, but check to make sure that the iron is **cool** or **warm,** rather than hot. Using a **hot** iron on relaxed hair will cause damage! Also be careful to use **only a minimum amount of tension.** Be careful not to stretch the hair too much. It is also important to remember not to overrelax the hair.

The safety precautions for a regular chemical relaxer also apply to the chemical blowout service. These include wearing protective gloves and applying protective bases and scalp creams, gels, hair conditioners, and other preparations. You should not shampoo or brush the hair (stimulate the scalp) before either of these chemical services.

Cosmetologists and their clients sometimes use the terms **chemical straightening** and **chemical relaxing** to mean the same thing, but they are actually two different chemical processes (Figure 21.1). **Chemical straightening** is relaxing naturally waving hair with products that contain ammonium thioglycolate. **Chemical relaxing** usually refers to relaxing super-curly hair with products that contain **sodium hydroxide** (SOH-dee-uhm high-DRAHK-sighd).

Ammonium thioglycolate (thio) and sodium hydroxide (**caustic** soda) have different effects on the hair. They differ in other respects as well. The hair should **not** be shampooed before using a sodium-based chemical relaxer, but **must** be shampooed before a thio-based relaxer. Read the manufacturer's directions before using either relaxer.

Thio can quickly relax naturally wavy hair without breaking it, but it is not strong enough to relax super-curly hair in a short time. If thio is left on super-curly hair long enough to relax it, the thio may also break it. Instead of thio, sodium hydroxide is most often used to straighten super-curly hair. This product, however, is too strong for naturally wavy hair. If you use a sodium-based relaxer on naturally wavy hair, it may dissolve or break the hair. Thus, thio is generally used for naturally wavy hair while sodium-based relaxers are used for super-curly hair.

A new type of mild relaxers called **acid chemical relaxers** is also available. These relaxers belong to a chemical family called **bisulfides.** Acid relaxers are similar to the acid waves discussed in Chapter 20 on permanent waving; they are milder than the thio- and sodium-based relaxers. However, some of the acid relaxers won't relax resistant hair satisfactorily.

Although you should understand the differences between chemical relaxing and chemical straightening, you should not be too concerned with the terms themselves. Use what feels comfortable for you. You may use the terms "chemical straightening" and "chemical relaxing" interchangeably as long as you remember their different chemical effects and applications.

Even the terms "straightener" or "straightening service" are not completely accurate. Chemicals make the hair straighter, but they should not make the hair completely straight. If you straightened the client's hair completely, it would not have enough curl (body) to hold the hairstyle. The professional terms that more accurately describe this process are chemical relaxing and chemical relaxer.

Hair relaxers are usually packaged in a kit that includes a variety of products (Figure 21.2). The **base cream** is an ointment that protects the scalp from irritation or burns that could be caused by

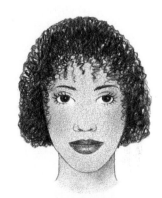

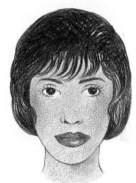

Figure 21.1
Before and after chemical relaxing

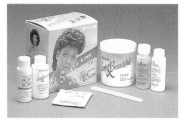

Figure 21.2
Relaxing kit; relaxing cream; neutralizing shampoo; hair conditioner; scalp conditioner; creme rinse and setting lotion.

the relaxer cream. The relaxer cream is a complex formula of sodium hydroxide or ammonium thioglycolate; however, most professional relaxers used today contain sodium hydroxide, which requires considerable instruction, supervision, and practice. With a pH of 11.5 to 14, a sodium hydroxide relaxer is very caustic. Nevertheless, it is preferred over ammonium thioglycolate (pH 8.5–9.5) for super-curly hair, because, as mentioned above, the thio products tend to break this type of hair if they are left on long enough to relax it. Ammonium thioglycolate also tends to allow the hair to revert to its original curliness in humid climates. As in most cases, you must make the decision as to which product to use.

Of course, hair varies from person to person, and you will need to control the relaxer. The **neutralizing shampoo** helps you achieve just the right effect. It stops the softening and straightening action of the thio or sodium hydroxide relaxer. It is also called the **neutralizer, stabilizer,** or **fixative.** This shampoo is made especially for stabilizing (stopping) the strong chemical process and is used only in chemical relaxing. No other process in the salon uses a shampoo in this way. The neutralizing shampoo not only stops the action of the thio or sodium hydroxide, but it also cleanses the scalp.

If the relaxing kit does not include a neutralizing shampoo, an **acid-balanced shampoo** is used, followed by a neutralizer or stabilizer. In any case, the main chemical that stops the straightening action is hydrogen peroxide, whether it is used in the form of a neutralizing shampoo or in a separate stabilizing preparation. It should be noted that the cystine disulfide bonds broken during chemical relaxing by sodium hydroxide are not re-formed chemically as they are in cold waving (Figure 21.3). Chemically, the bonds have been weakened too much to reharden or re-form in a straightened position.

The different effects of thio and sodium hydroxide on the cross-bonds can be summarized as follows:

Figure 21.3
Hair bonding

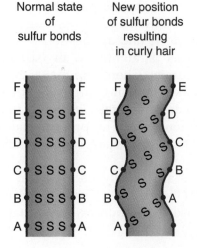

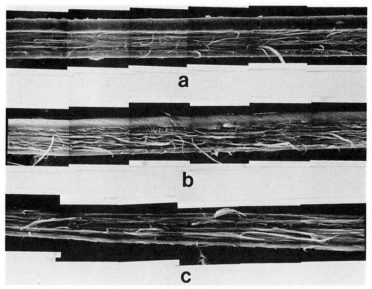

Figure 21.4
These scanning electron micrographs provide a dramatic illustration of the effect that chemicals have on the hair. (a) A normal hair magnified 500 times. Note that the cuticle still tightly adheres, forming a protective barrier against damage.
(b) This hair, which has been magnified 600 times, has been damaged by treatment with a thio permanent wave solution. Note how the cuticle has been partially eroded. This erosion allows the cementlike micropolysaccharide within the cortex to ooze out. The loss of this cement causes the fibers to become detached from their bundles.
(c) This hair, which is shown at a magnification of 550, has been treated with a sodium hydroxide relaxer. Note the total absence of cuticle. The fibers of the cortex, which have no cuticle to protect them, show excessive damage from the loss of the micropolysaccharide cement. The detaching of the fibers from their bundles is even more visible here than in (b), as is the loss of hair strength.

- **Thio.** When a **thio relaxer** is applied, the hair **swells** and **softens,** and the disulfide cross-bonds are broken. After you have worked the hair into a straighter position, you can neutralize it in the straightened position with an acid shampoo (stabilizer or neutralizer). The neutralizer stops the action of the thio relaxer on the cystine disulfide bonds and hardens them in a straighter position.

- **Sodium hydroxide.** Sodium hydroxide actually dissolves one of the cystine disulfide bonds (Figure 20.4). The cystine amino acid bond has two sulfur bonds attached to it in the polypeptide linkage; one of these bonds is not present in the hair after it has been re-formed by the stabilizer. Like thio, sodium hydroxide **swells** and **softens** the hair, but it acts **more quickly.** In the sodium hydroxide service, the stabilizer affects the salt bonds of the hair to a greater extent than it does in the thio relaxer.

Since chemical relaxers react strongly on the hair, many kits contain two conditioners to be applied after the neutralizer. One conditioner normalizes the hair. The other is a scalp conditioner that has an ointment-like consistency. This conditioner is applied by parting the hair into $\frac{3}{4}$-inch (1.88-centimeter) sections and gently rubbing a small amount onto the scalp. It relieves excessive dryness and gives the hair luster. This type of oil conditioner usually resists moisture.

The creme rinse/setting lotion lubricates the hair, which may be in a brittle condition from the relaxing treatment. Hair can break when it is combed during setting and styling. The creme rinse keeps it from breaking.

Theory Objective 2
Differences between a Base and a No-Base Relaxer

The manufacturers of professional products have research and development programs designed to improve existing products and develop new ones. A good example of the effectiveness of these programs was the introduction of the no-base chemical relaxer.

In a **no-base chemical relaxer,** the protective base cream is mixed into, or built into, the relaxing cream. This improvement eliminates one entire step—you do not have to apply the protective cream to the scalp. If you use the no-base kit, you can apply the relaxing-protective cream directly to the hair without applying a separate protective base, but you still have to be careful. Since the no-base relaxer eliminates one application, you will probably find it more convenient and time-saving for both yourself and your client. Doing a process faster gives you more time for other services and, therefore, more income.

Theory Objective 3
Safety Precautions Used in Chemical Relaxing and Straightening

Hair relaxers (straighteners) and their neutralizers are made in a very complicated way. Some of the other sophisticated chemicals contained in both could be listed here, but doing so might tempt some beginners to make relaxers and neutralizers themselves. This kind of experimenting is **very dangerous.** Only the manufacturers of professional products have the scientific knowledge needed to make **safe relaxers** and **safe neutralizers.** Relaxing products made in the school or salon often cause hair breakage and scalp burns. Today, the composition of the neutralizer is just as important as the composition of the relaxer itself. Doctors do not give out lists of chemicals so that anyone can fill a prescription; in the same way, professional cosmetologists should not make cosmetic hair relaxers for their clients.

Although the importance of reading and following label directions has been noted many times in this text, such safety measures must be stressed in chemical relaxing. The possibility of serious damage to the scalp and hair is great because of the strong chemicals used in this service.

Do not mix different chemical relaxing products. Mixing ◀ Safety Tip
different products can cause serious damage to the hair and scalp. This means that you must always check the relaxing kit **before** you start the service to make sure that all necessary supplies (and enough of them) are available to complete the service. **Brand A cannot be used to complete a relaxing service that was started with Brand B.**

Thio-based relaxers should **not** be applied to hair relaxed with a sodium hydroxide–based relaxer. Nor should hair that has been relaxed with a sodium-based relaxer have a thio-based relaxer applied to it.

Always select a relaxer that has the proper strength for your ◀ Safety Tip
client's hair texture. **Relaxers are made in different strengths: mild (for fine-soft hair), regular (for medium hair), and super (for resistant-coarse hair).**

Carefully read the directions for each strength of relaxer. One safe way to choose the right strength is to strand test a new client's hair.

In very warm climates, you should cool the temperature of ◀ Safety Tip
the client's scalp under a "cool" dryer before giving a relaxer!

The following list of specific safety precautions applies to all chemical hair-relaxing services:

1. Use $\frac{1}{4}$- to $\frac{1}{2}$-inch (.625- to 1.25-centimeter) subsections depending on the hair density.

2. Keep the relaxer cream off the scalp.

3. Begin applying relaxer cream in the most resistant section of the head (usually the crown). Apply the relaxer $\frac{1}{2}$ to 1 inch (1.25 to 2.5 centimeters) away from the scalp and up to $\frac{1}{2}$ inch (1.25 centimeters) away from the end of the hair strand.

4. The hair around the front hairline and nape sections is the most fragile, so apply relaxer cream to these sections last.

5. Apply the relaxer cream quickly. The ideal application standard for the relaxer is **2–3 minutes per section.** You should develop your skills so the time for application and processing does not exceed 25–29 minutes altogether.

6. As you apply the relaxer, do not tug or pull on the hair.

7. Use medium to low water pressure to prevent tangling the hair, and make sure that the water used to rinse the relaxer from the hair is warm, but **not too hot.** The scalp will be sensitive after the application of the chemical relaxing cream. After processing, thoroughly rinse all relaxer from the hair (until the water runs clear).

8. Shampoo the hair with the neutralizing shampoo at least **three times** to remove all traces of the relaxer cream.

9. During processing and neutralizing, frequently **change the neck towel** to prevent relaxer cream from coming in contact with the skin at the nape of the neck.

10. Use a timer to make sure you use the processing and neutralizing times recommended by the manufacturer.

11. **Do not leave your client unattended** during this chemical service. Do not permit relaxer cream or neutralizer to enter the client's eyes. Should that happen, **flush immediately** with lots of cool water, and take the client to a physician.

12. When giving a retouch relaxer, apply a protective conditioner to previously relaxed hair **before** making the application to the new growth.

Practical Objective 4
Applying a Base Chemical Relaxer to Virgin Hair

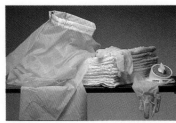

Figure 21.5
Always use a timer and wear gloves when giving a hair relaxing service.

Supplies

- client chemical services record form
- shampoo cape
- 3 laundered towels
- surgical or rubber gloves (Figure 21.5)
- rake comb and rat-tail comb (both hard rubber) (Figure 21.6)
- timer
- base chemical relaxing kit
- label directions
- protective base cream
- chemical relaxing cream
- neutralizing (stabilizing) shampoo
- hair conditioner
- scalp conditioner
- setting lotion with creme rinse qualities
- protective apron

Preparing Hair for Application of a Chemical Relaxer

Procedure

1. Drape the client for a chemical service. Using $\frac{1}{2}$-inch (1.25-centimeter) horizontal partings, examine the entire scalp. Put

Rationale

1. You must not use a chemical relaxer of any kind if the scalp has scratches, abrasions, or irregularities. If any of these conditions

protective gloves on both hands.

2. Review the client's chemical services record form and ask if any chemical services have been performed at home.

3. Carefully read the directions on the kit you have chosen. If you are unsure about which relaxing strength to use, strand test a 1-inch (2.5-centimeter) section of hair. To give the strand test, pull a small strand of resistant, wiry hair through a 4-by-4-inch (10-by-10-centimeter) piece of aluminum foil. Apply relaxer, process, then neutralize. If results are satisfactory, apply conditioning cream to the strand for protection, and go on to the next step.

4. Apply protective base cream (precream) around the front hairline and neck (nape) hairline (Figure 21.7). Cover the top and back of each ear.

5. Divide the hair into four equal sections (Figure 21.8). Using $\frac{1}{4}$-inch (.625-centimeter) horizontal partings, begin applying the base cream in the right nape section (Figure 21.9). Work up to the top of the section.

6. Using $\frac{1}{4}$-inch (.625-centimeter) horizontal partings, apply the

exists, the sodium hydroxide or thio will cause extreme discomfort and **possibly cause a serious scalp burn.**

2. Since chemical relaxers are applied to dry hair, you should know what home products, if any, may still be in the hair.

3. This is the safest way to check the condition of the hair and choose the best strength of relaxer. Different kits have different directions, so read them carefully.

4. The protective base cream prevents strong chemical agents in sodium hydroxide or thio products from burning the client's scalp.

5. These partings ensure that the entire scalp area will be protected. The client's body heat will cause the base to become liquid and spread over the scalp. **Do not rub** the base cream on the scalp. **Rubbing** increases circulation, which may cause a scalp burn.

6. Same as step 5.

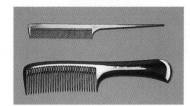

Figure 21.6
Rat-tail comb and rake comb

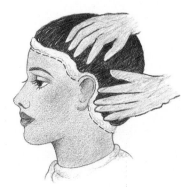

Figure 21.7
Protective base cream around hairline

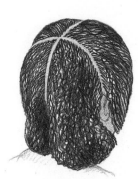

Figure 21.8
Applying base cream in section 1

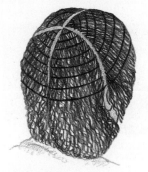

Figure 21.9
Subsectioning pattern for applying base cream

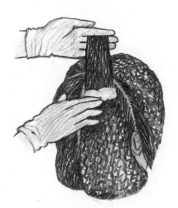

Figure 21.10
The base cream protects the scalp.

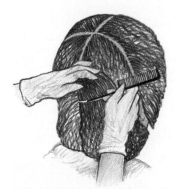

Figure 21.11
Apply relaxer using $\frac{1}{4}$-inch (.625-centimeter) partings.

base cream in the left nape section (Figure 21.10). Work up to top of the section. Then apply the base cream to the top left front section and work through the bottom of the section. Repeat for the right front section.

7. Check the bases of strands all over the head.

8. Put protective gloves on both hands. The relaxer cream may be applied by using fingers, brush, or comb. Here we will use the comb for the application. Do not permit relaxer cream to come in contact with the eyes (remove contact lenses), ears, or neck of the client. Keep relaxer off clothing—it will stain and discolor it.

Applying the Hair Relaxer

Procedure

1. Use the handle of the rake comb or the comb part of the rat-tail comb to stir the relaxer cream gently. Apply a base and a no-base cream in the same way. Do not permit relaxer cream to come in contact with eyes, ears, neck, and so forth!

2. Apply relaxing cream in $\frac{1}{4}$-inch (.625-centimeter) horizontal partings to the right nape section (Figure 21.11). Use the little finger of one hand or the rat-tail part of the comb to make

7. This ensures that the scalp is well protected before the relaxing cream is applied.

8. All sensitive areas of the skin must be protected from the caustic relaxing material.

Rationale

1. Some of the heavier chemicals in the relaxing cream tend to settle to the bottom of the container while it is sitting on the shelf. Stirring with the rake handle or a rat-tail comb blends the chemicals together so they will work more effectively on the hair.

2. Even distribution of cream is needed to ensure uniform relaxing. Holding the strand in your opposite hand helps you see better.

partings; then with your other hand, hold the strand above where you are going to apply the relaxer.

3. Apply the relaxer $\frac{1}{4}$-inch (.625 centimeter) from the scalp. Use your rat-tail comb to "set" the relaxer cream across the hair strand (Figure 21.12). **Do not use pressure.** Work in $\frac{1}{4}$-inch (.625-centimeter) horizontal partings toward the top of the section (Figure 21.13).

4. Apply the relaxing cream in the same way to the left nape section. Using $\frac{1}{4}$-inch (.625-centimeter) horizontal partings, set the relaxing cream $\frac{1}{4}$-inch (.625-centimeter) away from the scalp. Do not use pressure when you apply cream to a hair strand.

5. Apply relaxing cream from the left nape section through the top crown section.

6. Apply cream to the left front section. Begin application at the top center and work toward the hairline around the ear. Use $\frac{1}{4}$-inch (.625-centimeter) diagonal partings to set relaxing cream on the hair strands.

7. Go on to the right front section and apply the relaxing cream to the rest of the hair as described in the previous procedure.

8. Set the timer for 15 minutes. Spray any irritated parts of the scalp with water.

3. The relaxing cream does not work until you apply pressure (friction) to it with your hands and the comb. The cream should not be activated yet.

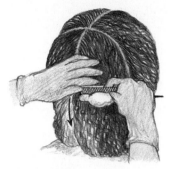

Figure 21.12
Use the back of the rat-tail comb for application. A brush applicator may also be used.

4. This is standard procedure. Do not use pressure (friction), which would activate the relaxing cream.

5. This is standard procedure.

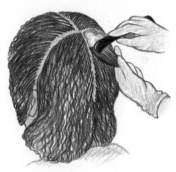

Figure 21.13
Use the back of the rake comb or your thumb or finger.

6. Diagonal partings make the hair lie back rather than toward the face. This reduces the chances of dripping relaxing cream into the client's face or eyes.

7. This is standard procedure.

8. Once the sodium hydroxide has been activated by the pressure of the hand and comb, it straightens the hair very quickly. You may find

the following timetable helpful: fine hair, 3 to 6 minutes; medium hair, 7 to 13 minutes; and coarse hair, 8 to 15 minutes. After you have started the hair relaxer, never allow it to remain on the hair for more than 15 minutes. Water slows or stops the action of the relaxer.

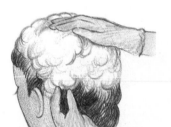

Figure 21.14
Friction (pressure) activates the relaxing cream.

Processing the Relaxer

Procedure

1. Using pressure (friction) with the hands and/or comb, begin in the nape section and work the relaxing cream down the hair strands toward, but not through, the ends (Figure 21.14).

2. Smooth the relaxing cream carefully, but quickly, through both back sections, from the nape through the crown.

3. Saturate each strand with relaxing cream. Add cream where necessary.

4. Activate the relaxing cream on the left front and then on the right front sections. Smooth (spread) the cream along the strands. Work from the top of the sections through the bottom hairline over the ears.

5. Work the relaxing cream through the hair. Use moderate pressure. **Strand test** at intervals of 3–5 minutes.

Rationale

1. Wait until later to work the relaxer through the ends and the hair next to the scalp. The hair will relax faster there due to porosity and body heat.

2. If you stretch the hair too much while you are smoothing the cream, **the hair will break.** Speed is necessary so that the hair will be relaxed evenly.

3. Long or very thick hair may require additional relaxing cream to cover all strands.

4. This is standard procedure to activate the relaxing cream in all four sections of hair.

5. As you work the relaxer through the hair, the "feel" will tell you how much relaxing is taking place on the head. As the bonds within the strands are softened and broken, the

hair will have a soft, mushy feel. The hair will also have a silky, shiny appearance. When strand testing, carefully stretch a small strand out, then release it. If the hair **reverts** (forms **beads** or sharp little bends) back to its natural curliness, continue processing 3–5 minutes and check again.

6. Watch the timer and compare your time to the timetable in step 8 of the preceding procedure. (If the client is allergic to the relaxer or experiences other extreme discomfort, rinse immediately with lukewarm to tepid water and neutralize according to directions. If only a very small area [less than "dime" size] stings, spray the area with water and continue.)

6. If you leave the relaxer on for more than 15 minutes, the hair may break. Be sure that the temperature of the water is comfortable for the client. Cool water stops the action and the stinging.

7. When the hair "feels" soft enough, work the relaxing cream onto all the hair next to the scalp and through all the ends quickly and thoroughly.

7. Working the relaxer carefully but quickly avoids hair breakage or discoloration.

8. **Immediately** escort the client to the shampoo area. Using the outside of your gloved thumb, immediately smooth hair around the front hairline. Use firm pressure and work quickly until hairs in that area are straight.

8. Reducing the curl around the hairline without breaking the hair is a standard part of this service.

Neutralizing the Relaxer

Procedure

1. Use a medium spray of tepid water to rinse the

Rationale

1. If the water is too cool, therelaxing cream, which is

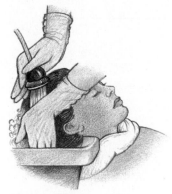

Figure 21.15
Rinse all relaxer from the hair.

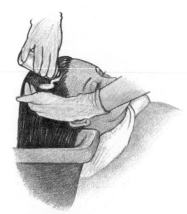

Figure 21.16
Apply neutralizing shampoo.

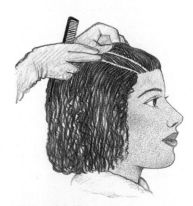

Figure 21.17
Apply scalp conditioner.

relaxer thoroughly from the hair (Figure 21.15).

2. Shampoo hair two or three times with the neutralizing shampoo and rinse until the water runs clear (Figure 21.16). The application of a separate neutralizer may also be required. Follow the manufacturer's directions.

3. Inspect the scalp for protective cream or relaxing cream; shampoo again if necessary.

4. Rinse the hair thoroughly. Then apply the hair conditioner according to directions. Apply scalp conditioner if needed.

5. Allow the conditioner to remain on the hair according to label directions; then rinse the hair, towel-dry, and apply creme rinse or setting lotion.

6. Apply scalp conditioner in 1-inch (2.5-centimeter) partings (Figure 21.17).

heavy, will not rinse out of the hair. On the other hand, if the water is too hot, the client will be very uncomfortable. The force of the water spray removes the relaxer and prevents the hair from tangling.

2. The procedure does five things for the hair and scalp: (1) cleanses the scalp, (2) removes protective base from the scalp, (3) removes the relaxing cream from the hair, (4) neutralizes (stabilizes) the sodium hydroxide or thio, and (5) hardens the hair in the straightened position (hardens the cuticle in the re-formed position). If the rinse water is milky rather than clear, chemicals are still in the hair.

3. All traces of protective and relaxing creams should be removed from the hair and scalp, or irritation may result.

4. The rinse water should look clear, not milky. Application of conditioners varies from one brand to another. **Foam will only appear if all the base and relaxer have been removed from the hair.**

5. The creme rinse or setting lotion reduces the chance of breakage from combing when the hair is brittle from the relaxing service.

6. Chemicals used in the relaxing service remove natural oils from the scalp;

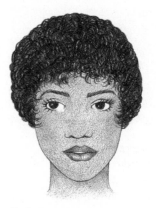

Before

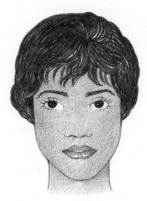

After

Figure 21.18
Before and after chemical relaxing

conditioners replace some of these oils so that the scalp returns to a healthy, supple condition.

7. On the client's chemical service form, record the product used, the date, timing, and suggestions for the next treatment (Figure 21.18).

7. Accurate records should be made so that both you and the client can refer to them for dates and products.

8. Shape hair with scissors only.

8. Super-curly hair that has been relaxed is very fragile; razor shaping will scrape bits of cuticle from the hair shaft because the hair may be very brittle.

Relaxer Retouch

As in a tint or lightener retouch, a relaxer retouch is applied only to the **new growth.** Use the base protective cream if the kit contains one. For added protection against overlapping, a conditioner may be applied over the hair that has already been relaxed. Otherwise, just apply a no-base relaxer and proceed as previously described. **Relax the new growth only.** Retouches every three or four months are recommended. The hair must not be thermally silked **(pressed),** or breakage will result. The hair can be **either** chemically relaxed **or** thermally pressed and curled, **but not both!**

 Safety Tip

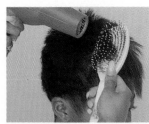

Figure 21.19
After the chemical relaxing service, dry the hair.

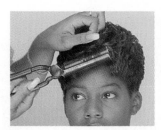

Figure 21.20
Curl the hair toward the face. Be careful not to burn the client's forehead.

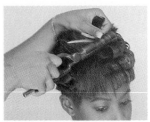

Figure 21.21
Continue to curl the hair in the top section.

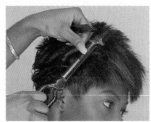

Figure 21.22
Curl the side sections.

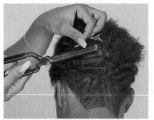

Figure 21.23
Use a smaller-diameter iron to curl shorter hair. Place a comb between the iron and the head to protect the scalp.

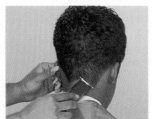

Figure 21.24
Use the clipper to touch up the hairline in the nape as needed.

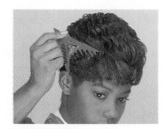

Figure 21.25
Arrange curls into desired finished hairstyle.

Sanitize your area as follows:
1. Wash, wipe, and store bottles and supplies.
2. Discard used supplies.
3. Clean and sanitize the cape and apron.
4. Sanitize the work area; wash your hands.

Supplies

- client chemical services record
- shampoo cape
- 3 laundered towels
- rake comb (or other wide-toothed comb)
- blowout kit with hair conditioner, scalp protective base, relaxer, and neutralizer

- electric clipper
- scissors
- hand hair dryer
- pick
- nonalkaline shampoo
- timer
- protective gloves
- manufacturer's directions
- protective apron

Procedure	*Rationale*
1. Put on protective gloves. Apply base to protect scalp.	**1.** This is standard procedure.
2. Begin application of mild relaxer following normal procedure.	**2.** This is standard procedure.
3. Process hair, but do not overstraighten.	**3.** Remember there should still be some degree of curliness and waviness in the hair to be picked out during styling.
4. Rinse, towel-blot, neutralize, rinse again, condition, and trim (with scissors if hair is wet; with the electric clipper if the hair has already been dried) to the desired shape, pick out the hair as it is dried.	**4.** This is standard procedure. A special, motor-driven clipper may also be used on wet hair.

Chemical Relaxing—Retouch and Hairstyling

The relaxing cream used for retouch is the same as for the virgin chemical relaxing service. Since the ends of the hair have already been relaxed, remember to apply the relaxing cream only to the new growth of hair.

1. Divide the hair into four sections. Apply protective scalp conditioner.
2. Begin in the crown of the head where the hair is usually more resistant. Use a brush or the back of a rat-tail comb to apply relaxing cream to the top and bottom of the hair strand on the new growth of hair. Don't overlap onto the previously relaxed hair.

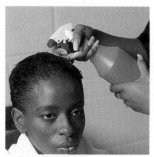

Figure 21.26
Apply styling lotion/conditioner.

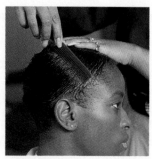

Figure 21.27
Comb hair (wrap) in a circular direction.

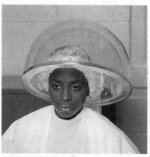

Figure 21.28
Thoroughly dry the hair.

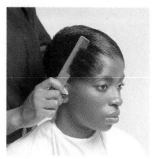

Figure 21.29
Comb hair in toward the face.

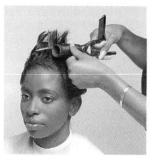

Figure 21.30
Use a large-diameter thermal iron to curl hair in the top section.

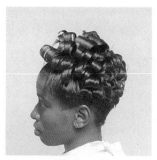

Figure 21.31
Continue to curl hair in the side section.

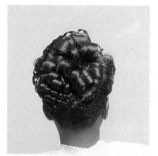

Figure 21.32
Use an iron with a smaller diameter for curling hair in the crown and nape sections.

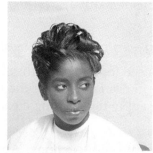

Figure 21.33
Brush hair into desired hairstyle.

3. Continue application to the front side section.
4. Apply relaxing cream to the other front side section. Process until the desired degree of straightening is achieved.
5. Blend relaxer throughout all of the hair before rinsing.
6. Thoroughly rinse all relaxer from the hair using tepid water. All relaxer should be removed from the hair. Remember the scalp will be sensitive, so ask the client whether the water temperature is too hot and adjust accordingly.
7. Apply neutralizing shampoo and leave on the hair for the time indicated by the manufacturer. Rinse.
8. Apply protein conditioner according to the manufacturer's directions.
9. Towel-dry and proceed with styling.
10. This is the procedure for finishing the hairstyle.

Sanitize your area as follows:
1. **Wash, wipe, and store bottles and supplies.**
2. **Discard used supplies.**
3. **Clean and sanitize the cape and apron.**
4. **Sanitize the work area; wash your hands.**

Glossary

Acid chemical relaxers A new type of chemical relaxers that are milder than others.

Base cream (petrolatum) An ointment that protects the scalp from irritation or burns that can be caused by relaxer creams.

Beads Sharp bends of curls that indicate the hair is reverting back to its natural curliness.

Bisulfides A family of chemicals used in the new acid chemical relaxers.

Blowout A procedure that includes applying a milder acid chemical relaxer and picking out (or lifting) the hair away from the head with a pick as the hair is dried and styled.

Caustic soda Sodium hydroxide, used in some chemical relaxing products.

Chemical relaxing Relaxing super-curly hair with products that contain sodium hydroxide.

Chemical straightening Relaxing naturally wavy hair with products that contain ammonium thioglycolate.

Hair relaxers Products that straighten curly hair by either swelling and softening or dissolving cystine disulfide bonds in the hair.

Method of applying chemical relaxers The use of fingers, brush, or comb to apply chemical relaxers.

Neutralizing shampoo A shampoo, usually containing hydrogen peroxide, that stops the softening and straightening action of thio or sodium hydroxide in hair relaxers.

No-base chemical relaxer A hair relaxer that comes with the protective base cream mixed into the relaxing cream.

Petrolatum See **Base cream.**

Pick An instrument used to lift the hair away from the head during the drying and styling process; used in a blowout.

Pick out The process of lifting the hair away from the head with a pick during drying and styling; performed in a blowout.

Sodium hydroxide (SOH-dee-uhm high-DRAHK-sighd) Fast-acting, caustic alkali used in chemical relaxers.

Thermal silking Temporarily straightening the hair with pressing combs; also called pressing.

Questions

1. What basic chemical is used in professional chemical relaxers?
2. Name three terms used for the chemicals that stop the action of the chemical relaxer.
3. After chemically relaxing the hair, would you thermally press and curl it? What if you did?
4. Is sodium hydroxide the same as sodium bromate?
5. What is the difference between a base and a no-base chemical relaxer?
6. When you straighten the hair, do you want to make it completely straight?
7. Is there any difference between sodium hydroxide and ammonium thioglycolate?
8. What is another term that is sometimes used for chemical straightening?
9. What are the pHs of sodium hydroxide and ammonium thioglycolate, respectively?
10. Why would a neutralizing shampoo be used following a chemical relaxer?
11. Does the neutralizing shampoo "fix" the hair in the straightened position?
12. Will sodium hydroxide straighten the hair faster than ammonium thioglycolate?
13. Do chemical relaxers generally come in one strength?
14. Is it necessary to wear gloves when applying a chemical relaxer?
15. True or false. If a chemical relaxer cream should drip into the client's eye(s), remove it by wiping with a towel.
16. Should a protective base be applied around the client's hairline and in back of the ears?

17. Does the application of a chemical relaxer begin in the top of the section?
18. Is the relaxer applied in $1\frac{1}{2}$-inch (3.75-centimeter) subsections?
19. Is the relaxing cream activated by exposing it to air?
20. What activates the straightening action once the relaxer has been applied to the hair?
21. True or false. After the application of the chemical relaxer, a plastic cap is put over the client's hair; then, the client is placed under the dryer for 15 minutes.
22. True or false. When giving a blowout to a client with fine hair, you should use a stronger relaxer.

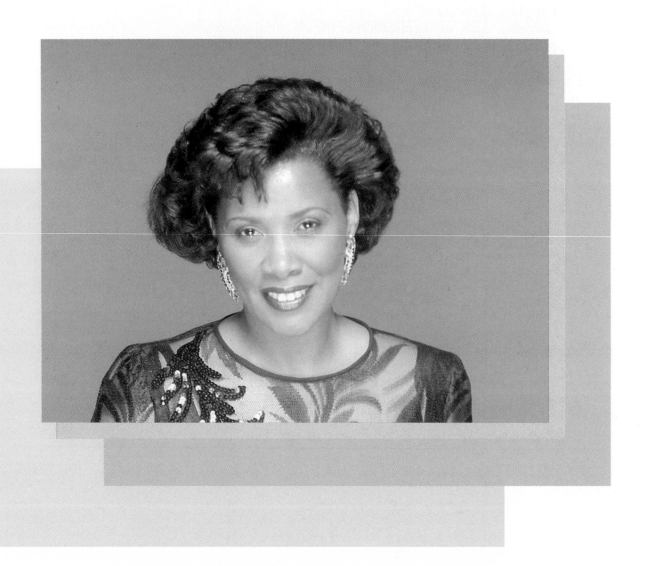

Thermal Pressing

Provided with a set of professional thermal irons and supplies, straighten the hair with the pressing comb, curl the hair with the marcel-type curling iron, and comb the curls into a hairstyle. Use the proper steps and safety precautions to press the hair in 30 to 45 minutes; then curl and style the hair in 45 to 60 minutes. Score 85 percent or better on a multiple-choice exam on the information in this chapter.

In order to achieve the above level of competence, you should master the following chapter objectives.

Theory Objectives

1. Describe the equipment and supplies used for pressing and curling super-curly hair.
2. Explain the use of the pressing iron.
3. Describe the techniques used to produce thermal curls.

Practical Objectives

4. Press the hair.
5. Curl the hair with marcel-type irons.

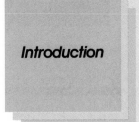

Introduction

The last few chapters have been concerned with the methods used to chemically straighten or curl the hair. Although these methods also involved a physical action on the hair, the chemical treatment was the most important part of the procedure. This chapter presents a process that **physically** straightens and curls the hair. You may be wondering how the thermal curling discussed here differs from the thermal curling covered earlier in the book. Well, there is not much difference. The basic difference is that the iron used for curling super-curly hair is designed so that the heat is spread more evenly across the iron. The iron also is hotter because more heat is needed to curl super-curly hair. The iron is heavier as well; the weight of the iron against the strand helps straighten the super-curly hair and control it during the curling service. Since thermal irons are very hot, you will need to be very careful when working with them on your client. If you are not cautious, you may severely burn your client.

Theory Objective 1
Equipment and
Supplies Used for
Pressing and Curling
Super-Curly Hair

Thermal pressing combs are used for straightening the hair. The **pressing comb** used today is made of copper and brass and has a wooden handle (wood is cooler than plastic when held in the hand). The copper and brass comb heats and holds heat better than combs made of other metals. Pressing combs generally come in three sizes. The smaller, or midget, comb is used to straighten shorter hairs around the front hairline and nape (Figure 22.1). The larger combs (with wide or narrow teeth) are used to straighten hair in the crown, top, and upper side sections.

Thermal curling irons are made of very fine-quality steel so that they can be heated evenly (Figure 22.2). These curling irons have circular barrels and handles made of nonflammable hard plastic or rubber. Like pressing combs, they may be purchased in three sizes.

Historically, a small gas burner was used specifically for heating the marcel-type iron and the pressing comb. This burner has now been replaced by an **electric heater** (also called a **stove** or **oven**). Most modern pressing combs are heated by placing them inside an electric heater (Figure 22.3). Thermal curling irons for use on super-curly hair are heated in much the same way by placing them in an electric heater. Some of the newer curling irons, however, plug into an electric outlet and become hot enough to curl hair that has been pressed. A **thermostat** is used to regulate the temperature of the iron for different hair textures. Remember that the **fine hair around the**

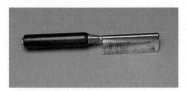

Figure 22.1
Pressing comb (midget)

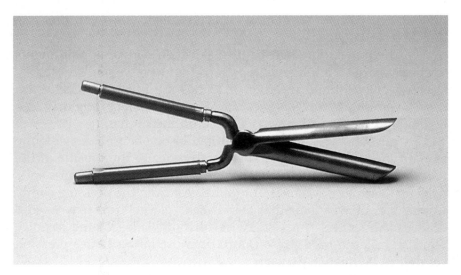

Figure 22.2
Curling iron

hairline is more fragile and can easily break if too much heat and pressure are applied.

The comb used for thermal pressing is a nonflammable (heat-resistant) hard rubber rake comb with wide teeth. Some of the newer plastics are heat-resistant, but ordinary plastic combs will melt. A nonflammable hard rubber styling comb is used for thermal curling and waving the hair after it has been straightened. To protect the client's scalp from the heat of the iron, the cosmetologist places this comb between the hair and the scalp as the iron is wound toward the head.

Special supplies are required for thermal pressing and curling. **Pressing oils,** such as creams, brilliantines, and lusterizing sprays, are applied to protect dry hair from breaking, scorching, or burning. Burned hair cannot be conditioned back to a normal condition; it should be cut off. Most of these protective preparations have a lanolin oil base, which is made from sheep wool.

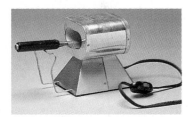

Figure 22.3
Electric heater

Theory Objective 2
Use of the Pressing Iron

In **thermal pressing** (also called **silking**) and curling, a thermal comb is used to straighten super-curly hair; then a curling iron is used to curl the hair. This service is usually given as part of the hairstyling service for black clients. First, the hair is straightened, using a heated pressing comb; then, a circular thermal curling iron (marcel-style iron) is used to make different kinds of curls in the hair. The hair can then be brushed or combed into a finished hairstyle. How long the style will last is determined by the amount of moisture (humidity or water) to which the hair is exposed. Moisture causes the hair to revert to its natural curl. Normally, however, pressing lasts about two weeks.

Thermal curling may be used between regular appointments to correct parts of a hairstyling pattern that have been disturbed by sleeping or by humid weather or to put the finishing touches on air-waved or blow-waved styles. Pressing and iron curling may also be done on wigs and hairpieces made of human hair.

In a **soft press, normal, medium, or fine** hair is pressed quite straight by applying the pressing comb **twice** to the topside of the hair strand and once to the underside of the strand. This process is used on hair that is not resistant to the heat from the pressing comb. **Coarse** hair or wiry hair that has a slick "glassy" feel may need a double comb press (pressed twice on both sides of the strand), which is called a **hard press.** More pressure and a hotter pressing comb may be needed as well.

Theory Objective 3
Techniques Used to Produce Thermal Curls

As Chapter 14 explained, three techniques can be used to style hair with a curling iron: the roller, croquignole, and spiral techniques. Since these techniques have already been explained, they need only be briefly reviewed here.

In the **roller technique** (round), a short hair strand is wound from the end of the strand to the scalp. Place the comb between the iron and the scalp for protection. When the heat penetrates the strand to the outside hair, slip the iron out of the curl. Then clip the curl into place and allow it to cool at room temperature.

For the **croquignole technique,** rotate the handle and turn your wrist to wind the strand in small or large sections from the scalp to the ends.

The **spiral technique** (poker curling) is really a combination of the spiral and croquignole methods. Wind the strand from the scalp in a spiral fashion (Figure 22.4). The resulting curl looks like a

Figure 22.4
The spiral technique

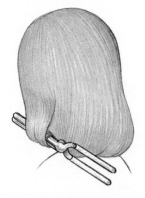 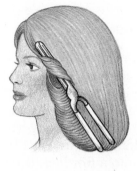 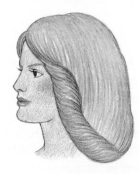

(a) Curl the hanging length. (b) Curl the hair around the face. (c) Completed hairstyle.

spiral candle, so this technique is sometimes called candlestick curling.

Supplies

- pressing cream or oil
- cloth cape and neck strip (Figure 22.5)
- hard rubber (heat-resistant) combs (rake, rat-tail, styling)
- pressing combs (regular and midget) (Figures 22.6 and 22.7)

- shampoo supplies and cape
- curling wax (optional)
- hair spray
- white tissue paper
- electric heater for combs
- duck-bill clips
- client record card

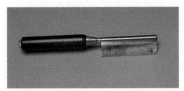

Figure 22.5
Use a heat-resistant cape.

Preparation for Pressing

Procedure

1. Use a heat-resistant cape to drape the client.

2. Examine the scalp for possible irregularities and tightness; analyze the condition and texture of the hair. Rotate the scalp with the cushion of your fingertips. **To avoid breakage,** condition tinted, lightened, brittle, or dry overporous hair as needed.

Rationale

1. A plastic shampoo cape would melt from the heat of the pressing comb. The cloth cape, which is made of cotton, rayon, and the like, will not melt. It is also cooler and is therefore more comfortable for the client.

2. By rotating different areas of the scalp you will see how flexible the scalp is. A scalp that is **very flexible** and supple is hard to press because it will move as the pressing comb moves through the hair. A **normal scalp** usually moves a little, and the hair has a medium

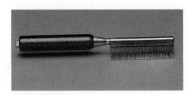

Figure 22.6
Pressing comb (regular)

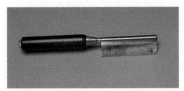

Figure 22.7
Pressing comb (midget)

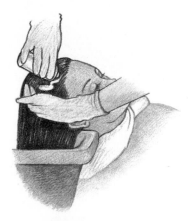

Figure 22.8
Rinse the hair thoroughly.

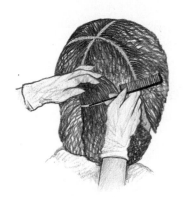

Figure 22.9
Apply lanolin to dry areas of the scalp.

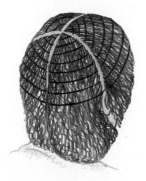

Figure 22.10
Divide the hair into four equal sections. Before pressing, a protective scalp cream is applied.

3. Carefully check the condition of the scalp. If flakes are present, carefully lift them with your comb.

4. Ask the client if the hair has been chemically relaxed within the last 12 months.

5. Shampoo the hair thoroughly.

6. Rinse the hair thoroughly and check it for shampoo residue (Figure 22.8). Towel-dry the hair.

7. Apply a small amount of lanolin cream or oily-scalp conditioner to dry areas on the scalp (Figure 22.9).

8. Use your fingertips to spread the cream or oil through the strands.

9. Divide the hair into four equal sections and hold each in place with a duck-bill clip (Figure 22.10). Dry the hair thoroughly with a dryer.

texture, elasticity, and porosity. A **tight scalp** moves very little. The hair is overporous, brittle, and dry. **To avoid hair breakage,** a tight scalp must be pressed in the direction in which the hair grows.

3. This helps you see how flaky or dry the scalp is. A scalp treatment and the proper shampoo will help control this condition. **If the scalp has open cuts, abrasions, or disease, refuse to perform the service.**

4. Hair that has been chemically relaxed within the last 12 months cannot be pressed. Pressing will **break** hair that has been **chemically relaxed** recently!

5. It is easier to press clean, thoroughly dry hair. If the hair is wet, the hair will be **scorched.**

6. The hair should be visibly free of lather and oils.

7. This helps keep the scalp moist.

8. This lubricates brittle hair and protects it from the extreme heat and pressure of the pressing comb. The hair is easier to handle with the wide-toothed rake comb.

9. The hair is very thick next to the scalp. It is easier to section when wet than when dry, but the actual pressing is done on dry hair.

Pressing the Hair

Procedure	*Rationale*
1. Plug in or turn on the electric heater and place the pressing comb inside it.	**1.** This is the best time to begin heating the combs. The heat keeps the combs **sanitized** too.
2. Stand behind the client. Remove the clips and carefully comb the hair from the ends to the scalp.	**2.** The rake comb's wide teeth will make it easier to comb tangles from the hair. **Remove the tangles** by combing the hair from the ends toward the scalp.
3. Part and secure the hair into four equal sections. Leave one crown and nape section free.	**3.** Start pressing the section that is hanging free.
4. Remove the pressing comb from the heater and touch it to white tissue paper. Stop if the tissue paper discolors in a yellow or brown pattern.	**4.** Discoloration of the tissue paper indicates that the comb is too hot for the hair. Let the comb cool. Test a second time. Remember, **to avoid discoloration and breakage** of tinted, lightened, and gray hair, use a lower temperature than is used for normal or wiry hair.

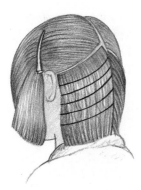

Figure 22.11
Thermal pressing subsections

5. Begin pressing the nape. From the **bottom** of the nape hairline, subdivide the hair into horizontal partings (Figure 22.11).	**5.** This is standard procedure. Smaller sections are easier to press than larger ones depending on hair density. Subsection width will vary from ½ inch (1.25 centimeters) to 1½ inches (3.75 centimeters). **Be careful not to burn the neck.**
6. Secure the hair above the subsection out of the way with a duck-bill clip.	**6.** The clip holds the hair out of the way.
7. Insert the teeth of the pressing comb into the top of each $\frac{1}{2}$-inch (1.25 centimeter) subsection as	**7.** The pressing comb is very hot; be very **careful not to burn** the client's skin, which may cause scarring.

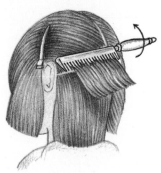

Figure 22.12
Insert the teeth of the comb into the top of the subsection.

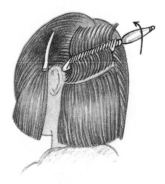

Figure 22.13
Always move the comb away from the client.

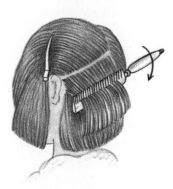

Figure 22.14
Pressing the underside of the subsection

close to the scalp as possible (Figure 22.12). Do not touch the scalp with the pressing comb. For fine hair, use large subsections; for coarse hair, use smaller subsections. Some subsections may be as large as 1½ inches (3.75 centimeters) or as small as ½ inch (1.25 centimeters). One-inch (2.5 centimeter) subsections are normal.

8. Rotate the handle of the pressing comb downward so that the teeth of the iron are pointed directly away from the client (Figure 22.13). Pull the hair through the comb so that the back of the comb presses against the hair as it is moved away from the scalp. Do not pull the comb through the hair too quickly. Repeat **twice** on the top of the hair strand.

8. Always move the pressing comb away from the client. The heat and pressure you put on the pressing comb straighten the hair.

9. Insert the teeth of the pressing comb into the **underside** of the **same** subsection, as close to the scalp as possible (Figure 22.14). **Do not** touch the scalp with the pressing comb. It is only necessary to do the underside once.

9. This is standard procedure. Press both sides of the strand to get maximum straightening.

10. Rotate the handle of the pressing comb **upward** and **away** from the client's scalp while you draw the hair **against** the **back** of the pressing comb.

10. The rotation causes the hair strand to be "pressed" against the back of the comb and straightened.

11. Repeat this procedure for each ½-inch (1.25-centimeter) to 1½-inch (3.75-centimeter)

11. This is standard procedure. Straightening all hair once is called a **soft press.**

horizontal subsection of each section of the head until all the hair has been straightened. Do the sections in the same order you use for tinting.

Repeating the entire procedure (straightening all hair twice) is called a **hard press.**

12. Proceed to curl the hair with your iron.

12. This is standard procedure.

Practical Objective 5
Curling the Hair with Marcel-Style Irons

Supplies

- curling irons of various sizes (Figures 22.15 and 22.16)
- brush
- white tissue paper

- duck-bill clips
- heat-resistant styling comb(s)
- marcel-style curling iron
- electric heater

Procedure

1. Heat the iron(s).

2. Select an iron with a large, medium, or small circumference.

Rationale

1. This is standard procedure.

2. The circumference of the iron is determined by the length and texture of the hair. Short, fine hair (especially strands around the hairline) requires an iron with a smaller circumference than longer, coarse hair does.

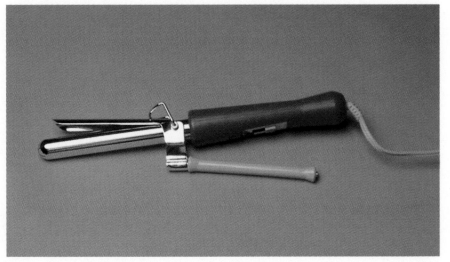

Figure 22.15
Small electric curling iron

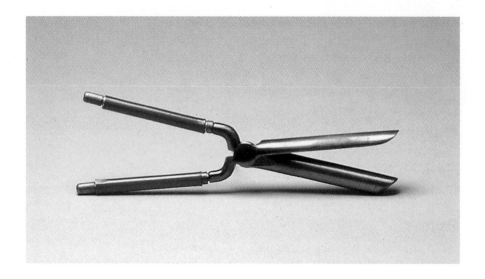

Figure 22.16
Larger curling iron

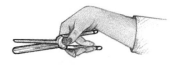

Figure 22.17
Control the iron with your ring finger and little finger.

3. Pretest the temperature on white tissue paper. Carefully use the little and ring fingers of your hand to control the iron (Figure 22.17).

4. Begin curling the hair in the same sequence you used to set the hair.

5. Hold the hair strand and comb in one hand and hold the iron in your other hand.

6. Practice holding the iron and clicking it (opening and closing the clamp) while rotating the comb. The barrel, not the clamp, of the iron curls the hair. The clamp merely holds the hair between movements.

7. Hold the strand away from the scalp and put the barrel of the iron to the hair next to the scalp. Push the iron against the scalp hair and bring the end of the strand

3. This helps you avoid applying too much heat to the hair. **Be careful not to burn the client's hair or scalp!** Be careful not to burn your fingers.

4. This is the easiest way to curl if a roller-type hairstyle is desired.

5. This is standard procedure.

6. Effective thermal waving takes practice. You can practice by using a cold iron on a mannequin.

7. This directs the base of the hair strand to give it the same height and strength as a curl formed in a wet setting.

toward you. **Rock** the iron against the base of the strand to form the base of the curl.

8. Open the clamp and wind the hair strand around the barrel of the iron (Figure 22.18). The strand should be placed between the barrel and the clamp. Then close the clamp to where it pivots next to the handle.

8. This is standard procedure.

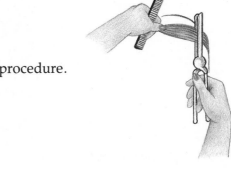

Figure 22.18
Wind the hair strand around the barrel of the iron.

9. Hold the end of the strand with your left hand. Curl this part of the strand (next to the head) by rocking the iron against the strand in a movement horizontal to the head. Spiral the strand between the clamp and the barrel next to the first part of the strand. Slowly "feed" hair around the iron (Figure 22.19). Repeat until the entire length of the strand has been curled.

9. This procedure gives an even curl to each section of the strand.

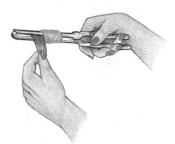

Figure 22.19
Slowly "feed" the hair around the iron.

10. Place the comb between the iron and the scalp (Figure 22.20). Place the fingertips of your hand on the hair that is wound around the iron.

10. You must place the comb between the iron and the scalp to avoid burning the scalp.

11. Slide the iron horizontally from one side of the curl and **hold the curl** with the edge of your comb as you slide the iron. Clip the curl to the scalp in the same way you would clip a roller. If you need assistance, consult your instructor.

11. The hair is quite warm when the iron is removed. A more durable curl is formed if the hair is allowed to cool in a clipped rather than an unclipped and unwound position.

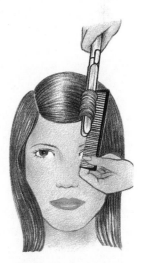

Figure 22.20
Use the comb to protect the scalp.

12. Use the curling iron on all of the hair strands.

12. This is standard procedure.

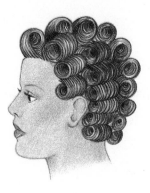 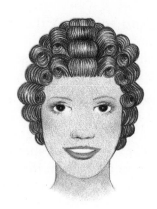

Figure 22.21
The completed curling pattern

13. Clip the curls and let them cool. All curls should be allowed to cool before the clips are removed for styling (Figure 22.21).

14. Clean the residue off your pressing comb.

13. This is standard procedure.

14. Residue from heated pressing oil and other carbon-scorched material may be removed by using "000" steel wool, very fine sand paper, or an emery board file.

Comb-Out

Procedure

1. Remove the clips and arrange the hair.

2. To make a wave pattern, insert the iron diagonally in the hair to the outside corner of the left eyebrow (Figure 22.22).

3. Close the clamp and rotate the iron one turn forward. Rest it on the comb (which is on the scalp) until the heat penetrates the hair evenly (Figure 22.23). Place your fingertips across the wound hair.

Rationale

1. This is standard procedure.

2. This is how you should begin to form the wave ridge.

3. Placing your fingertips on the hair helps you take the iron out quickly after you have finished heating the hair.

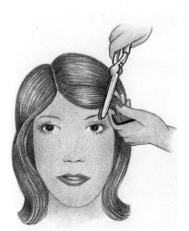

Figure 22.22
To make a soft wave, place the iron diagonal to the front hairline.

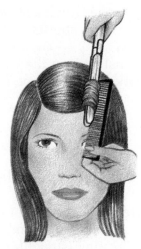

Figure 22.23
The comb protects the scalp as you rotate the iron.

4. Reverse the rotation of the iron, but return it to the original position.

5. Place the iron across the ridge, but do not close the clamp. Shift the hair beneath the iron with the comb to make the wave pattern (Figure 22.24).

6. Repeat steps 2, 3, and 4 until the hair on the bottom of the side hairline has been waved (Figure 22.25).

4. This gives you an even ridge.

5. This is standard procedure.

6. This is standard procedure.

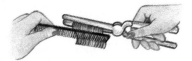

Figure 22.24
Shift the hair beneath the iron to form a wave.

Sanitize your area as follows:
1. Wash, wipe, and store bottles and supplies.
2. Discard used supplies.
3. Clean and sanitize the cape and apron.
4. Sanitize the work area; wash your hands.

Thermal Pressing the Hair

1. After the hair has been pressed, begin thermal curling in the top section of the hair.

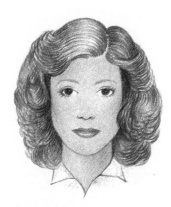

Figure 22.25
The finished thermal wave

2. As you curl the crown and nape sections, remember that when the hair becomes shorter, you may have to use a smaller-barrel curling iron.
3. Place thermal curls in the nape section.
4. When working in the nape section, be careful not to burn the client's neck.

Glossary

Croquignole technique A method of curling the hair from the scalp to the ends.

Electric heater A heater used to heat nonelectric marcel curling irons and pressing combs.

Hard press Pressing (straightening) the hair twice on both sides of the hair strand using a thermal pressing comb.

Poker curling See **Spiral technique.**

Pressing comb An instrument used to straighten hair with heat; usually made of copper and brass with a wooden handle.

Pressing oils Protective preparations such as creams, brilliantines, and lusterizing sprays used in thermal pressing and curling.

Roller technique A method of thermal curling in which a hair strand is wound from the end toward the scalp.

Silking A method of physically straightening super-curly hair; also called thermal pressing.

Soft press Pressing (straightening) the hair twice on the topside of the hair strand and once on the underside of the strand.

Spiral technique A combination of the spiral and croquignole methods of thermal curling; the hair is wound from the scalp in a spiral fashion.

Stove/oven See **Electric heater.**

Thermal curling irons Irons made of very fine-quality steel so that they can be heated evenly to curl the hair.

Thermal pressing A method of physically straightening super-curly hair; also called silking.

Tight scalp Scalp that moves very little when rotation with the pressing comb is attempted.

Questions

1. What does it mean to press the hair?
2. How long does a press last?
3. What do you use to press the hair?
4. Is it necessary to use a heat-resistant comb?
5. How is a pressing comb heated?

6. What effect does pressing have on the hair?
7. Once the hair is pressed, what will cause it to become curly again?
8. If the hair is pressed once, but remains quite wavy, what can be done?
9. Is pressing a style by itself, or must something else be done?
10. Is it necessary to use a lower temperature on lightened hair?
11. What can be used to remove carbon residue from the pressing comb?
12. Should a heat-resistant cape be used for thermal waving?
13. Before using the marcel-style iron on the hair, what safety precaution should you take?
14. Write a short definition of the croquignole, spiral, and roller techniques, respectively.
15. Is it necessary to examine the scalp before pressing the hair?
16. To avoid discoloration, what temperature should be used when pressing gray hair in comparison to wiry hair?
17. Should the hair be shampooed before the pressing service?
18. If the hair has been recently chemically relaxed, should you double press it?
19. Can towel-dried hair be pressed, or must the hair be thoroughly dried with a dryer?

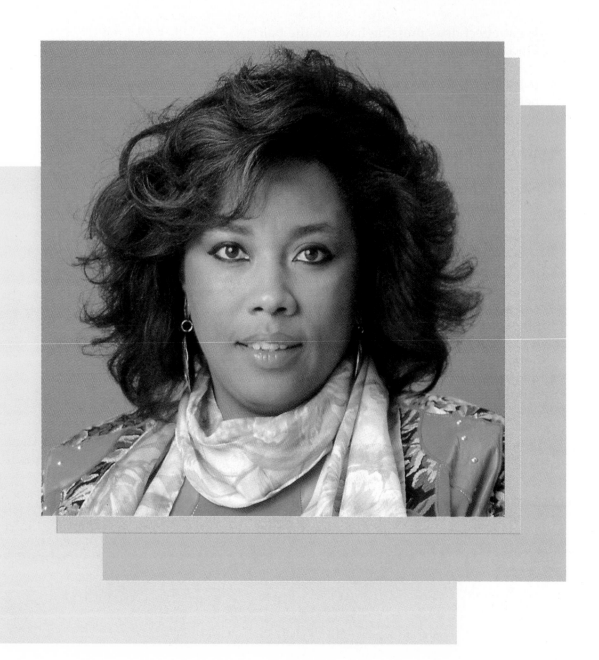

Recurling the Hair (Soft Curl Perm)

Learning Objectives

Using professional curl re-formation chemicals and implements, relax and re-form (recurl) super-curly hair to make it more manageable and durable from one styling to the next. Observing safety precautions and following label directions, use the proper steps to relax, then re-form (recurl) the hair. Use a chemical relaxing product to relax the hair in 30–45 minutes. Then, wrap the client's hair on permanent wave rods in 45–75 minutes. Score 85 percent or better on a multiple-choice exam on the information in this chapter.

In order to achieve the above level of competence, you should master the following chapter objectives.

Theory Objectives

1. Define the basic curl re-formation service and its advantages.
2. Describe the chemical processes of the curl re-formation service.
3. Evaluate the condition of the hair and scalp.
4. Identify important safety and after-care considerations for the curl re-formation service.

Practical Objectives

5. Analyze the hair and apply the chemical curl relaxer.
6. Section and subsection the client's hair and wrap it on cold-wave rods.
7. Process and neutralize the curl re-formation.

Introduction

The recurl service is very popular for clients with super-curly hair because it provides them with more hairstyling choices. Of all the services performed by a cosmetologist, the soft curl perm or recurl service requires the most skill. The soft curl perm not only requires mastery of artistic skills, but mastery of safety practices too. The recurl service is performed on super-curly hair to reshape the natural pattern of curl in the hair into a larger pattern. The larger curl pattern enables the cosmetologist to use more hairstyling techniques and to offer clients a greater variety of hairstyles.

The soft curl perm is actually two major chemical services merged together into one service. Special products have been developed just for the recurl service. In the first part of the service, the hair is chemically relaxed. The second part of the service involves permanent waving the hair around rods that are larger than the natural curl pattern of the client's hair. Since strong chemicals are used in both processes, extreme care should be taken not to irritate the skin around the hairline and the nape of the neck. The cosmetologist should also be sure to apply protective creams and change the neck towels frequently. This chapter will explain all the procedures and safety practices required for this service.

Theory Objective 1
Basic Curl Re-formation Service and Its Advantages

The **curl re-formation** service is also known as a **curl rearranger** (or recurl). These terms will be used interchangeably through this chapter. A **curl re-formation** is a double-application service, in which the hair is treated with two different chemical processes. The curl re-formation service is given to a client with super-curly hair. The service involves first straightening the hair, then recurling it in a larger curl pattern.

In the first stage of this process, a chemical relaxer (presoftener) is used to **straighten** the hair. The relaxer is usually an **ammonium thioglycolate** (thio) product. Other chemicals are also used, but generally, most salons use thio-based relaxers. The relaxer you use, however, will be determined by your school or salon.

Remember to read and follow the manufacturer's directions for the product you are using!

During the second stage of the process, the hair is wound around cold-wave rods, and another thio-based chemical is applied. The hair is processed until the desired degree of curl is achieved; then it is neutralized. The most common type of neutralizer used for a curl re-formation is **sodium bromate.** Although a few manufacturers use a peroxide neutralizer, the vast majority use sodium bromate. **Read the product** directions **carefully.**

The basic product used to relax the hair is called the **chemical rearranger.** As noted above, this is usually a thio-based relaxer. Since this product has a pH that is alkaline, gloves must be worn to protect the hands. Of course, irritation may result if the relaxer comes into prolonged contact with the client's skin and scalp, so care must be taken to protect them by working as rapidly as possible.

The chemical rearranger generally comes in different strengths: mild, for fine or tinted hair; regular, for average hair; and super, for very curly to resistant hair. Different manufacturers may recommend other strengths however, so **read the directions carefully.** After the chemical rearranger has been applied, it may be left on the hair from 17 to 30 minutes, depending on the resistance or texture of the client's hair. Fine, tinted hair will probably require less time; super-curly, coarse, virgin hair may take a little longer. To be on the safe side, check the rearranger every 3–5 minutes. Unlike a hair color strand test, the curl re-formation strand test uses a strand about the size as that used for wrapping a cold-wave rod (Figure 23.1).

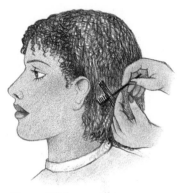

Figure 23.1
Strand test for re-formation (recurl) service. An applicator bottle or brush may be used.

After the chemical rearranger has been rinsed from the hair, the **curl booster** (waving solution) is applied. The curl booster is a thio product that is used to wrap the hair and then process it for the desired degree of curliness, based on the size of the rods used during wrapping. If the hair dries out during the wrapping process, in most cases you should apply only the curl booster, not water. Water would dilute the curl booster and might prevent the hair from curling. Although water is generally not used during wrapping, it can be used in some situations; follow your instructor's and the manufacturer's directions.

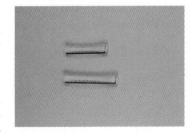

Figure 23.2
Two concave, medium-diameter rods in different lengths

Generally, **smaller rods** are used for the curl re-formation services (depending on the texture of the hair). For a curly hairstyle that can simply be "picked out" (lifted), small-diameter yellow or blue rods achieve the results preferred by some clients (Figure 23.2). If the hair is quite coarse, blue rods are used. However, if the client wishes to blow-comb/iron curl or wet set the hair, larger pink, gray, or white rods may be used. Thus, the rod used will be determined by the condition and texture of the hair and the amount of curl and the hairstyle desired by the client.

For several reasons, **wrapping** is somewhat different for a curl re-formation service than for cold/acid waving. First, the subsection of hair that is wound around each rod must be very thinly parted. Because small subsections of hair are used, many rods are needed to wrap the entire head. A curl re-formation will usually require 10 to 12 dozen (120–144) rods, whereas a typical cold wave or heat wave would most likely use 4 or 5 dozen (48–60) rods.

The **tension** used in wrapping the hair for re-formation is also a little different. The hair **must be wrapped with a firm, even**

tension across each rod. Another important part of the wrapping procedure is the technique for winding the rods and positioning them in the subsection. The individual strand should normally be wrapped as though you were making a no-stem roller. When wound, the rod should rest on the subsection of hair from which it was taken. Remember that **too much tension on the elastic rod strap will cause breakage.**

Safety Tip ▶

Furthermore, the best results are achieved when the right side, left side, and top sections are wrapped forward—toward the face.

Curl re-formation offers many advantages for super-curly hair, including the following:

1. The hair is more manageable.

2. More hairstyles can be achieved.

3. The hair can be easily blow-combed and iron curled.

4. The hair can easily be wet set in rollers.

Theory Objective 2
Chemical Processes of the Curl Re-formation Service

As noted earlier, the curl re-formation processes are not really new to you since you have already learned how to use thio products in several services. The thio found in the chemical rearranger used for relaxing the hair is **alkaline,** with a pH of 9.6. When this is applied to the hair, it softens and swells the cystine disulfide bonds (sulfur bonds). Smoothing the hair with your hands or the back of your comb causes the sulfur peptide linkages to ''slip'' into a straighter position (Figure 23.3). The hydrogen and salt bonds are also af-

Figure 23.3
Effect of the chemical rearranger on sulfur (cystine disulfide) bonds

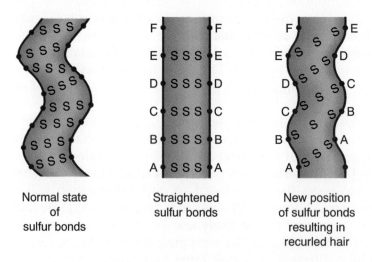

Normal state
of
sulfur bonds

Straightened
sulfur bonds

New position
of sulfur bonds
resulting in
recurled hair

fected, but to a lesser extent. Rinsing the hair with tepid water stops the action of the chemical rearranger because water has a pH of 7.0. This is an effective way to stop the chemical action of the rearranger.

The curl booster is also alkaline, with a pH of 9.6. The curl booster continues softening (or breaking down) the sulfur bonds, helping the hair to re-form around the shape of the permanent wave rod. Once this new shape has been achieved, it can be said that the hair has been "re-formed." You will need to take a test curl to determine how long the curl booster should be left on the rods after the hair has been completely wrapped. Take the test curl by unwinding a rod or two in each section of the head. Each rod should be unwound only $1\frac{1}{2}$ to 2 turns to check for the classical "S" pattern; then the rod is refastened, and another rod is checked (Figure 23.4). (However, some hair may not be long enough for two complete turns.)

Heat is used to accelerate (speed up) a **chemical process.** Heat also enables whatever chemical is used to better penetrate the hair. The heat generated naturally by the client's body is used by simply placing a plastic cap over the hair to capture the heat. The artificial heat of a hair dryer or infrared light can also be used. Different manufacturers recommend various uses of natural and artificial heat. Read each product's directions carefully to determine when to use which source of heat with which part of the service.

Coarse hair will normally require placing the client under the dryer for at least 5 minutes. Children under 12 years of age should not be put under the dryer at all because their bodies generate enough heat without the dryer. As a general rule, process the rearranger without the dryer for 20 minutes on all clients before using the hair dryer for heat!

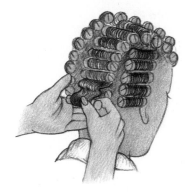

Figure 23.4
Definite "S" pattern. To take a test curl, unwrap rod a maximum of two turns, towel-blot, test, rewind, and reapply solution.

◀ Safety Tip

Theory Objective 3
Evaluating the Condition of the Hair and Scalp

When you are applying chemicals that penetrate the cuticle and cortex layers of the hair, you must take extra precautions before beginning the service. This is an important step. It is your responsibility to protect the client and yourself before, during, and after the curl rearranging service.

◀ Safety Tip

First, ask the client if the hair has been chemically relaxed in the previous 12 months. **Hair that has been relaxed with a sodium hydroxide relaxer must not be given a curl re-formation. That hair will not curl. The sodium hydroxide–treated hair must be cut off to avoid straight ends or hair breakage.** Explain this to the client during the evaluation process. A curl re-formation can be given over hair that has been treated with other ammonium thioglycolate products.

Figure 23.5
Degrees of curliness

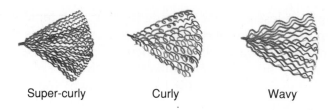

Super-curly   Curly   Wavy

Next, determine if the scalp has any open cuts, scrapes, or abrasions. If the scalp has any of these conditions, the curl re-formation service will **irritate** the condition; inflammation, blisters, or open sores will result. **Do not give this service to a client with any of the foregoing conditions!**

Now, you will want to determine the texture and condition of the client's hair. Coarse hair will be harder to curl than medium or fine hair. Porosity of the hair is also a factor. **Hair that is very porous will curl more easily** than hair that is not overporous because the softening and curling chemicals penetrate (enter) the hair faster (Figure 23.5). Porous or brittle hair should be conditioned with a **polymer conditioner** or other high-quality **protein conditioner** weekly for 2 to 3 weeks **before** the curl re-formation service or until the hair has regained its tensile strength. This also applies to hair that has been tinted with permanent hair color or lightened. Lightened hair will break easily! To sum up, the curl re-formation service should **only be given on strong, healthy hair.**

Safety Tip ▶

Finally, a personal, but brief medical history about the client may be very helpful. For example, if the client has high blood pressure (**hypertension**) or a heart condition, you may create a problem if you put the client under a hot dryer. **Allergies** are also an important consideration. Ask the client whether he or she is allergic or sensitive to thio products. Of course, **don't give this service to anyone who has had a chemical reaction as a result of this service in the past.** If the client already has a service record, check it. Make a record for a new client.

If the client's hair has been given a curl rearranger before, simply apply the straightener to the new growth only.

Theory Objective 4
Important Safety and After-Care Considerations for the Curl Re-formation Service

Since curl re-formation involves harsh chemicals, it is important to protect your client and yourself. The products in this service, which are strong enough to soften and curl the hair, can also soften and irritate your skin and the skin of your client.

To avoid chemical burns and irritation to the skin, eyes, ears and nose, **keep all products away from these areas.** If you accidentally drop or drip a product into one of these areas, **rinse with cool water immediately.** If the irritation continues, ask the client to contact a physician or dermatologist. Since you must depend on your hands in making a living, **protect them by wearing rubber or surgical gloves** during this service. Remember—failing to wear gloves on a long-term basis will result in damage to your hands. Even though you may be able to give this service today without gloves, tomorrow you may develop an allergy and be out of the school or out of a job!

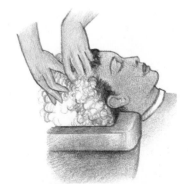

One other precaution must be observed. **Do not brush** the hair before this service. Doing so can cause the client to suffer scalp irritations or burns.

After Care

Care for the hair after the curl re-formation service is of the utmost importance! As the hair is softened by the thio, the inner bonds of the hair are softened (broken), then rehardened (rebonded) during the neutralizing process. Since natural oils are also removed from the hair and scalp along with moisture, they must be replaced to keep the hair looking shiny and strong.

Immediately after the hair has been neutralized, it must be conditioned with a keratin-type protein conditioner. Then a **curl activator** should be applied to the scalp. An **instant moisturizer** should be applied after the activator is used. At this point in the service, the hair may be shaped (cut). If the scalp still seems to be dry, an instant curl moisturizer may be sprayed near the scalp. Now the hair is ready for styling.

The hair and scalp moisturizers may be applied every other day or as directed. Read and follow label directions. If after-care recommendations are not followed, the client will have problems with a dry/itchy scalp and brittle hair that will have a tendency to break.

If the client does not have time for or cannot afford the prescribed after-care steps, recommend that he or she do the following:

1. Shampoo the hair at least weekly, using the shampoo suggested by the curl rearranger manufacturer (Figure 23.6). The shampoo must have a neutral or acid pH in order to protect the new curl formation.

2. All conditioners used should have a pH of 7.0 or less.

3. It is important to use a curl activator (oil) on the scalp.

4. Moisturizers should be sprayed on the hair before styling. If the hair is to be a "pick-out," the moisturizer can be sprayed on after styling.

Safety Tip

Safety Tip

Figure 23.6
Use a neutralizing shampoo to maintain the hair in good condition.

If the client does not follow these steps, he or she will note the following changes after one or two days: the hair will be excessively dry and brittle and will break easily, and the scalp will be overly dry.

The client should use a plastic cap to protect his or her clothing after applying a moisturizer or curl activator. Of course, the cap also improves the penetration of the hair/scalp. However, the client must not sleep in the plastic cap because the elastic around the cap will cause breakage around the hairline. Prolonged use of the plastic cap may also cause a bacterial scale infection.

Practical Objective 5
Analyzing the Hair and Applying the Chemical Curl Relaxer

Supplies

- shampoo cape
- towels
- cotton coil
- neutralizing bib
- rat-tail comb
- rubber or surgical gloves
- dryer
- end papers
- large-toothed comb
- timer
- sectioning clips
- cold-wave rods (10–12 dozen)
- plastic cap
- applicator brush (if applying to new growth)

- thio relaxer (chemical rearranger)
- waving solution (curl booster)
- neutralizer (sodium bromate)
- protein conditioner (keratin base)
- instant moisturizer
- curl activator
- conditioning shampoo
- polymer pretreatment
- protective base
- protective apron

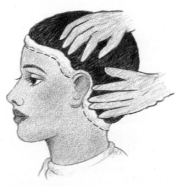

Figure 23.7
Apply protective base cream (petrolatum) around the hairline.

Procedure

1. Remove all neck and ear jewelry and double drape the client. Apply protective base cream around the hairline (forehead, ears, and neck) (Figure 23.7). Put on protective gloves.

2. Give several test curls (Figure 23.8).

Rationale

1. Metal jewelry may react with different solutions and cause a chemical burn on the skin. Draping protects the client's clothing. The base is needed to protect the client's skin. Protect your hands at all times.

2. You will be able to determine how long curling will take on hair that has been curled, tinted, or

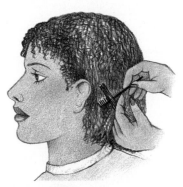

Figure 23.8
Take several test curls

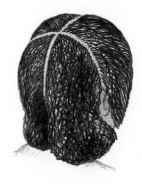

Figure 23.9
Sectioning pattern for recurl

3. Analyze the porosity, texture, and condition of the hair.

4. Part the hair into four sections, and begin applying the rearranger (relaxer) in the bottom of the right nape section (Figure 23.9). Use $\frac{1}{4}$- to $\frac{1}{2}$-inch (.625- to 1.25-centimeter) subsections (Figures 23.10 and 23.11). Continue to work to the top of the section until done. Go to the bottom of the other back section and repeat the application steps. Now apply rearranger to each front section, working from the bottom to the top of each section.

5. Begin in one nape section and work to the top of the section (Figure 23.12). Use the back of the comb or your fingers to smooth the hair firmly into a straighter

lightened, or whether the hair should be curled at all.

3. This will help you determine which strength of thio relaxer to apply to the hair.

4. This is standard procedure. Small subsections are needed so that the rearranger saturates each strand (subsection) of hair.

5. The dryer speeds up the relaxing process by allowing the relaxer to better penetrate the hair shaft.

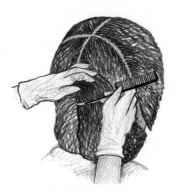

Figure 23.10
Use $\frac{1}{4}$- to $\frac{1}{2}$-inch (.625- to 1.25-centimeter) subsections.

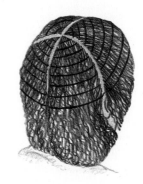

Figure 23.11
Subsectioning pattern for recurl

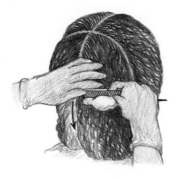
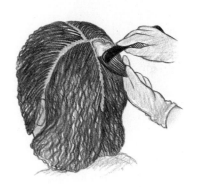
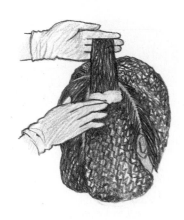

Figure 23.12

Begin application in the nape subsection and work to the top of the section.

position. Repeat on each section. Clients over the age of 12 may be put under a warm-hot dryer for 17–30 minutes with a plastic cap over the hair, if necessary.

6. Test the rearranger for straightness every 3–5 minutes. Be careful not to overprocess. Use a timer to check processing.

6. Rarely will the hair process take more than 30 minutes. In general, the following timetable will apply: tinted hair, 15 to 20 minutes; average hair, 20 to 25 minutes; and coarse hair, 25 to 30 minutes. A timer eliminates the need to guess the correct time.

7. Strand test the rearranger. Towel-dry a strand about the size of a cold-wave rod subsection to check for straightness of hair (Figures 23.13 and 23.14).

7. A section this size will give an accurate indication of the degree of straightness achieved. A larger section would not. The hair must be straight for successful curl re-formation.

8. Rinse the hair with tepid (lukewarm) water for 3 to 5 minutes until all rearranger has been rinsed from the hair (Figure 23.15).

8. Hot water would irritate the scalp. Water has a pH of 7.0 so it stops the chemical action of the relaxer.

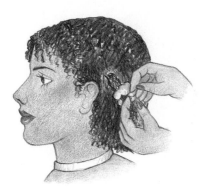

Figure 23.13
Dry the strand to test for the degree of straightening.

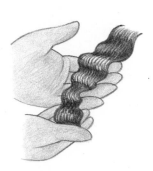

Figure 23.14
Note how the second strand test shows hair relaxing.

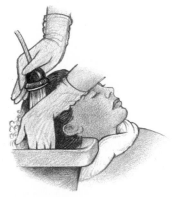

Figure 23.15
Rinse all rearranger from hair until the water runs clear.

Procedure

1. Select the rod diameter to be used. Now section the head for wrapping (Figure 23.16). Put on gloves.

2. Apply waving solution (curl booster) to the whole section you are about to wrap. Reapply as needed if the hair dries out. Begin wrapping in the top of the center crown section (or whichever system your

Rationale

1. Remember, you will need 10 to 12 dozen rods. The smaller rods will give a tighter curling pattern than larger rods.

2. The waving solution softens the hair so that it will "re-form" around the rod. It is important to keep the hair wet with the waving solution for good penetration of the hair shaft. **Do not use water.** Water

Practical Objective 6
Sectioning and Subsectioning the Client's Hair and Wrapping It on Cold-Wave Rods

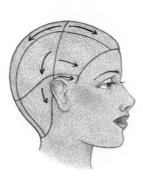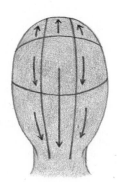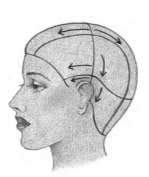

Figure 23.16
Many sectioning patterns are available. Your instructor will tell you which pattern to use.

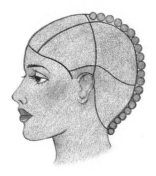
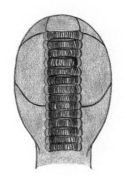

Figure 23.17
Begin in the center crown section. Continue to the bottom of the nape. Use small subsections.

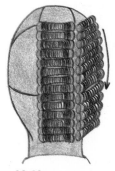

Figure 23.18
Wrap the right crown section, then the right nape section.

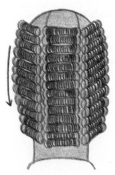

Figure 23.19
Wrap the left crown section, then the left nape section.

instructor advises) (Figure 23.17). Use protective gloves at all times and avoid contact with the client's face, eyes, and ears.

3. Wrap the hair using very thin subsections (one-fourth to one-half) the diameter of the rod used). Wrap with firm, even tension.

4. Apply waving solution to each section as you wrap. Wrap the right crown section, then the left crown section, working from the top of the section to the bottom (Figures 23.18 and 23.19). Apply waving solution to keep the hair wet at all times. Do not drip on the client's ear or face!

5. Apply waving solution to the center front top section. Begin wrapping from the back of the section and work toward the forehead (Figure 23.20). Rods are wrapped forward. Do not let solution drip in the client's eyes or

slows down the curling action. **If any waving solution drips onto the client's face, ears, or eyes, rinse with cold water immediately!**

3. **If large subsections are used, the hair bonds won't be broken enough to re-form around the rod you have selected.** Neat rods with tension evenly applied across the rod are needed to curl the hair uniformly.

4. **Dry hair won't process evenly.** Precautions are needed throughout the chemical application.

5. It is easier to wrap the hair by working from the back of the section toward the front.

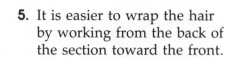

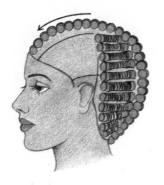
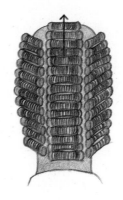

Figure 23.20
Wrap the top center section forward toward the face.

on the face! Stand in front of the client when you wrap this section.

6. Apply waving solution to the right front side section and wrap the rods forward. Begin wrapping at the back of each section and wrap the rods toward the face (Figure 23.21). **Do not drip solution on the client's face!** Apply waving solution to the left front side and wrap like the right side.

6. Since the hairs around the front hairline may be uneven, or thin and sparse, you will find it easier to roll the rods toward the face using a brick pattern to avoid splits.

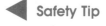 **Safety Tip**

Figure 23.21
Wrap the top right side sections toward the face; then wrap the top left side sections, also toward the face.

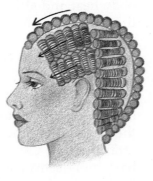
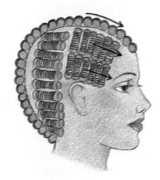

Practical Objective 7
Processing and Neutralizing the Curl Re-formation

Procedure

1. Check all rods for neat, even wrapping. Place cotton coil

Rationale

1. Cotton stops the waving solution from dripping onto

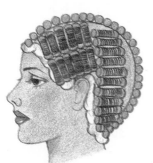

Figure 23.22
Place cotton coil around hairline. Remove after application of waving solution to prevent chemical burns.

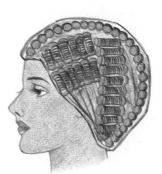

Figure 23.23
Place plastic cap over rods.

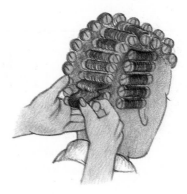

Figure 23.24
A definite "S" pattern. Unwrap the rod a maximum of two turns.

Safety Tip ▶

around the entire hairline and reapply waving solution to all rods (Figure 23.22).

2. Allow the cotton to become saturated for 1 or 2 minutes, then replace it with a new, dry piece of cotton coil. Replace towel(s) used to drape the client. Place plastic cap over rods and secure with clip or rod (Figure 23.23).

3. Place **adults** (over the age of 12) **under the tepid hair dryer for 10 to 30 minutes** if the cap alone hasn't relaxed the hair enough. **Always process children with the cap only!** After 10 minutes, test curl the hair by unwrapping a rod in each section **two turns;** check for the "S" pattern (Figure 23.24).

the skin, face, and ears. Resaturation with waving solution makes the hair process evenly. Some of the solution probably has evaporated since you started.

2. If the hair is allowed to process with the wet cotton or wet neck towel in place, **a chemical burn will result.** The plastic cap captures body heat and also prevents the waving solution from drying out. If the solution dries out, it won't curl the hair.

3. Normally, children have enough body heat to process the curl without the use of artificial heat. Children also have more sensitive skin than adults. Because everyone's hair is different, test curls are needed to protect against **overprocessing.** Using the cap alone is better for the condition of the hair and scalp.

4. When an "S" pattern has been achieved, remove the plastic cap and rinse the hair thoroughly with tepid water for 3 to 5 minutes (Figure 23.25). Use a timer. Gently towel-blot **each rod.**

4. Rinsing with water removes the waving solution and stops the re-formation process. Tepid water is used because hot water may irritate the scalp. Towel-blotting the rods removes excess water and "makes room" in the hair shaft for the neutralizer.

5. Attach the neutralizing bib around the hairline. Apply neutralizer thoroughly to each rod. Allow excess to drip into the bib.

5. The neutralizing bib stops neutralizer from dripping onto the client's neck, ears, and forehead.

6. Remove neutralizing bib. Allow hair to neutralize for at least 10 minutes or according to the manufacturer's directions. **Use a dryer only if required by the manufacturer** (Figure 23.26).

6. **Caution!** Some manufacturers require the use of a **sodium bromate neutralizer! Do not substitute neutralizers.** Read directions carefully. **Do not allow neutralizer to drip onto the client's mouth,**

◀ Safety Tip

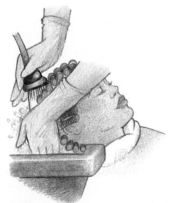

Figure 23.25
Thoroughly rinse the hair with tepid water for 3–5 minutes.

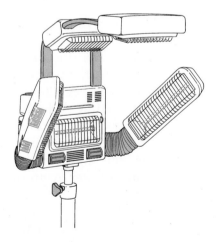

Figure 23.26
Infrared lamp for drying recurled (reformed) hair.

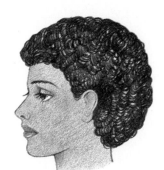

Figure 23.27
The completed hairstyle

eyes, or ears. If a drip occurs accidentally, rinse immediately with cool water. A dryer may cause scalp burns.

7. Rinse thoroughly with tepid water for 3 to 5 minutes. Use a timer. Gently towel-blot. Apply protein conditioner and allow it to remain on the hair for 5 minutes. Gently unwind all rods. Next apply activator to the scalp, follow with the curl moisturizer, shape, and then style the hair (Figure 23.27).

7. Rinsing with water removes the neutralizer from the hair. The hair should be unwound gently. Pulling may relax the curl.

Sanitize your area as follows:
1. Wash, wipe, and store bottles and supplies.
2. Discard used supplies.
3. Clean and sanitize the cape and apron.
4. Sanitize the work area; wash your hands.

Glossary

Allergies Extreme sensitivities to factors or substances in the environment.

Chemical rearranger The basic product used to relax the hair in a curl re-formation service.

Curl activator An oily product used in the curl re-formation service.

Curl booster The thio product that is used for wrapping the hair on rods, then processing.

Curl rearranger See **Chemical rearranger** and **Curl reformation.**

Curl re-formation A double-application service in which super-curly hair is straightened and then recurled in a larger curl pattern.

Hypertension High blood pressure.

Instant moisturizer A product that puts moisture back into the hair.

Polymer conditioner A high-quality protein conditioner.

Sodium bromate The main ingredient used in the most common type of neutralizers in the curl re-formation service.

1. What is another name for the curl re-formation service?
2. Is a curl re-formation a single- or double-application service?
3. Is a curl re-formation usually given to naturally straight hair?
4. True or false. In a curl re-formation, the chemical used to relax the hair is usually sodium hydroxide.
5. Is the basic chemical used in the neutralizer for a curl re-formation service generally peroxide?
6. Is it necessary to wear gloves when using the chemical rearranger?
7. Should the chemical rearranger be left on the hair more than 5 minutes?
8. Does the curl re-formation service require a strand test?
9. Are the wrapping subsections for a curl re-formation service the same as those used in wrapping a permanent wave?
10. True or false. In giving a curl re-formation, light, even tension should be used when wrapping the hair on the rods.
11. Would the curl re-formation service allow the hair to be set more easily in rollers for a bouffant hairstyle?
12. Does the curl re-formation process break down the cystine disulfide bonds?
13. Is the pH of the chemical rearranger 6.6?
14. Why is chemical rearranger used?
15. Can the processing of the chemical rearranger be speeded up by putting the client under the dryer?
16. Will porous hair take longer to process?
17. True or false. The curl re-formation service obtains the best results when given immediately after a sodium hydroxide chemical relaxer.
18. Should protein conditioners be avoided when giving a curl re-formation?
19. If the chemical rearranger comes in contact with the client's eyes or ears during the curl re-formation service, should you rinse with hot water immediately?
20. Is it important to brush the hair before giving a curl re-formation service?

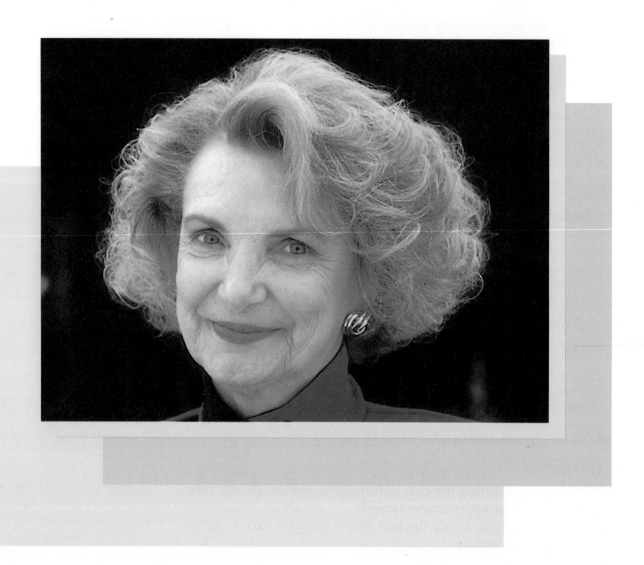

464

Describing the Skin

Using the information in this chapter, recognize common skin disorders that may be helped in the salon and diseases that should be referred to a medical doctor or dermatologist. Score 85 percent or better on a multiple-choice exam on the information in this chapter. In order to achieve the above level of competence, you should master the following chapter objectives.

Theory Objectives

1. Explain the structure and function of the skin.
2. Describe the layers of the epidermis and explain their functions.
3. Classify the appendages of the skin by name and function.
4. Describe the diseases of the sweat gland.
5. Explain skin pigmentation and its abnormalities.
6. Explain skin keratinization.
7. List the more common primary and secondary lesions.

Introduction

The word **esthetician** refers to someone who uses massage, skin preparations, facial devices, and the related arts and sciences to preserve and beautify the skin. Some states license estheticians separately from cosmetologists or manicurists. Other states, however, include the esthetician practice as part of the basic cosmetology program. Your instructor will explain how your state regulates the practice of skin care.

Since these services are performed directly on the skin of the client, it is important that they be done safely. In order to do that, the **practitioner** (esthetician or cosmetologist) must have a thorough understanding of the **histology** (microscopic study) of the skin, including its structure and functions.

The practitioner should also be familiar with some of the more common disorders and diseases of the skin. A doctor who specializes in disorders and diseases of the skin is called a **dermatologist,** and the scientific study of the skin is called **dermatology.** Part of your job is knowing when you **cannot** safely give a service to a client and must refer the client to a physician or dermatologist. This chapter describes the disorders and diseases of the skin that you may encounter and explains what action you should take.

Theory Objective 1
Structure and Functions of the Skin

The skin is the largest and one of the most efficient **organs** of the human body. It grows, reacts to sensation, and constantly renews itself. The skin is divided into three layers:

1. Epidermis
2. Corium (dermis)
3. Subcutaneous tissue

The **epidermis** is the thinnest and outermost layer of the skin (Figure 24.1). It is about as thick as this page. Although you can only see these skin cells through a microscope, they are very active.

The **corium** (KOHR-ee-uhm) or **dermis** is the true skin. It is 20 to 30 times thicker than the epidermis and rests upon a thick pad of fatty or **adipose** (AD-eh-pohz) subcutaneous tissue. This **subcutaneous tissue** below the corium is the third layer of the skin. It serves as a shock absorber and heat insulator for the body.

The protein, collagen, is produced in the dermis or corium layer of the skin. This protein gives skin its elasticity and prevents

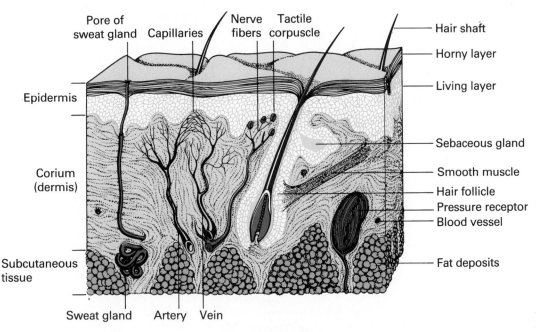

Pore of
sweat gland   Capillaries   Nerve   Tactile
              fibers   corpuscle   Hair shaft
                                                      Horny layer
Epidermis   Living layer

                                                      Sebaceous gland
Corium
(dermis)   Smooth muscle
                                                      Hair follicle
                                                      Pressure receptor
                                                      Blood vessel

Subcutaneous   Fat deposits
tissue

Sweat gland   Artery   Vein

Skin cross section

the wrinkling of the skin associated with aging and overexposure to harmful ultraviolet light from the sun or tanning beds.

Recently, dermatologists have discovered that a drug called **Retin-A** is very effective in preventing wrinkling of the skin; it also reduces wrinkles and stretch marks that have already appeared. Originally, Retin-A was prescribed to treat acne, and its initial approval by the Food and Drug Administration (FDA) was for that purpose. Now, however, although it is still used to treat acne, it is used against wrinkles as well. Retin-A seems to slow down the aging process and normalize skin functions by increasing the amount of collagen in the upper part of the dermis. In addition, Retin-A makes the skin smoother by reducing the production of melanin (the coloring pigment in the skin). Studies have shown that the drug can be effective in reducing wrinkling around the corners of the eyes (known as crows' feet) and that it reduces the formation of dark liver spots on the skin. Although Retin-A is used mainly on the face, some patients have used it successfully on their arms and legs as well.

Retin-A makes the skin **much more** sensitive to ultraviolet light from the sun and from tanning lamps. Thus, the skin will **burn** much more easily. Therefore, anyone who is being treated with this drug **must use a sunblocking product** to protect the skin.

In general, the skin serves as a barrier between the organs inside the body and the rest of the world. Specifically, the skin has several important functions:

Figure 24.1
Skin cross section

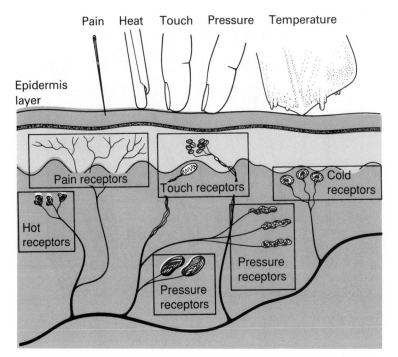

Pain   Heat   Touch   Pressure   Temperature

Epidermis layer

Pain receptors

Touch receptors

Cold receptors

Hot receptors

Pressure receptors

Pressure receptors

Figure 24.2
Sensor points of one square inch (2.5 square centimeters) of skin. The areas indicated by bold circles are controlled by the pituitary gland.

1. **Protection.** Healthy skin is soft and elastic. It protects the body from physical or chemical injury and from bacteria. Thus, it is both a shock absorber and a barrier against bacteria and viruses.

2. **Heat regulation.** The **sudoriferous** (sweat) **glands** and blood vessels of the skin keep the body's internal temperature at 98.6°F (37°C). Blood flows in the vessels to keep the body warm, while the sweat glands serve as the cooling system. Perspiration from the sweat glands increases as the temperature outside the body increases.

3. **Sensation.** The body feels heat, cold, pain, and touch through a network of nerve endings that are located all over the surface of the skin (Figures 24.2 and 24.3).

4. **Secretion.** The skin does not remove much body waste. Perspiration secreted by the sweat glands is practically the only waste removed by the skin. The kidneys are the primary excretory organs of the body.

5. **Absorption (permeability).** Some people believe that water and most other substances can go through the skin, but this is not true. Most liquids will not pass through the skin unless the layers have actually been destroyed, punctured, or penetrated. Gases and many volatile substances, however, easily pass through the skin. If liquids or other substances do penetrate

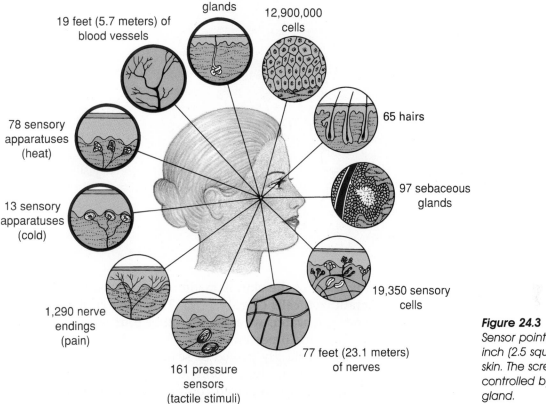

Figure 24.3
Sensor points of one square inch (2.5 square centimeters) of skin. The screened areas are controlled by the pituitary gland.

the unbroken skin, they do so partly through openings of the hair follicles and sebaceous (oil) glands. Scientists believe that only small quantities of substances enter the skin through the sweat ducts.

Theory Objective 2
Layers of the Epidermis and Their Functions

As objective 1 explained, the epidermis is the outermost layer of the skin. It has five distinct layers:

1. Horny layer or stratum corneum (STRAYT-uhm COR-nee-uhm)

2. Lucid layer or stratum lucidum (loo-SID-uhm)

3. Granular layer or stratum granulosum (gran-yoo-LOH-suhm)

4. Prickle layer or stratum malpighii (mal-PIG-ee-igh)

5. Basal layer or stratum germinativum (germ-in-ay-TIGH-vuhm)

Each of these layers needs some further explanation:

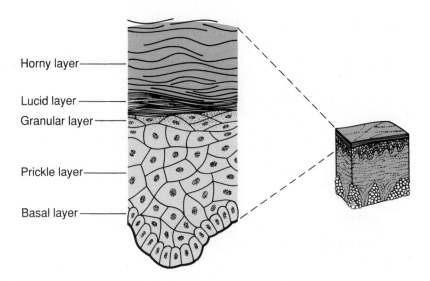

Horny layer

Lucid layer

Granular layer

Prickle layer

Basal layer

Figure 24.4
Layers of the epidermis

1. The **horny layer** of the skin is made up of several layers of dead, keratinized cells (Figure 24.4). This layer contains only 10 to 20 percent water, whereas the other four layers of the epidermis contain 70 percent water. The microscopic cells of this layer are constantly peeled or scaled off by washing/cleansing and by rubbing against clothing and bed linens. Surface skin is replaced completely every month. **Keratin** helps the skin hold water, which makes it soft and supple. It also prevents water from leaving the body and bacteria from entering the body. When the water content of the horny layer falls below 10 percent, the skin becomes chapped and visibly dry and scaly. Many people think that dry skin is due to a lack of skin oil (sebum), but it actually is caused by a lack of moisture. Humidity affects the amount of water the horny layer absorbs or loses. For example, dry skin is frequently a problem in heated homes and offices during the winter months because the inside humidity is lowered by heating units. Installing a humidifier or using moisture lotions helps remedy this problem. Drinking lots of water helps, too.

2. The **lucid layer** (clear layer) of the skin is evident only on the palms of the hands and the soles of the feet where the epidermis is thick. The lucid layer lies directly above the granular layer of the skin; these two layers are the skin's most important barriers against penetration.

3. The **granular layer** (cells look like granules) is strongest in the areas where the lucid layer is absent. In these areas, the granular layer protects the body from physical and chemical penetration.

4. The **prickle layer** is made up of several layers of epidermal cells that connect four or more keratin or melanin cells.

5. The **basal layer** of cells lies above the corium (dermis). The cells located here form **keratin** and **melanin.** The melanocytes, which form melanin, are sandwiched between the more numerous keratin-forming basal cells. As you know, keratin is the soft cornified tissue of the skin, while melanin is the pigment that gives skin its color. The basal and prickle layers work together to make pigment and skin.

Theory Objective 3
Appendages of the Skin Classified by Name and Function

An **appendage** is something that is added to or extended from something else that is larger or more important. The skin has two types of appendages: cornified appendages made of keratinized protein and glandular appendages. The cornified appendages are the hair and nails. Since they are discussed elsewhere, this chapter will deal only with the glandular appendages of the skin.

Glands are groups of cells that take certain substances from the blood, make new substances out of them, and then release the new substances, which are called **secretions.** Skin glands fall into two general categories—**sebaceous** and **sudoriferous.**

The **sebaceous** (sih-BAY-shuhs) **glands** are present all over the body except in the palms of the hands and the soles of the feet (Figure 24.5). They secrete an oily fluid called **sebum** through a duct to a follicle that may contain a hair. The sebum is actually material

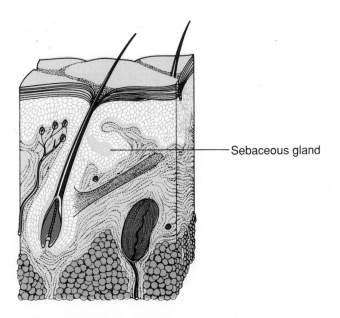

— Sebaceous gland

Figure 24.5
Sebaceous gland with hair follicle and hair

from cells that have broken down. When a sebaceous gland secretes sebum through its duct, the entire gland falls apart and is pushed out through the duct. Sebaceous glands are much larger and more numerous on the scalp and face than elsewhere on the body.

The oily **sebum** covers the skin with a film that helps fight bacteria and fungus. It also slows the evaporation of moisture (water) from the skin and protects against bacteria. The amount of sebum secreted depends on several factors:

- **Individual differences.** Some people have small, underdeveloped sebaceous glands, while others have numerous large glands that cause greasy, oily skin.

- **Age.** In infancy, people produce little or no sebum, but as they grow older, the sebaceous glands become more active, particularly at puberty. After a person reaches the age of 50, sebum production usually decreases.

- **Race.** Black persons usually have larger and more numerous sebaceous glands.

- **Climate.** Persons living in warm climates secrete more sebum than those living in cooler climates.

Scientists have not yet figured out how to increase or decrease the production of sebum. Drugs, hormones, and special products do not seem to affect its flow, but some prescribed drugs change the composition of the sebum and make it less irritating to the skin.

Sudoriferous (sood-ah-RIF-ah-ruhs) **sweat glands** are found everywhere in the human skin and are controlled by the nervous system. Sudoriferous is a general term that refers to both the apocrine and eccrine sweat glands.

Apocrine (AP-ah-krehn) **sweat glands** are found in the ear canal, under the arms, and in the genital region of the body. Each apocrine sweat gland opens into a hair follicle as does each sebaceous gland (Figure 24.6a). Although the sweat is sterile when excreted, it becomes contaminated by bacteria on the surface of the skin. This contamination causes "body odor." The gland secretes continuously into a reservoir beneath the skin; when the reservoir overflows, the sweat is excreted to the surface (sometimes this is set off by the adrenal glands, which can be activated by emotional stress). The overall importance of these glands has not been determined. Apocrine sweat is a whitish fluid containing water, salt, uric acid (found in urine), lactic acid (formed from sugar), proteins, and carbohydrates. The pH of sweat is 5.4–5.6 and the body secretes 2 pounds/2 pints (.9 kilograms/.94 liters) per day.

The **eccrine** (EK-rehn) **sweat glands,** by contrast, are the body's heat regulators (Figure 24.6b). Although they are much

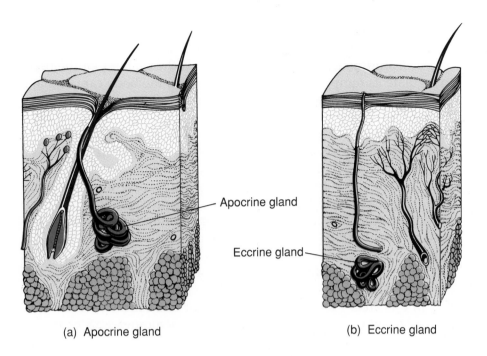

(a) Apocrine gland   (b) Eccrine gland

Figure 24.6
Apocrine and eccrine glands

smaller than the apocrine sweat glands, there are many more of them. Eccrine sweat glands are found all over the surface of the skin, but are most heavily concentrated in the areas of the forehead, underarms, palms of the hands, and soles of the feet. The eccrine sweat glands are regulated by the **hypothalamus** (high-poh-THAL-eh-muhs). The eccrine sweat glands secrete sweat into a duct or tube from which it is excreted directly onto the surface of the skin.

Unlike the apocrine sweat glands, eccrine sweat glands remain inactive unless something, such as heat or emotional stress, stimulates them to cool the body. Heat is the main activator of the eccrine sweat glands. These glands are not important for excreting body waste.

Cosmetic companies manufacture many products for underarm perspiration, which have a common ingredient called aluminum chloride. This substance shrinks the openings of the sweat pores. A fragrance is often added to mask any odor that does occur.

Theory Objective 4
Diseases of the Sweat Glands

Hyperhidrosis (high-per-high-DROH-siss) is an abnormal increase in the amount of sweat. It may be caused by something that affects the entire body, such as hot, humid weather or increased body heat due to work or exercise. It can also be localized sweating, such as from the palms of the hands, soles of the feet, underarms, or face. Sweating that affects only one part of the body is often caused by emotional stress. Hyperhidrosis may also be caused by menopause in women, overweight, gout, alcoholic intoxication, or a reaction to drugs. This condition should be treated by a doctor.

Anhidrosis (an-high-DROH-siss) is the inability of the body to regulate its temperature. In this condition, the body cannot make or send sweat to the skin's surface (sweat retention). Since the body's temperature cannot be controlled (cooled), a doctor should be consulted.

Bromhidrosis (brom-hi-DROH-siss), also called osmidrosis (oz-mi-DROH-siss), is abnormal, or foul-smelling, sweat. Eating garlic or onions or taking certain drugs may cause this condition. Some diseases, including diabetes, gout, and typhoid fever, also produce sweat that has a peculiar odor. Bromhidrosis is caused by surface skin bacteria coming in contact with secretions from the apocrine sweat glands. Keratin, bodily secretions, and bacteria that can cause odor on contact with sweat often collect in the underarm hair. Therefore, odor can be reduced by shortening or shaving the hair in this area. Carefully washing under one's arms with an ordinary antiseptic soap in the mornings and evenings and changing clothes regularly will also help.

Miliaria rubra (mil-ee-AR-ee-ah ROOB-rah), also called prickly heat or heat rash, occurs when the openings of the sweat ducts are blocked. It is common in very hot, humid climates. The blockage causes sweat ducts to rupture into the midepidermis. Itching and burning result. Mild powders and lotions will stop the itching and burning, but the best treatment is an air-conditioned environment.

Theory Objective 5
Skin Pigmentation and Its Abnormalities

As mentioned earlier in this chapter, **melanin cells (melanocytes)** are made in the basal layer of the epidermis. The chemical that activates the production of pigment or melanin is a basic amino acid called **tyrosine** (TIGH-roh-sin). Tyrosine causes the melanocytes to make melanin. Once the melanin is formed, it works its way through the epidermis to the horny layer. Melanin itself is colorless, but when it is exposed to oxygen, it becomes darker in color. Thus, it is the substance that gives color to the skin and causes the skin to tan when it is exposed to sunlight (Figure 24.7a).

Tanning and Sunscreens

Tanning occurs because ultraviolet rays from the sun cause the release of **tyrosinase** (tigh-ROH-sin-ayz), an enzyme that acts on the tyrosine to start the process of melanin formation. The sun emits two kinds of ultraviolet rays: **ultraviolet A** rays (UVA), which are in the wavelength of 320–340 nanometers, and **ultraviolet B** rays

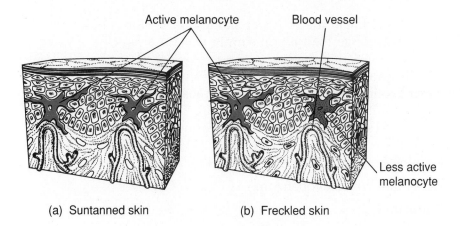

Active melanocyte

Blood vessel

Less active melanocyte

(a) Suntanned skin

(b) Freckled skin

Figure 24.7
Melanocytes in suntanned and freckled skin

(UVB), which are in the wavelength of 280–320 nanometers. Knowing the exact wavelengths is not as important as understanding that both types of rays are harmful to the skin.

In fact, melanin tans the skin in order to protect it from the sun's burning rays. Scientists generally agree that overexposure to sunlight over a number of years causes the skin to thicken and wrinkle (age). Overexposure to sunlight also causes **skin cancer.** Therefore daily use of a sunscreen that will protect your skin from both UVA and UVB rays is strongly advised.

Note that black skin can be sunburned just like white skin. White skin and black skin contain the same number of melanocytes, although black skin contains more pigmentation than white skin. The pigment granules in black and white skin also differ somewhat in size and shape. Nevertheless, black persons as well as whites are advised to use sunscreens when they are going to be outdoors.

How much sun is too much? The amount of sun to which you can be exposed without burning depends on several factors:

Natural pigmentation. If your skin is naturally quite dark, you will be able to absorb more sunlight without burning than someone who is very light. The darker skin will still be subject to sunburn, but a longer period of exposure will be needed before it will burn.

Location. If you live near the equator where the sun is closer to the earth, you will burn much faster than if you live in a northern city. For example, the sunlight is much stronger in Florida than it is in Minnesota.

Height. Following the same logic with regard to sun, if you live 5,000 feet (1,524 meters) up in the mountains, your skin will be more exposed to sunlight than if you live at sea level.

Water and snow. Water and snow both reflect the rays of the sun, so your skin will be exposed to more sunlight if you spend the day at the beach or skiing on the slopes of a mountain range than if you simply walk in a park.

Safety Tip ▶

To protect your skin from the sun, you should use a sunscreening lotion. These lotions block or absorb the harmful sunlight and prevent it from penetrating the skin. The following four chemicals are used separately or together in various sunblocking formulas:

- P-amino benzoic acid (PABA)
- Parsol (known as avobenzone)
- Padimate-O
- Benzphenon-3

The Food and Drug Administration (FDA) recognizes the importance of sunscreening lotions as a simple way to prevent skin cancer. The FDA requires all sunscreen lotion manufacturers to label their products with a number that indicates the amount of the sun's ultraviolet rays that can penetrate through the product and reach the skin. Protecting the skin is important not only to prevent skin cancer but also because wherever the skin is burned by the sun, a form of **herpes simplex,** a severe and very painful skin condition, can develop. The sun triggers the herpes virus, which causes the nerve endings in the skin to become inflamed and irritated. This condition must be treated by a physician and can be difficult to clear up in some cases.

The labeling system that is used is called the **sun protection factor (SPF).** The **SPF** is a numbering system from 1 to 15 (Figure 24.8). A rating of "1" indicates that almost all of the sun's rays are allowed to penetrate through the lotion to your skin. On the other hand, a lotion with an **SPF** of "15" would act as a **"sun block."** A **sun block** doesn't allow any of the sun's rays to reach your skin. People with average skin color and sensitivity should start with a tanning lotion with an SPF in the range 8 to 10. Individuals with a very light complexion should begin with a product that has an SPF of at least 12.

Some sunscreen lotion manufacturers claim their product has a sun protection factor greater than 15, e.g., "SPF 33," but this statement is not entirely correct. What the maker may mean is that the product has such a thick consistency that it remains on the skin longer—it doesn't rub off on clothing or towels as easily, or it doesn't evaporate as quickly as a sunscreen with an SPF of 15.

A sunscreen with a higher SPF may also expose the skin to a stronger concentration of chemicals that may **irritate** the skin. The stronger concentrations of chemicals may be worth the risk of irritated skin for people who plan to spend many hours in the sun

Examples of reading from this bar chart:
SPF-15 screens out 100% of ultraviolet rays
SPF-8 screens out 50% of ultraviolet rays

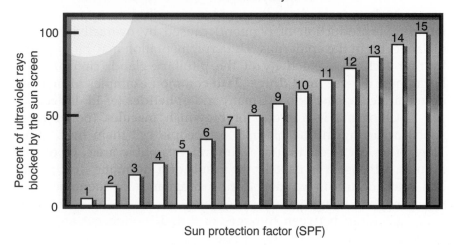

Figure 24.8
To read this chart, find the SPF you are interested in at the bottom, and look at the numbers at the left to find the percentage of ultraviolet rays it blocks.

rather than just an hour or so. These stronger products also protect the skin from both ultraviolet A rays and ultraviolet B rays (from the sun and tanning booth lamps).

Any sunscreen should be **water-proof** so that it will not be washed off too easily by perspiration or a quick dip in the swimming pool.

Since no one wants his or her skin to wrinkle prematurely, thicken, or develop cancer, it is best to begin tanning on a gradual basis. **Avoid sun tanning** between the hours of 10:00 A.M. and 2:00 P.M. Limit exposure time at the beginning of the season to 15–20 minutes. If you live near the equator, where the sun is closer to the earth, be especially careful to use a sunscreen **daily.** Individuals who live near water or snow should also be very careful because water and snow reflect the ultraviolet rays, and you will receive a double dose of sunlight.

Read the label directions carefully to see whether the product needs to be reapplied after swimming or perspiring heavily. Perspiration usually waters down a sunscreen by 50 percent. A few sunscreening lotions will stain clothing, so read the label to be sure the one you are purchasing does not stain.

Abnormalities Involving Melanocyte Activity

The pigmentation of the skin can change for a variety of reasons. A few of the more common conditions that cause changes in pigmentation will be discussed here.

Before scientists discovered how melanocytes work, they called the overproduction of pigment **melanoderma** (mel-an-oh-

DER-mah) and the underproduction of pigment **leukoderma** (loo-koh-DER-mah). Although more specific terms can be applied now, these terms are still basically correct.

Melanoderma is a term used to describe any hyperpigmentation (overproduction of pigment) caused by overactivity of the melanocytes in the epidermis. Hyperpigmentation may be triggered by four factors: overactivity of the pituitary gland, circulation of hormones, disease, and drugs. Two common examples of melanoderma are **chloasma** (klo-AZ-mah) and **ephelides** (ef-EE-li-deez).

Chloasma is a group of brownish macules (nonelevated spots) occurring in one place. Most people call them liver spots. They often occur on the face, around the pubic area, or on the nipples. Chloasma is usually the result of a hormone disturbance and often occurs in women during pregnancy or menopause or when they are using oral contraceptives.

Children between the ages of 2 and 5 often get **ephelides (freckles)** (Figure 24.7b) The freckles appear more in summer than winter. Freckles are also called **lentigines,** although technically these are different from freckles.

As noted earlier, sunlight is the most effective activator of melanocyte activity. An inflammation of the skin called **photodermatitis** is caused by the ultraviolet light in sunlight and sun lamps, internal or external drugs, and cosmetics, shaving lotion, and perfume.

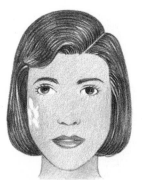

Figure 24.9
Vitiligo pigmentation

Leukoderma refers to **hypopigmentation** (underpigmentation) of the skin, caused by a decrease in the activity of the melanocytes. Hypopigmentation can be either the result of a congenital defect, such as albinism, or an acquired condition, such as vitiligo.

Albinism is a congenital failure of the skin to form melanin pigment. Persons with albinism have pink skin, white hair (sometimes it may be reddish), and pink eyes. Albinos have a marked hypersensitivity to light. Their skin ages very early, sometimes in early adulthood.

Vitiligo is characterized by oval or irregular patches of white skin that do not have normal pigment. It usually occurs on the face, hands, or neck as patches of depigmentation (Figure 24.9). The patches may slowly enlarge. Skin with vitiligo must be protected from overexposure to sun or any exposure to ultraviolet lamps. Gradual exposure to sunlight, ultraviolet lamps, or Wood's light (cold quartz light) may restore pigment, but a doctor should be consulted before these procedures are tried.

Miscellaneous Pigmentation Abnormalities

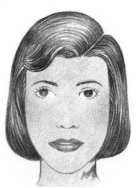

Figure 24.10
Nevus flammeus

A **nevus flammeus** (NEE-vuhs FLAM-ee-uhs) is a birthmark or congenital mole (Figure 24.10). The nevus birthmark is a reddish purple, flat mark that may look like a stain (port wine stain) on the face.

The stain is caused by dilation of the small blood vessels in the skin. Cosmetic makeup is the only remedy for a nevus birthmark. Sometimes a nevus birthmark disappears shortly after birth, but if it doesn't, it is permanent.

Moles or **melanocytic nevi** (mel-an-oh-SIT-ik NEE-vigh) are the most common tumors of the skin; almost everyone has one or more of them. These brown pigmented nevi first appear as macules, but may become elevated after a period of time. Hair often grows through moles, but this hair should not be removed. Any change of color in a mole should be reported to a dermatologist.

Melanotic sarcoma (fatal skin cancer) begins with a mole. Its main characteristic is an overabundance of pigment.

The term **verruca** (veh-ROO-kah) is assigned to a variety of warts (Figure 24.11). Warts are caused by a virus. They can be contagious and may spread all over the body. Dermatologists can easily remove one wart or a cluster of them through a variety of methods.

Callus or **hyperkeratosis** (high-per-ker-eh-TOH-siss) is a thickening of the cornified layer of the epidermis, which results from physical trauma, e.g., very heavy work involving the hands or feet (Figure 24.12) A callus occurs when pressure or friction is applied to the skin.

Wrinkles are caused by the breaking down of the elastin and collagen fibers below the surface of the skin. When the fibers become broken and lumpy, they cannot support the epidermis, and the skin loses its resiliency (elasticity). Grooves, lines, and wrinkles are the results.

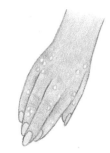

Figure 24.11
Verruca

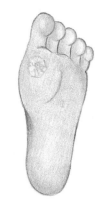

Figure 24.12
Callus

Theory Objective 6
Skin Keratinization

Keratin is a very tough and elastic layer of protein that protects the underlying skin. It is the main (but not the only) ingredient in the horny layer of the epidermis. Keratin is not **easily penetrated** or dissolved by diluted alkalis, weak acids, organic solvents, or water.

There are two kinds of keratin. **Soft keratin** is produced by the epidermis all over the body. This type of keratin is present throughout all five layers of the epidermis, although mature hard scales (protective keratin) are found only in the horny layer of the skin.

Hard keratin is found in the nails and hair (Figure 24.13). It forms compacted and hard scales. By contrast, soft keratin is continually shed in fine loose scales.

The process of **keratinization** (ker-eh-tin-eh-ZAY-shun), or the formation of keratin, begins in the **basal** and **prickle** layers of the epidermis and is completed in the horny layer, where the keratin appears as a tough elastic substance that forms the outer layer of the skin. The elasticity of the horny layer and the chapping of the skin

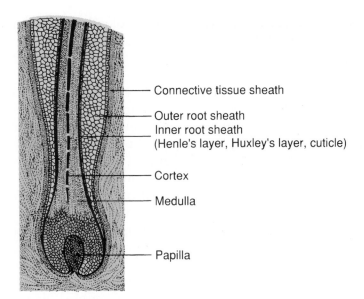

Connective tissue sheath

Outer root sheath
Inner root sheath
(Henle's layer, Huxley's layer, cuticle)

Cortex

Medulla

Papilla

Figure 24.13
*Vertical cross section through a
hair and root sheath*

depend mainly on the water content of the keratin, not on the amount of sebum produced by the sebaceous glands.

Theory Objective 7
Primary and Secondary Lesions

Since you will be offering some services involving the skin, you should know the basic terms used to describe the skin. Most of the time, if you see a client who has an abnormal skin condition, tell him or her to see a dermatologist, a doctor who specializes in treating diseases of the skin. The dermatologist can determine the **etiology** (ee-tee-AHL-eh-jee) (cause) of a skin disorder, **diagnose** (identify) a specific skin disease, treat it, and offer a **prognosis** (prediction of the chance for improvement and the time it will take). The dermatologist may even take a skin sample and send it to a **pathology laboratory** (a place where the origin, nature, cause, and development of disease are studied) for examination.

A **lesion** (LEE-zhun) is any abnormal or harmful change in the structure of an organ or tissue. Lesions are classified as primary and secondary according to when they develop.

As the name implies, "primary" means first. So primary lesions develop on the skin first. A secondary lesion often **results** from an untreated primary lesion. For example, you may develop a "patch" of dry skin at the corner of your mouth. This would be a primary lesion. If you didn't moisturize that area, it would become so dry that a fissure (crack) would result. The crack would be an example of a secondary lesion.

The following are 12 of the more common **primary lesions:**

1. **Macules** (MAK-yoolz) are discolorations on the skin's surface that can be as large as $\frac{2}{5}$ inch (1 centimeter) (Figure 24.14). They are flat and have **distinct (circumscribed) edges.** Freckles and tatoos are examples of macules.

2. **Patches** are macules that are larger than $\frac{2}{5}$ inch (1 centimeter). They are circumscribed, flat discolorations of the skin (Figure 24.15).

3. **Papules** (PAP-yoolz) are circumscribed, elevated, solid lesions up to $\frac{2}{5}$ inch (1 centimeter) in size (Figure 24.16). Warts are papules.

4. **Wheals** (WEELZ), or hives, are a type of papule. Sharply circumscribed, they are solid and rise above the skin (Figure 24.17). An insect bite, such as a mosquito bite, is a wheal.

5. **Nodules** (NAHJ-yoolz) are also referred to as tumors, but they are smaller than true tumors. Nodules are up to $\frac{2}{5}$ inch (1 centimeter) in size. They are solid lumps and may be above or beneath the skin's surface (Figure 24.18).

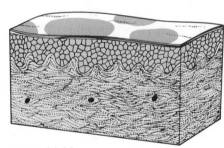

Figure 24.14
Macules

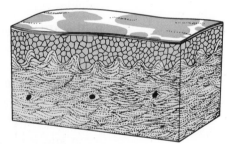

Figure 24.15
Patches

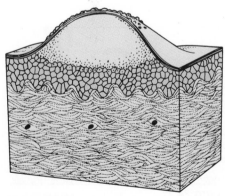

Figure 24.16
Papules

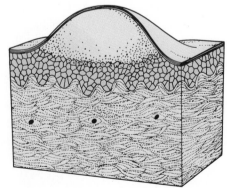

Figure 24.17
Wheals

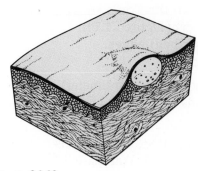

Figure 24.18
Nodules

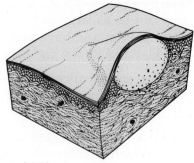

Figure 24.19
Tumor

6. **Tumors** are larger than $\frac{2}{5}$ inch (1 centimeter) and are deeper than nodules. They are circumscribed penetrations of the skin and subcutaneous tissue (Figure 24.19). Tumors extend both above and below the skin's surface.

7. **Vesicles** (VES-ih-kehlz) can be as large as $\frac{2}{5}$ inch (1 centimeter). They are circumscribed elevations of skin containing a clear, watery liquid (Figure 24.20). Examples are chicken pox, contact dermatitis, and blisters.

8. **Bullae** (BULL-ee) are larger than $\frac{2}{5}$ inch (1 centimeter). They are circumscribed lesions above and below the skin that contain a clear, watery fluid (Figure 24.21). Second-degree burns are characterized by bullae.

9. **Pustules** (PUHS-chyoolz) vary in size. They are circumscribed elevations of skin containing puslike fluid (Figure 24.22). Acne and impetigo are examples of pustules.

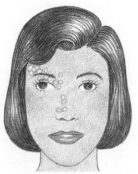

Figure 24.20
Vesicles

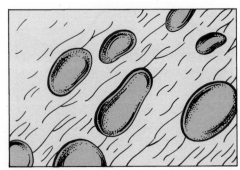

Figure 24.21
Bullae

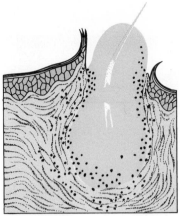

Figure 24.22
Pustule

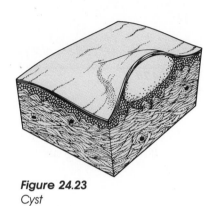

Figure 24.23
Cyst

10. **Cysts** are semisolid or fluid lumps above and below the skin (Figure 24.23). An example is a sebaceous cyst.

11. **Furuncles** (boils) are large localized infections of hair follicles, usually caused by staphylococci (Figure 24.24). They appear above the surface of the skin.

12. **Carbuncles** are extreme infections of several adjoining hair follicles that drain onto the skin's surface from multiple openings (Figure 24.25). They extend above and below the skin.

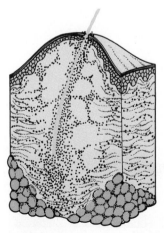

Figure 24.24
Furuncles (boils)

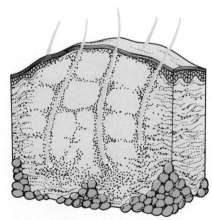

Figure 24.25
Carbuncles

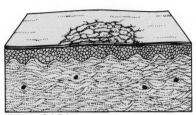

Figure 24.26
Scales

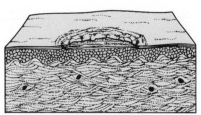

Figure 24.27
Crusts

The following are five of the more common **secondary lesions:**

1. **Scales** are shedding, dead cells of the horny layer of the epidermis (Figure 24.26). The cells may be dry or greasy, as in dandruff or psoriasis.

2. **Crusts** (scabs) are the dried remains of an oozing sore (Figure 24.27). They may consist of dried blood, dried pus, dried sebum, or a combination of these substances.

3. **Excoriations** are lesions of the skin that are usually superficial and traumatic (Figure 24.28). They occur in scratched insect bites and scabies.

4. **Fissures** are almost straight-line breaks in the skin (cracks) that are sharply defined (Figure 24.29). They are commonly seen around the fingertips and heels.

5. **Scars,** also called **cicatrices** (sik-eh-TRIGH-seez), are formations of connective tissue that replace tissue lost through injury or disease (Figure 24.30). Scars occur when the corium is damaged.

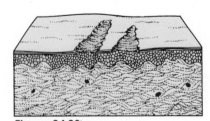

Figure 24.28
Excoriations (scratches)

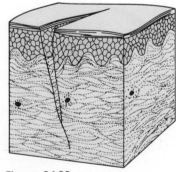

Figure 24.29
Fissure

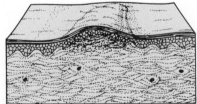

Figure 24.30
Scar

Adipose (AD-eh-pohz) tissue Fatty tissue beneath the epidermis and the corium. See also **Subcutaneous tissue.**

Albinism (AL-beh-niz-uhm) A congenital failure of the skin to form melanin pigment.

Anhidrosis (an-high-DROH-siss) The inability of the body to regulate its temperature through perspiration.

Apocrine (AP-ah-krehn) sweat glands Sweat glands in the ear canal, under the arms, and in the genital region. Each gland opens into a hair follicle.

Basal layer The layer of the epidermis where cells form keratin and melanin.

Birthmark See **Nevus flammeus.**

Boils See **Furuncles.**

Bromhidrosis (brom-hi-DROH-siss) Abnormal, or foul-smelling, sweat. Also called osmidrosis.

Bulla (BULL-ah) A circumscribed lesion, such as a second-degree burn, that occurs above and below the skin and contains a clear, watery fluid. See also **Vesicles.**

Callus See **Hyperkeratosis.**

Carbuncles Extreme infections of several adjoining hair follicles that drain from multiple openings onto the skin's surface.

Chloasma (klo-AZ-mah) An overpigmentation producing brownish macules (nonelevated spots) occurring in one place; caused by a hormone imbalance. Also called liver spots.

Cicatrices (sik-eh-TRIGH-seez) See **Scars.**

Corium (KOHR-ee-uhm) The layer of the skin between the epidermis and the subcutaneous layers; sometimes called the true skin.

Crust The dried remains of an oozing sore on the skin; commonly called a scab.

Dermatology The scientific study of the skin.

Eccrine (EK-rehn) sweat glands Heat regulators of the body.

Ephilides (ef-EE-li-deez) Freckles.

Epidermis The outermost and thinnest layer of the skin.

Esthetician A practitioner who specializes in the preservation and beautification of the face and neck.

Etiology (ee-tee-AHL-eh-jee) The cause of a disease or a disorder.

Excoriations (ek-sko-ri-AY-shunz) Abrasions of the skin.

Fissures Almost straight-line breaks (cracks) in the skin that are sharply defined; commonly seen around the fingertips and heels.

Furuncles Large, localized infections of hair follicles caused by staphylococci; commonly called boils.

Glands Groups of cells that take certain substances from the blood, make new substances from them, and then release the new substances, which are called secretions.

Granular layer The layer of the epidermis that protects the body from physical and chemical penetration.

Histology Microscopic study; the histology of the skin includes its functions, diseases, and disorders.

Horny layer The outermost layer of the epidermis; it is made up of several layers of dead keratinized cells.

Hyperhidrosis (high-per-high-DROH-siss) An abnormal increase in the amount of sweat.

Hyperkeratosis (high-per-ker-eh-TOH-siss) A thickening of the cornified layer of the epidermis that results from pressure or friction applied to the skin; commonly called a callus.

Hypothalamus (high-poh-THAL-eh-muhs) The gland that regulates the eccrine sweat glands.

Keratin A very tough and elastic layer of protein that protects the underlying skin; it is found in two forms: soft keratin, which is present through all five layers of the epidermis, and hard keratin, which is found in the nails and hair.

Keratinization (ker-eh-tin-eh-ZAY-shun) The process of forming keratin in the skin.

Lesion (LEE-zuhn) Any abnormal or harmful change in the structure of an organ or tissue.

Leukoderma (loo-koh-DER-mah) Underpigmentation of the skin that can be either congenital (albinism) or acquired (vitiligo).

Liver spots See **Chloasma.**

Lucid layer The layer of the epidermis that is directly above the granular layer; it is evident only on the palms of the hands and the soles of the feet.

Macule (MAK-yool) A flat discoloration with distinct edges that appears on the skin's surface.

Melanocytic nevi (mel-an-oh-SIT-ik NEE-vigh) Tumors of the skin that may become elevated and often have hair growing from them; commonly called moles.

Melanoderma (mel-an-oh-DER-mah) Overactivity of the melanocytes in the epidermis caused by overactivity of the pituitary gland, circulation of hormones, disease, or drugs.

Miliaria rubra (mil-ee-AR-ee-ah ROOB-rah) A heat rash caused by blockage of the openings of the sweat ducts; common in hot, humid climates.

Moles See **Melanocytic nevi.**

Nevus flammeus (NEE-vuhs FLAM-ee-uhs) A birthmark or congenital mole.

Nodules (NAHJ-yoolz) Solid, tumorlike lumps above or beneath the skin.

Osmidrosis (oz-mi-DROH-siss) Abnormal, or foul-smelling, sweat. Also called bromhidrosis.

Papules (PAP-yoolz) Circumscribed, elevated, solid lesions, such as warts.

Patches Macules that are larger than $\frac{2}{5}$ inch (1 centimeter).

Photodermatitis (foh-toh-der-meh-TIGH-tis) An inflammation of the skin caused by ultraviolet light, drugs, cosmetics, shaving lotion, or perfume.

Prickle layer A layer of the epidermis made up of several layers of cells that connect four or more keratin or melanin cells.

Prickly heat See **Miliaria rubra.**

Pustules (PUHS-chyoolz) Circumscribed elevations of the skin containing a puslike fluid; examples are acne and impetigo.

Retin-A A drug used in preventing and reducing wrinkling of the skin.

Scales Shedding, dead cells of the horny layer of the epidermis that may be dry or greasy. Scales occur with dandruff and psoriasis, for example.

Scars Formations of connective tissue that replace tissue lost through injury or disease; occur when the corium is damaged.

Sebaceous (sih-BAY-shuhs) glands Glands located over most of the body that secrete a lubricating and bacteria-fighting substance called sebum.

Sebum (SEEB-uhm) An oily substance that helps fight bacteria and slows evaporation of moisture from the skin.

Secretions Substances made and released by glands.

Stratum corneum (STRAYT-uhm COR-nee-uhm) See **Horny layer.**

Stratum germinativum (STRAYT-uhm germ-in-ay-TIGH-vuhm) See **Basal layer.**

Stratum granulosum (STRAYT-uhm gran-yoo-LOH-suhm) See **Granular layer.**

Stratum lucidum (STRAYT-uhm loo-SID-uhm) See **Lucid layer.**

Stratum malpighii (STRAYT-uhm mal-PIG-ee-igh) See **Prickle layer.**

Subcutaneous tissue Layer of tissue beneath the epidermis and corium.

Sudoriferous (sood-ah-RIF-ah-ruhs) glands Sweat glands.

SPF See **Sun protection factor.**

Sun protection factor A numbering system from 1 to 15 that indicates the level of screening from the sun's rays provided by the product.

Tumors Solid lumps, larger than nodules, that penetrate the skin and subcutaneous tissue and extend above or below the skin's surface.

Tyrosinase (tigh-ROH-sin-ayz) An enzyme that activates the production of pigment.

Verruca (veh-ROO-kah) Warts that are caused by a virus and may be contagious.

Vesicles (VES-ih-kehlz) Circumscribed elevations, smaller than ⅖ inch (1 centimeter), of skin containing a clear, watery fluid; examples are chicken pox, contact dermatitis, and blisters. See also **Bulla.**

Vitiligo (vit-i-LIGH-goh) Oval or irregular patches of skin that lack normal pigment. The cause is unknown, but may involve mental or physical trauma.

Wart See **Verruca.**

Wheals (WEELZ) Sharply circumscribed, solid, elevated papules. A mosquito bite is a wheal.

Questions

1. Explain briefly how each of the following relates to the skin: epidermis, dermis, adipose tissue, corium, keratin, lesion.
2. What is another name for miliaria rubra?
3. What is a break or crack in the skin called?
4. What does the word etiology mean?
5. What does subcutaneous mean?
6. What is the technical name given to the study of the skin?
7. What is a lesion?
8. Is the epidermis the outermost layer of the skin?
9. Does perspiration (sweat) help to regulate the temperature of the body?
10. Is it true that anything you rub on the skin will penetrate into the areas below the skin?
11. How often is the outer layer of the skin replaced?
12. Does the skin act as a barrier to prevent bacteria from entering the body?
13. What is another name for the corium?
14. Do you have sebaceous glands on the palms of your hands and the soles of your feet?
15. What is the name given to substances that are released from glands?
16. Do sweat glands empty directly onto the skin, or do they empty into a hair follicle?
17. What is the technical term for excessive perspiration?
18. What does the abbreviation SPF stand for?
19. True or false. For the most beneficial type of sun tan, it is best to tan from 12:00 P.M. to 2:00 P.M.
20. True or false. If a sunscreen has a rating of "10," it will provide very little protection.

21. What is the coloring substance in skin called?
22. Can overexposure to the sun cause premature wrinkling and possibly cause skin cancer?
23. What is the technical name for a mole?
24. What form of protein gives skin its soft elastic quality?

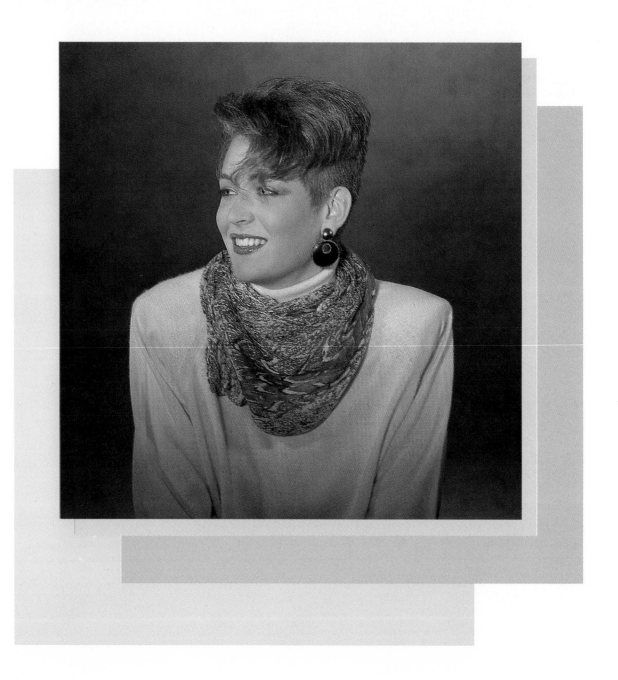

Facial Treatments

Learning Objective

Use the information in this chapter and the knowledge you gain in class to give a facial massage and skin analysis. Follow the prescribed steps of your school procedure or the steps in this chapter to give a facial treatment in 45 minutes. Score 85 percent or better on a multiple-choice exam on the information in this chapter.

In order to achieve the above level of competence, you should master the following chapter objectives.

Theory Objectives

1. Describe the five basic massage movements.
2. Explain the basic considerations when giving a facial.
3. Describe the nature and benefits of light therapy.

Practical Objective

4. Use the proper steps and safety precautions to give a facial treatment for normal skin, dry skin, and oily skin.

Introduction

The beauty industry is placing increasing emphasis on developing three types of beauty salons: "full-service salons," specialty "esthetician salons," and "nail salons." Full-service salons provide a complete shopping list of services from which the client can select. **Esthetician salons** specialize in the preservation and beautification of the face and neck. (A person who specializes in the care, preservation, and beautification of the skin is an **esthetician.**) Nail salons specialize in the preservation and beautification of the nails and hands.

Cosmetologists at all types of salons have come to realize that skin care is as important as hair and nail care. As a result, many of them are attending skin-care seminars to develop their skills in this area. If you learn some of the basic procedures used for facial treatment services, you will have the knowledge and skills needed to be employed at either a full-service salon or a specialized esthetician salon.

The major effect of facial massage is to stimulate the skin. This stimulation normalizes the skin and makes it healthy. Although cosmetologists cannot treat minor skin conditions, such as acne, the services they offer can correct and improve skin tone (which will reduce wrinkling of the skin), balance moisture levels, remove dirt and impurities, and remove oil from the skin. All of these measures reduce some of the causes for skin blemishes, such as blackheads.

On the psychological side, cosmetology services relax the client, which reduces stress.

Theory Objective 1
Five Basic Massage
Movements

Most people want to have an attractive appearance, but no amount of makeup can really give the "natural look" of healthy skin. Facial massages help to keep the skin fresh and smooth and keep the muscles firm. Massages are one of the best ways to enhance facial beauty.

Facial massages should not be performed on **diseased, broken** (sores that are open), **bruised,** or **scraped** (abrasion) skin or on skin that is extremely inflamed with acne. You should analyze and examine the client's skin and determine its condition **before** the facial.

Facial massages benefit the skin in several ways:

■ The skin, muscles, and nerves are stimulated. This causes the blood vessels to dilate (open), which increases the blood supply to the skin.

■ The facial muscles are stimulated, which improves muscle tone and reduces wrinkles.

■ The adipose (fatty) tissue in the subcutaneous layers is reduced, giving the skin a firmer texture.

■ The facial nerves are relaxed and soothed, and the metabolism of the skin glands and the keratinization process are normalized.

The following are the **five basic massage movements:**

1. **Effleurage** (ef-fler-AZH) is a light, stroking movement applied with either the palm of the hand or the ball of the finger. This manipulation has a soothing effect on the skin. Effleurage is used mainly in the smaller areas of the face, such as around the jawline (mandible), mouth (orbicularis oris), eyes (corrugator), and forehead (frontalis).

2. **Petrissage** (peh-tri-SAHJ) is a kneading or rolling movement applied with both the palm and the fingers. It has a stimulating and tightening effect on the skin in the same way that pinching it would affect it. Petrissage is used over larger areas of the face, neck, and shoulders. The rotating and sliding of the skin in this movement stimulate the muscles and increase the circulation of the blood to the skin.

3. **Tapotement** (ta-poh-MAHN) is a light tapping or slapping movement applied with the fingertips. It creates a slight stimulating effect on the skin. Tapotement is also used over larger areas of the face. For example, tapotement is applied to each cheek to stimulate the muscles and nerves.

4. **Friction** is a rubbing movement applied with either the fingertips or the flat of the hand. It has a stimulating effect on the skin and is used over a larger area of the face.

5. **Vibration** is a shaking movement done with the fingertips and arm. Because it is very stimulating, it should be done for only a few seconds in any one location. Vibration is used over smaller areas during the facial. Remember that facial movements should always be made in up **upward** direction to prevent dragging, sagging muscles and wrinkling of the skin.

Theory Objective 2
Considerations When Giving a Facial

Emollient creams used in the facial service lubricate and soften normal skin. Use a cold cream for normal skin and a cleansing cream, lotion, or gel for **oily skin.**

When giving any facial manipulations, remember to apply enough cream on the face so your fingers slide over the surface of the skin. Add more cream if the skin dries out. This is particularly true when you are massaging the forehead (frontalis muscle). You are attempting to "iron" (smooth) out wrinkles with your hands, and you will need enough cream to slide across the skin. Any excess cream that is not needed during the facial should be removed, however. A **facial sponge** is a good way to remove excess cream (and impurities) from the face.

It is also important to use sufficient cream when you are working with the skin around the eyes and nose because the skin is **thinner** in these areas than elsewhere on the face. Avoid excessive pressing, pulling, and stretching of the skin in these areas. The muscles and nerves of these tissues are also closer to the surface of the skin.

During the facial, keep your fingers on the face to help maintain an even, relaxing rhythm and tempo throughout the massage service.

Theory Objective 3
Nature and Benefits of
Light Therapy

Although you do not need a sophisticated understanding of light, you should have some basic knowledge about how light is used in facial treatments and therapy.

Light is a form of energy. Its energy is related to wavelengths, which have two ranges or spectrums: visible and invisible. Ordinary light, which is visible, can be seen in a spectrum (array of different colors) when sunlight passes through a prism. The spectrum of visible light can also be seen in a rainbow. This **visible light** comprises about 12 percent of sunlight (Figure 25.1). In addition to visible light, sunlight is made up of 80 percent **infrared** (in-frah-RED) rays and 8 percent **ultraviolet** rays (also called **actinic rays**). Both the infrared and ultraviolet rays are part of the **invisible spectrum.**

In light therapy, cosmetologists use four types of light: infrared and ultraviolet, which are in the invisible spectrum, and white and blue light, which are in the visible spectrum (Table 25.1). In the school or salon, it is possible to obtain the benefits of these different types of light by using a **therapeutic lamp.** This is an electrical device containing a light bulb (called a lamp) that artificially duplicates the wavelength of the type of light you wish to use.

The infrared lamp uses a large glass bulb in combination with a large metal reflector to produce infrared heat for giving facials. The ultraviolet lamp uses a hot quartz lamp to produce ultraviolet rays for services such as tanning the skin. The ultraviolet rays are also used to sanitize implements in a dry sanitizer.

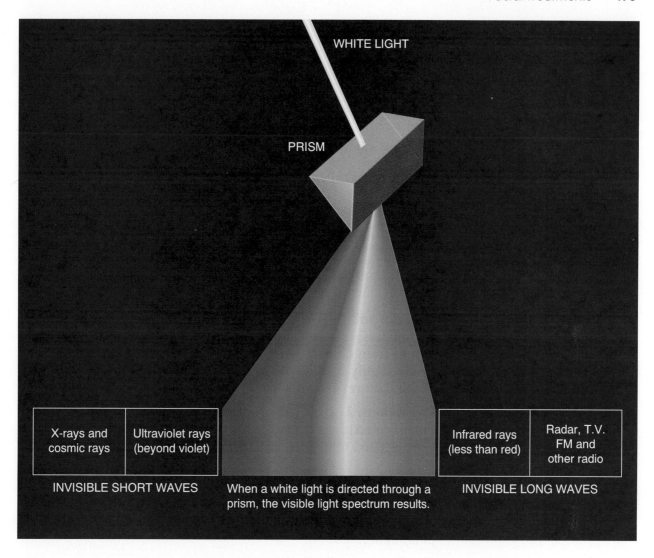

WHITE LIGHT

PRISM

X-rays and cosmic rays	Ultraviolet rays (beyond violet)		Infrared rays (less than red)	Radar, T.V. FM and other radio
INVISIBLE SHORT WAVES		When a white light is directed through a prism, the visible light spectrum results.	INVISIBLE LONG WAVES	

Figure 25.1
The visible spectrum

The white and blue lamps are used with either a **cold quartz bulb** or a **hot quartz bulb.** These lamps have moderate chemical and germicidal effects and can also soothe the nerves and relax muscles.

Remember to read the manufacturer's directions before using any of these lamps.

Since infrared and ultraviolet light are particularly important in the salon, their characteristics are summarized here. **Infrared** rays have long wavelengths—7,700 angstroms and longer—that are capable of deep penetration. (An **angstrom** is a unit used to measure the wavelength of light.) Knowing the following characteristics of infrared light will help you use it effectively in the school or salon:

■ **Source.** A therapeutic lamp made especially to produce these rays.

Table 25.1
Light Used in the Salon

Type of Light	Wavelength	Sunburn Skin?	Effects and Use
Infrared	7,700 Å*	No	Therapeutic, penetrating, soothing to muscle tissue, source of heat. Used with a facial cream or oil when giving a facial.
Ultraviolet	2,800–3,000 Å	Yes	Chemical/germicidal, nonpenetrating. Used for tanning, acne, and scalp treatments.
White	2,537 Å	No	Chemical/germicidal, nonpenetrating. May relieve pain and relax muscles of the upper torso; used on normal skin.
Blue	2,500–2,800 Å	No	Chemical/germicidal, nonpenetrating. Soothes nerves and tones skin; also used for oily skin.

*Å is the abbreviation for angstrom, a unit used to measure the wavelength of light.

- **Distance and time.** The lamp should be placed 30 inches (75 centimeters) from the client for about 5 minutes. To protect the tissues from damage, expose the skin intermittently to the light by constantly turning the base of the lamp so that the pattern of the light rays is broken.

- **Precautions.** Use only the recommended distance and exposure time. Protect the eyes with cotton saturated with water. If the lamp is used to dry the hair, be careful not to burn it.

- **Effects.** Infrared light relieves pain by providing soothing heat, increases circulation by causing the blood vessels to dilate, increases the metabolism of skin cells and causes other chemical changes within tissues, and stimulates the production of perspiration and oil.

Ultraviolet rays have shorter wavelengths (about 1,850 to 3,900 angstroms) and do not penetrate as deeply as infrared. Ultraviolet light is helpful in controlling acne. **Ultraviolet rays can be very dangerous.** Always follow the directions for the specific lamp being used. The following summary of ultraviolet light's characteristics will help you use it effectively:

- **Source.** A therapeutic lamp designed to produce these rays.

- **Distance and time.** The lamp should be 12 to 36 inches (30 to 90 centimeters) from the client, depending on the effects desired. The initial exposure should be 1 to 2 minutes, which can be increased gradually to 8 minutes in later treatments, depending on the sensitivity of the client's skin.

- **Precautions.** Use only the recommended distance and time (overexposure can damage the skin severely). Protect your eyes and the client's eyes by using cotton saturated with cool water. The eyes must not receive any exposure to ultraviolet rays.

■ **Effects.** Ultraviolet rays stimulate several chemical effects on the skin including an increase in **vitamin D** and an increase in blood and lymph circulation. Ultraviolet light also stimulates the pigmentation process in the skin cells, resulting in tanning of the skin.

Practical Objective 4
Facial Treatment for Normal Skin, Dry Skin, and Oily Skin: Proper Steps and Safety Precautions

Facial Treatment for Normal Skin

Remember to practice safety and sanitation procedures when giving a service on the face and around sensitive areas, such as the eyes and nose. These practices should include the following:

1. Wash your hands before giving the service.
2. Use only sanitized cotton pledgets, cotton balls, facial sponges, and laundered towels.
3. Drape the client properly, and use linens to protect the hair and clothing (Figure 25.2).
4. Give an allergy test behind the client's ear before using facial packs and masks. If no reaction occurs, proceed with the service.
5. Be careful when working around the client's eyes with pointed implements, such as scissors. Keep your fingernails filed smoothly, so that you don't scratch the client's skin.
6. Avoid contamination of cosmetics by using a new cotton swab or spatula each time it is necessary to remove a product from a container or bottle. This method will allow you to give many services from a large container of a cosmetic preparation. Powder should be dispensed from a shaker.
7. Dispose of used materials in a covered waste container.
8. Recap bottles and jars of cream and other facial preparations immediately after each use.
9. Follow the manufacturer's directions for the use of each product.

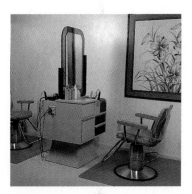

Figure 25.2
Adjustable facial chair. Change the head rest covering after each client.

Preparation

Supplies

- cleansing lotion
- cold cream
- alcohol (for hands)
- emollient cream
- astringent lotion (witch hazel)
- facial machine (with high frequency)
- towels for head band
- skin freshener
- cotton
- spatulas
- cotton pledgets or tissue
- protective gown (smock)

*Basic Facial Manipulations**

Procedure

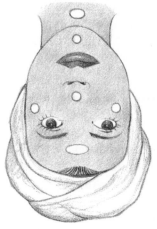

Figure 25.3
Follow this pattern in applying cleansing cream to the face.

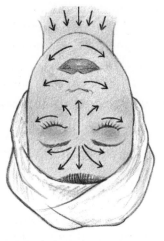

Figure 25.4
Spread the cream evenly across the face and neck.

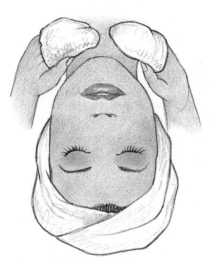

Figure 25.5
Remove excess cleansing cream using a clean tissue or a towel moistened with warm water.

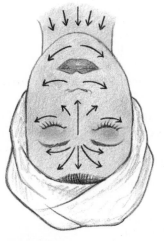

Figure 25.6
Apply emollient cream in the same way the cleansing cream was applied.

*These figures are turned upside down to assist you in performing facials.

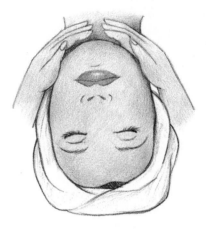

Figure 25.7
Use moderate pressure to lift the chin. Repeat each movement four times.

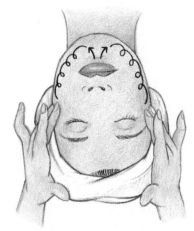

Figure 25.8
Mandible-effleurage. Work from the center of the lower lip toward the ears.

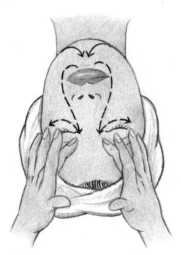

Figure 25.9
Orbicularis oris—effleurage. Starting at the center of the chin, slide your fingers up to the nose and around the eyes. Use a rotating movement at the corners of the eyes.

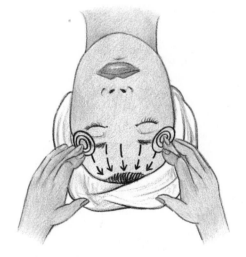

Figure 25.10
Frontalis-effleurage. Draw your fingers upward from the eyebrow toward the hairline. Work from one side of the forehead to the other.

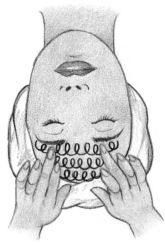

Figure 25.11
Frontalis-friction. Begin just above the eyebrows and work in a circular motion from the center of the forehead toward each side.

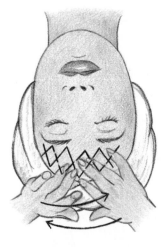

Figure 25.12
Frontalis-friction. Use a semirotating, criss-cross movement across the forehead.

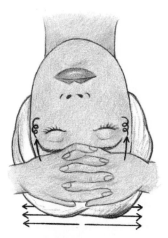

Figure 25.13
Frontalis-effleurage. Interlace your fingers, and slide them firmly from the forehead.

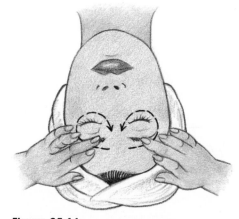

Figure 25.14
Corrugator-effleurage. Using your index and middle fingers, gently press and slide around the eyes in a circular manner.

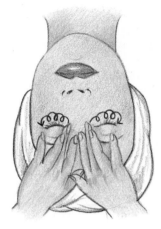

Figure 25.15
Corrugator-effleurage. Slide down along the client's nose and along the cheekbones. Then rotate gently beneath the eyes to the outside corners. Slide back to the brows.

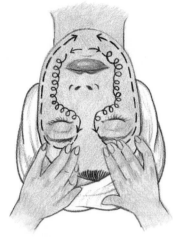

Figure 25.16
Zygomaticus/orbicularis oris—effleurage. Starting at the corners of the mouth, rotate fingers up along the cheekbones and around the eyebrows.

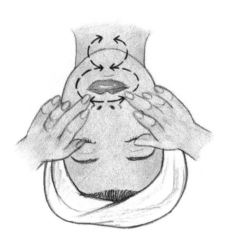

Figure 25.17
Orbicularis oris/mentalis—effleurage. Slide your fingers from the nose downward around the lower lip, then under the chin.

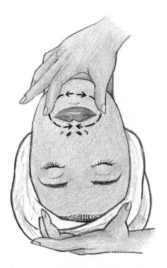

Figure 25.18
Orbicularis oris—effleurage. Support the head with one hand while you perform a circular drawing movement with the other hand.

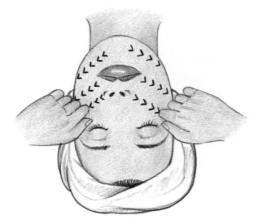

Figure 25.19
Zygomaticus-petrissage. Lightly pinch the skin along a row from the mouth to the sideburn area. Continue with two more rows.

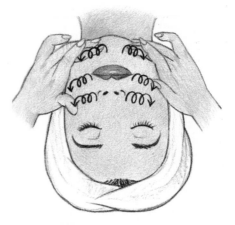

Figure 25.20
Zygomaticus-friction. Use the index, middle, and ring fingers in a rotating movement over the rows worked in the previous step.

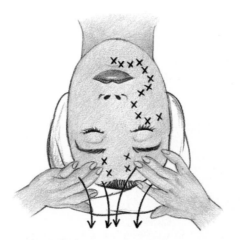

Figure 25.21
All–light tapotement. Work in an upward direction from the chin to the eyes. Now work from the eyebrows to the top of the forehead.

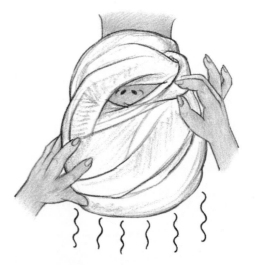

Figure 25.22
Place a moist towel over the face for a few minutes.

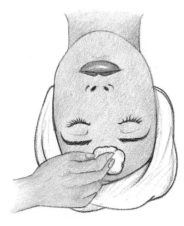

Figure 25.23
Using a cotton pledget, or sterilized cotton ball, saturated with astringent (squeeze out the excess), remove cream from the surface of the skin.

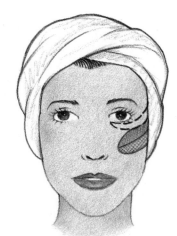

Figure 25.24
Apply makeup as desired.

Figures 25.25, 25.26, and 25.27 illustrate the location of the important nerves and muscles with which you will come in contact when giving facials.

Figure 25.25
Nerves of the facial area—front view

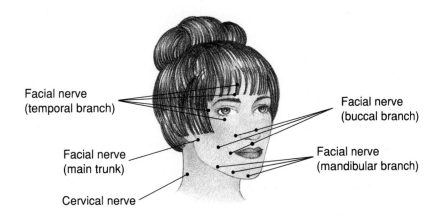

Facial nerve (temporal branch)

Facial nerve (buccal branch)

Facial nerve (main trunk)

Facial nerve (mandibular branch)

Cervical nerve

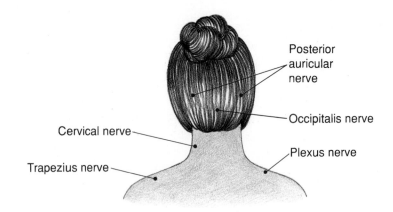

Figure 25.26
Nerves of the facial area—back view

Posterior auricular nerve

Occipitalis nerve

Cervical nerve

Plexus nerve

Trapezius nerve

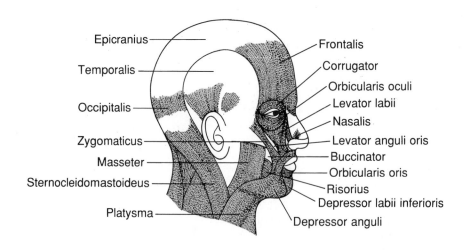

Figure 25.27
Muscles of the facial area

Epicranius

Temporalis

Occipitalis

Zygomaticus

Masseter

Sternocleidomastoideus

Platysma

Frontalis

Corrugator

Orbicularis oculi

Levator labii

Nasalis

Levator anguli oris

Buccinator

Orbicularis oris

Risorius

Depressor labii inferioris

Depressor anguli

Facial Treatment for Dry Skin

Supplies

cleansing lotion
dry-skin lotion
emollient cream
cotton pledgets or tissue
towels for head
smock (cape), linens

hot oil mask, gauze material
and scissors, and oil heater
infrared or red dermal lamp
high-frequency electrode
spatulas

Procedure

1. Follow the procedural steps
for a plain facial, but use a
lotion formulated for dry

Rationale

1. This is standard procedure.

skin. Or you can apply the gauze material and then use the formula for that process.

2. Sponge the client's face with a cleansing lotion formulated for dry skin. Avoid using a product that has a high alcohol content. Next apply the emollient cream. Apply a hot oil **mask** to the dry skin. Remove the gauze following the manufacturer's directions.

2. Alcohol will have a drying effect on the client's skin. A hot oil mask is recommended for dry skin and is followed with the dermal light. The **mask** should be used for **dry skin.** Be sure to check the temperature of the mask before applying it.

3. Cover the client's eyes with cotton pads moistened lightly with cool water.

3. The client's eyes must be covered before light therapy begins (contact lenses should be removed, too). If the cotton pads are moistened, they will stay in place. This is a safety precaution.

4. Expose the client's face to an infrared lamp for 5 minutes. Do not put the infrared lamp closer than 24 inches (60 centimeters) to the client's face. Cover the rays with a towel from time to time so that exposure is not constant. Do not exceed the recommended time.

4. The heat from the lamp will help the skin absorb the oil.

5. After removing the mask, apply **witch hazel** (astringent).

5. The skin will absorb only a small amount of oil, so it is necessary to remove the excess. Witch hazel has a soothing effect on the skin. It is made from witch hazel bark and alcohol.

6. Sponge the face with skin lotion formulated for dry skin. Pat dry.

6. Sponging the skin will remove impurities along with traces of excess oil.

Facial Treatment for Oily Skin

Supplies

cleansing cream	medicated soap
mildly abrasive facial cleanser	antiseptic lotion
astringent	facial steamer
cotton pledgets or tissue	comedones extractor
towels for head	Wood's light
extra towels	spatulas
facial pack	

Note: Use of the Wood's light has been prohibited in some states.

Procedure	Rationale
1. Give the client a hand mirror. Warn the client not to look into the Wood's light (Figure 25.28).	**1.** The mirror will allow the client to see what you see during the examination. The client must never look into any ultraviolet instrument for long periods.
2. Turn off the light in the work area. Following the manufacturer's directions, turn on the Wood's light. Allow 2 to 3 minutes for the Wood's light to **warm up.**	**2.** Directions may vary from one manufacturer to another. The Wood's light is always used in a darkened area for best viewing results.
3. Show the client in the mirror the points that appear coral, orange, or red. The Wood's light, which was developed by Robert	**3.** Any of these colors is a sign of overactive or inflamed oil glands and indicates the need for corrective measures, such as medicated

Figure 25.28
Using Wood's light

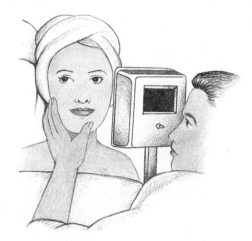

Williams Wood, is used to help detect skin conditions. Its deep violet rays cause substances to become luminous so that blemishes that cannot be seen by the naked eye become visible. The shades of color indicate different conditions: blue to white is a sign of normal healthy skin; violet indicates dehydrated skin; yellow to pink indicates oily areas; and brown indicates pigmentation and dark spots. The thicker the skin, the whiter the light.

soap, abrasive facial cleansers, or a steamer treatment. Use of the steamer will flush the oil ducts and allow oil to flow normally.

4. Turn on the light in the work area and turn off the Wood's light. Proceed to apply abrasive cleanser to the areas identified by the light. Use a facial steamer if desired, following the manufacturer's directions.

4. This completes the analysis and corrective procedure.

5. Remove excess cleanser from the skin with a tissue folded like a mitten, and apply the facial pack.

5. This will also remove excess oil and impurities. The facial **pack** is used for normal to oily skin, or skin that has a tendency to wrinkle.

6. Apply an astringent skin lotion to the skin and pat dry.

6. The astringent lotion will dry the skin and close the pores.

Treating Minor Problems of Oily Skin: Acne

Procedure

Rationale

1. Cleanse the client's face with medicated soap and apply acne cream (or a pack) to the face.

1. Medicated soap will help prevent the spread of infection. The cream will allow the facial electrode to glide smoothly over the skin.

2. Apply direct high-frequency current for 3 to 5 minutes. Watch the affected areas closely.

2. High-frequency current has a germicidal and drying effect on skin.

3. Remove the cream with a tissue folded like a mitten or a towel moistened with warm water.

3. This will remove excess cream and impurities.

4. Saturate cotton pads with astringent lotion and apply them to the skin.

4. Astringent lotion will help dry the skin and close the pores.

5. Apply antiseptic lotion to cotton pads and place them on the affected areas.

5. Antiseptic lotion will help reduce the spread of infection.

6. Do not apply makeup unless it is medicated.

6. Makeup has a tendency to clog the pores, which causes the acne condition to spread.

Treating Minor Problems of Oily Skin: Comedones/Milia

Procedure

Rationale

1. Apply the abrasive cleansing cream and remove it with a cool, moist towel.

1. This is standard procedure.

2. Apply a **clay pack** formula, allow it to dry, and peel it off.

2. Comedones (blackheads) or milia (whiteheads) are an indication of oily skin. A clay mask breaks up and removes oil from the skin. Keep the **pack material away from the mouth, nose, and eyes.** Packs may also be made from lemon gel or some other mixture, such as an oatmeal formula.

3. Reapply the abrasive cleansing cream and steam the face with warm towels, a facial steamer, or a direct high-frequency current for 3 to 5 minutes.

3. The warmth and moisture will open the pores.

4. Remove comedones or milia with a sanitized comedones extractor (Figure 25.29).

4. The extractor must be sanitized to prevent infection.

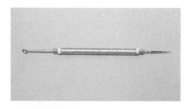

Figure 25.29
Comedones extractor

5. Sponge the face with an antiseptic lotion, and apply towels moistened in cool water.

5. This will prevent the spread of infection and cause the skin to contract and the pores to close.

6. Apply an astringent lotion to the face, concentrating on the affected areas; pat dry.

6. This will dry the oils and close the pores.

Sanitize your area as follows:
1. **Wash, wipe, and store bottles and supplies.**
2. **Discard used supplies.**
3. **Clean and sanitize the cape and apron.**
4. **Sanitize the work area; wash your hands.**

Glossary

Absorption The process by which one substance takes in (soaks up) another.

Auriculotemporal nerve A nerve located in front of the ear.

Depressor labii inferioris A muscle that affects the muscles of the lower lip.

Effleurage (ef-fler-AZH) A light, stroking movement used in massage to soothe the skin.

Friction A rubbing movement used in massage to stimulate the skin.

Frontalis (frahn-TAH-liss) Part of the epicranius muscle located in the eyebrow area.

Infrared (in-frah-RED) light Light with long wavelengths (7,700 angstroms or longer) used in light therapy on the skin.

Levator labii superioris A muscle that affects the upper lip.

Mask A treatment applied to dry skin that tends to wrinkle easily.

Mentalis muscle A chin muscle that makes the lower lip protrude.

Mental nerve A nerve serving the skin of the lower lip and chin.

Orbicularis oris A circular band of muscle surrounding the mouth.

Pack A treatment applied to the face to remove oil and impurities from the skin.

Petrissage (peh-tri-SAHJ) A kneading or rolling movement used in massage to stimulate the skin.

Risorius A mouth muscle used in smiling.

Supratrochlear (soo-pra-TROK-lee-ar) nerve A subdivision of the ophthalmic branch involved in facial massage.

Tapotement (ta-poh-MAHN) A light tapping or slapping movement used in massage to stimulate the skin.

Triangularis A muscle that stimulates the muscle that pulls down the corners of the mouth.

Ultraviolet light Light with wavelengths of 1,850 to 3,900 angstroms that is used in light therapy on the skin. This is the type of light that causes the skin to tan.

Vibration A shaking movement used in massage to stimulate the skin.

Witch hazel A mild astringent solution that has a soothing effect on the skin. It is made by combining witch hazel leaves and bark with alcohol.

Wood's light A light with deep violet rays that is used to help detect various skin conditions.

Zygomaticus A muscle in the area of the cheekbones.

Questions

1. For sanitation purposes, how often should the head rest covering for the facial chair be changed?
2. What should be used to remove facial cream (creams) from a jar?
3. Are most facial movements upward away from the neck or downward toward the neck?
4. Should facial treatments be given using an even rhythm and tempo?
5. Is the frontalis muscle located in the jaw area?
6. Is the supratrochlear nerve located between the eyes on the upper part of the nose?
7. Is tapotement a facial massage movement?
8. Is the trapezius muscle located along the forehead?
9. Is the Wood's light used to identify scars?
10. Does high-frequency current have a germicidal effect on the skin?
11. Would a clay mask temporarily cleanse the face of excessive oil?

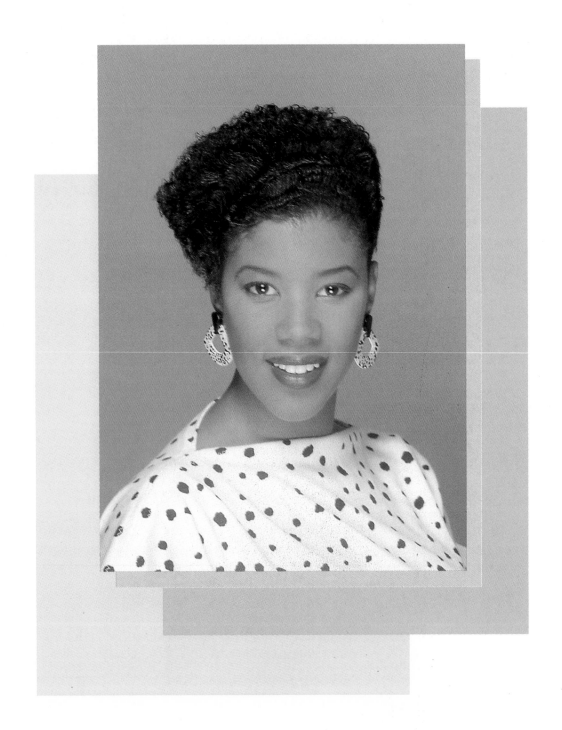

Applying Makeup

Learning Objective

Using professional cosmetics and implements and the proper principles and techniques, apply makeup that enhances your client's particular facial features and meets the client's other needs. Use the proper steps to apply makeup on the client in 40 to 60 minutes. Score 85 percent or better on a multiple-choice exam on the information in this chapter.

In order to achieve the above level of competence, you should master the following chapter objectives.

Theory Objectives

1. Describe the basic cosmetics used on the face.
2. Explain how to select an appropriate color of foundation (base).
3. Describe the cosmetics and techniques used to enhance facial features and correct specific problems.
4. Describe the techniques used to apply false (strip) eyelashes and semipermanent lashes (eye tabbing) and to tint lashes and brows.
5. Describe the basic cosmetics used for black clients.

Practical Objective

6. Apply makeup for a black client.

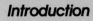

Introduction

One of the most challenging areas of cosmetology is the selection and application of makeup. Many products and techniques are available to choose from—and new ones are being introduced all the time. Because of the artistic nature of this service, however, it is very difficult to claim that one product or method is better than another. This chapter will introduce you to basic products and techniques used in the makeup service. Keep in mind, however, that your instructor will show you the best method for the application of makeup.

In applying makeup, you will be working near three orifices (openings) of the body—the eyes, nose, and mouth. Bacteria or viruses can enter the body through these openings and cause a disease to develop. Therefore, state boards of cosmetology and other regulatory agencies concerned with health and safety issues have established a number of guidelines for the safe application of makeup. Table 26.1 lists important safety practices that you should follow in performing the makeup service.

Theory Objective 1
Basic Cosmetics Used on the Face

In order to apply makeup properly, you need to be familiar with the products used in facial care and makeup. The following list describes some of the basic cosmetics you are likely to use, but does not include such products as eye and night creams because they usually are not applied in the salon (Figure 26.1):

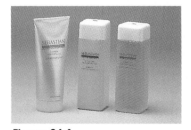

Figure 26.1
Basic facial cosmetics

1. **Cleansers,** usually in cream or emollient form, clean the epidermal layer of the skin. They remove makeup and unsightly matter that could cause skin eruptions and then prepare the face for a new application of makeup. Cleansing products usually come in formulas for oily and dry to normal skin.

2. **Liquid** and **bar soaps** can also be used to cleanse the skin. You must consider the pH rating of a soap that you are going to use. Alkaline products are very drying to the skin, so you should not use soap that has a pH of more than 6.5. Doctors often suggest medicated soaps and those with a low pH rating for blemishes and acne. Superfatted soap is sometimes recommended for very dry or sensitive skin. Castile soap can be used on almost any skin.

Table 26.1
Safety Practices for Applying Makeup

Do	Don't
Sanitize your hands before and after a makeup application.	Share makeup.
Properly drape the client using clean, sanitized linen.	Reuse items that cannot be sanitized easily, such as Q-tips.
Use the client's makeup.	Reuse cotton balls or pledgets.
Use only sanitized makeup applicators, such as brushes and sponges.	Use products from professional, large (gallon or quart) containers. Pour the product into a smaller container, and label it properly.
Properly discard items that cannot be sanitized.	Drip or splash lotions, antiseptics, astringents, or other liquids into the client's eyes.
Sanitize tweezers.	Share makeup applicators that have not been sanitized.
Sanitize all sponges immediately after the service, and store in a sanitary container.	Place used implements with clean ones until they have been sanitized.
Use a brush to apply cream or liquid lip color.	Reuse eyebrow pencils. Discard them so that they won't be used on another client.*
To prevent infection, apply antiseptic to any area of the client's skin that has been tweezed.	Mix clean linen with soiled linen.
Place used implements in a container until sanitized.	Put your fingers into bottles and jars.
Place soiled linen in a separate container.	Work with rough fingernail edges—keep them smoothly filed.
Dispense products by pouring or by using a spatula or a special applicator.	Work in a messy, cluttered area.
Use a shaker to dispense powder.	Apply makeup to hair—use a clean hairline strip.
Keep your work area clean, neat, and orderly.	Allow the client's head to rest against unprotected facial chair upholstery.
Pour liquids from bottles.	Use implements that have not been sanitized.

*In some states, pencils can be sharpened and used on another client. Your instructor will explain the proper procedure in your state.

3. **Skin fresheners (toners)** usually come in liquid form. They are used to remove traces of cleansing creams and to close the pores of the skin. They are preferred for normal and dry skin.

4. **Astringents,** which contain alcohol, are available in liquid and cream form. They can be used on oily skin to close the skin pores and help dry excessive sebum. Because of their drying effect, however, they are not used as widely as fresheners.

5. **Moisturizers,** usually in emulsion or a thicker cream form, are needed for all types of skin. They help the skin retain moisture and give it a fresh appearance.

6. **Emollient creams** contain lanolin, which lubricates the skin. They are used in facial massages.

7. **Foundation** (base) comes in a variety of forms, including liquid, cream, cake, and stick. All of these forms help to cover blemishes. They also protect the skin from unsightly matter in the atmosphere. Some manufacturers have made bases especially for black skin. These or dark shades of other foundations can be employed for black clients.

8. **Corrective sticks** (both white and dark) are used to create the illusion of an oval-shaped face. White contour is used to give fullness to sunken areas, and dark contour is used on areas that need to be toned down.

9. **Blusher** is used to enhance and add color to various areas of the face, especially the cheekbones. It comes in many forms, including liquid, cream, creamy cake, and powder cake. The powder cake types can be used to add color to the forehead, cheekbone, and chin areas.

10. **Lipstick** is available in a number of forms, including gloss, liquid, cream, creamy stick, and crayon. In the salon, this cosmetic must be applied with a lip brush that can be sanitized with 70 percent alcohol.

11. **Powder** is used over the foundation to set the makeup and keep it from rubbing off on clothing. Powder also provides a matte (dull rather than shiny) finish for the face.

12. **Eye shadow** is used both to highlight and shadow the area of the eyes. With eye shadow, small eyes can be made to look larger, and large eyes can be made to look smaller. Eye shadow comes in powder cake, creamy cake, cream, and stick forms.

13. **Mascara** is used to make lashes look darker and thicker. It is available in cake, cream, and liquid forms. (Some state boards do not allow cake mascara to be used in salons.)

14. **Eyeliners** are employed to outline the eyes. They come in liquid, cream, and cake forms. (Some state boards do not allow cake eyeliner to be used in salons.)

15. **Eyebrow pencils** are pencil-like waxy products that are used to fill in and/or darken the brows.

Theory Objective 2
Selecting an Appropriate Color of Foundation (Base)

As with many of the skills you have learned in this book, the first step in applying makeup—the step no one actually sees—is the most important. In the makeup service, selecting the right foundation—one that is an appropriate color for your client—is crucial to the client's overall appearance.

After you have prepared your client's skin with a cleanser, moisturizer, and freshener (or astringent), the skin is ready for the application of a foundation. This cosmetic will be partially absorbed into the epidermal layer, enhancing the individual's skin tone.

Since you want a **natural** rather than a painted look, select a color that is one shade darker than the client's natural skin tone. Natural skin tones are usually classified as **pink, florid, cream white, sallow, olive,** and **dark.** They can also be grouped more simply as light, medium, and dark. These classifications are helpful, but you can use an additional factor in choosing a color: your knowledge of pH.

The **natural pH of skin** ranges from 4.5 to 5.5, but agents used in cleansing, toning, and the like can alter this value. Cleansing with soap and water (and some cleansers) can change the skin's pH to about 7.

If the skin has a pH of more than 7, foundation makeup tends to **stand** out from the natural skin tone. When you find that foundation stands out on your client's skin, you should select a color that is one shade lighter than the skin tone itself. When the skin is acidic, foundations have a tendency to disappear on (be absorbed into) the face. For this type of skin, you should use a darker than normal color.

Although knowledge of basic skin tones and pH factors can help you choose a likely color, you will still need to try one or more colors on the client before making your final decision. Apply a small amount of the foundation to the lower jawbone on the skin just in front of the ear. If the color is too light or dark, remove the foundation with cleansing cream, and try a different color.

Theory Objective 3
Using Cosmetics and Techniques to Correct Specific Problems

As you know, an **oval face** is considered to be the ideal shape. Corrective makeup techniques can be applied to other facial types to create the **illusion** of an oval shape. In applying these techniques, you use the contours of the face to give the optical illusion of an oval shape. You can use corrective makeup to enhance an oval face (Figure 26.2), make an oblong face look shorter (Figure 26.3), make a round face look thinner (Figure 26.4), and make a square face look softer (Figure 26.5).

This chapter will concentrate on these four basic facial shapes. If you learn the principles involved in applying makeup to these shapes, you should be able to handle any problems that might arise for any shape.

You can use a simple rule when applying corrective or contour makeup: "lights in the valley—shadows on the hills." In other words, **highlighting** is used to add width while shadowing is used

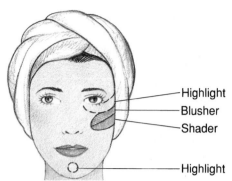

Figure 26.2
Using makeup to enhance an oval face

Highlight
Blusher
Shader

Highlight

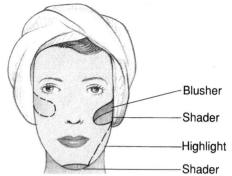

Figure 26.3
Corrective makeup for an oblong face

Blusher
Shader
Highlight
Shader

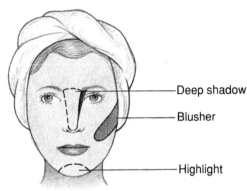

Figure 26.4
Corrective makeup for a round face

Deep shadow
Blusher
Highlight

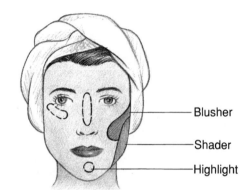

Figure 26.5
Corrective makeup for a square face

Blusher
Shader
Highlight

to narrow and play down prominent features. **Highlighting in this sense is not accenting.** For an oval face, follow the general procedures shown in Figure 26.2. Figures 26.3, 26.4, and 26.5 show how highlighting and shadowing can be used to create the illusion of an oval shape.

The rest of this objective illustrates corrective techniques that can be used for specific facial features. Figure 26.6 shows how to make a short nose look longer and a protruding nose look less prominent. Note that highlighting is applied down the center of a short nose while shadowing is applied to the sides of a protruding nose.

You can use the same principles in applying makeup on the chin:

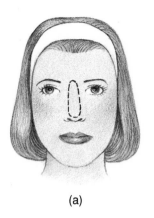
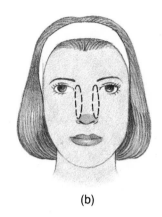

(a)   (b)

Figure 26.6
Corrective makeup for (a) a short nose and (b) a protruding nose

1. For a protruding chin, apply shadow to the areas to be played down (Figure 26.7a).

2. For a receding chin, use highlighting in the shallow area (Figure 26.7b).

3. For a sagging double chin, play down the extra chin by applying darker foundation (Figure 26.7c).

   Corrective makeup can also be applied to the jawline:

1. Use highlighting to add width to a narrow jawline (Figure 26.8a).

2. Play down a broad jawline by applying shadowing (Figure 26.8b).

   Corrective techniques for the lips are shown in Figure 26.9.

Figure 26.7
Corrective makeup for (a) a protruding chin, (b) a receding chin, and (c) a sagging double chin.

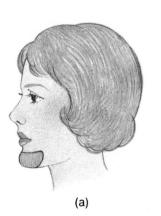
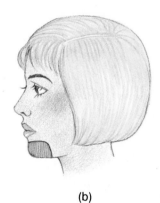
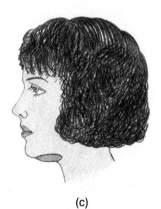

(a)   (b)   (c)

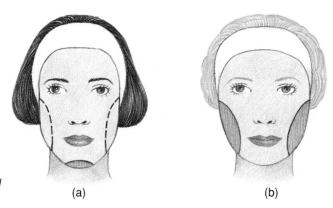

Figure 26.8
Corrective makeup for (a) a narrow jawline and (b) a broad jawline.

(a) (b)

A client's eyebrows may sometimes be an incorrect shape for the size of the eyes and other facial features. Use the following rules to determine the proper shape for your client's eyebrows:

1. Place the eyebrow pencil in a straight line at the side of the nose (Figure 26.10a). Start the eyebrow at this point.

2. To find where the eyebrow should end, measure a 45-degree angle from the outside corner of the eye (Figure 26.10b).

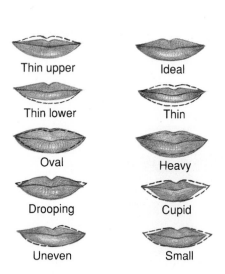

Thin upper   Ideal

Thin lower   Thin

Oval   Heavy

Drooping   Cupid

Uneven   Small

Figure 26.9
Corrective makeup for the lips

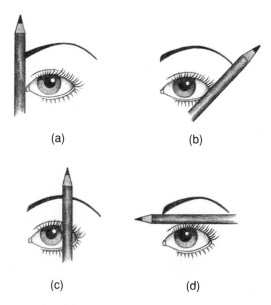

(a) (b)

(c) (d)

Figure 26.10
Determining the proper shape for the eyebrows

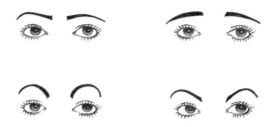

Figure 26.11
Eyebrow shapings to avoid

3. Hold the pencil parallel to the nose along the outside edge of the iris of the eye (Figure 26.10c). The arch of the eyebrow should be at this point.

4. Hold the eyebrow pencil horizontally just above the eye (Figure 26.10d). The pencil should connect the beginning and the end of the eyebrow in an evenly curved arch.

Shaping eyebrows requires a good deal of practice, but these rules will help you avoid improper shapings (Figure 26.11). Once you have determined the correct shape, tweeze the eyebrows as shown in Figure 26.12.

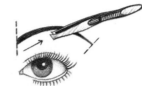

Figure 26.12
Always work in the direction the hair grows when tweezing eyebrows. Use a "quick" movement of the tweezers.

Applying False Eyelashes

Use the following steps to apply false strip eyelashes:

1. Measure the false lash on the client by placing it so it extends from the inside corner of the eye to the outside corner; cut off any extra lash at the outside corner (Figure 26.13).

2. Using tweezers or your fingers, put the center of the false lash directly above the center of the left eyelash (Figure 26.14).

Theory Objective 4
Techniques for Applying False (Strip) Eyelashes and Semipermanent Lashes (Eye Tabbing) for Tinting Lashes and Brows

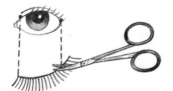

Figure 26.13
Trim eyelashes to fit the client's eye.

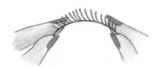

Figure 26.14
Apply false strip eyelashes using tweezers or your fingers.

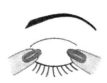

Figure 26.15
Press the inside corner of the eyelashes with your thumb and the outside corner with your index finger.

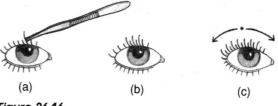

(a)   (b)   (c)

Figure 26.16
Applying semipermanent lashes (eye tabbing)

3. Press the inside corner of the false lash with your thumb; then press the outside corner with your index finger (Figure 26.15). Hold for 1 minute.

   Apply semipermanent lashes (eye tabbing) using the following steps:

1. Use tweezers to take the lash bulb from the tray. Dip the bulb in the glue.

2. Start in the center of the lashes of the right eye (Figure 26.16a). Stroke the lash bulb from the beginning (at the lid) to the end.

3. Place the semipermanent lash on the client's glued lash (Figure 26.16b); continue this procedure to the inside corner and then to the outside corner of the eye (Figure 26.16c).

Tinting Lashes and Brows

To tint lashes and brows, follow these four basic steps:

1. Apply petroleum jelly around the eyes and on paper shields (Figure 26.17a).

Figure 26.17
Tinting lashes and brows

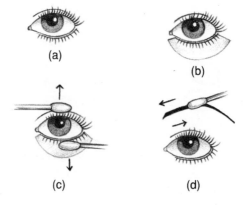

(a)

(b)

(c)

(d)

2. Apply paper shields under the bottom lashes on both eyes where the skin and lashes meet (Figure 26.17b).

3. Use an upward stroke to apply tinting solution on the upper lashes (Figure 26.17c). Apply the solution several times. Stroke the lower lashes of both eyes from the eyelid to the tips of the lashes.

4. Stroke the eyebrows first in the direction of growth and then against it (Figure 26.17d).

Theory Objective 5
Makeup Techniques for
Black Women

Analysis and Diagnosis

When conducting an analysis of a client's skin, the cosmetologist must be careful with black skin because the dark pigmentation makes imperfections more difficult to detect than on white skin. Darker skin also has more and larger sebaceous glands. Because light is reflected more easily on dark skin, the skin may be incorrectly diagnosed as oily.

Since inflammations of the skin, such as acne, may cause lightening or darkening of the skin, avoid using abrasive sponges and strong soaps or squeezing the skin. These practices tend to cause continued irritation of the skin.

Combination skin is a condition that usually is located in the "T zone" of the face. It occurs when the skin in this location is oily in some places but dry in others. This condition is very common among black clients. Therefore, it is important to normalize these areas through the correct selection and use of makeup products.

Black clients should be encouraged to schedule regular appointments for skin care. For example, facial treatments using corrective masks are available to normalize the skin and keep the complexion free of blemishes.

Basic Cosmetics for Black Women

The following are the basic cosmetics used for black clients. Remember that the skin should be thoroughly cleansed and moisturized before makeup is applied.

- **Blusher or rouge.** Blushers are used to complement the skin tones in the cheek area. The most popular colors for blushers are plum, wine-bronze, and medium brown. For vibrant and avant-garde looks, choose from the reds, pinks, teal, oranges, and gold. Never apply blusher on the cheeks lower than the tip of the nose. Use brown tones for contouring along the jawline.

■ **Eye shadow.** Black clients tend to use eye shadow in deep and vibrant blue, green, or wine shades. Some black clients may want to experiment with pastel colors. Powdered eye shadow is recommended for clients with oily skin because it lasts longer.

■ **Mascara.** Black mascara is the usual color of choice, although you may suggest brown for a softer, more subtle look. Sometimes pastel mascara is used to match the selected eye shadow. Skin tone should also be taken into consideration.

■ **Eyeliner.** Eyeliner is used to accentuate the eyes, change their shape, and make the eyelashes appear thicker. Black, charcoal gray, blues, greens, and dark brown are very popular. When applying a pastel shade, cake eyeliner works the best.

■ **Eyebrow powder.** Eyebrow powder is applied with an eyebrow brush to achieve a more natural look. The most popular shades are brown and sable brown.

■ **Lip color.** The most popular shades of lipstick are wine, dark red, mahogany, and oranges.

Selecting an Appropriate Foundation Color

As we noted earlier, foundation is used to even out the tone of the skin and enhance its appearance. It is important to test the foundation color along the jawline before proceeding with a full application. A foundation that is too light for a particular skin tone will make the client's face and neck appear ashy.

Table 26.2 lists seven basic categories of skin colors for black clients. Some 20 to 30 shades of dark skin are found with various undertones. These shades range from a cream color with yellow undertones to ebony with undertones ranging from deep red to blue. Use this table as a basic guideline to help you select a foundation color, but remember to consider the color of the client's eyes and hair as well as the skin color. It is usually necessary to use two

Table 26.2
Skin and Foundation Color Chart for Black Women

Skin Color	Undertones	Foundation Color
Cream	Yellow	Rosy beige
Tan	Yellow	Match or coordinate with natural skin tones.
Olive	Yellow	Beige to even out the color
Copper	Red	Medium to dark beige
Earth brown	Yellow	Match or coordinate with natural skin tones.
Dark reddish brown	Red	Natural or beige to tone down red
Ebony	Deep red into blue	Match or coordinate with natural skin tones.

different colors of foundation on various parts of the face to even out the client's complexion.

Preparation

1. Drape the client to allow for complete cleansing of the face and neck area. The head drape should not interfere with the facial cleansing or the application of makeup.

2. Analyze the client's skin; then cleanse, tone, and moisturize (Figure 26.18).

Procedure

1. Use your fingers or a makeup sponge to apply the foundation. Dot the foundation on the face (Figure 26.19), and then stroke the foundation sparingly and evenly over the entire face and neckline. In Figure 26.20, two different colors were mixed together due to yellow and red undertones in the client's skin. To set the foundation, sprinkle translucent powder on a soft brush and dust the face.

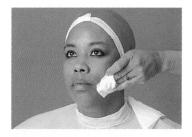

Figure 26.18
Remove cleanser with a tissue.

2. Use a soft brush to sweep powder blusher in a triangular motion up and onto the cheekbone toward the temple (Figure 26.21). Next, apply contouring (usually darker or an earth tone) blusher below the color to define the bone structure (Figure 26.22).

3. Using a brush, washable sponge-tipped applicator, or Q-tip, apply powdered eye shadow from the base of the lashes to the crease of the eyelid (Figure 26.23). For contouring, apply a highlighting color directly under the eyebrows, and blend with the first color so there is no line where the colors meet (see Figure 26.25 below for completed highlighting).

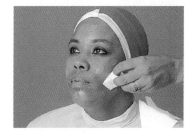

Figure 26.19
Apply dots of foundation in a triangular pattern on the cheeks. Blend up, out, and down using a makeup sponge or your fingers.

4. Apply mascara to the eyelashes first by stroking outward while the client looks down and then by stroking upward while the client looks at the ceiling (Figure 26.24). Always stroke away from the client's eyeball. Use cake mascara to protect the client and to give you more control over the amount being applied.

5. Make sure the eyelids are dry and free of oil before applying the eyeliner.

6. Using an eyebrow brush, brush the eyebrows upward and then across in the direction of the hair growth (Figure 26.25). Since many black clients have abundant facial hair, you may suggest facial waxing to remove excess hair.

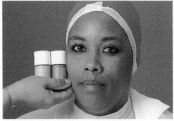

Figure 26.20
If the client's skin has undertones of two colors, blend two colors of foundation together. Test your color selection on the fold of the client's upper forearm before the final application.

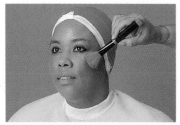

Figure 26.21
Using a soft brush, stroke blusher up toward the temple in a triangular sweeping motion on the cheekbone.

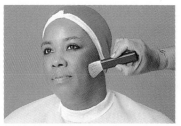

Figure 26.22
Apply contouring blusher below the color to define the bone structure; again, use a triangular stroking motion.

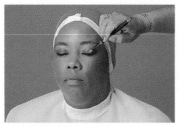

Figure 26.23
Apply powder eye shadow with the client's brush, a Q-tip, or a sponge-tipped applicator.

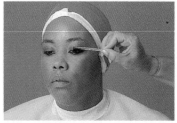

Figure 26.24
A mascara brush is washable and allows more control during application. Ask the client to look down while you stroke outward.

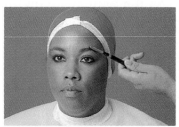

Figure 26.25
Use an eyebrow brush to control and direct brow hair. Brush upward and outward toward the temple area.

7. Apply lip liner with a sharpened lip liner pencil, and then fill in the outline with a lighter shade of lip color (Figures 26.26 and 26.27). Apply the lip color with a Q-tip or the client's lip brush. To provide an even base for the color, you may often have to apply foundation to the lip area before applying lip color.

    Facial waxing may be needed on upper lip hair because it is so dark. Usually, facial hair on black clients cannot be lightened because the contrast with the skin would be too obvious.

8. Figures 26.28 and 26.29 show the completed makeup application.

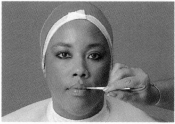

Figure 26.26
Use the client's lip brush or a Q-tip to apply lip color. The lip color will usually be a lighter shade than the lip liner.

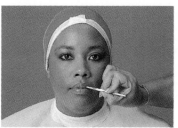

Figure 26.27
Color is developed throughout the face, including the eyes, cheeks, and lips.

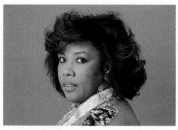

Figure 26.28
The colors blend and balance each other in the completed application.

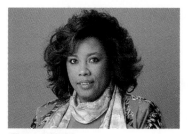

Figure 26.29
The completed makeup application

Glossary

Astringent A liquid or cream containing alcohol that is used on oily skin to close skin pores and help dry excessive sebum.

Blemish stick See **Corrective stick.**

Blusher A product available in a variety of forms that is used to add color to an area of the face. It may be applied to the forehead, cheekbones, and chin.

Cleanser A cream or emollient used to clean the epidermal layer of the skin.

Contour makeup See **Dark contour makeup** and **White contour makeup.**

Corrective stick A makeup stick used to help cover blemishes and scars.

Dark contour makeup A dark stick or thick cream used to tone down areas on the face.

Emollient cream A cream containing lanolin, which lubricates the skin; used in facial massage.

Eyebrow pencil A pencil-like, waxy product that is used to fill in and/or darken the eyebrows.

Eyeliner A product available in liquid, cream, or cake form that is used to outline the eyes.

Foundation A makeup product available in a variety of forms that helps cover blemishes and protects the skin from matter in the atmosphere.

Lipstick A product available in a variety of forms that is used to add color or gloss to the lips.

Mascara A product available in cake, cream, or liquid form that is used to make eyelashes look darker and thicker.

Moisturizer An emulsion or cream that helps the skin retain water.

Powder A product used over makeup foundation to keep it from rubbing off and to give the face a matte finish.

Skin freshener A liquid product that removes traces of cleansing creams and helps close the pores of the skin.

White contour makeup A white stick or thick cream used to give the illusion of fullness in sunken areas of the face.

Questions

1. How does an astringent affect the skin pores?
2. Does an emollient lubricate the skin?
3. How is an eyeliner used?
4. What name is given to a product that is used to remove makeup and other matter from the face?
5. What product containing alcohol is used to remove oil from the skin and close the pores?
6. What product lubricates the skin and helps it retain moisture?
7. What makeup is used to enhance the eyes by highlighting or shading them?
8. What is the natural pH of the skin?
9. What facial shape is considered the "ideal"?
10. Should tweezing be performed with a slow movement or a quick movement?
11. Is tweezing normally done in the same direction as the hair growth or in the opposite direction?
12. When applying artificial eyelashes, are the false lashes glued only to the natural lashes?
13. When tinting eyelashes, is it necessary to use protective eye shields?
14. Is eyelash tint usually applied with a cotton ball?

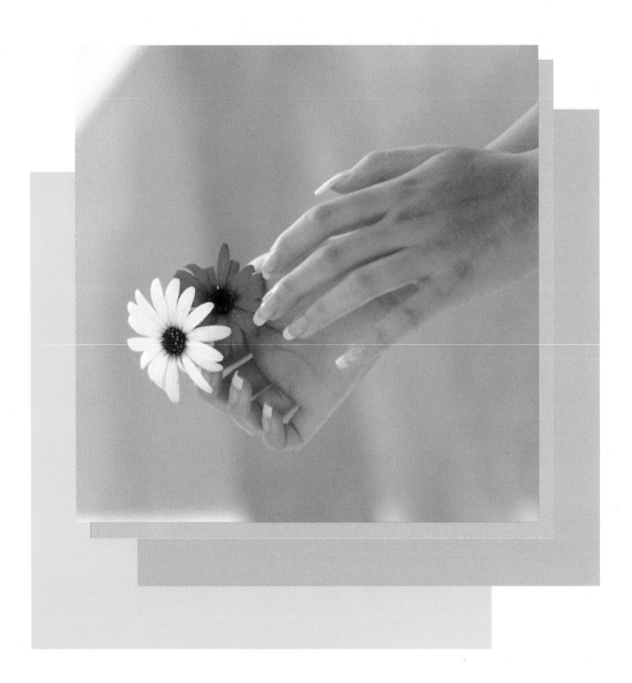

Nail Anatomy, Disorders, and Diseases

Use the information in this chapter to recognize, describe, and label nail shapes, disorders, and diseases as well as the main bones of the arms, hands, feet, and legs. Score 85 percent or better on a multiple-choice exam on the information in this chapter.

In order to achieve the above level of competence, you should master the following chapter objectives.

Theory Objectives

1. Describe four basic nail shapes, the anatomy of the fingernail, its surrounding structures, and nail growth.
2. Describe nail irregularities.
3. Identify nail diseases.
4. Identify and label the main bones of the arms, hands, feet, and legs.
5. Describe the disorders and diseases of the feet.

Introduction

This chapter presents important information about human fingernails and toenails, including their shapes, growth, structure, disorders, and diseases. Knowing this information will help you give manicures and pedicures successfully. You will need to be able to recognize certain nail disorders and diseases so that you can answer clients' questions about them and also so that you can protect yourself from performing services on clients who have a highly contagious disease. If you give a service to a client who has a contagious disease, you may become affected with the disease yourself and spread it to other clients visiting the salon. Therefore, the information about the nails in this chapter will serve as preparation for the next chapter, which describes how different nail services are given.

Theory Objective 1

Four Basic Nail Shapes, Anatomy of the Fingernail, Its Surrounding Structures, and Nail Growth

Although nail shapes may vary, four shapes are generally recognized: square, round, oval, and pointed (Figure 27.1). The **oval shape** is usually the most complimentary, but current fashions, finger shape, and the needs of the client should be considered. Rather long nails can interfere with a client's work or recreation. For example, a client who plays basketball may experience frequent nail breakage unless the nails are somewhat short and rounded, instead of long and oval.

The fingernail is an **appendage** (ah-PEN-dij) **of the skin.** It includes the nail plate and the tissues that surround it.

The **nail plate** (nail body) is the visible (almost clear) hard keratin portion on the top of the finger (note that, like hair, the nail is made of keratin). The tissue directly under the nail plate is called the **nail bed.** A healthy nail looks **pink** because the blood that flows to the nail bed can be seen through the nail plate.

The **free edge** of the nail is that part that extends beyond the end of the fingertip and can be seen from both above and below the hand.

Figure 27.1
Nail shapes

| Square | Round | Oval | Pointed |

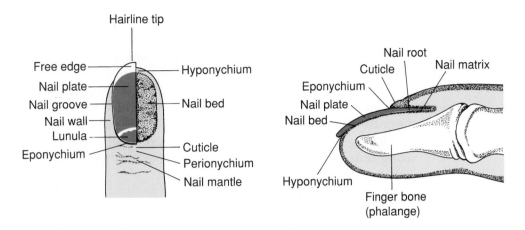

Figure 27.2
The fingernail and its surrounding structures

The nail is surrounded by the cuticle, eponychium, nail wall, nail groove, nail mantle, hyponychium, and perionychium. Each of these structures is described here and illustrated in Figure 27.2:

- The **cuticle** is a thin semicircular piece of skin that overlaps the nail.

- The **eponychium** (ep-oh-NIK-ee-uhm) is the inside point where the nail enters the skin.

- The **nail wall** is a semicircular fold of skin that overlaps the nail plate on either side and extends to the first knuckle.

- The **nail groove** is the channel (slit) on each side of the nail plate. This is where the nail moves when it grows.

- The **nail root** is beneath the skin at the base of the nail in a deep fold of skin called the **nail mantle.**

- The **hyponychium** (high-poh-NIK-ee-uhm) is the skin located directly **beneath** the nail's free edge.

- The **perionychium** (PER-ee-oh-nik-ee-uhm) is the skin that surrounds the entire nail.

The **matrix** (MAY-triks) is the inner part of the nail. It affects the nail's shape, size, regeneration, and growth. The matrix contains the lymph, blood vessels, and nerves that help the nail grow. Keratin grows and hardens in the matrix. This process produces the **nail body.** A bacterial infection in which pus is produced in the matrix is called **onychia** (ON-ik-ee-ah).

The light arc at the base of the nail is called the **lunula** (lu-NOO-lah). It has a half-moon shape. The light color results from an air pocket between the nail plate and the nail bed at the base of the nail.

If the matrix is injured, the nail's growth and shape can be distorted. Unlike hair, nails grow continuously at the rate of .1 millimeter per day ($\frac{1}{8}$ inch per month). (They grow faster in summer than in winter.) If a nail is lost or removed, it will take about 3–4 months to restore a fingernail and 9 months for a toenail. The middle fingernail grows fastest, the thumbnail slowest.

Nails may grow more slowly during serious illnesses and old age. Nail biting from nervous tension may cause nails to grow faster because the blood flow to the matrix is increased by the trauma of the biting. Because the nails are affected by illness and stress, the condition of the fingernails may reflect the individual's general physical and emotional condition.

Theory Objective 2
Nail Irregularities

Although there are only four basic nail shapes, you probably will encounter nails of many different appearances. If you know the basic shapes, you will be able to suggest services that will improve the appearance of the client's hand, but even more important, you will be able to recognize disorders. **You must refuse service to clients who have contagious diseases.** Advise them to consult a doctor. Remember that a **disease** is a disorder that interferes with the normal state and/or function of the body.

This objective describes various irregularities and diseases of the nail, using a simple, easy-to-follow format. First, each disease is described, followed by its cause, prognosis, and treatment. The **prognosis** (prahg-NOH-siss) for a disease (or irregularity or some other condition) is the outlook, or forecast, for recovery from it. **Treatment,** of course, is the procedure needed to avoid or stop the disease.

You will notice that many of the diseases begin with onych-. This comes from **onycho,** the Greek word for fingernail. (The word **onyx** [ON-ix] comes from onycho.) **Onychosis** (on-ee-KOH-siss) is a term used to describe any nail disease.

Figure 27.3
Onychophagy

Onychophagy (on-ee-KOF-aj-ee) is the technical term for nail biting. The condition involves slightly deformed nail shapes, with no inflammation (redness) or other abnormal signs (Figure 27.3).
Cause It is a nervous habit of many individuals.
Prognosis The condition will subside if the person stops biting the nails. If the habit is continued, the individual risks getting a disease from bacteria found on the nails or an infection of the cuticle from bacteria in the mouth.
Treatment Having regular manicures helps many people stop biting their nails because nail polish has an unpleasant taste. Other distasteful chemicals may be applied to discourage the habit, but will power is the only effective solution to the problem.

Onychatrophia (on-i-kat-ROH-fi-ah), also called **onychia,** is characterized by the **atrophy,** or wasting away, of the nail plate. The nail loses its sheen; the plate becomes smaller and may separate from the nail bed (Figure 27.4).

Cause Injury to the nail matrix or internal disease can result in onychatrophia.

Prognosis Nail regeneration depends on the extent of the injury to the matrix or the illness of the client.

Treatment Use only a fine emery board. Do not use a metal pusher or file during the manicure service. Advise the client to avoid highly alkaline soap or detergents.

Figure 27.4
Onychatrophia

Hangnails (also called **agnails**) involve small skin tears or nail splits (Figure 27.5). The skin may bleed and be painfully raw.

Cause Dryness, injury, or sometimes improper manicuring techniques cause the skin in the cuticle area to tear.

Prognosis If the affected area is very small, the skin rebuilds quickly. Larger areas require more treatment and time for healing.

Treatment Soaking in an antiseptic solution and application of antiseptics are in order for small areas. A large area of skin should be treated only by a doctor since surgery may be required. If caution is not exercised, bacterial infection may result.

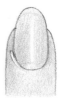

Figure 27.5
Hangnail

Leukonychia (loo-koh-NIK-i-ah) is characterized by white spots on the nail plates on fingernails or toenails (Figure 27.6).

Cause Heredity or minor injury may cause leukonychia. One theory suggests that the white spots are tiny air bubbles caused by incompletely keratinized cells.

Prognosis The spots may disappear when the nail grows out.

Treatment None.

Figure 27.6
Leukonychia

Onychorrhexis (on-ee-koh-REX-iss) is a condition in which the nails are split and brittle. Long parallel splits occur on one or more fingernails (Figure 27.7). No inflammation is present around or under the nail.

Cause The condition may result from heredity and, in some cases, from use of permanent-type polishes or strong solvents for removing nail polishes. Injury to the nail may also cause splitting.

Prognosis A 3-month treatment will usually improve the condition of the nails.

Treatment Advise the client to see a doctor to make sure that no disease is present. Hot oil manicures may also help.

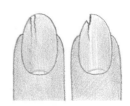

Figure 27.7
Onychorrhexis (brittle nail)

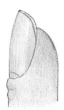

Figure 27.8
Onychauxis

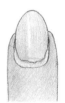

Figure 27.9
Pterygium

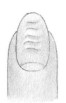

Figure 27.10
Corrugations

Onychauxis (on-ee-KAWK-siss) is a thickening, or hypertrophy, of the nail plate. It results in overgrowth in the thickness or depth of the nail (Figure 27.8).

Cause The condition may result from internal disorders or minor injury to the nail.

Prognosis The client should be advised to see a doctor for a prognosis.

Treatment Advise the client to see a doctor. If no infection is present, a manicurist may buff the nails with pumice powder.

Pterygium (ter-IJ-ee-uhm) is a condition in which the cuticle adheres (sticks) to the surface of the nail base (Figure 27.9).

Cause Usually this condition is caused by dry skin around the fingernail.

Prognosis The condition may recur.

Treatment Hot oil manicures will soften the cuticle and make unneeded growth easy to remove. Carefully remove it with a sanitized cuticle nipper.

Corrugations (kor-uh-GAY-shuhnz), also called beau's lines or transverse furrows, are characterized by wavy horizontal lines across the nail (Figure 27.10).

Cause The condition may result from heart disease, pregnancy, emotional shock, or some acute infections. It may also be caused by minor injury to nails.

Prognosis The nail usually grows out normally in 3 months, but this may vary with the individual's condition.

Treatment Advise the client to see a doctor to determine the underlying cause of the nail condition. Buffing may improve the appearance somewhat, but it cannot completely smooth most corrugated nails.

Blue nails appear bluish instead of healthy pink. A client with blue nails can receive a manicure.

Cause The condition results from heart trouble or other circulatory (blood flow) problems.

Prognosis and treatment The client should ask a doctor about the internal cause of blue nails.

Bruised nails have dark spots caused by dried blood beneath the nail plate.

Cause The condition is caused by an injury to the nail.

Prognosis Whether the new growth will be normal depends on the extent and nature of the injury.

Treatment A client with a badly bruised nail may need to see a doctor. In manicuring, the nail must be handled carefully to avoid further injury or pain.

Theory Objective 3
Nail Diseases

In general, you can recognize nail diseases by **inflammation** of the skin surrounding the nail, soreness causing extreme discomfort, and other signs of infection.

A client may not realize that the disease exists until you point it out. Tell the client to ask a doctor about the condition. **Do not treat diseased nails.** By referring a client to a doctor, you will protect yourself and your clients from the possible spread of contagious or infectious disorders.

When manicuring, you should be extremely careful not to damage the nail or surrounding tissue. Damaging the nail can cause a local infection. If bleeding should occur from accidental improper use of a manicuring implement, apply an antiseptic immediately. If an antiseptic is not applied to an injured matrix, bacteria may enter the matrix and cause onychia. Note: When applying nail wraps or acrylic nails, always keep the nail dry, otherwise, moisture may cause a green-colored fungus to grow under the nail plate. The cosmetologist may encounter some of the following diseases.

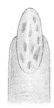

Onychomycosis (on-ee-koh-migh-KOH-siss), also known as **tinea unguis** (UNG-gwis), is **ringworm of the finger or toenails.** In this condition, a vegetable fungus (parasite) disturbs the nail growth. Onychomycosis is not very common, but it is very contagious. The condition is characterized by thickening and deformity and finally loss of the nail (Figure 27.11).

Cause Heredity can be a factor, but this disease usually results from a nail injury coupled with an invasion by a fungus.

Prognosis The nail usually requires 3 months to grow back if it is treated by a doctor. Although the condition is resistant to treatment, competent dermatologists treat it with success.

Treatment Tell the client to obtain a doctor's advice immediately.

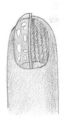

Figure 27.11
Onychomycosis

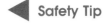 Safety Tip

Tinea of the hands affects the skin rather than the nails, but you should be aware of it. It is a rare infection that is sometimes called the **one-hand-two-foot disease** because it affects only one hand but both feet. Its acute (short-term) form is characterized by blisters at

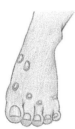

Figure 27.12
Tinea

Figure 27.13
Onychocryptosis

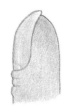

Figure 27.14
Onychogryposis

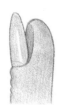

Figure 27.15
Onycholysis

the edge of inflamed areas on the palm and fingers. In its chronic (long-term) state, it can be identified by dry, scaly lesions, which usually occur in one large patch instead of several areas (Figure 27.12).

Cause It is a fungus infection.

Prognosis It is resistant to treatment.

Treatment Tell the client to see a doctor for treatment.

Onychocryptosis (on-ik-oh-krip-TOH-siss) is the technical term for an **ingrown nail.** It is characterized by the lateral growth of the nail plate into the edge of the nail groove (Figure 27.13). Usually, it occurs in the big toe, but it may also occur in the other toenails and fingernails.

Cause Improperly fitting (tight) shoes and incorrect trimming can cause the condition.

Prognosis It may recur after treatment.

Treatment It may be remedied by trimming the nail in a semilunar (crescent-shaped) manner so that the corner of the nail is raised above the skin surface. In cases of extreme discomfort, a doctor should be consulted for surgical relief and/or advice about bacterial infection.

Onychogryposis (on-ee-koh-gri-POH-siss), also called **claw nails,** involves marked thickening of the nail (Figure 27.14). The nail plate becomes elongated and twisted (curved).

Cause The condition results from trauma (shock); other causes are unknown.

Prognosis and treatment Tell the client to get a doctor's advice.

Onycholysis (on-ee-KOHL-eh-siss) involves a spontaneous separation of the nail plate from the nail bed, without actual shedding (Figure 27.15).

Cause Local or general infections and treatment with certain types of antibiotic drugs may cause the condition.

Prognosis and treatment Tell the client to consult a doctor.

Paronychia (par-on-NIK-ee-ah), or felon, is a bacterial infection of the tissue around the nail. It is characterized by pain, redness, and swelling of the skin around the nail plate, without nail loss (Figure 27.16). This condition is very contagious, so it is not treated in the school or salon.

Cause People who have their hands in water for long periods of

time may develop this condition. Dishwashers and cosmetologists are particularly likely to have it.
Prognosis The condition usually responds well when treated by a doctor.
Treatment Tell the client to ask a doctor for advice.

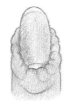

Figure 27.16
Paronychia

Eggshell nails or **hapalonychia** (hap-palo-NIK-ee-ah) involves very thin, fragile nails that are white in color. These nails split and break easily. A defect in the nail matrix causes this condition.
Cause This condition is rare, but it can result from aging and/or the use of acetone or hydroxide solutions in manicuring.
Prognosis and treatment Using nail hardeners or polish (enamel) strengthens these nails and prevents splitting.

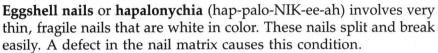

Theory Objective 4
Main Bones of the Arm and Hand

To understand the manicuring task, you need to be familiar with the main bones of the arm and hand (Figure 27.17). The arm has three bones, and the hand has many small bones, which can be classified into three types.

The three bones in the arm are the humerus, ulna, and radius. The **humerus** (HYOO-meh-ruhs) is the **large bone** in the upper part of the arm. The **ulna** (UHL-nah) and **radius** are the two bones that form the forearm. The ulna, which is attached to the wrist, is on the same side as the **little finger.** The **radius** (RAYD-ee-uhs) is the bone that attaches to the wrist on the **thumb side.**

The wrist is the flexible joint between the forearm and the hand. The wrist is made of eight bones called carpals (KAHR-puhlz). The **metacarpals** (met-ah-KAHR-puhlz) are the long bones that form the palm of the hand (Figure 27.18). The **phalanges** (FAY-lanj-ez) are the bones that form the fingers **(digits)** of the hand. There are 14 digits, 3 for each finger and 2 for the thumb.

Theory Objective 5
Disorders and Diseases of the Feet

Care of the feet and toenails is very important because the feet are subjected to many shocks and germs every day. Sports and other exercise, such as tennis, jogging, racquetball, roller/ice skating, aerobic dancing, and walking, leave the feet open to many different disorders and diseases. Some of the more common disorders and diseases that appear on the feet are calluses, ingrown nails, athlete's foot, and plantar warts.

A **callus** is an abnormal thickening of the skin commonly found on the heels and around the edge of the foot. (Calluses also

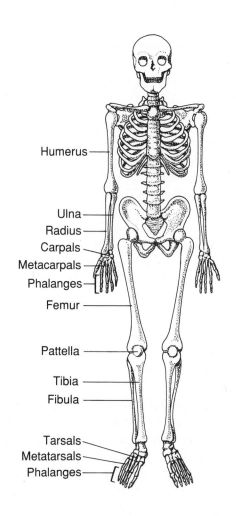

Figure 27.17
The main bones of the arm, hand, leg, and foot

Humerus

Ulna
Radius
Carpals
Metacarpals
Phalanges

Femur

Pattella

Tibia
Fibula

Tarsals
Metatarsals
Phalanges

commonly occur on the elbows, knees, or somewhere on the hands.) A callus is caused by repeated shocks to a particular area of the skin. For example, these "shocks" may be caused by a shoe that doesn't fit properly and rubs against the skin of the foot in the wrong way. In order to protect itself, the skin "thickens." Extra thick socks or even two pairs of socks will often prevent calluses from forming.

An **ingrown nail** occurs when the side of the toenail overgrows into the fold of skin along the edge of the toe. This condition is usually caused by cutting the nail too deeply into the corner of one or both sides of the nail. If the nail is left more square at the corners, ingrown nails may be avoided.

Safety Tip ▶   Diseases of the foot are very common because feet create a natural environment for the growth of bacteria, funguses, and viruses. Particularly during exercise, the feet become hot and perspire. In addition, shoes shield the feet from the germicidal affects

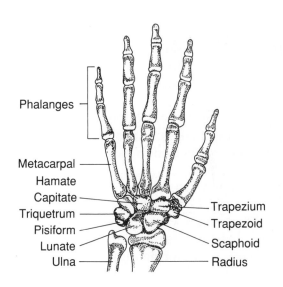

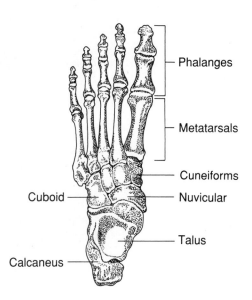

of the sun's ultraviolet rays. Therefore, the feet require special care during and after bathing. After they have been washed, feet must be thoroughly dried, particularly between the toes.

Athlete's foot is a common fungus-type disease that can be particularly bothersome (Figure 27.19a). It is caused by a type of fungus known as **ringworm.** Since it is very contagious, it is important that a **client who has this disease not be given a pedicure.** The symptoms of athlete's foot are itching and the appearance of one or more clear, watery blisters. White scaling and thickening of the skin, as well as cracks (fissures) between the toes, may also be seen. Athlete's foot should always be treated by a doctor.

Plantar warts, which are caused by a virus, are found on the sole of the foot. These warts are contagious. For example, when a person with a plantar wart walks through a shower area, the virus causing the wart is left behind on the floor. If another person walks on the spot on the floor where the virus is present, that person probably will develop a plantar wart, too. A plantar wart looks like a circle within a circle—like a small circular target (Figure 27.19b). Thus, these flat warts have a small spot right in the center. Plantar warts are painful, and removing them is not always easy because their roots can penetrate deep into the skin. A doctor must always treat plantar warts. Different treatments are used, depending on where the warts are located. Pedicures should **not be given to a client with plantar warts.** Refer the client to a dermatologist.

Disorders and diseases of the feet are so common that this is a major field of study called **podiatry.** A doctor who specializes in disorders and diseases of the feet is called a **podiatrist** (PEH-dightrehst).

Figure 27.18
The bones of the hand and foot

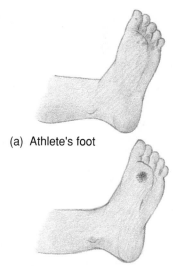

(a) Athlete's foot

(b) Plantar wart

Figure 27.19
Athlete's foot and plantar warts are both contagious disorders of the foot.

Agnail See **Hangnails.**

Athlete's foot A highly contagious fungus-type disease.

Atrophy Wasting away or withering of a part of the body, as atrophy of the nails.

Blue nails A condition in which the nails appear bluish instead of healthy pink; caused by circulatory problems.

Bruised nails Nails with dark spots underneath the nail plate; caused by injury to the nail.

Callus An abnormal thickening of the skin.

Carpals (KAHR-puhlz) The eight bones in the wrist.

Corrugations (kor-uh-GAY-shuhnz) Wavy lines or furrows across the nail; caused by heart disease, pregnancy, emotional shock, acute infection, or minor nail injury.

Cuticle The thin semicircular piece of skin that overlaps the nail.

Disease (diz-EEZ) A disorder that interferes with the normal state and/or function of the body.

Eggshell nails (hapalonychia) Thin, white, fragile nails resulting from a defect in the nail matrix.

Eponychium (ep-oh-NIK-ee-uhm) The inside point where the nail enters the skin.

Free edge The part of the nail that extends beyond the edge of the fingertip.

Hangnails Skin tears or splits in the cuticle area due to dryness of the skin, injury, or improper manicuring.

Humerus (HYOO-meh-ruhs) The large bone in the upper part of the arm.

Hyponychium (high-poh-NIK-ee-uhm) The skin located directly beneath the nail's free edge.

Ingrown nail A toenail that has grown into the fold of skin along the edge of the toe.

Leukonychia (loo-koh-NIK-i-ah) White spots on the nail plates caused by heredity or minor injury.

Lunula The light arc (half-moon) at the base of the nail.

Mantle The deep fold of skin at the base of the nail that contains the nail root.

Matrix (MAY-triks) The inner part of the nail that contains the lymph, blood vessels, and nerves.

Metacarpals (met-ah-KAHR-puhlz) The long bones that form the palm of the hand.

Nail bed The tissue directly under the nail plate.

Nail body See **Nail plate.**

Nail plate The visible (almost clear) hard keratin portion on the top of the finger.

Nail root The place where the nail begins beneath the skin; it is located at the base of the nail in the mantle.

Nail wall The semicircular fold of skin that overlaps the nail plate on either side and extends to the first knuckle.

Onychatrophia (on-i-kat-ROH-fi-ah) The wasting away of the nail plate due to injury of the nail matrix. Also called onychia.

Onychauxis (on-ee-KAWK-siss) A thickening of the nail plate caused by internal disorders or a minor injury to the nail.

Onycho (on-IK-oh) A prefix that means pertaining to the nail.

Onychocryptosis (on-ik-oh-krip-TOH-siss) An ingrown nail caused by improper trimming or tight shoes.

Onychogryposis (on-ee-koh-gri-POH-siss) Elongated, twisted, thickened nails caused by trauma. Also called claw nails.

Onycholysis (on-ee-KOHL-eh-siss) A spontaneous separation of the nail plate from the nail bed, without actual shedding; caused by local or general infections or certain types of antibiotic drugs.

Onychomycosis (on-ee-koh-migh-KOH-siss) Ringworm of the nails; it is caused by a vegetable fungus.

Onychophagy (on-ee-KOF-aj-ee) A slight deformation of the nails caused by nail biting.

Onychorrhexis (on-ee-koh-REX-iss) A condition in which the nails are split and brittle; caused by heredity, permanent polishes, or strong polish-removing solvents.

Onychosis (on-ee-KOH-siss) Any nail disease.

Onyx From the Greek word for fingernail, onycho.

Paronychia (par-on-NIK-ee-ah) A bacterial infection of the tissue around the nail.

Pedicuring (ped-eh-KYUR-ing) Care of the feet and toenails.

Phalanges (FAY-lanj-ez) The bones that form the fingers.

Plantar warts Warts that appear on the sole of the foot; caused by a virus.

Podiatrist A doctor who specializes in the disorders and diseases of the feet.

Podiatry Study of the disorders and diseases of the feet.

Prognosis (prahg-NOH-siss) The outlook, or forecast, for recovery from a disease.

Pterygium (ter-IJ-ee-uhm) A condition in which the cuticle adheres to the surface of the nail base; caused by unusually dry skin.

Radius (RAYD-ee-uhs) The bone of the arm that attaches to the wrist on the thumb side.

Tinea unguis (UNG-gwis) Ringworm of the nails. See **Onychomycosis.**

Ulna (UHL-nah) The bone of the arm that is attached to the wrist on the same side as the little finger.

Questions

1. What is the part of the nail that extends beyond the fingertip?
2. What is the name for the skin directly beneath the free edge of the nail?
3. What is the channel on either side of the nail called?
4. What part of the fingertip affects nail growth and regeneration?
5. Can nail growth slow as a person grows older?
6. Are contagious diseases treated in the salon?
7. What term is used to refer to any nail disease?
8. Does onychophagy mean ingrown nail?
9. What is the condition in which the nail plate wastes away?
10. Is the forearm bone that leads to the thumb called the radius?
11. What condition is characterized by a thickening of the nail plate?
12. Should tinea of the hand and nail be treated in the salon?
13. Is paronychia a bacterial infection of the tissue around the nail?
14. What are the bones called that make up the wrist?
15. What name is given to the abnormal thickening of the skin in the areas of the elbows and the heels of the feet?
16. What is the name given to a contagious foot disease caused by a virus?

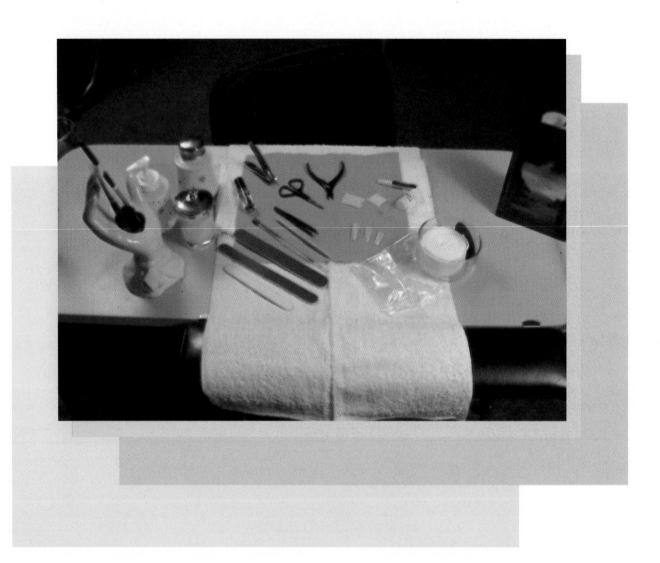

Manicuring and Pedicuring

Learning Objective

Using professional manicuring implements, supplies, and procedures, shape and apply polish to the nails. Your instructor may also require you to be able to give special nail services. Using the proper safety precautions and sanitation methods, manicure the fingernails. Give a plain manicure in 25–40 minutes and an oil manicure in 45–50 minutes. Score 85 percent or better on a multiple-choice exam on the information in this chapter.

In order to achieve the above level of competence, you should master the following chapter objectives.

Theory Objective

1. Identify different nail services and explain when they are given.

Practical Objectives

2. Give a plain or oil manicure (including hand and arm massage).
3. Give a nail wrap.
4. Apply different types of artificial nails.
5. Give a sculptured nail repair with fills.
6. Give a pedicure.

Introduction

Most people like to have a total "look." Some things are obvious; they set the style. Others, like the details in a picture, fill in the overall impression and make it complete. These details could be eliminated, but the total effect, the total "look," would not be the same. Manicuring and pedicuring are two of these details. **Manicuring is the art of caring for the hands and fingernails.** Manicuring completes the appearance of a well-groomed client and complements high-fashion hairstyling and clothing. While most full-service schools and salons offer manicuring, some also provide pedicuring. **Pedicuring is the art of caring for the feet and toenails.**

Many state licensing agencies or boards have a special separate license for persons who have been trained to be manicurists (nail technicians). Therefore, in these states, a person who is not taking the entire cosmetology program can obtain a license as a nail technician. Most states automatically allow a licensed or registered cosmetologist to perform manicuring services.

Nail care has become an important part of the beauty world. Many new products and services have been developed to enhance, beautify, or strengthen the nails. Of course, these new services will bring many more dollars and profit to the person performing them, as well as to the schools and salons.

Theory Objective 1
Different Nail Services and When They are Given

The **basic manicure** service is given to men and women whose fingernails are in a normal condition. "Normal" in this case means that the nails grow normally and do not have any unusual problems, such as brittleness or cracking. The skin surrounding the nails is also healthy. This service usually includes removing nail polish, cleansing, filing, nipping excess skin around the cuticle, applying cuticle/nail builder, applying polish, and applying a sealer coat to protect the polish.

The service usually differs, depending on whether the client is a man or a woman. For example, a man would probably have either a clear polish, a clear paste polish, or a powder polish that simply adds sheen to the nails. A nail buffer is used with the nail paste or **powder pumice polish.** Buffing is done from just below the nail cuticle to the free edge of the nail. By contrast, a woman would probably request polish with color.

The **oil manicure** service is similar to the basic manicure, except that a special skin moisturizing cream or lotion is used to supply or keep moisture in the skin surrounding the nail. The oil manicure prevents hangnails from occurring or will help heal them if they are present.

The **nail wrapping** service strengthens the fingernails. Various fibers, such as very thin sheets of linen or silk, are glued to the nail and then shaped. The fiber is sealed over the free edge of the nail. **Nail wrapping protects the nails** and is helpful for the client who has trouble growing longer nails because of splitting. Clients believe that longer nails will make their fingers look longer, thinner, and more graceful—and they are right! When a fingernail is cut or filed too far down into either side of the nail groove, the free edge of the nail is weakened; breakage or cracks may result. The nail wrap must be done every 2 to 3 weeks, depending on the growth rate of the nail and how much "wear and tear" the nails receive.

Artificial wraps is a general term that is used to describe any one of three or more services. These services include, but are not limited to acrylic sculptured nails, nail tips, nail caps, and artificial nail shells made from porcelain, plastic, or nylon.

For example, **acrylic sculptured nails** really aren't nails at all. They are made from a powder mixed with a special chemical hardener to make a paste. Then, a special form is secured around the nail. The acrylic paste is applied to the nail and then shaped and molded with a brush into a nail shape before it dries. After the acrylic paste has completely dried, the form is removed, and the nail is filed into the desired shape.

◀ Safety Tip

A few words of caution should be kept in mind when you are using artificial nail supplies as well as regular manicuring supplies. **Most nail polish removers (acetone),** hardeners, glues (adhesives), and so forth **are very flammable.** To avoid the threat of fire, **do not smoke and do not allow clients to smoke** during any of these manicuring services!

Sanitation precautions and procedures for manicuring must be followed for the protection of the cosmetologist and the client. For example, orangewood sticks must be discarded after use on each client. All protective and sanitation procedures involving blood-borne infection must be strictly followed. Your state's regulatory body is the authority on these procedures.

Practical Objective 2
Giving a Plain or Oil Manicure (Including Hand and Arm Massage)

Equipment, Supplies, and Materials

- manicure table (Figure 28.1)
- cosmetologist's chair
- client chair
- finger bowl (Figure 28.2)
- closed cotton container
- manicure tray
- small glass or plastic implement container
- hot oil heater
- 2 new emery boards (Figure 28.3)
- metal pusher

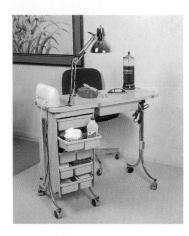

Figure 28.1
A manicure table

- manicure scissors
- buffer (Figure 28.4)
- orangewood stick
- cuticle nipper and scissors (Figure 28.5)
- nail brush
- spatula
- new paper cup for the hot oil heater
- 2 laundered towels
- cotton
- cuticle softener
- cuticle remover (solvent)
- base coat
- sealer (top coat)
- hand lotion or cream
- absorbent tissue
- enamel/polish thinner
- enamel/polish remover
- disposable plastic bag
- 70 percent alcohol
- soap
- nail builder
- nail enamel
- aerosol enamel dryer
- powder or paste nail polish
- manicure oil
- pumice powder

Removing Polish and Shaping the Nails

Procedure

1. Examine the client's nails for irregularities or disease.

2. Help the client decide on a nail shape and an enamel color. Sanitize the client's hand with antiseptic.

3. Saturate a small piece of cotton with the correct nail polish remover. Hold the cotton between the middle and index fingers of your right hand.

4. Hold the client's wrist in one of your hands. Hold the client's finger between your thumb and index finger. Apply the remover to one of the client's nails for 5 seconds; then move the cotton firmly down the

Rationale

1. Never work on a client with an infectious or contagious nail disease. Ask your instructor or manager if you are unsure about the condition of the client's hands.

2. Some clients may select a clear or neutral enamel rather than a color. **Nonacetone remover** must be used on artificial nails.

3. If you hold the cotton this way, you will protect your own nails from the polish remover.

4. Polish (enamel) will dissolve in 5 seconds. Moving the cotton toward the free edge is the easiest way to remove old polish. Polish must be removed from all nails prior to shaping.

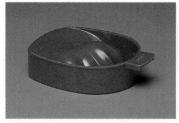

(a)

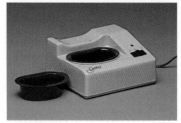

(b) and (c)
Figure 28.2
(a) Finger bowl, (b) electric heater, and (c) paper or plastic cup for lotion (oil).

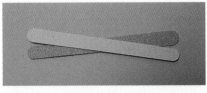

(a)

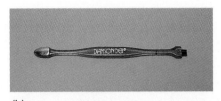

(b)

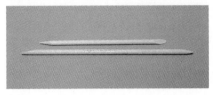

(c)

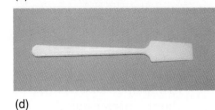

(d)

Figure 28.3
(a) Emery boards, (b) metal pusher (c) orangewood sticks, and (d) spatula.

nail toward the free edge (Figure 28.6). Repeat until all enamel has been removed from each nail.

5. Use a small piece of cotton rolled onto an orangewood stick and saturated with enamel remover to remove polish around the edge of the cuticle of each nail. **Keep the remover away from heat or clients who are smoking.**

6. Make any necessary recommendations to the client regarding the best

5. The cotton protects the client's skin, yet allows for complete removal of old enamel. Nail polish remover is **very flammable.**

6. Consider the client's occupation, leisure activities, age, and finger

 Safety Tip

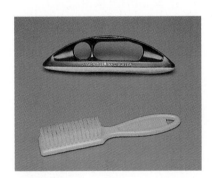

Figure 28.4
Nail buffer (top) and nail brush (bottom)

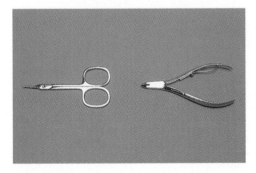

Figure 28.5
Cuticle scissor (left) and cuticle nipper (right)

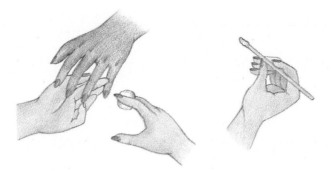

Figure 28.6
Removing polish

nail shape. Discuss the client's preferences.

7. Using a coarse emery board, begin shaping the nail on the little finger of the left hand (Figure 28.7). Always shape the nail from one side toward the center, then from the other side toward the center. Never use a back-and-forth sawing technique. Begin with the little finger and move toward the thumb.

8. Tilt the board slightly so that it touches the bottom side of the nail's free edge (Figure 28.8).

shape. Usually, the shape of the nail should conform to the shape of the finger.

7. If the nails are in good condition, the coarse side of the emery board will shape them quickly. Filing from each side to the center of the nail helps the nail grow evenly. Filing back and forth can cause the nail edge to split or crack as it grows from the finger.

8. If you hold the emery board this way, any mistakes you make will be beneath the free edge.

Figure 28.7
Shaping the nails with an emery board

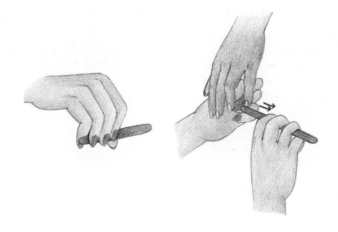

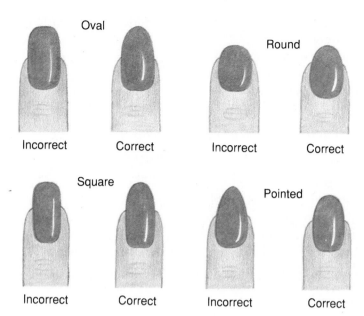

Oval

Incorrect   Correct

Round

Incorrect   Correct

Square

Incorrect   Correct

Pointed

Incorrect   Correct

Figure 28.8
Correct and incorrect nail shapes

These errors can be corrected and will not be visible when enamel is applied.

9. Always file from the corner to the center of the nail. Use quick, smooth, short strokes.

9. Filing in one direction at a time avoids splitting nails.

10. Use the fine side of the emery board to lightly file the edge of the nail downward.

10. The fine side neatly completes the shaping of each nail. The coarse side of the emery board will shred the free edge.

11. When you have finished the nails, place the client's left hand in a bowl containing warm soapy water. If you are giving an oil manicure, check the temperature of the oil in the heater cup. Place the fingers of the client's left hand in the oil cup.

11. The soapy water or hot oil softens the cuticle so that it can be shaped more easily. It is possible for the heater to overheat, so **check the temperature of the oil or lotion.**

◀ Safety Tip

12. Shape the nails of the right hand.

12. This is standard procedure.

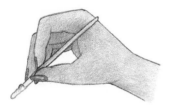

Figure 28.9
A cotton-tipped orangewood stick

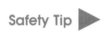

Safety Tip ▶

13. Remove the left hand from the finger bowl and towel-dry each finger. Place the right hand in the soapy water or heated oil.

13. Since both hands will not fit into the finger bowl or cup at once, soak the hands one at a time.

Applying Cuticle Remover and Shaping the Cuticle

Procedure

1. Use a cotton-tipped orangewood stick to apply cuticle remover to each free edge and the cuticle to the left hand (Figure 28.9).

2. Gently push the cuticle back to the fold of the skin (Figure 28.10). Apply styptic powder if the nail bleeds.

3. Reapply cuticle remover as needed.

4. Use a metal pusher to loosen the dead cuticle

Rationale

1. The cuticle remover softens the cuticle and dead skin beneath the free edge. Once softened, they can be removed easily.

2. The cuticle is fragile, so sharp metal instruments must be used carefully. **Styptic** (STIP-tik) **powder** (with alum) or antiseptic astringent will stop minor bleeding. Never use styptic pencils because they are **not sanitary:** they may carry bacteria from one client to another.

3. Cuticle remover may dry out.

4. Shaping the cuticle is easier with the metal pusher. The

Figure 28.10
Soaking the hand softens the cuticle so it can be pushed back more easily.

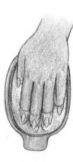

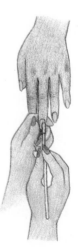

around each nail of the left hand. Return the pusher to the alcoholized cotton in the glass container.

5. Use a cotton-tipped orangewood stick to clean under the nails of the left hand.

6. Use a towel to remove excess cuticle remover from the left hand (Figure 28.11).

7. Using a clean orangewood stick, apply a small amount of nail builder (cuticle cream) to the back of your left hand or directly to the nail.

8. With your index finger, apply cream to each nail. Using the thumb and index finger of both hands, massage the cream into the nails.

9. Massage the client's thumbnail with your left hand. Use your right hand to massage the client's little finger. Use circular movements to massage the nail builder into the nails.

10. Massage all the nails of the left hand.

11. Use an orangewood stick to gently shape the softened cuticle.

12. Carefully use the manicure nipper to remove the

70 percent alcohol keeps metal implements sanitized and prevents the spread of pathogenic bacteria.

5. Cotton protects the skin from the sharp orangewood stick. The cotton also absorbs the cuticle remover and soil from the nails.

6. This will keep the client's hands from becoming too slippery.

7. The orangewood stick must be clean and free from bacteria.

8. This works the cream into the nail plate and surrounding tissue.

9. The nail builder, or cuticle cream, strengthens the nail and surrounding tissue. Circular movements help the nail builder penetrate the nail. Nail builder discourages the development of hangnails.

10. Nail builder, or cuticle cream, must be worked into the surface of each nail plate.

11. This prevents injury.

12. This is standard procedure.

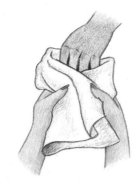

Figure 28.11
Thoroughly dry the fingers and nails.

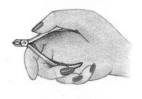
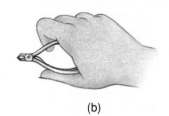

(a)   (b)

Figure 28.12
Using the manicure nipper

ragged cuticle of each nail (Figure 28.12). Put the nipper in alcoholized cotton at the bottom of the implement container.

13. Remove the client's right hand from the finger bowl and towel-dry it.

13. This is standard procedure.

14. Place the client's left hand in the finger bowl or heated oil and repeat steps 1 through 12 on the right hand.

14. The same procedure must be followed on both hands.

15. After you have manicured the client's right hand, apply hand lotion to the client's hand, and work the lotion from the fingertips to above the elbow. Begin the massage at the elbow. Use both hands in a circular motion toward the wrist.

15. This service is added to a manicure.

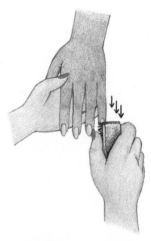

Figure 28.13
Brush in one direction toward the free edge of the nails.

16. Massage down each fingertip and push back the cuticle around each finger.

16. It is easier to push back the cuticle at this point in the manicure.

17. Repeat steps 15 and 16 on the left hand.

17. This is standard procedure.

18. Use a nail brush to scrub the nails of the left hand (Figure 28.13); towel-dry the fingers. If an oil

18. The nail brush removes bits of dead skin and the creams or oils that have been applied.

manicure is given, a finger bowl and warm soapy water will be needed now. Repeat this procedure on the right hand.

19. Check the appearance of the cuticle and the shapes of the nails. Reshape if necessary. Apply cellophane tape to torn or split nails (Figure 28.14).

20. Apply a small amount of nail polish remover to a piece of cotton. Use nail lightener or peroxide to remove any stains. Wipe the nails of both hands.

19. Nail cuticles and free edges should be shaped the same. Tape is applied and trimmed to repair split or broken nails. A cold-wave end paper also works well for patching split nails.

20. The base coat and enamel will not stick unless all traces of oil and creams are removed.

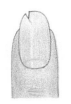
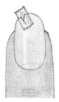

Figure 28.14
Use a nail patch if artificial epoxy-type nails are not available.

Applying Base-Coat Polish

Procedure

1. Apply a clear base coat to the nails of the left hand. Start with the little fingernail and work toward the thumbnail.

2. Hold the base-coat brush between your thumb and index finger (Figure 28.15). Place your little finger on the manicure table. Hold the client's other fingers with your left hand.

3. Apply the base coat in three strokes—from just below the cuticle down the center to the free edge and then along each side of the nail from just below the cuticle to the free edge (Figure 28.16).

Rationale

1. The base coat serves as a primer, or foundation, for the nail enamel.

2. Placing your little finger on the manicure table will steady your hand so that you will not apply the base coat to the cuticle of the nail.

3. Applying the base coat in this way minimizes the possibility of streaking and promotes even drying.

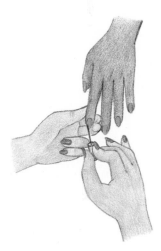

Figure 28.15
Hand positions for applying polish

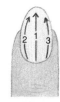

Figure 28.16
Polish strokes

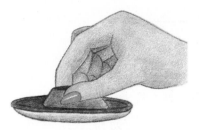

Figure 28.17
Position of the buffer

4. Repeat steps 1 through 3 until you have put a base coat on all nails.

4. This is standard procedure.

5. Roll the enamel bottle between the palms and fingers of both hands.

5. This movement mixes the enamel.

6. Begin applying liquid enamel polish on the little fingernail of the left hand. If clear dry polish is used, apply it and buff the nails (Figure 28.17).

6. Most enamels are lacquers, which give a shiny, varnish-like coating. They are made of a variety of compounds. Many new ones are being developed that give translucent, frosted, and pearl effects. Buffing the nails helps circulation.

7. Follow steps 2 and 3 to apply polish to the nails of the left hand.

7. This is standard procedure.

8. Repeat steps 2 and 3 to apply polish to the nails of the right hand.

8. This is standard procedure.

9. Apply additional coats of polish as needed.

9. Deep colors may require two or three separate applications to produce the proper color or shade.

10. Use a cotton-tipped orangewood stick and nail polish remover to remove polish from the cuticle or the surrounding skin of each finger.

10. Do not allow the client to leave with enamel on the nail's cuticle or surrounding skin.

11. Carefully spray the nails as directed with aerosol enamel dryer.

11. Aerosol drying products shorten the drying time ordinarily required for nail enamel.

12. After the nails are dry, apply a top, or sealer, coat. Use the procedure employed for enamel application.

12. A top coat, or sealer, will prevent the enamel from chipping or cracking between manicures.

13. Sanitize the work area, implements, all bottles, and your hands.

13. This is standard procedure.

Hand and Arm Massage

Manicuring usually includes hand and arm massage. The purpose of hand and arm massage is to increase the circulation of the blood in those areas and to stretch the muscles of the hand and arm. This service also moisturizes the skin, helping it retain its elasticity and flexibility.

The hand and arm massage is performed **after** the filing, soaking, cleaning, and nipping, but **before** polish is applied to the nails. Because the objective is to increase circulation in the arm and hand, the procedure begins at the elbow and ends at the hand. Since the accompanying figures are easy to follow and the steps should not be hard to perform, a rationale for each step has been omitted. Each **manipulation of the hand and arm may be repeated three times.** For example, if the procedure calls for the elbow to be massaged, you may massage it three times before going on to the next step. The exact procedure you use will be determined by your instructor.

1. Sanitize your hands.
2. Pour a small amount of lotion into your hands and rub it around to warm it to a comfortable temperature.
3. Apply lotion along one of the client's arms from the elbow to the hand. Add more lotion, if necessary.
4. Hold the client's wrist with one hand and cup the client's elbow with your other hand. Use a circular motion to massage the client's elbow (Figure 28.18).
5. With both of your hands, use a circular thumb motion in alternating directions to work around the arm from the elbow to the client's wrist (Figure 28.19).
6. Use a **chucking movement** on the forearm and elbow (Figure 28.20). This movement is similar to the movements you would make in wringing out a large **wet** bath towel. Pay

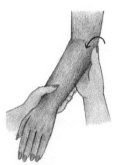

Figure 28.18
Use a circular motion to massage the elbow.

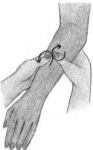

Figure 28.19
Use a circular motion in alternating directions from the elbow to the wrist.

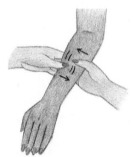

Figure 28.20
Chucking movement

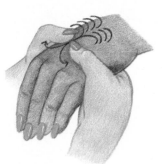

Figure 28.21
Use circular movements down the back of the hand to the knuckles.

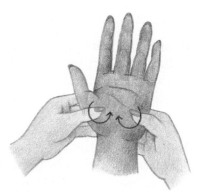

Figure 28.22
Massage from the wrist to the knuckles on the palm of the hand.

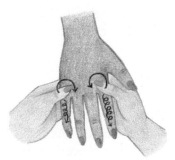

Figure 28.23
Massage each finger.

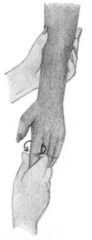

Figure 28.24
Finger rotation

particular attention to massaging the elbow because the skin is often very dry there, and a callus may be forming.

7. After massaging the elbow and forearm, begin a circular chucking movement on the wrist. Then, with the thumbs of both hands, use circular movements to work your way down the back of the hand to the knuckles (Figure 28.21).

8. Repeat the circular thumb movement from the wrist to the knuckles on the palm of the hand (Figure 28.22).

9. Continue the circular thumb movements of both your hands along each side of the client's hand until all the fingers have been massaged (Figure 28.23).

10. Rest the client's elbow on the manicure table; then support the wrist with one of your hands, and gently rotate each finger (Figure 28.24).

11. Take each of the client's fingers (one at a time) between your thumb and index fingertips. Using a gentle squeezing action, slide along the finger about $\frac{1}{4}$ inch (.625 centimeters), and squeeze again. Repeat until all fingers on this hand are done.

12. Gently flex the hand back and forth to relax and limber up the muscles of the hand.

13. Repeat steps 1–12 on the other hand.

Practical Objective 3
Giving a Nail Wrap

The supplies used in the nail wrapping process will depend on the particular "kit" or products used by your school. The following is a partial list of supplies that different manufacturers would be likely to include in a kit:

Supplies

- fast-drying glue (usually 5-second type)
- linen or silk wrapping fiber
- round file/buffer
- emery board
- small scissors
- orangewood stick

Your instructor will tell you the exact steps you will use for a nail wrap. Unless strict sanitation practices are followed, the nail can develop a **fungus** from moisture.

◀ Safety Tip

    When a client is having a regular manicure as well as a nail wrap, the nail wrap is done before the application of a base coat and/or nail polish. A rationale has not been given for each of these short nail wrapping steps.

1. Apply adhesive (glue) across the tip of a **dry** fingernail (Figure 28.25).
2. Apply linen or silk fiber to the nail. The fiber should be applied only to the first ¼ inch (.625 centimeters) of the nail's tip (Figure 28.26).
3. Apply glue to the top of the fiber covering the nail, and briefly hold each side of the fiber across the nail—the glue will "set up" in 5–10 seconds and is called "5-second glue" (Figure 28.27).
4. Trim excess fiber, but leave enough to tuck under the free edge of the nail (Figure 28.28). If you are using a silk fiber, remember **not** to tuck it under the free edge. Apply more glue under the free edge of the nail. Use the flat end (some prefer the pointed end) of an orangewood stick to smooth the line under the free edge.
5. Use downward strokes of your emery board to shape the excess fiber to match the shape of the nail's sides and free edge (Figure 28.29).

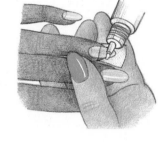

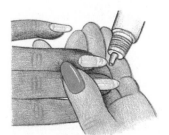

Figure 28.25
Make sure the fingernail is dry before applying adhesive across the tip.

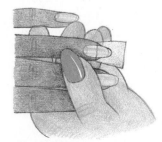

Figure 28.26
Apply fiber (linen or silk) only to the first ¼ inch (.625 centimeters) of nail.

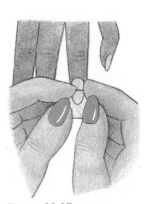

Figure 28.27
Apply glue to the top of the fiber and hold until it is "set up."

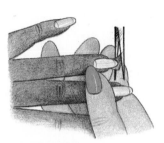

Figure 28.28
Trim the fiber per the manufacturer's instructions.

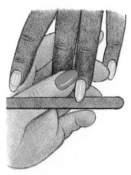

Figure 28.29
Shape with an emery board.

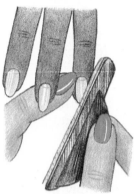

Figure 28.30
Shape and smooth with a round file/buffer.

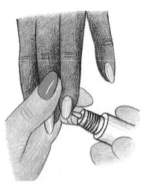

Figure 28.31
Apply additional glue as necessary, filing after each application.

6. Using the round file/buffer, shape and smooth the nail seam on the top of the nail and the nail tip (Figure 28.30).
7. Apply additional glue to ensure proper bonding between the nail and the fiber (Figure 28.31).
8. Repeat the application of glue/filing procedure until the seam becomes almost invisible. The seam should "feather" from below the seam through the nail tip.
9. Repeat steps 1–8 for each nail.
10. Your client has the option of having polish applied or simply leaving the nails natural.

A variety of artificial nail products are available for professional use. This objective will explain two types: **acrylic sculptured nails** and **nail tips** (also called caps). **The main purpose of both products is to extend the length of the fingernails,** giving the fingers a more slender, graceful appearance. This service would normally follow the basic manicure, except that no polish or base coat would be applied before the application of either type of artificial nails.

Remember that many of these products are flammable! Do not allow smoking in the immediate area in which you are working! Store supplies away from heat.

◀ Safety Tip

Since most of these nails come in a "kit" from the manufacturer, it is difficult to identify a supply list for these services. One kit may include a powder or hardener that another kit does not. At least a partial list of supplies would be as follows:

Supplies

- manicure scissors
- nail forms or tips
- adhesive (glue)
- brush
- round nail file/buffer
- emery board
- orangewood stick
- solvent

Note: Your instructor will have the best list of supplies for the particular procedure you should follow. Always follow the manufacturer's directions.

Acrylic Sculptured Nail Procedure

1. Use the emery board to roughen the surface of the nail plate (Figure 28.32).
2. Apply nail forms and secure along the side of the fingertip (Figure 28.33). Be careful not to slant the tip of the forms in a downward direction. If you do, the finished nail will have an unnatural downward slope that will be unattractive.
3. **Carefully read and follow the manufacturer's directions on mixing the acrylic paste.** Apply the acrylic paste with a clean brush, beginning at the free edge and working to the end of the nail form.
4. Apply the acrylic paste to the center of the nail plate and smoothly work it across the entire natural nail, blending it into the nail form (Figure 28.34). Allow nails to dry for 5 minutes, or as directed.
5. Carefully remove forms.
6. File each nail to the desired length and shape. Seal and apply nail enamel, or buff and allow nails to appear natural (Figure 28.35).

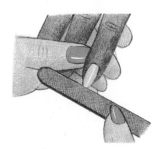

Figure 28.32
Roughen the surface with an emery board.

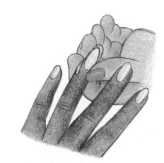

Figure 28.33
Apply nail forms and secure.

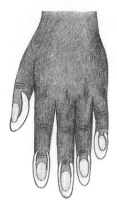

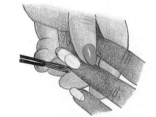

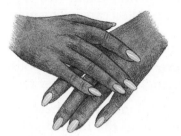

Figure 28.34
Start in the center of the nail plate, and work across the entire nail. Blend the acrylic paste into the nail form and dry.

Figure 28.35
File, seal, and apply enamel, or buff for "natural" nails.

Safety Tip ▶

Note: Use regular polish remover (acetone) to **remove a sculptured nail. Follow the manufacturer's directions.** Use a rolling motion to peel the sculptured nail away from the natural nail. Don't pry off the artificial nail. Pulling may injure the nail permanently! Clean the brush and mixing container immediately after use, or they will become unusable. Tightly cover all bottles.

Practical Objective 5
Giving a Sculptured Nail Repair with Fills

If an existing acrylic nail is badly damaged, you may want to simply clip to the right the free edge end; then fill from the base of the nail to the free edge and blend to a smooth, even surface.

1. Remove any nail polish.
2. Clip any loose material from the nail bed; using a rolling motion in a clockwise direction to remove any broken material.
3. Lightly roughen the new nail growth or exposed area with an emery board; then dust the nail to remove any residue.
4. Apply primer to the prepared area, following the manufacturer's instructions.
5. Saturate the tip of your brush with liquid nail forming material; then dip the brush into the powder formula and form the mixture into a small "ball."
6. Place the ball on the exposed area and mold it into the space between the cuticle and the artificial nail. Be sure to shape the material with your brush so that it blends smoothly into the artificial nail. Let this nail dry and go on to the next nail that you will be repairing.

7. Use the emery board to reshape the nail as needed; then buff so that the nail has a smooth look and feel.

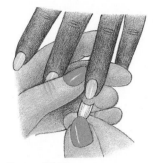

1. Work only in an area that has good ventilation.

2. Avoid contamination (by germs) of the nail after the antiseptic nail primer has been applied.

3. Carefully label all bottles and keep them tightly capped to avoid spills.

4. Examine nails for discoloration (green or gray nail spots could indicate the presence of a fungus growth), which may require medical treatment.

5. Do not apply artificial nails over a fungus growth.

6. Store nail chemicals away from heat or sources of open flame.

7. Thoroughly clean all brushes and mixing containers as directed by the manufacturer.

Figure 28.36
Match the tip to the client's nail and file to fit.

Nail Tip Procedure

1. Give a basic manicure up to the base coat/polish step.
2. Match the nail tip to client's nails (Figure 28.36). File to adjust small differences.
3. Apply glue to the nail groove of the nail tip to be used (Figure 28.37).
4. Place the tip across the free edge of the nail and adjust the placement with an orangewood stick (Figure 28.38). Hold the client's finger in a downward position so that the glue doesn't run onto the cuticle. Polish remover on the end of a cotton-tipped orangewood stick can be used to clean up small amounts of glue.
5. Use your manicure scissors to trim straight across the tips from the corner to the center (Figure 28.39).

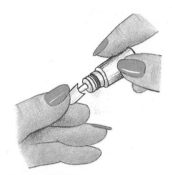

Figure 28.37
Apply glue to the nail groove of the nail tip.

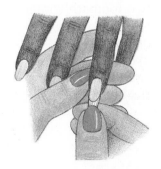

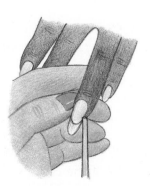

Figure 28.38
Place the nail tip across the free edge and adjust with an orangewood stick.

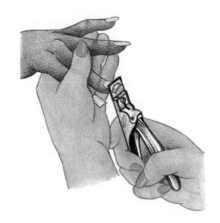
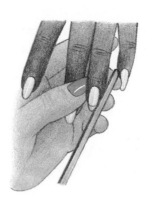

Figure 28.39
Trim the tips with manicure scissors and shape with an emery board.

6. Use an emery board to shape the nail to the contour of the client's finger.
7. Pay particular attention to the nail seam when buffing to achieve a "natural" look from the nail plate to the sculptured extension.
8. Apply glue to the seam and tip for added durability, strength, and smoothness. Repeat as needed.
9. Proceed until all nails have been done.

Note: Patches are available to fix a tip that has split or cracked. An acrylic "overlay" may also be used to extend the life of a nail tip.

Practical Objective 6
Giving a Pedicure

Since the steps in pedicuring are similar to those in manicuring, the rationales have been omitted.

Supplies

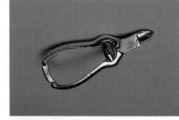

Figure 28.40
Toenail clipper

- 3 terry towels
- disposable emery board (nail file)
- antiseptic/disinfectant
- toenail clipper (Figure 28.40)
- cuticle remover
- nail polish
- cotton
- nail polish remover

- nail massage cream
- moisturizing lotion
- two footbath containers
- orangewood stick or plastic pusher
- plastic refuse bag
- nail builder cream
- alcohol

Preliminary Steps of a Pedicure

1. Soak both of the client's feet in disinfectant solution for 4–5 minutes (Figure 28.41). (The solution should cover the ankle.) Then dry with a terry towel (Figure 28.42).

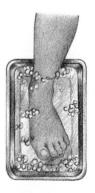

Figure 28.41
Make sure the disinfectant covers the ankle.

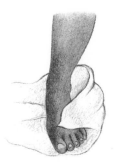

Figure 28.42
Soak feet in disinfectant for 4–5 minutes and dry with a towel.

2. Use nail polish remover to remove polish from the toenails (Figure 28.43).
3. Shape the toenails with an emery board and/or toenail clipper, depending on how long the nails are (Figure 28.44). Remember not to file or clip the nails too far into the corners, or the client may develop an ingrown nail. Shape the nails straight across, then gradually round the corners.
4. Check the other foot, which is still soaking in the footbath, at this time.
5. Apply cuticle remover and use an orangewood stick or plastic pusher to carefully remove unneeded cuticle. **Be careful** not to injure the matrix of the nail. **Do not** use metal pushers.
6. Apply nail cream around cuticle and massage. Then, clean the free edges of the nails, using a cotton-tipped orangewood

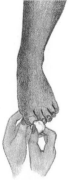

Figure 28.43
Remove old nail polish.

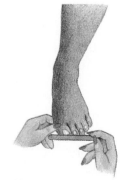

Figure 28.44
Shape with an emery board or toenail clipper.

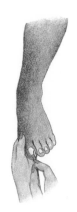

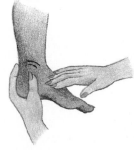

Figure 28.45
Massage around the cuticle with nail cream; then clean the free edge with a cotton-tipped orangewood stick.

Figure 28.46
Apply moisturizer and massage.

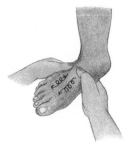

Figure 28.47
Massage from the instep to the first toe digit.

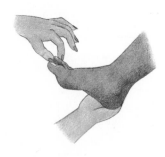

Figure 28.48
Rotate each toe three times.

stick (never re-use an orangewood stick) and polish remover and solvent (Figure 28.45).

7. Apply moisturizing cream to the foot and massage (Figure 28.46). Give extra manipulations to the heel and sides of the foot.

8. Remove the other foot from the footbath and dry thoroughly. Nip cuticle as needed.

9. Repeat steps 2, 3, 5, 6, and 7 on the foot you have just dried.

10. Using the footbath and nail brush, remove excess moisturizing lotion, massage cream, and cuticle cream from the nails of each foot. Dry each foot.

Foot Massage

1. Rest the heel of the foot on a footstool.

2. Apply a small amount of massage cream evenly from the ankle to the toes.

3. Using your thumbs in firm rotating movements, massage the skin from the instep of the ankle down to the first digit of the toes (Figure 28.47).

4. Return to the instep and repeat the massage three times.

5. Continue until the entire top area of the foot has been massaged.

6. Support the client's heel with one hand and rotate each toe with the thumb and index finger of the other hand (Figure 28.48). Repeat three times.

7. Now rotate the foot from the ankle (Figure 28.49). Repeat three times.

8. Massage the entire sole of the foot, using a rotating manipulation with your thumbs (Figure 28.50).

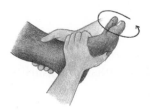

Figure 28.49
Rotate the foot from the ankle.

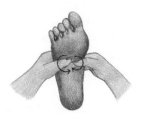

Figure 28.50
Massage the sole of the foot.

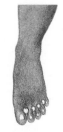

Figure 28.51
Separate toes with cotton.

9. Repeat steps 1 through 8 on the other foot.
10. Sanitize the work area.

Application of Nail Polish

1. Place cotton between the toes to separate each toe for the application of polish; otherwise, the nails may smear (Figure 28.51).
2. Double-check each nail to make sure all cream films(s) have been removed, or the polish won't stick to the nail. Remove any residues with cotton dampened with alcohol. Place new cotton strips between the toes.
3. Apply a base coat to the toenails of one foot (Figure 28.52).
4. Repeat steps 1 through 3 on the other foot.
5. Apply nail enamel (polish) to one foot; then the other. Allow at least 20 minutes for the enamel to dry before permitting the client to put on footwear.
6. Sanitize your work area and discard soiled supplies, such as used cotton, orangewood sticks, refuse bags, and so forth. Sanitize footbath containers and other equipment.

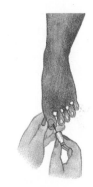

Figure 28.52
Apply the base coat, then enamel.

Glossary

Acetone The chief ingredient of some nail polish removers for natural nails.

Acrylic sculptured nails Artificial fingernails that are formed from acrylic paste and shaped on the client.

Alum Used in styptic powder to stop bleeding.

Artificial nails Materials shaped to look like fingernails.

Artificial nail shells A type of artificial nails made from porcelain, plastic, or nylon.

Chucking movement A massage technique similar to wringing out a towel.

Manicuring Care of the hands and fingernails.

Nail caps A type of artificial nails used to extend natural fingernails.

Nail tips See **Nail caps.**

Nail wrapping A service to protect the fingernails from breakage.

Nonacetone polish remover Used to remove polish from artificial nails.

Pedicuring Care of the feet and toenails.

Powder pumice polish Very fine powder used to polish (shine) fingernails and toenails, resulting in clear, shiny nails.

Styptic (STIP-tik) powder A powder that will stop minor bleeding.

Questions

1. What is the art of caring for the hands and fingernails?
2. What is the art of caring for the feet and toenails?
3. True or false. Manicures are given exclusively to men.
4. Is a special skin moisturizer used in an oil manicure?
5. Does nail wrapping weaken the nail?
6. Are acrylic sculptured nails made in different sizes?
7. Are nail polish removers and adhesives likely to catch fire when exposed to a spark or flame?
8. Would you normally use a cotton-tipped orangewood stick and polish remover to remove polish from around the cuticle?
9. Before shaping the nails, should you remove all polish?
10. Should nails be filed from one side to the center?
11. Should you use quick, smooth strokes when filing the nails?
12. Are styptic pencils a sanitary way to stop bleeding?
13. Is using 70 percent ethyl alcohol (99 percent isopropyl alcohol) to sanitize metal manicure implements an effective way to control germs in the salon?
14. Is it a good idea to leave a thin film of polish around the cuticle to protect it?
15. Is nail lightener or peroxide used to remove stains from the nails?
16. Will nail polish adhere properly to a nail that is **not** thoroughly dry?
17. Is "chucking" a massage movement?
18. Are nail tips sometimes called nail caps?
19. If you aren't careful during the application, can an acrylic sculptured nail end up sloped in an unnatural downward direction?
20. True or false. Manicure scissors are never used to shorten nail tips that are too long. The tips should only be filed.
21. Are small toe towels used between the toes during the application of nail polish when giving a pedicure?
22. Is a base coat used on the toenails as well as the fingernails?

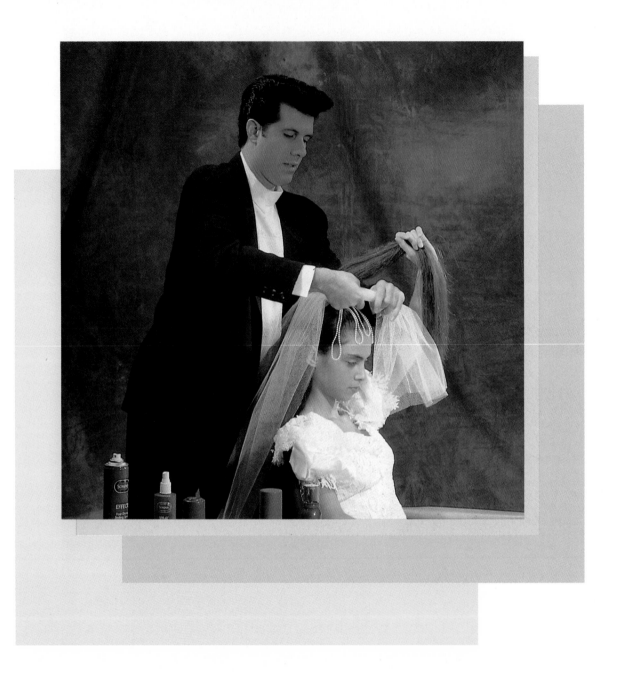

Wigs and Hairpieces

Learning Objective

Use professional wiggery supplies and implements to fit, shape, clean, set, and style a wig and hairpiece. Using the proper steps and safety precautions, clean a wig in 20 minutes, set it in 25 minutes, and comb it into a finished hairstyle in 20 minutes. Also, clean a hairpiece in 15 minutes, set it in 10–20 minutes, and comb it into the client's hair in 15–30 minutes. Score 85 percent or better on a multiple-choice exam on the information in this chapter.

In order to achieve the above level of competence, you should master the following chapter objectives.

Theory Objectives

1. Describe the various types of wigs and hairpieces, and explain how they are made, colored, and styled.
2. Explain how wigs are measured and altered.

Men and women have worn wigs and hairpieces for thousands of years. Until only 20 to 25 years ago, hairpieces were something of a status symbol. They were very expensive, and only very wealthy people could afford to buy them. Recently, modern manufacturing methods have lowered the cost of hairpieces so that many more people can afford them.

Today, people wear wigs for many different reasons. Some wear wigs to cover baldness. Others feel that a hairpiece gives them a new look and improves their appearance. Many people who lead fast-paced lives find that wearing a wig is the only practical way they can look good and meet the demands of a busy schedule.

Making hairpieces has become such a large industry that many states have separate licenses for the care and styling of hairpieces. Cosmetologists usually receive instruction on hairpieces and practice caring for them as **part** of their training, so additional licensing and training are not really necessary.

Since most salons try to offer a full range of services to their clients, knowledge and skill in servicing hairpieces are an important part of any basic training program. The demand for people who can care for and style hairpieces has created a new source of income for schools and salons.

Theory Objective 1
Types of Wigs and Hairpieces and Their Construction, Coloring, and Styling

Types of Wigs and Hairpieces

The terms **hairpieces** and **hairgoods** are used to describe any of the following: wigs, toupees, postiches, wiglets, cascades, chignons, switches, and falls (or minifalls).

Wigs usually are hairpieces that cover 80 to 100 percent of the head. A **toupee** is also a wig, but it is considered a special kind of hairpiece. It ordinarily covers **less** than 80 percent of a client's head.

Postiches (pos-TEESH-ez) are small hairpieces made from angora and yak hair. They are round at the base and are used in an ornamental way, usually in competition hairstyling. Pastel colors can be applied to them for "fantasy" styling effects.

Wiglets vary in size and length. They are put on different areas of the head to complement or enhance the hairstyle. Often an individual will use more than one wiglet in the hair for "cocktail" or "evening" styles.

Cascades have oval-shaped bases. They vary in length from 4 to 8 inches (10 to 20 centimeters) and are worn in the upper and lower crown sections (Figure 29.1). A cascade is larger than a wiglet, but smaller than a fall.

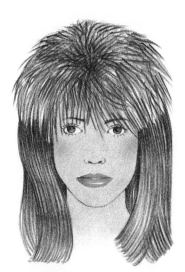

Figure 29.1
A cascade

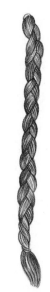

Figure 29.2
A chignon

Chignons (SHEEN-yahnz) and **switches** are long tresses of hair secured at one end that are used to add height or volume to hairstyles. They are arranged in knots, braided, or woven through the hair (Figures 29.2, 29.3, and 29.4).

Falls are long hairpieces of varying size. A fall has a base that is larger than a cascade but smaller than a wig. Usually secured in the crown section of the head, a fall may be arranged casually or set and combed into a very elaborate "haute coiffure." Minifalls are simply small falls (Figure 29.5).

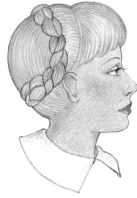

Figure 29.3
A chignon in a hairstyle

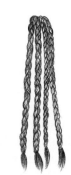

Figure 29.4
Braids

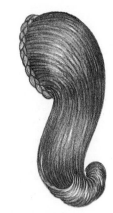

Figure 29.5
A minifall

Hairpiece Construction

Hairpieces are made from human and synthetic hair. **Human hair** is classified as European, Oriental (Asiatic), and, less often, West Indian. The consensus seems to be that **European hair** is the easiest to arrange. It also is the most expensive. Oriental or Asiatic hair is usually coarser and has a tendency to curl too much unless rather large rollers are used. Although Oriental and West Indian hair are somewhat more difficult to style than European hair, they are also less expensive. Most hairpieces are made in Japan, Korea, or Europe.

Hairpieces made of **synthetic** (human-made) **fibers** are much less expensive than pieces made from human hair. In the past, the synthetic fibers used in hairpieces were too shiny and looked unnatural; today, however, modern technology has improved their appearance so much that many professional synthetic hairpieces are sold in schools and salons. Some people prefer synthetic hairpieces because they are made with a permanent curl. Unlike hairpieces made from human hair, which must be set/styled, synthetic hairpieces only have to be cleaned, dried, and then combed.

Professional hairpieces made from either synthetic fibers or human hair may be purchased directly from the manufacturer or from a professional beauty and barber supplier.

You can use a simple test to find out if a wig is made of human or synthetic hair. Cut a single hair from the hairpiece, and burn it with a lighted match. If it is synthetic, it will melt, and a bead will form on the end. You will notice very little odor. If the hair is human, you will notice a strong sulfur odor (from the sulfur in the hair).

Human and synthetic hairpieces are made in one of two ways—hand-tied or machine-wefted. **Hand-tied hairpieces** are usually quite expensive because, as the name implies, each hair is sewn by hand one at a time to a mesh (netting) cap that forms the base. Machine-made hairpieces are less expensive because a machine sews the hair to a strip of material called a **weft.** The wefts are then sewn in ¼-inch (.625-centimeter) lengths to a mesh cap.

In the 1960s, at the beginning of the modern wig boom, many people preferred hand-tied wigs because machine-tied wigs often were bulky, heavy, and difficult to style. Modern technology, however, has developed "ventilated," light, natural-looking machine-made wigs.

Safety Tip ▶ Hand-tied hairpieces **must** be cleaned with a special **dry cleaning** fluid made just for hair. The dry cleaner is necessary to prevent the mesh in the cap from loosening, which could lead to hair loss from the wig. You should be very careful when you use dry cleaning fluids because many of them are **flammable.** Do not work around anyone with a lighted cigarette or any other flame that could start a fire. Try to use this fluid only in open, well-ventilated areas of the salon. Synthetic wigs are cleaned with a nonflammable cleaner that is similar, but not identical, to shampoo.

Coloring of Hairpieces

Hairpieces are colored (dyed) to match the 70 color choices on the **JL color ring.** All hairpieces have "processed" colors rather than natural ones. Human hair (regardless of color) is boiled many hours in chemicals that clean and take out its color. When the hair is pure white, it is dyed with a fabric color **(not a tint)** that matches one of the colors on the JL color ring. Synthetic hair is also dyed with a fabric color to match one of the colors on the ring. **Hairpieces need conditioning** because the sun causes those processed colors to become lighter, in the same way that natural hair can become "sun lightened."

Human hairpieces can be colored with professional temporary, semipermanent, or permanent products. However, since the hair has already been "processed," **coloring is risky** and the results are unpredictable. If a hairpiece requires a drastic color change, you should warn the client that the results cannot be guaranteed. Since mass production has substantially lowered the cost of hairpieces, advise the client to purchase a new hairpiece. Considering the cost of supplies and the cost of your time, coloring a hairpiece may be a very expensive service for the client.

Synthetic hairpieces may be dyed with over-the-counter fabric or vegetable colors. Professional tints and lighteners **should not** be used on synthetic hairpieces.

When any type of hairpiece is colored, you must be sure to protect the mesh cap or wefting from any contact with tint, lightener, or toning material. Oxidizing tints, lighteners, and toners will cause the wefting fabric to deteriorate (weaken).

Theory Objective 2
Measuring and Altering

Several basic pieces of equipment that are used in measuring and altering hairpieces are shown in Figure 29.6. The wig is placed on a

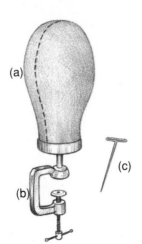

Figure 29.6
(a) The canvas block (head) holds the wig for styling; (b) a wig clamp supports the canvas block; and (c) the T-pin secures the wig to the canvas block. Note: a plastic bag is usually put over the canvas block to protect it from water, setting lotions, and the like.

canvas block (a) that is held in place on the styling station by a **wig clamp** (b). A **T-pin** (c) is used to hold the wig on the canvas block. The block is usually covered with a plastic bag to protect the canvas cloth from water and setting lotions.

A client's head can be measured for a hairpiece in several simple steps. Measure the distance from the **front** center hairline to the center **nape** hairline (Figure 29.7a). Measure from each hairline to the beginning of the crown (Figure 29.7b), then from each side hairline to the beginning of the nape section (Figure 29.7c). Transfer the measurements to the canvas block. Use a pencil to write on the plastic cover. Now measure the distance around the head (Figure 29.7d) and the width of the nape hairline (Figure 29.7e). Transfer both measurements to the canvas block.

Figure 29.7
Measuring the client's head size

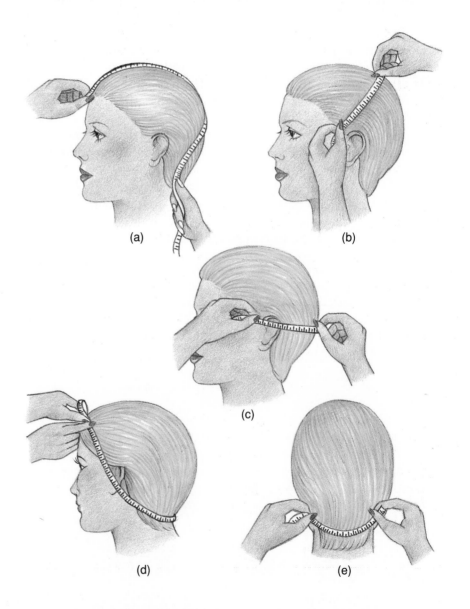

(a)

(b)

(c)

(d)

(e)

Figures 29.8 through 29.12 show how you can alter a hairpiece that is too large for the client's head. Figure 29.13 shows some examples of styled wigs and hairpieces.

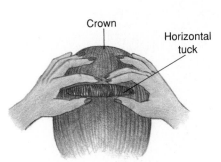

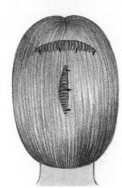

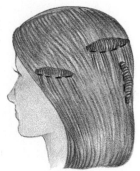

Figure 29.8
Gather the extra wefting in the crown section first, and carefully mark it horizontally with T-pins.

Figure 29.9
Gather the extra wefting and mark a vertical tuck.

Figure 29.10
If the wig comes down over the tops of the client's ears, put horizontal tucks on each side of the wig.

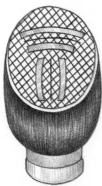

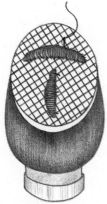

Figure 29.11
Remove the wig and place hair-setting tape on the inside of the wig along the fold of each tuck. Pull the T-pins from the outside of the wig. Turn the wig inside out again, and pull the tuck to the inside of the wig. The base of the tuck should come between the strips of hair-setting tape.

Figure 29.12
Use a needle and special thread to stitch the base of the tuck. Then sew the top of the tuck flat against the wefting of the wig.

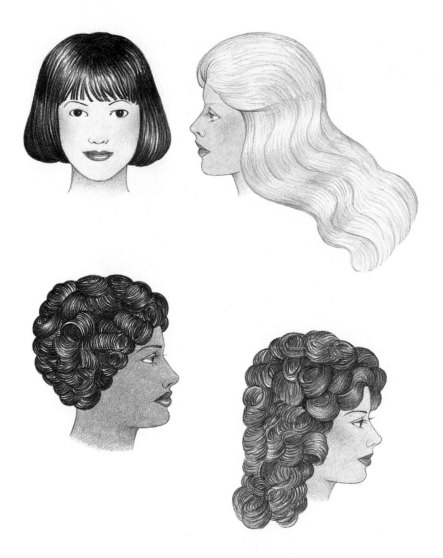

Figure 29.13
Some examples of wigs

Glossary

Cascade A hairpiece from 4 to 8 inches (10 to 20 centimeters) long with an oval-shaped base that is worn in the upper or lower crown section.

Chignon (SHEEN-yahn) A long tress of hair secured at one end; used to add volume or height to a hairstyle.

Fall A long hairpiece with a base larger than a cascade but smaller than a wig.

Hand-tied hairpiece A hairpiece in which each hair is sewn individually to the mesh cap.

JL color ring The 70 standardized colors that are used to dye human and synthetic hairpieces.

Postiche (pos-TEESH) A small hairpiece that is made from angora and yak hair; used as an ornament.

Switches Long tresses of hair secured at one end.

Synthetic fibers Fibers made of materials other than natural animal or human hair; used to make wigs.

Toupee A hairpiece that covers less than 80 percent of a client's head.

Weft The strip of material to which the hair is sewn in a machine-made hairpiece.

Wig A hairpiece that covers from 80 to 100 percent of the head.

Wiggery The services of fitting, shaping, cleaning, setting, and styling wigs and hairpieces.

Wiglet A hairpiece that may vary in size and length and may be put on different areas of the head to complement or enhance a hairstyle.

Yak hair Animal hair that is used to make postiches.

Questions

1. What should you use to clean a wig made with human hair?
2. What is a weft?
3. What is the difference between a wig and a toupee?
4. In a hand-tied hairpiece, is the hair actually sewn entirely by hand to the mesh base?

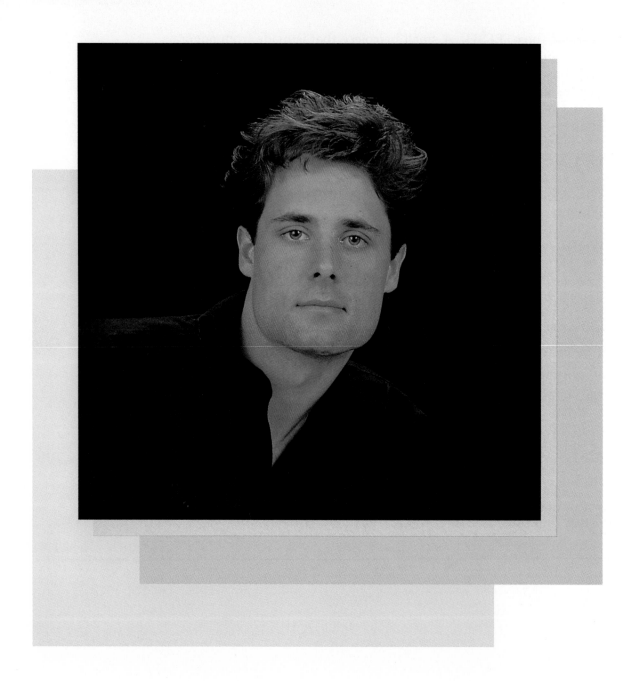

Shaving

Learning Objective

Given the material in this chapter, score 85 percent or better on a multiple-choice exam on the information in this chapter.

In order to achieve the above level of competence, you should master the following chapter objectives.

Theory Objectives

1. Describe the supplies, implements, and equipment used in shaving.
2. Identify shaving safety precautions.

Practical Objective

3. Shave the client.

Introduction

The one personal grooming service that most men perform daily is the shaving of their face. Although this service is usually not given in the beauty salon, shaving is performed in barber shops and barber styling salons. Because some states have combined cosmetologists and barbers under one licensing board, the shaving service has been included in this book.

Theory Objective 1
Shaving Supplies,
Implements, and
Equipment

Shaving the client's face requires supplies and equipment that are not typically found in the salon. Among the special equipment needed for shaving are a barber chair, hot lather machine (**electric latherizer**), straight razor, hone, and strop.

The most expensive equipment used in the shaving service is the **barber chair.** This chair differs from a hydraulic hairstyling chair in that it not only goes up and down, but also has an adjustable back. Because men tend to weigh more than women, barber chairs are also made of heavier materials to support the extra weight.

Lather is basically soap suds. In a barber salon, lather may be dispensed from a regular barber **latherizing** machine, which preheats the lather before it is dispensed (Figure 30.1). Preheated lather softens the facial hair faster and feels more comfortable to the client. Lather may also be used from an aerosol can or even the old-fashioned "shaving mug." In the mug method, a small bar of special soap is placed at the bottom of the mug. Hot water is added (Figure 30.2). Then, a brush is used to stir the mixture into a lather before it is applied to the face. A disposable paper liner should be placed in

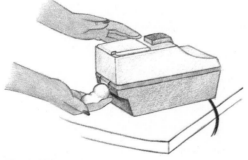

Figure 30.1
A latherizing machine
dispenses preheated lather.

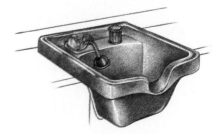

Figure 30.2
A barber bowl

the mug for each client. A new, sanitized bar of soap should also be used for each client.

Using a circular motion, you work the lather into the beard with your fingertips or a shaving brush. The lather softens the beard and provides a protective surface on which the blade of the razor "floats" as it cuts the beard hair.

Although disposable razors are available, in a barber salon, the **straight razor** is the shaving implement of choice (Figure 30.3). It must be used with extreme caution because it is extremely sharp and can cut the skin merely by touching it. For this reason, it is important that the blade and handle of the razor be correctly balanced. This means that the weight of the blade (metal cutting part) of the razor should be the same as the weight of the handle. A properly balanced razor will be safer and easier to use. To determine a **razor's balance,** open the razor and lay its center across one finger. The razor should "balance" there rather than tipping to one side or the other. Note that with a straight razor there is no cutting "guard" to protect you or your client as there is with the razor shaper used for hair cutting (Figure 30.4). Be careful!

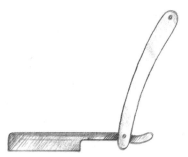

Figure 30.3
A straight razor

Since most beard hair has a very coarse texture, the razor must have an extremely sharp edge so it can remove the hair without a painful drag (scrape) across the client's face. Be careful not to use too much pressure. Remember the point of the razor goes before the rest of the blade (Figure 30.5).

The cutting edge of the straight razor is made of very high quality tempered steel. Since the blade is not replaceable, it will need to be sharpened from time to time. A straight razor is sharpened in two steps: first, by using a **hone** and then by using a **strop.**

The **hone** is a natural or manufactured piece of stone about the size of a pocket calculator. It has an abrasive surface that is harder than the steel of the blade. Drawing the edge of the razor across the hone in a figure-eight pattern grinds the edge of the blade

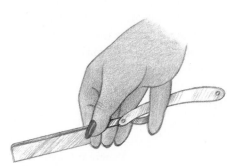

Figure 30.4
Hold the razor as shown to avoid injuring yourself or your client.

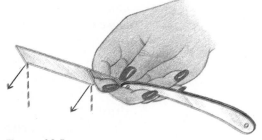

Figure 30.5
The point of the razor should go before the rest of the blade.

to the desired degree of sharpness. The hone is usually dampened with water before the razor is sharpened; then after the sharpening, the water is wiped off along with any tiny bits of metal from the razor.

The **strop** is a specially tanned strip of leather used to make the edge of the razor keener, smoother, and sharper. The strop feathers the edge of the razor. To use a strop, hold the blade of the razor perpendicular to the strop, then drag the razor across the strop with a long back-and-forth motion.

Theory Objective 2
Shaving Safety
Precautions

Before shaving the client, you should carefully examine the condition of the skin. Note any irritation, inflammation, or suspected contagious lesions. If the skin is simply irritated, you should advise against the use of a steamer towel before the shave. The **steamer towel** is usually soaked in hot water, wrung out, then wrapped around the client's face after the lather has been applied. If the skin appears irritated, skip this step. If you suspect that the client has a contagious or infectious skin disease, explain the condition to the client, stop the service, and recommend that the client see a dermatologist or family doctor.

Special note should also be made of **ingrown hairs.** Often this condition is the result of being shaved too close. In shaving, you hold the area of the skin to be shaved taut with the fingertips of one hand and stroke with the razor with the other hand. If too much pressure is applied to the razor, the shave will be "too close" and will actually cut the hair below the surface of the skin. This causes the hair to become **ingrown** or to grow beneath the surface of the skin rather than through it. Curly hair, in particular, when shaved too close, tends to grow to the side—beneath the skin and alongside the epidermis rather than out to the surface of the skin.

Usually, an ingrown hair can be treated by applying a drying agent such as a benzol peroxide lotion. The lotion dries the skin and causes it to flake open enough for the hair to come out. Otherwise, the client may have to go to a dermatologist who will make a tiny cut (incision) or tiny burn to form an opening that will allow the hair to come out from beneath the skin, rather than grow inside it. You should not remove any ingrown hairs for the client.

Just as you would be careful when using sharp implements during the haircutting process, you should be careful not to cut the client's skin, particularly around the eyes, ears, nose, mouth, and the Adam's apple area of the neck. Also, be careful not to scrape the skin.

If you accidentally "nick" the client, you can control **bleeding** from a small cut by applying pressure, an antiseptic, and then a styptic powder (see Chapter 3). Remember to wash your hands and sanitize your razor with 70 percent alcohol before and after each client. To protect the client from possible infection, some barbers prefer to shave the face with a disposable razor.

Supplies

- cape/chair cloth
- neck strip
- lather
- towels
- razor
- shampoo cape or chair cloth

Drape the client as shown in Figures 30.6 through 30.10. In shaving, the face and neck are divided into 14 sections. Figures 30.11 and

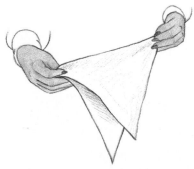

Figure 30.6
Fold the towel as shown.

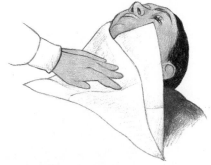

Figure 30.7
Place the towel at the base of the client's neck.

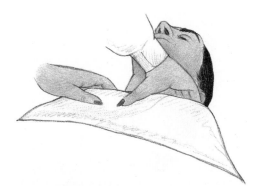

Figure 30.8
Tuck the towel under the cape and the client's shirt to protect the clothing.

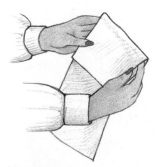

Figure 30.9
Another towel will be used to remove lather and beard hair.

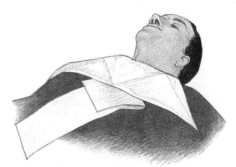

Figure 30.10
Place the lather towel underneath the first towel.

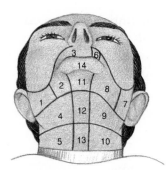

Figure 30.11
Sections for right-handed barbers

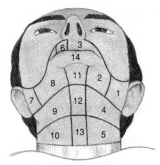

Figure 30.12
Sections for left-handed barbers

30.12 show the order in which right-handed and left-handed barbers, respectively, would shave the sections. Figure 30.13 through 30.26 illustrate the proper strokes to use throughout the shave.

Figure 30.13 (right)
*Use a freehand shaving movement beginning at the right sideburn. Remember to **stretch** the skin with the other hand, so the razor strokes along a smooth path of skin.*

Figure 30.14 (far right)
Use a backhand movement from the cheek to the chin.

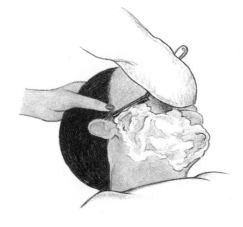

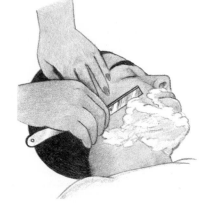

Figure 30.15 (right)
Use a downward stroke on the right side of the upper lip. Be careful not to scrape or cut the skin.

Figure 30.16 (far right)
Use a downward stroke below the chin.

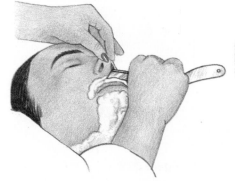

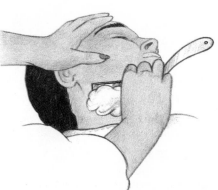

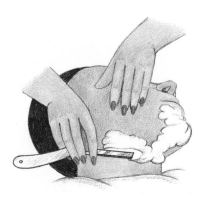

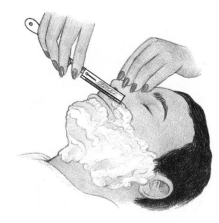

Figure 30.17 (far left)
The neck may be shaved with either an upward or a downward stroke. The important point to remember is to stroke in the direction of the hair growth.

Figure 30.18 (left)
Use a downward backhand stroke on the left side of the upper lip.

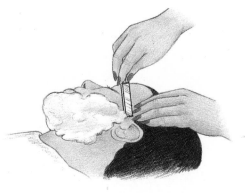

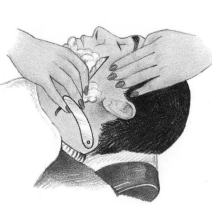

Figure 30.19 (far left)
Use a downward stroke at the left sideburn.

Figure 30.20 (left)
Shave downward across the cheek to the chin.

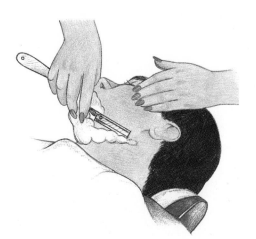

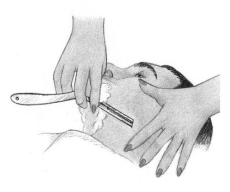

Figure 30.21 (far left)
Use a backhand stroke below the jaw.

Figure 30.22 (left)
Shave the neck in the same direction as the hair grows.

Figure 30.23
The razor should glide across the chin.

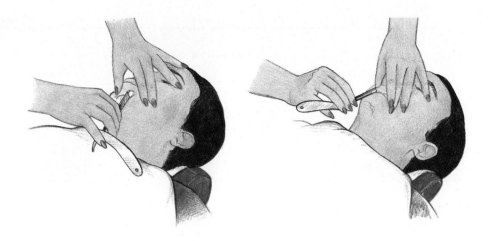

Figure 30.24 (right)
Shave downward below the chin.

Figure 30.25 (far right)
The final stroke should be in the same direction as the growth of the beard.

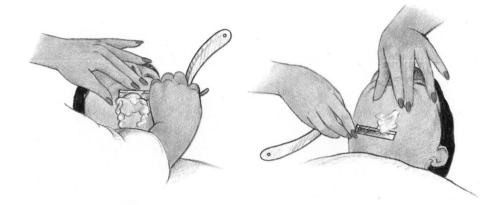

Figure 30.26
Finish the shave below the lower lip.

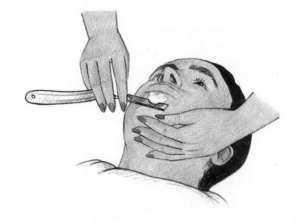

Balance (razor's) The weight of the blade (metal cutting part) of the razor should be the same as the weight of the handle.

Barber chair A sturdy, adjustable chair used by barbers.

Bleeding control Use pressure, apply an antiseptic, and then use styptic powder (see Chapter 3).

Hone A hard abrasive stone use for sharpening a straight-edge razor.

Ingrown hair A hair that grows beneath the surface of the skin rather than through it.

Lather Soap suds used to soften beard hair and provide a protective surface for shaving.

Latherizer An electric machine that dispenses warm soap suds for shaving.

Steamer towel A towel soaked in hot water, wrung out, then wrapped around the client's face after the lather has been applied.

Straight razor The haircutting implement used in a barber salon for the shaving service.

Strop A specially tanned strip of leather used in sharpening a straight razor; the strop brings the edge to a keener, smoother, and sharper point.

Styptic powder Alum powder used to stop bleeding from minor cuts.

1. What is the name of the machine that dispenses shaving lather in the barber salon?
2. What purpose does lather serve in the shaving service?
3. What term is used to describe the condition when a razor is equally weighted between the blade and the handle?
4. What two items are used to sharpen the straight razor?
5. What is the texture of most beard hair?
6. Under what conditions should you recommend **not** using a steamer towel?
7. Should you remove an ingrown hair for your client?
8. Where on the client's neck do you have to be particularly careful?
9. If you accidentally cut your client, what should you do first?
10. What should be applied to a minor cut on the skin?

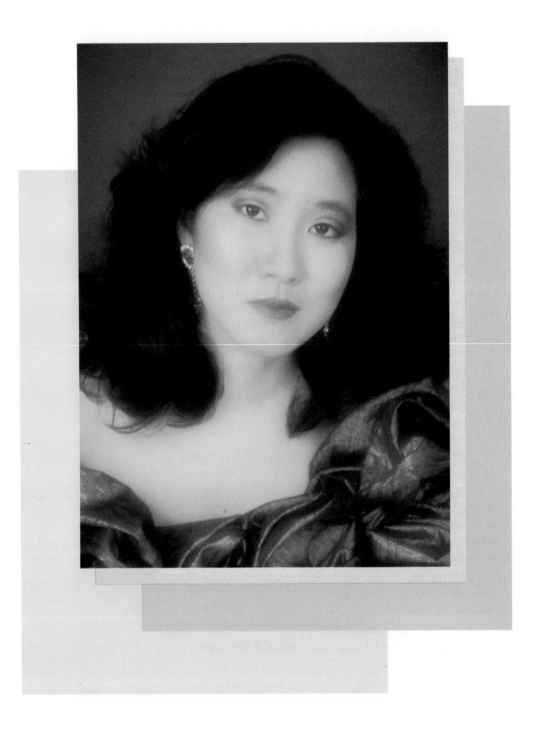

Planning a Salon

Learning Objective

Understand the basic principles needed to plan a salon as a successful business. Score 85 percent or better on a multiple-choice exam on the information in this chapter.

In order to achieve the above level of competence, you should master the following chapter objectives.

Theory Objectives

1. Identify the basic forms of business ownership.
2. Explain how to select a good salon site and building.
3. List points to consider in negotiating a salon lease.
4. Identify salon insurance needs.
5. Describe the importance of the salon reception area.
6. Explain the importance of retailing in the salon.

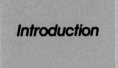

Introduction

Early in this book, we pointed out that cosmetology is an art, a science, and a business. At this point you may be thinking, "Now I know how an artistic imagination and creative flair will help me as a cosmetologist. I understand why knowing some science is helpful, and I realize how important it is to have technical skill. But what about business? Except for a few references to selling products to a client who comes into the salon, I haven't learned anything about starting my own business." This chapter will introduce you to some basic aspects of salon ownership.

You will need to know a great deal about salon planning before you will be ready to start your own business. Some of the things you will need to know can only be learned through experience, and working in a salon will give you the background you need. Nevertheless, you can learn some basic principles of salon planning now.

Theory Objective 1
Basic Forms of Business
Ownership

When one person owns a salon, the business is called a **sole proprietorship.** When **two or more persons** own a salon without issuing stock, the business is called a **partnership.** Sometimes a large salon or a chain of salons will be organized as a **corporation,** a form of business that is owned by one or many persons called **stockholders.** A **corporation** is a legal entity that can protect people against certain liabilities. It also has tax advantages for larger operations. Your lawyer can tell you more about the advantages and disadvantages of corporations when you are ready to open your own salon.

In a business organized as a **sole proprietorship,** the proprietor (or owner) is solely **responsible for all liabilities** (debts) of the business, but also is entitled to **all profits** from the business. In a **partnership,** the owners are liable for an **equal share of the debts** of the business and entitled to an **equal share of the profits.**

One difficulty with a partnership is that each partner may be held liable for debts incurred by the other partner(s). For example, A and B have formed a partnership. Partner B charges $1,000 worth of goods at a local department store in the name of the salon and leaves for another state to begin a business there. Partner A must pay for the goods charged to the business by partner B.

Another problem is that few partners take in exactly the same number of dollars for any given period of time, yet each partner is entitled to an equal share of the profits (unless the partners have agreed to divide the profits in some other way). For example, partner A takes in $500 per week from services, while partner B's take-in is $400. If the profit from staff covers all fixed and variable costs, would partner A receive $500 and partner B $400? No, they wouldn't. The take-ins would be added together and divided by 2 ($500 + $400 = $900 ÷ 2 = $450), so each partner would receive $450, less state and federal taxes and other deductions. If this pattern continues—and it often does—partner A will have to give $50 of his or her money to partner B every week.

Partnerships can operate smoothly (although few do) if a lawyer draws up a **partnership agreement** before the business opens. This document should spell out what partners A and B agree to do and not to do. All of the following will usually be included in the agreement:

1. The number of (and which) days and hours each partner will work per week.

2. The amount of money each will invest in the business.

3. A provision stating that profits will be divided on the basis of the amount each partner takes in.

4. A provision stating that **both partners must sign** all business checks.

5. A provision for dissolving the partnership in the event that one partner dies. The wife or husband of the deceased partner will be paid an amount of money equal to the value of the partner's share of the business.

A partnership should never be formed without a partnership agreement approved by a lawyer (Figure 31.1).

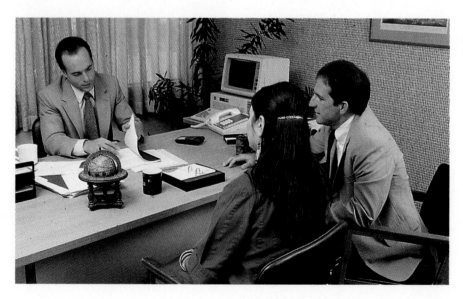

Figure 31.1
Consult an attorney before signing any agreements.

Theory Objective 2

Selecting a Good Salon Site and Building

You will have to make two important decisions when you plan a salon: Where should the salon be located? What kind of building is best?

When selecting a location, you should consider several things:

1. **Population density.** This means the number of people living in an area. A rule of thumb is that the more people there are in a given area, the more desirable it is as a salon location. A high-income neighborhood that has large apartment buildings is a good location, particularly if those buildings are within walking distance of the site you are considering. If there are only a few apartment buildings in the immediate area, a different location might be better.

   When choosing a location, you must consider more than the available buildings and your preferences (Figure 31.2). Most cities and towns have zoning restrictions (ordinances) that say how property in various locations can be used—that is, whether it can be used as residential or business property. You can obtain the ordinances for your area at your local city hall. A salon that will employ more than one person in addition to the owner must be located in an area that is zoned for commercial use.

2. **Accessibility.** This is an important factor. The location should be easy to find. Clients should not have to cross unusually

Figure 31.2
Selecting a possible salon location can involve many considerations.

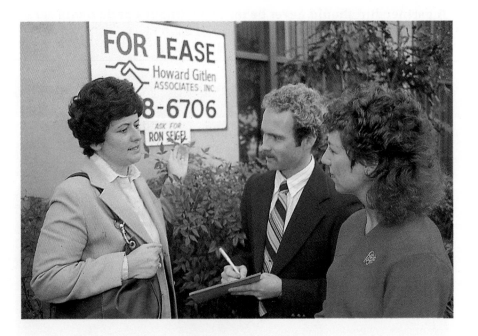

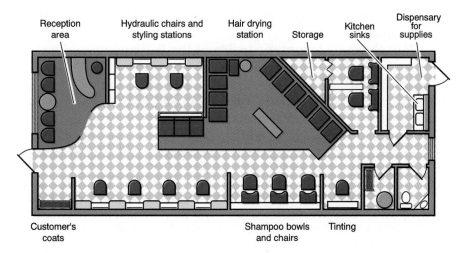

Reception area   Hydraulic chairs and styling stations   Hair drying station   Storage   Kitchen sinks   Dispensary for supplies

Customer's coats   Shampoo bowls and chairs   Tinting

Figure 31.3
A basic floor plan for a 6-station salon. Notice how the walls are used to define the main working areas: reception, styling, drying, shampooing, and tinting. Equipment and counters are placed against the walls so clients and employees can move from one area to the next in a direct line. Supplies are located out of the main traffic pattern, at the back of the salon. Note that only the reception and drying areas are carpeted.

busy streets or take complicated routes to reach the salon. The building should be visible from the street and should be near public transportation.

3. **Traffic patterns.** You should also consider the established routes people use to travel from one part of the community to another. These are the routes people follow when they are going to work, recreational facilities, grocery stores, church, and so on. The salon should not be located in an area that is "off the beaten track."

4. **Socioeconomic factors.** These factors are important. Consider the average income level of possible clients who live in the area. If the income level for these potential clients is very low, you should select a different location.

5. **Physical advantages.** The building you select should have adequate plumbing for shampoo bowls and a 100-gallon (380-liter) fast-recovery hot water heater. It should also have good lighting and an adequate number of electrical outlets for hair dryers, air wavers, curling irons, and thermal heaters (Figure 31.3).

The most successful salons are always located on the ground level of the building. **Second-floor** or **basement** locations have been far less successful than street-level salons because clients dislike walking up or down stairs.

The name of the salon and its phone number should be visible from the street so that clients can call for appointments. In most cities, ordinances restrict the size, height, shape, and location of outside business signs. In some cases, you may have to appear before the local zoning board to describe the sign you want to put up and get permission to display it. If the type of sign you want to put up is prohibited, you can ask for, and sometimes receive, an **exception** (called a **variance**) to the ordinance.

Both the outside and the inside of the building should be attractive and in good condition.

Ample parking for clients is a must for almost any salon. A recent survey showed that few people will walk more than about 900 feet (275 meters) to conduct any kind of business.

The building owner should agree to maintain a year-round temperature of 72°F (22.2°C) in the salon. Air conditioning is important because of the heat generated by the hair dryers.

6. **Existing businesses.** The businesses in an area provide clients for each other. A drugstore, for example, is an excellent neighbor for a salon because many shoppers will visit the salon after completing their business in the drugstore. Salons also do well near medical and dental offices.

Since you will probably remain in the same location for quite a few years, you should carefully consider all six of these factors before you select a location.

Theory Objective 3
Negotiating a Salon Lease

The legal agreement between the owner of a building and a renter is called a **lease.** The person granting the use of the building or space is called a **lessor.** The person using the space to operate a business is called the **lessee.** The **lessor** is also called the **landlord,** although this term will not appear on the lease agreement. Similarly, the **lessee** may casually be referred to as a **tenant,** but this term will not appear on the lease agreement either.

The desirable term (length of time) for a salon lease is 7 years with an option (chance) to renew the lease for 7 more years at the same monthly rent. A long lease serves several purposes:

1. It prevents the landlord from increasing the rent.

2. It prevents the salon owner from being evicted (legally ordered to move out).

3. The salon can continue to operate in the same location and establish a clientele.

4. The salon owner can sell the remaining term of the lease in the event he or she decides to stop operating the salon. The time remaining on a lease that has a low monthly rent can be valuable and can make a business very salable.

Most landlords will ask you to sign a "form" lease, but you should **not** sign this form until you have added amendments to it.

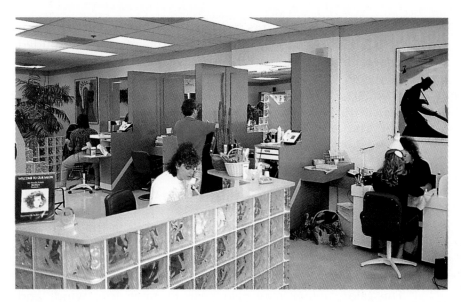

Figure 31.4
The landlord should agree to maintain the sidewalks and other areas outside the salon.

Amendments are written descriptions of items that the landlord agrees to provide at no charge. The amendments are part of the lease. Honest landlords (lessors) who say they will do certain things to make the property more usable for a salon will be willing to put the items in writing **if** they actually intend to do them. **Do not sign a lease agreement until your lawyer has approved it!**

As a minimum, you should add the following amendments to a lease to specify what **the lessor will do:**

1. Supply and maintain appliances that provide a year-round temperature of 72°F (22.2°C) in the salon.

2. **Provide** an adequate supply of **hot and cold** water for the efficient operation of the salon.

3. **Supply and maintain parking places** (whatever number is needed) for the exclusive use of the salon clients and post parking signs if needed.

4. **Maintain the sidewalks** and common areas that connect or are next to the salon (Figure 31.4).

5. **Supply and maintain necessary plumbing** (including a dispensary sink), electrical power, and outlets for a (*fill in number*)-operator salon (Figure 31.5).

6. **Repaint or wallpaper the interior** of the salon every three years.

7. **Supply and maintain shelving** for storage.

These amendments are **absolutely necessary;** changes in wording may cost you a great deal of money. Some landlords re-

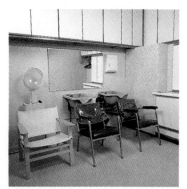

Figure 31.5
A shampoo/styling station

quire a deposit of three months' rent in advance to cover any damage to the building. At the end of the lease, this money is refunded if no damage has been done. Ordinary wear from use is **not** considered damage.

Most leases contain a **tax escalator clause,** which simply means that if the lessor's property tax increases, the rent will increase, but only in proportion to the tax levied for the space used.

Theory Objective 4
Salon Insurance Needs

Business **liability insurance** is necessary to protect the salon from a lawsuit brought by a person injured in front of or in the salon. For example, a client may trip on the sidewalk or fall on a slippery floor. Most leases specifically state that the **lessee** must carry liability insurance.

The salon owner may also wish to carry fire, wind, and glass-breakage insurance; these, too, are often required by the lease agreement.

The salon owner is expected to carry **malpractice insurance** for accidents that may result in injury to a client—for instance, cold-wave solution may drip into a client's eye or a scissor point may pierce a client's ear. People frequently sue others, sometimes for good reason and sometimes for **no** reason. Salon owners can spend a great deal of money proving their innocence. Therefore they must have the financial protection of good insurance that **covers all salon employees.** This type of coverage is usually available through the National Hairdressers and Cosmetologists Association.

Theory Objective 5
Importance of the
Salon Reception Area

The reception area is very important to the operation of any good salon. This area is really the "nerve center" of the salon. Consider the following points about the reception area:

1. The **client's first impression** of you and your business is based on this area.

2. The **appointment book is located in the reception area.**

3. The **telephone** is at the reception desk for receiving appointments.

4. The **cash register** is conveniently located here also.

5. Client color/permanent wave **record cards** are usually filed near the reception desk.

6. Shelves and displays for **retail items** are often located in the reception area.

The person who "directs traffic" by greeting clients, scheduling appointments, collecting money, handling complaints, and so forth at the reception area is the **receptionist.** As you might imagine, the receptionist must be enthusiastic, polite, diplomatic, and smart enough to keep things at the desk running smoothly. Of course, the receptionist should be neatly groomed at all times, as well as willing and able to assist the clients. Assistance may include (but is not limited to) explaining a new product, answering the phone, and handling a client's complaint.

Theory Objective 6
Retailing in the Salon

Retailing in the salon usually includes products such as shampoos, conditioners, hair sprays, nail-care items, unique hairstyling appliances (curling irons, hair dryers), combs/brushes, and cosmetics. Other retail products could include special hair ornaments, scarves, jewelry, and many other items that clients will buy on a regular basis. The following information will help you select and sell retail items in the salon. Some salon owners are so successful at retailing that they pay the salon rent with these profits.

- **Selecting a retail item.** It is much easier to sell an item that is **used in the salon.** For example, an excellent shampoo that is used every day in the salon can usually be sold successfully.

- **Packaging and labeling a retail item.** The item should be packaged neatly and attractively. Of course, **by law,** the **ingredients** in a product sold to a client **must be listed on the label.**

    After finding an excellent shampoo or other product, some salon owners **private label** it with their own name. In such cases, the label should be attractively designed and should include the salon name, address, and phone number. Private labeling protects the sale of the product since the client can be assured of getting exactly the same item only at the salon whose name appears on the label.

- **Pricing a retail item.** Price is a very important concern for clients. Therefore you should take special care when determining the price of an item. **Your retail item(s) should be priced competitively** with similar ones available to the client elsewhere. At the same time, the salon's goal is to make a profit so the selling price should include a markup.

- **Determining how much to retail.** The amount of retailing done in a salon will be determined by its size and location. A small one- or two-stylist salon may want to retail only 3 or 4 items, while a large, chain-type (10–20 stylists) salon may choose to retail 15 or more items.

■ **Retailing professional products.** Rather than selling private-label products, some salons successfully sell brand-name professional products. The rationale is that clients will be more willing to spend money for brands advertised in a magazine or on television. The only problem with this practice is that some manufacturers establish an identity for a product of being sold exclusively in professional salons. Later they begin selling the same product to drugstores and discount stores. When this happens, salons can't sell the product for a price that is competitive! Drugstores or discount stores can afford to sell the product at a lower price than salons because these stores buy large volumes at a lower cost.

As these points indicate, retailing is important, but it must be approached in an orderly, business-like way. It's best to begin retailing gradually until you can determine what will sell and what won't.

Glossary

Amendments Written statements added to a lease that describe items the landlord agrees to provide at no charge.

Corporation A business owned by a number of stockholders.

Lease A legal agreement between the owner of a building and a renter; the lease fixes the amount of rent, how long it will remain at that amount, and the rights and responsibilities of the owner and the renter.

Lessee The renter; the tenant.

Lessor The building owner; the landlord.

Liability insurance Insurance against loss that could result from liability for an injury or damage to persons or property.

Malpractice insurance Insurance that protects the cosmetologist against being sued for accidental injury to a client during the performance of a service.

Partnership A business owned by two or more people without issuing stock.

Partnership agreement A document outlining the rights and responsibilities of each partner in a business.

Private label The salon's name and address appear on a product that it is retailing.

Proprietorship The amount the business is worth.

Sole proprietorship A business owned by one person.

Stockholders People who have a partial ownership in a corporation through their purchase of one or more stock certificates.

1. What is the name given to a business that has two or more owners, but issues no stock?
2. Should two people start a partnership and open a salon without a partnership agreement?
3. Is it a good idea to consult a lawyer before signing important legal papers?
4. If you like a particular area for the location of your salon, should population density remain an important factor?
5. True or false. If a building is particularly well suited for a salon, accessibility really isn't important.
6. What is another name for local zoning restrictions?
7. What socioeconomic factor should be considered in selecting the location for a salon?
8. Are percentage rents desirable for salon owners?
9. Does rent tend to decrease over the years?
10. What is the term for a person who rents space in a building?
11. What is the term for a person who grants the use of space in a building for a particular purpose, such as a salon?
12. Name the legal document or agreement between the landlord and the renter.
13. Will a lease generally prevent increases in rent for the term of the agreement?
14. In the absence of a written agreement, must the landlord provide adequate air conditioning for a salon?
15. True or false. Plumbing and electrical work are the cheapest things you can have done in a salon.
16. What type of insurance covers the situation when a client slips on a puddle of water in the salon?
17. What type of insurance covers the situation when lightener blisters the client's scalp?
18. What name is given to the person who answers the phone at the front desk and schedules appointments?

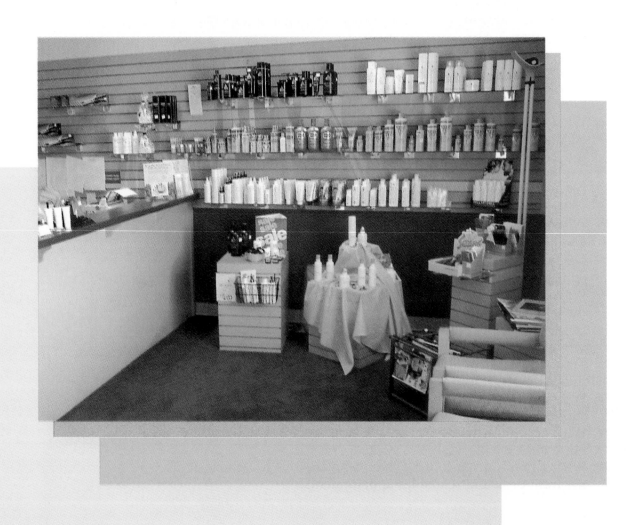

Salon Operations

Learning Objective

Describe the basic principles involved in the operation of a new salon. Score 85 percent or better on a multiple-choice exam on the information in this chapter.

In order to achieve the above level of competence, you should master the following chapter objectives.

Theory Objectives

1. Explain the factors to be considered in purchasing salon equipment and supplies.
2. Identify the considerations involved in developing salon operating policies, and describe the techniques used in interviewing prospective employees.
3. Describe how the salon's operating costs are computed.
4. Explain the client supply charge system.
5. Explain basic accounting and taxation principles.
6. List the advantages of accepting credit cards.
7. Explain the booth rental system.

Introduction

Now that you have some idea of what goes into planning a salon, it's time to discuss actually operating a salon. The objectives that follow are very thorough, but they cannot cover all possible salon operating situations. Your instructor may have additional information that is very important, too. Nevertheless, the information in this chapter will be very helpful and may well determine whether your salon is a success or a failure.

Theory Objective 1
Purchasing Salon
Equipment and
Supplies

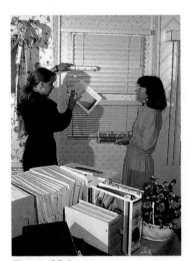

Figure 32.1
Selecting decorating samples
for the salon

The cost of operating a salon is normally figured in "per-operator" dollars. Usually, the cost per operator of opening a new salon is $3,000 to $3,500. This dollar range should easily include the usual operating equipment and supplies, such as the reception desk, dryer lounges, hydraulic styling chairs, shampoo bowls, shampoo chairs, and so on (Figure 32.1). Of course, custom-made equipment will be more expensive. Ordering standard equipment from catalogs will keep costs at or below $3,500 per operator. Always get bids for equipment from several beauty supply dealers. You can do this by submitting a written request for a bid to each dealer. Your request for a bid should include the following information:

1. The color, fabric, and style of the equipment you need.

2. How many pieces of each kind of equipment are needed.

3. The supplies needed to open the salon.

4. The date the bids will be opened.

5. The date the equipment is needed for the salon.

Dealers may give a discount if you pay for the equipment in cash. Some dealers give a discount if you make your first purchase through them. Study the bids carefully to select the best deal!

You may wish to purchase the equipment through an installation agreement with the dealer. After you make a down payment, you must make monthly payments, usually for a period of 1 to 5 years. There is usually a **service charge** for **late payments.** Under some sales agreements, if you miss more than three payments, the dealer may be able to call for all of the money to be paid immediately (usually referred to as a **balloon clause**)! If the balloon payment is not made in full, the dealer may repossess all of the equipment. **Never sign any legal agreement unless your lawyer has approved it!**

Equipment may also be financed through a bank, probably at a lower interest rate (the cost of using money) than a dealer will charge. Small loan companies usually charge the highest rate of interest and should be avoided.

Operating supplies are also called "consumable supplies" because they are **used completely** in the performance of a service. **They cannot be reused.** Consumable supplies will ordinarily be about **8 percent** of the total dollar sales for any given year. For example, if a salon spends $8,000 per year for supplies, its total sales are about $100,000. This can be determined as follows:

$$\text{Step 1: } 8\% = .08$$

$$\text{Step 2: } .08x = \$8,000$$

$$\text{Step 3: } \frac{.08x}{} = \frac{}{.08}$$

$$\text{Step 4: } x = \frac{\$8,000}{.08}$$

$$\text{Step 5: } x = .08 \overline{)\$8,000.00} \quad \$100,000.$$

Answer: $100,000

If another salon did $72,000 in sales and spent $12,000 on consumable supplies, something would be very wrong with their supply costs because $72,000 × .08 = $5,760; $12,000 is between 16 and 17 percent of $72,000, which is **too high!** This percentage is calculated as follows:

$$\text{Step 1: } \frac{\$12,000}{\$72,000} = \frac{\text{supplies}}{\text{sales}}$$

$$\text{Step 2: } \$72,000 \overline{)12,000.000} \quad .166$$

Answer: .166 or 16.6%

The answer can be rounded off to .17 or 17 percent.

Most salon owners find that salespersons call on them regularly. Although these salespersons may seem a bit of a nuisance, they are actually very **helpful.** The **supply salesperson** is the **important link** between the manufacturer and the salon owner. New products are advertised, but advertisements are not substitutes for discussing the advantages and benefits of a new product with a salesperson who can answer questions. The salesperson may also give advice on choosing a salon location.

Any reputable sales representative for a supply dealer will **guarantee** a product. New products that do not perform according to the salesperson's claims may be **credited** to the salon account if the empty container or unused portion of the product is returned. The dealer will issue a credit to the salon and return the product to the manufacturer.

A salon owner should **not divide** (split) the salon's **supply business** between more than two or three dealers for several reasons:

1. **Bookkeeping becomes difficult** as the number of dealers increases.

2. **Too much time** is spent chatting with sales representatives if you buy from many dealers.

3. If the volume of business is **large enough** and bills are paid **promptly, a discount** may be given. If your business is split among many dealers, you will be less likely to receive discounts.

4. With many dealers, you are likely to experience **product duplication;** that is, you will needlessly buy the same type of product from several dealers.

Each of these points needs further explanation:

1. **Bookkeeping becomes difficult** when many suppliers are used because detailed records must be kept on all products and the firms that are supplying them.

Some salons buy supplies on credit; but remember, a **charge account is a privilege** that should not be abused because doing so is both unethical and unwise. Credit ratings can be checked between almost any two cities in the world. If you cannot pay the full amount of a bill, explain the situation to the dealer's credit manager and make a partial payment.

Some salons prefer to pay for supplies **C.O.D. (cash on delivery).** This practice can be convenient, but remember there is a charge for handling a transaction in this way. Therefore, it is important to order weekly rather than every other day.

When the supplies are delivered to the salon, the invoice with them will state all of the following:

- Salon name

- Address

- Invoice number and date

- Quantity ordered

- Description of supply

- Price

Figure 32.2
Sample invoice from a beauty supply house

BEAUTY SUPPLY COMPANY

2000 Hairstyle Lane
Anytown, USA 00001

Ship to: Family Hair Care Salon 1305 Green St. Everytown, USA 00000	Bill to: *(if different)*	

Invoice No. 00000	Purchase Order No. XX	Terms Net

Qty.	Item No.	Description	Unit Price	Extension
12	QA1	Q hair color	$1.67 ea	$20.04
12	AA1	A hair color	1.67 ea	20.04
6	123	Shampoo	1.25 ea	7.50
6	876	Conditioner	1.42 ea	8.52

Total Items 36	Packed by MM	Total	$56.10
		Transportation *(if applicable)* Sales Tax	5.00
			2.75
Weight Shipped 15 lb		Please pay this amount	$63.85

- Tax
- Delivery charge

Always check **invoices against the supplies accompanying** them and pay only for the supplies that you actually receive (Figure 32.2). Sometimes part of an order will accidentally be left out of a shipment.

Salon owners **do not** pay for supplies from a **statement,** which usually comes at the end of each month, unless the invoice numbers listed on the statement and the corresponding dollar amounts coincide exactly with the invoices collected through the month.

It is good practice to always make checks **payable only to the company, not** the salesperson. The number of the invoice that the check is covering should **always** be written above the date in the upper right-hand corner of the check. Also, write the check number and date on the invoice(s). This system serves as an accurate cross-reference. Always write the date, company, invoice numbers, and the amount of the check on the check stub. Invoices, check stubs, and canceled checks should be kept on file.

2. Salespersons can be valuable resources for assisting the salon owner in solving problems, contacting schools for graduates,

learning about new products, and finding a new location if another salon is to be opened. Most experienced salespersons are quite knowledgable about the industry and are good sources of information. If many suppliers are used, however, talking to a large number of salespersons about legitimate concerns can become very time-consuming.

Always treat salespersons **courteously. Respect their time** as well as your own. If you cannot leave the work area, invite the salesperson to come over to that area and describe products or **write** the prices of items on the back of the order book. If you cannot stop to talk, explain this and ask the salesperson to return later.

3. Discounts, which are common among large-volume accounts, can be useful. However, an owner can spend too much time bargaining for lower prices. Some salon owners spend 20 hours a week trying to bring the unit price of an item down. Even if they are successful in getting a discount, they may have to tie up a great deal of money in supplies, and the discount will still have only a **small** effect on the percentage of dollars spent for supplies. The owner could probably make much more money spending that time dressing hair.

Regardless of the price, **no** supplies should be ordered that cannot be used within **90 working days.** Stocking supplies for longer than this ties up too much of your cash. The cost of borrowing money to pay dealers for a large discount may **be greater than** the saving made on that purchase.

4. **Product duplication** is the salon owner's worst enemy. Stick with the tried and proven products for **each** task. Avoid stocking many products that do **exactly** the same things. Purchase only small quantities of any new product for trial use.

Developing an index card system on products that are **ordered often** can be helpful. Each card will show the quantity ordered and the unit price of a product. Then you can compare the cards with each other to look for price differences and product duplication. Remember that nothing is "free." For example, if a supplier offers 6 cold waves for $60 and 6 cold waves free, you are actually getting 12 cold waves at a cost of $5 each. Use an inexpensive calculator for figuring such unit prices.

Theory Objective 2
Developing Salon
Operating Policies and
Interviewing
Prospective Employees

All salon owners, large or small, should have a list of **operating policies.** This list lets all employees know exactly what their responsibilities are and what they are expected to do. Operating policies also include the salon owner's responsibilities toward the employees. In making up the list, the owner must ask what he or she can offer a prospective employee. In turn, an owner must consider what an employee has to offer.

For example, an employee might be required to do all of the following:

1. Sanitize the work area at the end of each day to prepare for the next day's work so that clients will not be kept waiting.

2. Arrive 15 minutes before the first appointment to be ready for the client.

3. Be cheerful and courteous to all the clients in the salon.

4. Willingly help other employees and the owner in an emergency so that everyone remains on schedule for appointments.

5. Write legibly and accurately in the appointment book so scheduling does not become confused.

6. Stay late for a client on special occasions.

7. Consult the owner before ordering any supplies.

In exchange, an employee looks for a working arrangement that offers the following:

1. The salon is neat and clean and kept in good repair, and new equipment is purchased as needed.

2. The salon owner carries malpractice insurance and provides medical insurance for employees.

3. Paid vacations equal to half to three-fourths of the individual's average weekly take-in dollars are provided (also based on how long he or she has been employed).

4. The owner pays for professional seminars and has self-improvement styling classes once a month.

5. Only the best supplies are purchased for use in the salon.

6. Staff meetings are held to discuss and solve operating problems.

All professional businesses put their operating policies in writing—the salon is no exception. Employees and employers can avoid many misunderstandings if a list of operating policies is given to each new employee.

Interviewing New Employees

You will need to develop interviewing skills to use when you talk to prospective employees (Figure 32.3). Two techniques are particularly important: close observation and note taking.

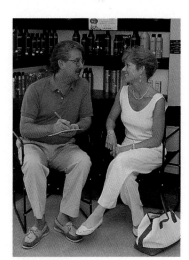

Figure 32.3
Interviewing a prospective employee

The following are some of the basic things you should look for at the interview:

1. Is the applicant on time?
2. Is the applicant's hair attractively styled?
3. Are the applicant's clothes neat and clean, and are his or her shoes shined or polished?
4. Is the applicant poised and alert?

You will need to ask the applicant a number of questions, including the following:

1. What school did you graduate from?
2. Where were you last employed?
3. What other salons have you worked for?
4. Why did you leave your last position?
5. Would you object if I called your last employer? If so, why?
6. Do you have a particular specialty?
7. What are your address and phone number?
8. How far do you live from this salon?
9. What commission do you expect?
10. What else do you expect?
11. Are the working days and hours acceptable?
12. Do you realize the importance of **working on Saturdays?**
13. Will you consent to cut, set or comb a model's hair to demonstrate your skills?
14. Do you have any questions about the salon's operating policies?

You may wish to type these questions as a questionnaire for the applicant to complete. Keep written notes of each interview, and file them carefully for future reference. You may interview several applicants over a several-week period and may have difficulty remembering the particular abilities of each applicant unless you have notes.

Theory Objective 3
Salon Operating Costs

As you are probably aware, one of the most important aspects of planning and running a business is keeping expenses under control.

You should keep two general categories of expenses in mind when you plan your salon:

1. Fixed costs

2. Variable costs

Fixed costs remain the same no matter how much business you do. Whether you have one client or a thousand, these expenses will be the same. And they will remain the same all year long. **Some good examples** of fixed costs are rent, insurance, membership dues for professional organizations, license fees, and basic legal fees. These expenses must be paid every month to keep the salon open for business. These expenses can change; for example, insurance rates, rent, or licensing fees may increase, but these increases will cover a specific period of time. For example, if your insurance is increased from $50 a month to $75 a month, you will know that insurance will cost $75 a month for the next six months or a year. Fixed expenses do not change from day to day or week to week.

Variable costs change according to the number of clients you have. As the number of clients you serve increases, so will your variable costs. Supply costs are probably the best example of variable costs. They change directly with the number of clients served. For example, if you serve 12 clients, you will use twice as much shampoo as you would use for 6 clients. Other examples of variable costs are commissions, laundry, utilities (water, light, sewer), interest, and repairs and maintenance.

You should be aware that in the salon business employees (other cosmetologists) are paid differently than in most other businesses. Think about this difference for a moment. If you buy a shirt in a department store, the clerk does **not** receive 50 percent of the price of the service.

For this reason, your decision to add new services must be based on what they cost. Although most salons must provide a fairly wide range of services to please their clients, you need to recognize which services are most profitable. You can develop your skill in those areas and become known as an expert.

As an example of the importance of costs, consider that giving a shampoo/hairstyle takes about the same time as a haircut. You charge $8 for the shampoo/hairstyle and $10 for the haircut. Obviously, the salon (and the stylist) can make more money giving haircuts than shampoo/hairstyles because the price is higher, and it **costs** the shop **less** to give haircuts. If you are good at cutting hair, you can provide 15 shampoo/hairstyles or 15 haircuts per day. Table 32.1 illustrates the possible gross income that you can earn from various combinations of these two services in an 8-hour day.

You will also need to think about other types of services as in the following **example:**

Table 32.1

Possible Combinations of Gross Income Earned by a Stylist in One Day

Combinations of Services				Income
Shampoo/Hairstyles @ $8		Haircuts @ $10		Total Service Dollars
15	$8	0	$ 0	$120
14	8	1	10	122
13	8	2	10	124
12	8	3	10	126
11	8	4	10	128
10	8	5	10	130
9	8	6	10	132
8	8	7	10	134
7	8	8	10	136
6	8	9	10	138
5	8	10	10	140
4	8	11	10	142
3	8	12	10	144
2	8	13	10	146
1	8	14	10	148
0	0	15	10	150

1. 15 shampoo/hairstyles at $8 = $120.

2. 6 shampoo/hairstyles at $8 plus 3 cold waves at
   $40 = $48 + $120 = $168.

Note that in this case, you served 6 fewer clients, but took in $48 more.

Table 32.2 shows the usual salon operating expenses. You can use the percentages of variable and fixed costs as a guide in planning your own salon.

Theory Objective 4
Client Supply Charge
System

Historically, salon owners paid hairstylists a commission based on the total amount paid by the client for a service. For example, if the client paid $50 for a permanent wave/hairstyle, the stylist received a 50 percent commission, which would amount to $25. The salon owner paid the cost of the perm and other costs, such as rent, advertising, and electricity, out of the other $25. This system worked well for many years. In the late 1980s and early 1990s, however, supply costs doubled, and the salon owners could no longer make a profit. As a result, many salons changed to a service charge program in order to stay in business.

To determine the supply charge, the salon calculates the cost of supplies required for the different services. Although the cost of

Table 32.2
Salon Operating Expenses

Costs	Percentage of Total Expenses
Variable costs	
Salaries and commissions (staff and owner)	52.50%
Service supplies	7.00
Retail supplies	1.00
Towel service	1.50
Utilities (water, heat, power, light)	3.50
Repairs and maintenance	1.00
Interest and carrying charges	.25
Legal services (including accounting)	.25
Taxes	4.00
Fixed costs	
Rent*	8.00
Advertising	2.50
Depreciation	.50
Insurance (malpractice, liability)	.50
Telephone	1.50
Association dues, magazines	.50
Education and travel	.50
Total costs	85.00
Profit	15.00
	100.00

*Note that rent is the highest fixed cost percentage.

a permanent wave varies with the product, an average price might be $5. If the salon has been charging $50 for a permanent wave/hairstyle under the old system, the price will be increased to $55 to include a client supply charge. The client's sales ticket is then coded with the supply cost of each service; in this example, the perm cost is coded as $5. Therefore, the stylist will be **paid a commission after the supply charge has been subtracted** from the service sales ticket. If the client pays $55 for the service, the supply charge of $5 is subtracted; then the stylist is paid a commission on $50:

Price charged client	$ 55
Cost of perm	− 5
	$ 50
	× 50% commission
	$ 25 amount paid to stylist

Subtracting the charge for supplies makes sense. Why should the stylist be paid for using a supply? The stylist is actually selling skills, talent, experience, and personality. After all, the salon owner is in business to make a profit!

If you don't realize how important record keeping is to a successful business, you will soon find out. You already know some of the reasons for keeping **accurate records.** All of us pay income taxes, and so will your business. If you have employees, you will have to know when to pay them. You will also have to pay Social Security and other items for your employees. You will have to know when to pay your rent and many other bills.

In addition, there are other important reasons to keep accurate records. Good records can **help** you **plan ahead** and help you operate your business more efficiently. For example, sometimes you can buy supplies for less at certain times of the year, and sometimes you can buy supplies for less if you buy larger amounts. Your records will show you the best times to buy supplies and the best amounts.

Also, your business may vary from time to time during the year. Records will show when you take in more money than at other times. If you know you are very busy during the spring or at Christmas but rather slow during the summer, you may want to hire temporary help for the busy periods.

Still, you may be wondering if records are really so necessary. After all, after you have been in business for a year or two, you will know about ordering supplies and when the busy seasons are. That's true, but operating a business involves many, many details. If you don't have complete records, you will have to remember all of them—and you probably won't. Good records are your memory. **Record keeping** is probably the most unpopular part of running a business, but it is also one of the most important. You may want to have a professional bookkeeper or accountant or, even better, a certified public accountant (CPA) to keep your records for you, but you still need to be able to read and interpret your records. An accountant or CPA will be able to help you understand your records.

In addition, there are a few simple formulas that you can use to interpret your records. They correspond to the two basic accounting statements. The first formula is called the **basic accounting equation:**

$$\textbf{Assets} = \text{Liabilities} + \text{Proprietorship}$$

These terms are very easy to understand. **Assets** are what the business **owns. Liabilities** are what the business owes. What is left over is **proprietorship,** or what the business is worth. You can see how this equation works by looking at a **balance sheet** (Table 32.3). The assets ($50,000) equal the total of liabilities ($15,000) and proprietorship ($35,000).

Table 32.3
Family Hair Care Center Balance Sheet, December 31, 19XX

Assets
Cash	$30,000	
Equipment	15,000	
Supplies	5,000	
		$50,000

Liabilities
Loan	15,000	15,000
Proprietorship	35,000	35,000
		$50,000

You can use this equation in several ways. For instance, you may know what you own (assets) and what you owe (liabilities), but you do not know how much you are worth. You can find out by subtracting your liabilities from your assets like this:

Assets	$ 50,000
Liabilities	− 15,000
Proprietorship	$ 35,000

The income statement and the formula that goes with it are also very important. The **income statement** shows how much money you made (Table 32.4). The formula is the basic income equation:

Gross Income − Expenses = Net Income

Gross income is the money you receive from clients. As you may know only too well, what you earn and what you get to keep are two very different things. You have rent to pay, clothes and food to buy, and other bills to pay. So the money that goes for those things is not really your own. The same thing is true for a business. Your business must use money it takes in to pay for salaries, supplies, and other items that are needed to run the business. These are called **expenses.** They are the cost of doing business. (Accountants make a technical distinction between an expense and a cost. Entire books have been written about the difference, but you don't need to worry about it here.)

If you subtract all expenses from gross income, you will get net income. **Net income** is the money you have left after you have paid the expenses of the business. You can do whatever you want with the net income. You can put it back into the business by hiring more employees, buying more supplies, or renting a bigger salon. Or you may save it as part of the business's proprietorship—in other

Table 32.4
Family Hair Care Center Income Statement, December 31, 19XX

Gross income		
Services—shampoos, etc.	$14,000	
Miscellaneous—manicures, etc.	1,000	
Total gross income		$15,000
Expenses		
Salaries	$ 3,500	
Benefits	1,500	
Total expenses		$ 5,000
Net income		$10,000

words, how much the business is worth. Or you may take it out of the business by paying it to yourself.

These two equations and statements should give you a basic idea of what accounting is about. But follow your own advice to your clients: get a professional to help you. A client might be able to give a shampoo and set, but he or she will be an amateur; there is no telling what the results will be. The same thing is true for you when it comes to record keeping and accounting. A professional will **know** what to do; a professional won't just "hope it's right" or "guess" at the solution to a problem.

Taxation

If you are planning to become a salon owner or manager, you should also know a few important facts about tax laws. **Tax laws are made by the state or federal legislature** (Congress). These laws are called **acts** because they are "enacted" (made) by a legislature. A violation of a tax law (failure to pay a tax) is a crime!

Certain taxes are paid by the employee in the form of a **payroll deduction** (subtracted from the employee's paycheck). The employer sends the employee's payroll deduction to the government monthly and reports the amount to the government quarterly (four times per year). Employers generally **pay federal taxes to a local bank.** The bank sends the tax money to the federal government. State taxes are sent directly to the state's department of revenue (or taxation).

The following tax laws require the **employer** (salon owner) to pay certain taxes out of his or her own pocket:

1. Federal Unemployment Tax Act (FUTA)

2. State Unemployment Tax Act (SUTA)

3. Federal Insurance Contribution Act (FICA)

4. Worker's Compensation Act

FUTA (FEW-tah) requires all employers to pay .7 percent of the first $6,000 the employee earns to a maximum of $42 per month to the federal government. This money is used to pay the employee should he or she become unemployed.

SUTA (SOO-tah) **requires all employers to pay a percentage** of the worker's earnings to the state government. This percentage tends to vary from state to state. SUTA funds are used by the state to pay unemployment benefits.

FICA (FI-ka) is the **Social Security** tax. **All employers are required to match (pay an amount of money equal to) what the employee contributes** to the Social Security fund. For example, if the employee's contribution is 6.13 percent of his or her earnings, the employer must pay an amount of money equal to that 6.13 percent. Therefore the **total money paid to FICA** will be an amount equal to 12.26 percent of the employee's earnings. The percentages change from year to year, so check with the **Internal Revenue Service (IRS)** or your accountant.

The Worker's Compensation Act requires all employers to pay for an insurance policy that **protects employees who may be injured** at work. The cost of this insurance policy will be different for various types of job categories. For example, insurance coverage for a hairdresser will most likely cost less than the coverage for a police officer because a hairdresser is less likely to be injured on the job.

The following taxes must be withheld from the employee's paycheck:

1. Federal income tax

2. State income tax

3. FICA tax

The actual amount of money withheld from your paycheck will be determined by numerous factors, such as your total earnings, your marital status and number of dependents, and the percentage owed to the government—remember this changes from year to year (Figure 32.4).

Remember that as an employee you must **declare all tips of more than $20 per month, and pay the added tax.**

The salon owner should also realize that he or she is **responsible** for **unpaid taxes of a hairdresser who rents** space in the owner's salon. For example, in the case *Wolfe v. United States*, No. 77-1434, the United States Court of Appeals for the Eighth Circuit (North Dakota) held that a person renting space from a salon owner

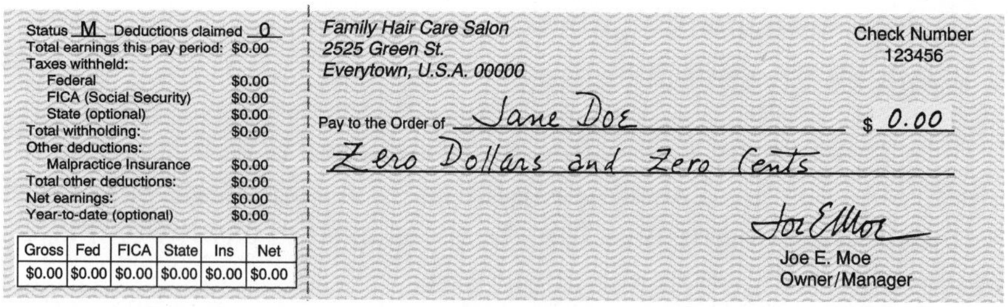
Status M Deductions claimed 0
Total earnings this pay period: $0.00
Taxes withheld:
Federal $0.00
FICA (Social Security) $0.00
State (optional) $0.00
Total withholding: $0.00
Other deductions:
Malpractice Insurance $0.00
Total other deductions: $0.00
Net earnings: $0.00
Year-to-date (optional) $0.00

Gross	Fed	FICA	State	Ins	Net
$0.00	$0.00	$0.00	$0.00	$0.00	$0.00

Family Hair Care Salon
2525 Green St.
Everytown, U.S.A. 00000

Check Number
123456

Pay to the Order of Jane Doe $ 0.00
Zero Dollars and Zero Cents

Joe E. Moe
Owner/Manager

Figure 32.4
Sample payroll check with stub attached. Withholding and "other" deductions vary from state to state, city to city, and salon to salon.

was **not** an independent contractor but was actually an employee of the owner. Therefore, the owner was liable (had to pay) the unpaid taxes owed by the hairdresser renting space in the salon. Note that courts in other areas have ruled that persons who rent space in a salon are **not** employees. Check your state's regulations to see which rule is followed in your area.

Theory Objective 6
Advantages of Accepting Credit Cards

Credit cards are now used for billions of dollars worth of purchases every year. We live in a "plastic world." Many people feel more comfortable charging services and products than paying for them in cash.

One reason credit cards have become so popular is that they are **convenient to use.** Charging a purchase to a credit card allows the individual to avoid the "hassle" of cashing a personal check. Furthermore, paying for a service or a purchase with "plastic" eliminates the need to carry large sums of money in a purse or billfold, which could be lost or stolen.

Another reason individuals like to use credit cards is that they can delay the actual payment until the transaction is processed by the credit card company. In other words, even though people could probably pay cash for a product or service, if they charge it, they **will have the use of the money** until the monthly credit card payment is due.

Developments in technology have also contributed to the growth of credit cards. **Satellite communications** make it possible for a person living in Minneapolis, Minnesota, to charge a jewelry purchase in Paris, France. The store owner makes a **credit check** simply by using the **telephone.** The store owner's call is relayed via satellite to the credit card company in Minneapolis. If the cardholder's credit is good, the purchase is approved.

Many salons have discovered that accepting credit cards is good for business. In particular, salons located in areas where there is lots of traffic, such as shopping malls, hotels, heavily populated areas, or tourist attraction/resort areas should probably have a credit card program. Figures clearly indicate that accepting credit cards **increases overall salon sales.** An added advantage to accepting credit cards is that unlike a personal check, which may be returned because of insufficient funds, payment for services charged on a credit card is **guaranteed** by the credit card company.

The only **disadvantage** to accepting credit cards is the **fee.** All credit card companies charge a user **fee,** which is usually a percentage of the amount that is charged. For example, a credit card company might charge an across-the-board fee of 8 percent. Therefore if a client pays for services costing $100 with a credit card, the credit card company would pay the salon $92. Of course, a salon that accepts credit cards usually adds the user fee into the cost of the service to the client.

When a client wishes to pay by credit card, salon personnel should check the expiration date on the card and ask the client for other forms of identification. If the salon has followed these procedures, the credit card company will pay the charges. It is assumed that the salon has given the cardholder a reasonable service or product in exchange for the amount charged.

Theory Objective 7
Booth Rental System

In the **booth rental system,** a stylist who has an established clientele **rents a booth** in a salon. The stylist agrees to pay the salon owner a set amount of money every week or month. In exchange, the salon owner allows the stylist to use the salon's equipment, such as shampoo bowls, styling stations, hydraulic chairs, telephone, and restrooms. The stylist must furnish his or her own operating supplies, including shampoo, permanent waves, conditioners, and the like. Under the booth rental agreement, the stylist keeps all money that the client is charged. A person renting from a salon owner under this kind of agreement is called a **renter.**

For example, suppose Mary rents a booth at the **Family Hair Care Center** for $200 per week. Mary collects only $150 from her clientele during the first week of her rental. She must pay the salon owner that $150, plus $50 from her savings account. But during the second week, Mary collects $800 from her clientele; she still pays the salon owner only the $200 specified in the booth rental agreement and keeps the remaining $600 for herself.

The booth rental system has several **advantages for the stylist:**

1. No money has to be paid out for equipment.

2. The stylist can set the working hours and working days he or she chooses.

3. The stylist can select his or her own uniform.

4. Less bookkeeping is required for phone, advertising, electricity, and so forth.

5. The stylist can control the prices charged for his or her services, regardless of the prices set for regular employees.

6. The stylist runs no risk of going out of business and losing an investment, because no investment has been made.

The booth rental system has many **disadvantages for the salon owner,** however, and may **not** be a good business arrangement for an otherwise successful salon. The following are some of the **disadvantages** for the salon owner:

1. Booth rental stylists don't have to follow salon operating policies.

2. Regular salon employees may have to answer the phone for the renter and/or schedule appointments.

3. Salon equipment receives additional use and will need replacement sooner.

4. Management is more difficult because the renter does not work a set schedule of hours/days per week.

5. Other staff members may resent the fact that renters don't have to follow the salon's operating policies.

6. Newly hired regular stylists (paid an hourly rate and/or commission) will have difficulty developing a clientele because the clients brought in by the renter have their hair done exclusively by the renter.

7. The salon owner may have to pay any tax due to the government that the renter has not paid.

8. If the renter moves to another salon in the neighborhood, most, if not all, of his or her clients will also move to the other salon.

Booth rental is not legal in all states. Check with your state regulatory office.

Glossary ▬▬▬▬▬▬▬▬▬▬▬▬▬▬▬▬▬▬▬▬▬▬▬▬▬▬▬▬▬▬▬▬▬▬▬▬▬

Assets What a business owns.

Balloon clause A statement in an installment purchase agreement that allows the dealer to demand full payment if more than three payments have been missed.

Basic accounting equation (assets = liabilities + proprietorship) A formula for interpreting the worth of a business.

C.O.D. (cash on delivery) A shipping arrangement in which full payment is made on delivery.

Expenses The costs involved in doing business, such as salaries and supplies.

Fixed costs Costs that remain the same and do not fluctuate with the number of clients served.

Gross income Money received from services and products before expenses are deducted.

Liabilities What a business owes.

Net income The money left after expenses have been paid.

Operating policies A list showing what the employee and employer can expect of each other in respect to salon operations.

Operating supplies Supplies that are completely used in the performance of a service.

Renter A stylist who rents a booth from a salon.

Supply charge The cost of a supply that is subtracted from the price of the service before the stylist's commission is figured.

Variable costs The costs that may change according to the number of clients served.

Questions

1. What type of supplies are completely used when giving the client a service?
2. What percentage of total sales should the operating supplies represent?
3. Name the communications link between the manufacturer, the dealer, and the salon.
4. Is there usually a handling charge for C.O.D. supply orders?
5. True or false. The best way to make sure you are paying accurately for supplies that are charged is to pay the amount indicated on the statement.
6. Is it a good idea to order enough supplies to last 6 months?
7. Should you attempt to avoid product duplication?
8. Should a prospective employee arrive at 8:00 A.M. for an 8:00 A.M. appointment?
9. Should all employees in the salon order supplies?
10. True or false. An applicant for a new job should arrive a few minutes late so the salon owner will know the applicant's time is also important.
11. Do variable costs remain the same?
12. Should a newly licensed person explain to a prospective employer that he or she likes to have Saturdays off?
13. Do fixed costs change, or do they remain the same?
14. What is the technical name for the description and analysis of the production, distribution, and consumption of goods and services?

15. Does it make sense for the salon owner to deduct the supply cost from the amount on which the stylist's commission will be based?

16. Is the total amount of money taken in by the salon called gross income?

17. True or false. Costs connected with doing business, such as supplies, are called expenses.

18. What are the exact abbreviations for the Federal Unemployment Tax Act, the State Unemployment Tax Act, and the Federal Insurance Contribution Act?

19. Under the Federal Insurance Contribution Act, what percentage must the employer pay compared to the employee's share?

20. True or false. You must report all tips that exceed $20 per month.

21. Name two disadvantages to the salon owner of renting a styling station.

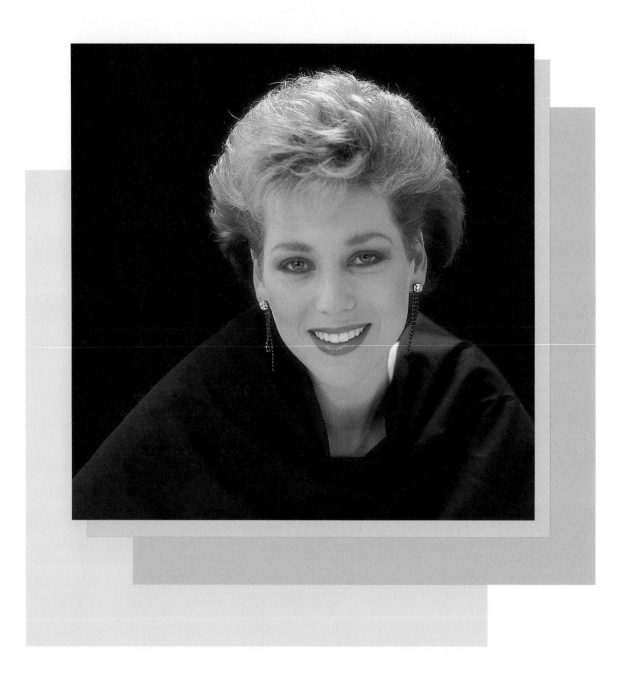

The Psychology of Interpersonal Skills and Retailing

Learning Objective

Use the information in this chapter to apply the techniques described here. Score 85 percent or better on a multiple-choice exam on the information in this chapter.

In order to achieve the above level of competence, you should master the following chapter objectives.

Theory Objectives

1. Understand the process for developing successful salon communications.
2. Use psychology to develop communication strategies and improve salon sales.
3. Identify four income-producing strategies.

Practical Objective

4. Recognize and use effective client-handling techniques.

Introduction

Combining technical skills in cosmetology with basic skills in behavioral psychology can bring you great success as a professional cosmetologist. Of course, success means different things to different people. To some, success is simply doing a job well. To others, it is achieving a certain position. In most cases, however, society measures success directly or indirectly by a person's ability to generate income. Despite this tendency to "keep score" in terms of income, success involves many other factors, such as happiness, fulfillment, and the ability to help others.

Fortunately, a good cosmetologist can combine the personal satisfaction of helping others with a high score in income generation. It is crucial to understand that you and your client have a common goal: improving the client's appearance. You can best achieve this goal by taking every opportunity to provide appropriate expert advice and services that meet the client's needs. In doing so, you will also be selling a full range of products and services that provide income for you and the salon.

Theory Objective 1
Developing Successful
Salon Communications

When you are working with a client, it is important for you to develop a rapport—a comfortable style of communication so that you and the client can share thoughts with each other. You and the client need to feel comfortable with each other because the client has to communicate to you what "look" would improve his or her appearance. You also have some ideas that will improve the client's appearance and need to be able to explain them to the client. In addition, it will be necessary for you to sell the client products and/or services, such as a retail shampoo or a permanent wave, that he or she will need to maintain the desired hairstyle. Combining these two sets of thoughts about the client's appearance will lead to satisfaction for both you and your client. This objective uses a systematic approach to communication skills that will help you be more successful in this psychological process.

Technical Skill Isn't Everything

Cosmetologists spend a great deal of time learning how to cut, perm, and color hair and perform other services. And well they should. One cannot achieve any level of success without these technical skills. But why is it that two people can

- attend the same cosmetology school,

- study with the same instructors,

- graduate at the same time,

- possess the same technical skills,

- be hired by the same salon,

- go through the same orientation process, and

- work on the same type of clientele,

and yet one stylist will outperform the other by a significant margin? The answer, of course, lies in the way the two cosmetologists treat their clients. In other words, a stylist's success depends in large part on his or her client-handling skills.

What Is Client Handling?

Good **client-handling techniques** involve treating customers in ways that make them feel good about the salon experience. For instance, all customers come into a new salon with a certain amount of fear. They know that something is going to happen to their looks, but they aren't sure whether the experience will be good or bad. If the stylist can say and do things that will relieve that fear, the clients will feel better about the outcome regardless of what it is.

Top Stylists Are "Salespeople"

Not many cosmetology students enter school thinking that they will come out as salespeople, and this is probably just as well. The term "salesperson" seems to have a negative meaning for many people. But a **salesperson** is simply a person who is attempting to provide solutions to a client's problems. It just so happens that the solutions are the services and products that the salesperson is selling. If you don't like the term salesperson, think of yourself as an educator, a helper, an adviser, or a beauty consultant. The result will be the same.

You may not be aware that you often act as a salesperson in your personal life when you use your ability to convince other people. For example, you are "selling" when you convince your friends to go to a movie you think they will enjoy rather than another movie. You are using the same tactic when you suggest a particular service or product that you believe will benefit a client.

Now that you have accepted that part of your job is to be a salesperson, you must learn how to overcome all the problems that the typical salesperson faces.

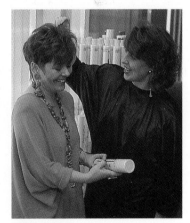

Figure 33.1
A salesperson is someone who is trying to find solutions to a client's problems.

Fear

All of us, even if we aren't salespeople, have a **fear of rejection.** We want people to like us. We are afraid that we may do something that will cause people not to like us. If we ask for something and our request is turned down, we feel rejected. Consequently, we may choose not to make a request to save ourselves the embarrassment of being rejected.

As a salesperson, you can overcome fear of rejection by realizing that, first of all, when a client says "no" to your recommendation for a product or service, the client is not rejecting you as a person. Secondly, the services or products that you are recommending might be the key to solving that client's problem. In that case, you would not be doing your job if you did not make the recommendation.

Many times your own notions about what a client is thinking may prevent you from being an effective salesperson. For example, you may not offer a product or service because you think that the client can't afford it. Or you say to yourself that if clients wanted this product or service, they would ask for it.

Years of experience in the salon industry, however, indicate that clients do not ask about a service or product for several reasons: (1) they are afraid to ask, (2) they are not aware of the service or product, or (3) they do not know that the salon carries that service or product. Instead, clients depend on their stylist to tell them about the services and products they need to maintain their appearance.

Since your clients are relying on you to tell them what they need, you will have to develop your communication skills so you can explain the products and services you offer in the most effective manner.

Methods and Process of Communication

Even though you communicate every day and in many ways, you probably never think about the process. Nevertheless, to communicate effectively, you need to understand what communication is. There are three basic **methods of communication.** You communicate **verbally** through the actual words you use when you speak. You communicate **extraverbally** through the tone of your voice, your inflection, and the rate and quality of your voice. And you communicate **nonverbally** through what is often called "body language." Each of these methods is important to the total communication process. This process is also known as **interpersonal communications.**

In any **communication process,** two people will be involved—the sender of the message and the receiver. The sender may sometimes give mixed signals to the receiver. For instance, when a friend asks you how you are feeling, you may reply, "Fine."

But your client doesn't believe you because your facial expression or posture or the tone of your voice may be saying that you are depressed or angry or hurt. Such "mixed signals" are very common, and your clients may sometimes send them. If you understand the importance of extraverbal and nonverbal communication, you will be able to interpret your client's messages and will also be able to send clearer messages to your client.

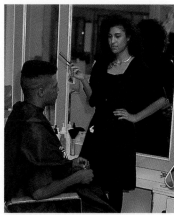

Figure 33.2
Even though your words may be friendly, if your expression and posture are hostile, the client will most likely believe the message sent by your body language.

The different types of communication vary in effectiveness. Most studies indicate that a receiver of a message relies only 10 percent on the verbal message (the actual words that are spoken), but relies 30 percent on the extraverbal message—the tone of voice, inflection, and so on. And the nonverbal aspect of communication accounts for a whopping 60 percent of the message. This means that if your facial expressions, posture, and bodily actions are saying one thing and your voice and words are saying something else, the receiver will most likely believe the message that is being sent by the nonverbal communication.

This concept applies in the salon as well. When a stylist says, "Now just relax, you're going to look great," but is frantically reading the directions on the perm box at the same time, the client does not receive a reassuring message.

A key to communicating effectively with a client is to be sincerely interested in him or her and in what you can do to help his or her appearance. If you are sincere, you will sound sincere and act sincere. You must also remember that the client comes to you to look and to feel better. Through effective communication, you can help the client feel better.

Communication works both ways; consequently, as a stylist you must be alert to the clues you receive from the client. Those clues (verbal, extraverbal, or nonverbal) will tell you what services and/or products might be appropriate for the client. As we pointed out earlier, often clients are not aware of the options that are available to them in your salon. The clients can always say no, so feel free to communicate the options.

The most effective way to sell services and products is to understand some of the psychological factors that influence the client during a sales presentation. This objective will look at some of those factors. A salon appointment usually includes several crucial communication opportunities. You can use these opportunities to develop good communication strategies. The first opportunity usually occurs when you meet the client for the first time.

Theory Objective 2
Using Psychology to Develop Communication Strategies and Salon Sales

Bonding

Bonding is the positive emotional connection that develops between you and a client. It begins when you greet the client in such a way that he or she feels that you are competent, trustworthy, and professional. If you shout at the client from your styling station, "Who's next?" the chances that he or she will get a good first impression of you are small.

If, on the other hand, you go out into the reception area to greet the client, shake hands, introduce yourself, and escort him or her back to the work area, that person will probably have a much better opinion of you.

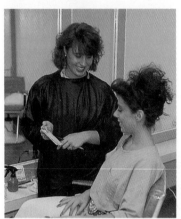

Figure 33.3
Discovering the client's needs and problems is an important part of the cosmetologist's job.

Discovery

Early in the appointment (as well as throughout the appointment), you will want to ask the client questions about his or her needs and problems. If you do this in a haphazard or intimidating way, the client may not be able to respond appropriately, and those needs or wishes won't be satisfied. But if you ask the right questions, listen to the client's answers, and pay attention to nonverbal cues that the client might send, the chances of the service being performed correctly and the client's being satisfied soar.

We like to call this question-asking process the **discovery** process. You are discovering what types of problems the client has so that you can perform services that will solve these problems.

Consultation

The next communication opportunity is **consultation**—the process in which you talk with the client about possible solutions to his or her problems. This is the point at which you might suggest appropriate services and/or products to maintain the service. The consultation process is usually carried on throughout the entire appointment. This aspect of the job can greatly affect your ability to generate more income. Consultation is the "added value" that a good stylist will give to a client. And it usually results in the client buying extra services or products or sending in referrals and coming back to the stylist again. Developing skills in consultation will be very important to your success.

Asking

You may provide the client with the information necessary to solve the problems, but the client has to decide to take your advice. Too often a stylist merely calls attention to the need for a product or service, but fails to **ask** the crucial question, "Would you like to have the service done today?" or "Would you like to take a bottle of that shampoo and conditioner home with you today?" If the question is not asked, the client's problem may not be solved, the salon will lose a potential sale, and the stylist will miss an opportunity to increase his or her income. Asking the specific question will be important to your success. Asking is necessary to **close the sale.**

Follow Through

When the client leaves, your job is still not finished. **Follow through** is the process of making sure that the service was satisfactory and that the client will book another appointment. You can use several techniques to accomplish this. A phone call asking the client if everything is all right accomplishes several objectives. It lets the client know you are concerned. It gives you a chance to correct any problems, and it provides an opportunity for you to book the next appointment. This technique is called a **follow-up phone call.**

Sending thank you cards through the mail is another way to accomplish the same thing. Handwritten notes are the most effective. Some salons provide thank you cards and pay for postage, but even if the salon where you are employed does not, it is in your best interest to send thank you cards to your clients.

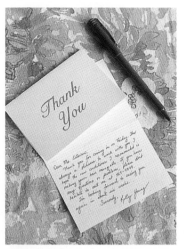

Figure 33.4
Sending a thank you note is an effective follow-through technique.

Rapid Growth in Business: Developing a "Full Book"

A cosmetologist may take up to five years to develop what is called **"full book."** A full book means the cosmetologist is booked so tightly that it is difficult to fit in new clients. Top cosmetologists tend to reach full book status much more quickly—often in one to two years. What do they do differently from the average stylist? The best cosmetologists treat the client in such a way that he or she chooses to take advantage of more of the services and products offered by the salon.

Theory Objective 3
Four Income-Producing Strategies

The "Big Four" Income-Producing Strategies

If you have good client-handling skills based on effective communications and sales techniques, you will be able to build and maintain a large clientele. You can also employ these skills to generate income through the four most important income-producing strategies, or the **"big four"** as they are called:

1. Extra services
2. Retail product sales
3. Referrals
4. Client retention

Extra Services

The first strategy is extra services. In most salons, the basic service is the haircut. In that case, **extra services** would be any service other than haircuts—perms, relaxers, colors, nails, and so forth. Every time the cosmetologist suggests an extra service to solve a client's problem, the cosmetologist has an opportunity to increase income.

It is important to understand that these extra services are recommended **only** when they are in the client's best interest. "Selling" a perm to a client who doesn't want or need one is an unethical tactic and can result in the loss of a client. But many clients are eager to hear a stylist's professional advice for additional ways to improve their appearance. Giving this advice is not only beneficial to the stylist, but it is also the stylist's duty to suggest and recommend appropriate services.

You will find that extra services are a good way to create more income per client.

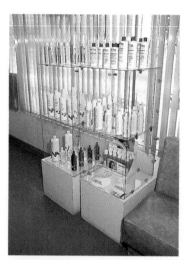

Figure 33.5
Since products sold in the salon are generally of higher quality than those sold elsewhere, recommending them can be beneficial for your clients.

Retail Product Sales

Another way to increase the number of dollars that the client spends is through **retail product sales**—providing the client with appropriate retail products. Evidence collected over the past few years indicates that most hair-care products manufactured for sale in professional salons are generally of higher quality than products sold over-the-counter in drug and grocery stores. Consequently, it can be argued that the products in most professional salons will be better for the client than products bought elsewhere. Thus, in effect, the stylist who promotes professional products is providing another valuable service to the client. If the client uses higher-quality products, the service he or she received will be better maintained.

Again, this does not mean that you should "force" the client to buy the product. But you should let the client know that the quality of the products used to maintain the hairstyle could make an obvious difference in the way it behaves.

It is also an economic fact that although many salons survive on the services that they promote, their profits come from their retail product sales. Retail product sales also provide the stylist with an opportunity to increase income. Many salons offer their stylists a commission for all retail product sales. This commission is usually in the area of 10 percent of the amount of the sale.

Referrals

As we mentioned earlier, the faster a stylist builds a "full book," the greater his or her earnings potential will be. As a stylist, you can accomplish this by getting more clients to come into the salon and specifically by getting more clients to come into your chair. Clients can be attracted in two ways:

1. Advertising and promotions by the salon.
2. Seeking **referrals**; that is, new clients who come to a stylist on the recommendation of a friend, relative, or acquaintance.

A referral can also be a new client who comes to the salon as a direct result of the efforts of a particular stylist. For example, if you pass out a business card at a party and that person comes into the salon for a haircut with you, that client is considered a referral.

You can't always depend on the salon or the salon owner to recruit new clients to the salon. Many factors may prevent the salon from getting more clients; for example, no funds may be available for advertising, or the salon may be in a poor location. However, the stylist who wishes to recruit referrals is limited only by his or her imagination.

Every satisfied client who leaves your chair is a potential "referral recruiter." If clients are satisfied with the service that they received, they will naturally tell others. If you give your clients a business card or a coupon, it will be easy for them to promote you to their friends and acquaintances.

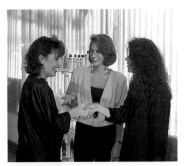

Figure 33.6
A satisfied client can be a very effective recruiter.

Generally speaking, stylists will generate about 4 to 6 percent of their income through referrals. Stylists who have less than 4 percent referrals will have a hard time building their business. In contrast, stylists who have more than 6 percent referrals, perhaps even up to 10 percent, will be able to build their business at a much faster rate than other stylists.

Client Retention

It doesn't really matter how many clients you have if you don't have a way to ensure that your clients will come back. **Client retention** is the art of keeping clients coming back to you. You retain clients in three ways:

1. Giving the clients the service they request
2. Listening to the client's needs and problems and responding to them
3. Giving each client special treatment

More than any other factor in the salon, retention depends on the emotional bond that develops between the stylist and the client. It is similar to the bond that develops between a doctor and a patient. Your professionalism can affect the client's self-esteem. The client will either look better or look worse once the service has been performed. But what the client thinks about the result is just as important, and this is often affected by how you treated him or her. Consequently, retention depends on your client-handling skills.

The following script shows how you can use good communications and sales skills in client-handling techniques that will result in client satisfaction and income generation.

Greeting

Objective: Help the client to feel good about doing business with you.

Stylist: Mrs. Johnson?
Client: Yes.

Stylist: (Handshake) Good morning, my name is Katie Sandstrom, and I'll be styling your hair today.
Client: It's nice to meet you, Katie. Please call me Linda.

Stylist: If you would follow me, I'm the fourth station on the right. Let me help you with your things, and we'll go over and sit down, and then you can tell me what you'd like me to do for you today. How's that sound?
Client: Fine.

Stylist: I understand this is your first visit to our salon, Linda.
Client: Well, yes it is.

Stylist: Welcome. I hope your visit is a pleasant one. (Stylist escorts the client to the work station and turns the chair around.)

Stylist: Here we are, Linda. Have a seat and make yourself comfortable.
Client: Thank you!

Stylist: By the way, may I get you a cup of coffee before we begin?
Client: That would be great.

Stylist: How do you take it?

Discovery

Objective: Find problems.

Stylist: (With client record card) Linda, it's important to me that two things happen before you leave. First, that you get a hairstyle that you like and feel good about, but more importantly, that you have a hairstyle that you're going to be able to do yourself—what we call a self-help hairstyle.
Client: Sounds good to me.

Stylist: Before we do anything, I'd like to ask you a few simple but very important questions about your hair. Is that okay?

Client: Fine.

Stylist: I'll also be jotting down some notes on the card you filled out when you came in so that the next time you come I'll have some history on what we did today. Okay?

Client: That's fine.

Stylist: How would you describe your hair condition ("Got" question)

Client: My hair is so fine . . . I can't do a thing with it. It takes me forever to style it in the morning, and I can't get it to stay in place.

Stylist: I see. What kinds of styling tools are you using? ("Cause" question)

Client: First, I blow it with a brush and dryer. Then I use a curling iron, but the curl doesn't last.

Stylist: What is your history with chemical services?

Client: Two or three times a year, I get a perm. That's about it.

Stylist: What is your daily hair-care routine?

Client: Every morning, I use that Goop Coop shampoo and conditioner that they advertise on television.

Stylist: What do you think is causing the manageability problems you're having?

Client: I don't know. I think I'm one of those people who are born with unmanageable hair.

Stylist: Oh, I don't think so at all, Linda. I think there's a lot we can do for you today.

Client: You really think so? You're the first stylist who's ever told me that.

Stylist: Well, let me ask you this: What qualities are you looking for in your hairstyle? ("Want" question)

Client: I wish my hair would look fuller because my face is so wide, and I'd like it to be easier to style because I don't have time to fuss with it.

Stylist: I'll tell you what, Linda. When I'm styling your hair today, I'll give you a couple of easy "tips" for things that you can do at home that will make your hair look a lot fuller. It'll also be easier for you to style.

Client: Really? That would be great!

Consulting

Objective: Solve the problems.

Stylist: Linda, after your hair is . . . gently roll the hot brush through the top and sides of your hair as I'm doing right now. This is what gives it that fuller look.

Client: Oh, and it looks so simple.

Stylist: It is! Now the key to locking in the fullness so it stays is to spray a little mist set into your hair right before you use the brush. Then, spray again right after you use the brush for double holding power.

Client: So that's how you get it to look that way. This is the first time anyone has ever taken the time to show me how to do that!

Stylist: There's really nothing to it. . . . By the way, Linda, be careful with the Goop Coop stuff you're using. Although it's a fairly good over-the-counter product, it may not have the ingredients you need for the control and the fullness you want.

Client: Really, I thought so, too, but I wasn't sure.

Stylist: Remind me to show you what I use on my hair when we go up front. My hair is similar to yours, and I've found something that works well for me. I think you'll like it. In fact, we used it today.

Client: Well, my hair does feel as though it has more body.

Asking

Objective: Close the sale.

Stylist: Let's take a look. What do you think, Linda? Doesn't it look a lot fuller than it did when you can in?

Client: It looks super! This is the nicest my hair has looked in a long time!

Stylist: I'm glad you like it. A lot of what you see is due to that tip I showed you with the hot brush and the mist I used. And, by the way, those are the keys to keeping it looking this good. I can't stress that enough.

Client: And I think I should stop using the Goop Coop, don't you?

Stylist: It certainly wouldn't hurt.

Client: Will you recommend something for me?

Stylist: Certainly. Let's go up front and I'll show you what I use.

Stylist: (At the display counter) Here, Linda (hand bottle to client), this is the spray you can use to lock in the hold, and here are the shampoo and conditioner that will build more fullness into your style.

Client: Well, if you think I need these products, I should probably get them, but I'm not sure I can afford them. After all, if they don't work, I'll be out a lot of money.

Stylist: You really can't afford not to try them, Linda. Not only are these products highly concentrated so they cost about the same per application as products like Goop Coop, but these products are also guaranteed. If you're not satisfied for any reason, simply bring back the unused portion, and we'll refund your money.

Client: I guess I really can't lose. Okay, I'll take them all. As I said before, you're the first stylist I've ever had who took the time to explain things to me. I appreciate it.

Stylist: I'm glad you're happy. By the way, Linda, do you know anyone else who would enjoy my services? If I promise to take good care of the friends you send my way, would you give them my card? I certainly would appreciate it.

Client: Why yes, I do. My sister needs a haircut, and I'm sure she'll come when she sees what you did for me.

Stylist: Thank you. I'll also be calling you in about six weeks or so to remind you of your next appointment—it's all part of our service.

Client: Oh, how nice.

Stylist: Thanks again, and I'll be in touch.

Where Do You Go from Here?

You are learning how to perfect the skills of cosmetology. You will be able to make a living with those skills. But technical skills alone won't assure your success in terms of either how much money you make or how much fulfillment you get from your job. To be a success, you will have to learn many other valuable lessons about how to treat your customers appropriately. The purpose of this chapter has been to make you aware of what is necessary to become a successful stylist. Now you must take every opportunity that arises to learn more about the client-handling techniques that will help you satisfy your clients and improve your chances of success.

Glossary

Asking The act of asking a specific question to close a sale.

Big four income-producing strategies Extra services, retail product sales, referrals, and client retention.

Bonding The positive emotional connection between the cosmetologist and the client.

Client retention The art of keeping clients coming back.

Client-handling techniques Ways of treating the customer that will make him or her feel good about the salon experience.

Close the sale The process of moving the client to a decision to buy; includes asking the specific question.

Communication methods Verbal, extraverbal, and nonverbal communication.

Communication strategies Communication opportunities involving bonding, discovery, consultation, asking, and follow through.

Consultation The process of discussing with the client possible solutions to his or her problems.

Discovery The process of asking questions about the client's problems so you can find possible solutions.

Extra services Any service other than haircuts.

Fear of rejection Being afraid to ask for something because you think the request may be turned down.

Follow through The process of making sure that the service was satisfactory and that the client will book the next appointment.

Full book Being booked so tightly that it is difficult to fit in new clients.

Interpersonal communications The process of communication through body language; also called nonverbal communication.

Nonverbal communication The process of communicating through body language.

Referral A new client who comes to a stylist on the recommendation of a friend, relative, or acquaintance.

Retail product sales Providing the client with appropriate retail products.

Salesperson A person who is attempting to provide solutions to a client's problem.

Selling The process of convincing another person to do something, such as buy a particular product.

Questions

1. To work effectively with your client, what should you try to develop?
2. In addition to technical skill, what factor will most likely determine whether you are successful in the salon?
3. What role are you playing when you are suggesting services and products that will solve a client's problems?
4. What is our biggest fear when we suggest products for clients?
5. How can you overcome the fear that a client will not accept your suggestion for a product or service?
6. Why don't clients ask for some salon products or services?
7. What are most people-handling skills related to?
8. What must clients communicate to you so that they are not disappointed?

9. What are the basic ways that you communicate with your client?
10. What term is used to describe the process of communicating with others?
11. What percentage of communication is accounted for by facial expressions, posture, and body actions?
12. How do you communicate effectively with a client?
13. What is "bonding"?
14. What strategy should you use to improve the chances that a service will be performed correctly and that the client will be satisfied?
15. What strategy should be practiced to communicate with the client about possible solutions to problems?
16. After you have communicated with your client and it is time for him or her to decide whether to buy a service or product, what should you do next?
17. After your client leaves the salon, what should you do to determine if he or she was satisfied?
18. What do you have when your scheduled appointments are so tight that it is difficult to fit in new clients?
19. List the "big four" income-producing strategies.
20. What is the difference between over-the-counter products and products sold in the salon?
21. What is the term used to describe a client who comes to you based on the recommendation of a friend, relative, or acquaintance?
22. How can new clients be attracted to a salon other than through referrals?
23. Approximately what percentage of your income in the salon will be generated through referrals?
24. What is the benefit of developing a bond between you and the client?
25. Practicing what skill will result in client satisfaction and income generation?

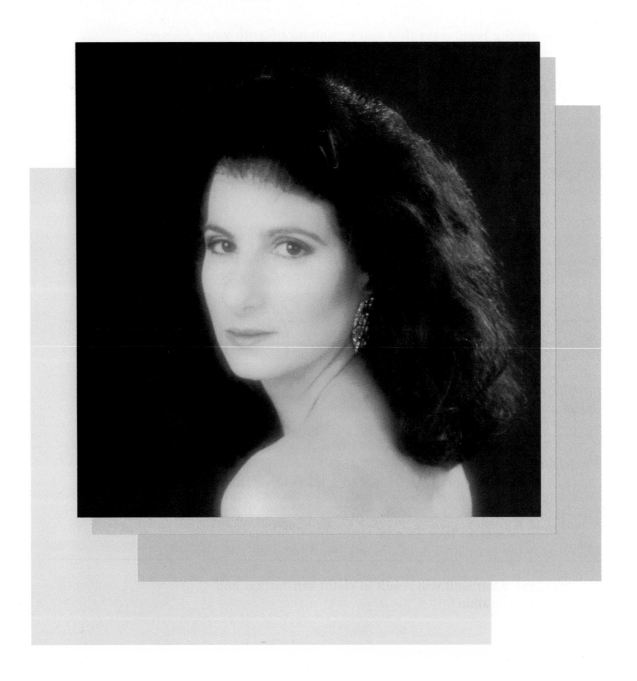

Principles of Electricity

Provided with the information in this chapter and help from your instructor, describe how electricity is used in cosmetology and define the terms related to this use. Score 85 percent or better on a multiple-choice exam on the information in this chapter.

In order to achieve the above level of competence, you should master the following chapter objectives.

Theory Objectives

1. Explain basic electrical concepts.
2. Explain how electricity is produced and controlled.
3. Describe the types of electrotherapy and the precautions needed when using it.
4. Describe the processes of electrolysis and thermolysis (diathermy).
5. Describe the benefits of a high-frequency scalp treatment.

Practical Objective

6. Give a high-frequency scalp treatment.

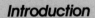

Introduction

You are undoubtedly already familiar with the word "electricity." After all, you have been using electricity all your life to run appliances from stereos and blow dryers to air conditioners and clothes dryers. Yet the principles underlying electricity may not be so familiar to you. Understanding electricity is important for you as a cosmetologist because many of the devices you will be using in both skin-care and hair-care services are electrical. For example, you cannot perform various skin-care services safely and effectively, unless you know which form of electrical current will give the best results for the service requested by the client. In order to do this, you will have to learn a small part of the "language of electricity."

Theory Objective 1
Basic Electrical
Concepts

Some of the basic concepts in the theory of electricity are: **current, voltage, resistance,** and **power.**

Current and Voltage

What actually happens when you plug an electrical appliance into a wall socket and turn it on? The wire that you plugged into the socket is **made** of **copper.** It consists of billions and billions of copper atoms strung together side by side. Each of these copper atoms can be thought of as a miniature sun with planets rotating around it (Figure 34.1).

The center of an atom is called the **nucleus;** a rotating particle is an **electron.** Both of these particles have a charge. The **nucleus is positively charged,** and the **electron is negatively charged.** The electrons in the atoms of copper and other metals are loosely bound to their nucleus and can easily leave the atom and move about. They always move according to a fundamental principle of electricity:

Figure 34.1

(a) The crystalline structure of copper wire. (b) The structure of a copper atom is like a miniature solar system with planets (electrons) rotating around the sun (nucleus).

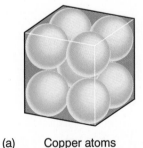

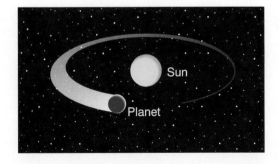

(a)   Copper atoms   (b)

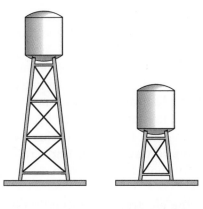

Figure 34.2
Just as water pressure is greater when the water must fall from a high tower, electrical power is greater when the voltage is larger.

High pressure   Low pressure   High pressure   Low pressure

similar charges repel, and **opposite charges attract.** In other words, two similar charges (two positives or two negatives) will repel (move away from) each other whereas two opposite charges (one positive and one negative) will attract (move toward) each other. When the electrons are moving through the wire, we say that **current** is flowing through the wire. Electrical current is measured in units called **amperes.**

The electrons start moving through the wire under the influence of a force called voltage. **Voltage** is the amount of **electrical potential that is available** for use in the form of electricity. It is measured in units called **volts.** Generally, the larger the **voltage,** the more electric power there is available. This situation is somewhat similar to water pressure. For example, if water falls a long distance from the top of a high water tower, the pressure will be greater than if the water falls a short distance (Figure 34.2). In other words, if the voltage is larger, more electrons will start moving, and more current will flow through the wire (Figure 34.3). If the voltage is smaller, fewer electrons will move, and the current will be lower.

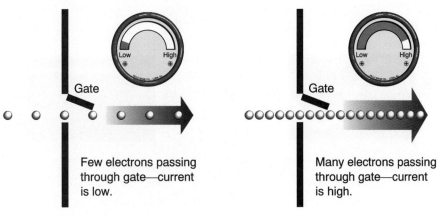

Gate
Few electrons passing through gate—current is low.

Gate
Many electrons passing through gate—current is high.

Figure 34.3
When the voltage is low, fewer electrons are moving, and the current is low. Increasing the voltage increases the number of moving electrons, and the current is high.

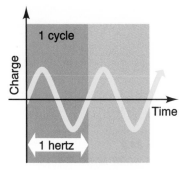

There are 60 cycles
in one second.

Figure 34.4
*Voltage alternates at a
frequency of 60 hertz (60 times
per second).*

The voltage that comes from a wall socket in your home or the salon is called **alternating voltage.** This means that the voltage is constantly changing from a positive charge to a negative charge and then back to a positive charge; this process is repeated over and over again. The change (or alternation) from positive to negative occurs 60 times each second in the United States and Canada (it occurs at other intervals in other countries). Each change or cycle is called a **hertz** (Figure 34.4). (A hertz used to be called cycles per second.) Therefore the voltage is said to alternate at a **60-hertz rate.** Another way of expressing this is to say that the **frequency** of the alternating voltage is 60 hertz.

As voltage alternates, it causes the electrons to move first in one direction and then in the other; therefore the current in the wire is called **alternating current** or simply **AC** (Figure 34.5). In contrast to this alternating current, a battery causes current to move in only one direction. Therefore this current is called **direct current** or **DC** (Figure 34.6). Direct current occurs because the negative end of the battery repels electrons (remember that electrons have a negative charge, and similar charges repel each other), while the positive end attracts electrons. Therefore the electrons flow through the wire from the negative end to the positive end. Note, however, that the direction of the current is the opposite of the direction of the electron flow.

Two voltages are used in homes and salons in North America: 110 volts and 220 volts. All small electric appliances, except those that operate on batteries, run on 110 volts. Very large appliances, such as electric clothes dryers, operate on 220 volts. If you were to connect an appliance requiring 110 volts to a 220-volt outlet, the appliance could be damaged, and more importantly, you or your client could receive an electrical shock. To prevent this from happening, appliance manufacturers use **different shaped plugs for each type of voltage** (Figures 34.7 and 34.8). Therefore you **cannot** plug a 110-volt appliance into a 220-volt outlet. If the plug fits the socket, the voltage will be safe for you to use.

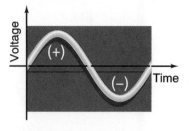

Figure 34.5
Alternating current (AC)

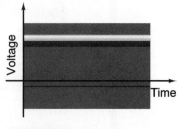

Figure 34.6
Direct current (DC)

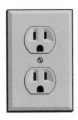

Figure 34.7
A 110-volt receptacle

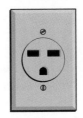

Figure 34.8
A 220-volt receptacle

Power

When voltage and current are considered together, they determine the electrical power, which is measured in **watts.** The term **"wattage"** is sometimes used to refer to the electrical power of appliances (Figure 34.9). A 1000-watt blow dryer works on the same AC voltage (110) as a 1500-watt blow dryer. The 1000-watt dryer has a smaller power rating because it uses fewer amperes of current when it is turned "on." At the same time, it produces **less heat.**

Conductors

Current and heat are closely related. The greater the current, the more heat an appliance will produce. As we have seen, current moves through wire as the electrons move. Any material that nor-

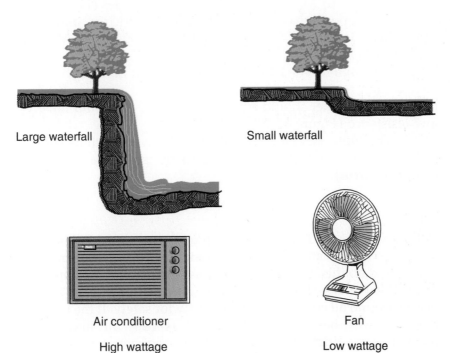

Large waterfall

Small waterfall

Air conditioner

High wattage

Fan

Low wattage

Figure 34.9
A high-voltage appliance will use more power (watts) than a low-voltage appliance. Thus, the difference between the amount of power used by the air conditioner and the fan, respectively, is similar to the difference between the power produced by a large waterfall and a small waterfall.

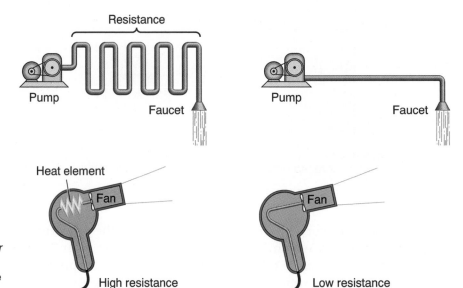

Figure 34.10
When water must flow up and down through a pipe rather than in a straight line, it is meeting resistance. Electrical current also encounters resistance to a greater or lesser extent when it flows through a wire. This resistance creates the heat expelled by the hair dryer.

mally allows electrons to move through it is called a **conductor. All metals and most liquids are conductors** of electric current, but not all conductors allow current to move through them with the **same** ease. No conductor is perfect. Even a good conductor like copper will offer some opposition to the current. In the field of electricity, opposition is called **resistance.** The amount of resistance in a conductor is measured in **ohms.** Therefore, conductors with the highest resistance (opposition) will have the highest ohms values (Figure 34.10).

The opposition can also be thought of as friction, and **friction causes heat.** Therefore, when current flows through a blow dryer or curling iron, heat is produced because of the resistance in the wire. The wire chosen for the heat-producing element in the dryer should have a high resistance, whereas the wire used to plug the device into the wall socket should not produce heat—it should have very low resistance (Figure 34.11).

The route that an electrical current travels from its source of generation via conductors and back to the source is known as a **complete circuit.**

Insulators

Safety Tips ▶

Conductors are used to move current from one place to another, but often we want to stop current from moving someplace. **Insulators** are used to do this. **Current cannot pass through an insulator. Plastic, rubber, glass,** and **air** are examples of insulators. They are placed around all conductors of electricity for safety. If the insulation around a wire becomes damaged and exposes the inner wire, a dangerous condition exists. If any other conductor comes into con-

High–resistance heating
element produce heat

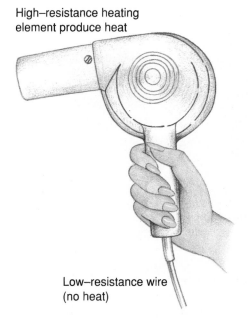

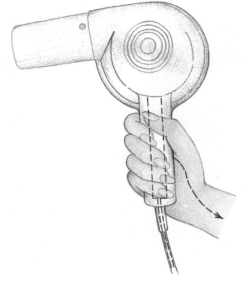

Low–resistance wire
(no heat)

Figure 34.11
*Since resistance produces heat,
a high-resistance wire is used in
the heating element of a blow
dryer, but a low-resistance wire
is used to plug the appliance
into an outlet.*

Figure 34.12
*In a short circuit, the current
leaves the wire and flows
through another conductor.*

tact with this uninsulated wire, current may leave the wire and flow through the conductor it contacts. This situation is called a **short circuit** (Figure 34.12). If you are the conductor, current flows through you, rather than through the appliance, and you will get a "shock!" **This is very dangerous and may be deadly to you.**

*Theory Objective 2
Producing and
Controlling Electricity*

Electricity can be produced in a variety of ways, but batteries and generators are the most common sources of electrical volts. They produce direct and alternating current, respectively.

Direct Current

As we have noted, **batteries** produce **direct current only** (Figure 34.13). They are either **wet cells** or **dry cells** (Figure 34.14). A 12-volt car battery is an example of a wet cell. An example of a dry cell would be a 9-volt portable radio battery. Both types of batteries contain two metal plates, which have a nonmetallic electrical con-

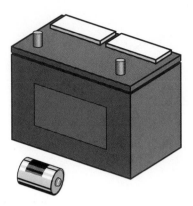

Figure 34.13
Batteries

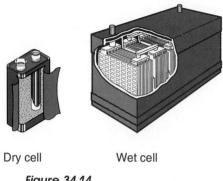

Dry cell   Wet cell

Figure 34.14
A dry cell and a wet cell

ductor between them called an **electrolyte.** Because of a chemical action, one plate becomes negatively charged, while the other becomes positively charged. The result is either a wet or a dry cell battery, which is a source of voltage.

Alternating Current

Generators are used to produce alternating current. Your local power supply company uses huge generators (as big as a semitrailer truck) to provide your home with 110 and 220 volts of electrical power. Alternating current is created when a conductor is rotated through a magnetic field (Figure 34.15). This action makes one end of the conductor positive, and the other end negative at the same instant in the voltage cycle. The conductor is rotated so the voltage alternates at 60 hertz, making it safe for use in all appliances.

Devices are available that will change alternating current into direct current. A **converter** is a mechanical electrical device used to change direct current so it can be used to power alternating current appliances. (This term is now obsolete and has had several other definitions in the past.) A **rectifier** is a device (generally electronic) that changes alternating current into direct current.

Thermocouples consist of two different metals joined together at one point. Voltage is produced between the two metals when the junction is heated. The amount of voltage depends on the metals used and the temperature at which the two metals are joined. A heating device, such as a furnace, is controlled by a thermocouple. It can produce only a small voltage of about one or two volts.

Photoelectric cells are made of materials that will produce a voltage when exposed to any light. The strength of the voltage depends on how strong the light is. These cells are used to turn streetlights on at night and off during the day.

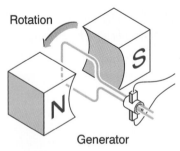

Rotation

Generator

Figure 34.15
In a generator, a conductor is rotated through a magnetic field.

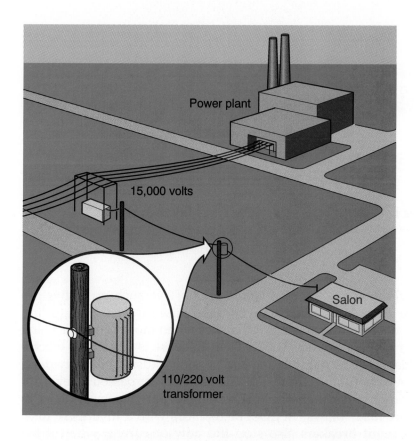

Power plant

15,000 volts

Salon

110/220 volt
transformer

Figure 34.16
*A transformer lowers the
voltage so it can be used by
the salon.*

Piezoelectric crystals will develop a voltage if pressure is applied to them in the form of twisting or bending.

As this brief survey of sources of electricity indicates, only alternating current line voltage and direct current battery voltage are strong enough for the needs of a salon. Although battery-powered devices are used in a salon, the primary power source will be the 110/220 volts of alternating current supplied by the local power company. It is not really practical, however, for the power company to supply 110 volts all the way from the generating plant, which may be located miles away, to the salon. Instead the power company generates thousands of volts at the plant and uses power lines to bring the voltage almost into the salon. Very close to the salon, the power company installs a **transformer** (Figure 34.16). This electrical device can "transform" alternating voltages. It can raise them if desired, but usually the voltages are lowered to 110 or 220 volts. Transformers only work on alternating current.

Fuses and Circuit Breakers

Since more than enough power is available from the power companies, safety devices have been designed and codes established to prevent consumers from drawing more current into the salon or

◀ **Safety Tip**

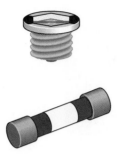

Figure 34.17
Fuses

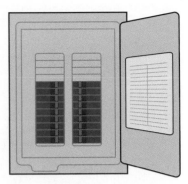

Figure 34.18
A circuit breaker

house wiring than they can handle safely. Two such protective devices are the **fuse** and the **circuit breaker. Fuses** are designed to **stop the flow** of current to an electrical device when more current is being used than is safe (Figure 34.17). Their purpose is to prevent electrical appliances from overheating and possibly causing property damage or personal injury. Fuses should never be bypassed. **Never install a larger fuse than the one you take out.** For example, if a 15-ampere fuse "blows," it must be replaced with a 15-ampere fuse!

Circuit breakers also stop the flow of current when it becomes too great (Figure 34.18). Unlike fuses, circuit breakers are **not replaceable.** Instead, they shut off power in much the same way as a light switch does. To reactivate the circuit breaker, you simply slip the breaker lever back on.

In most cases, an appliance's label will indicate how much current (amperes) it will draw. If this information is not on the label, you can calculate the amperage of the device by simply dividing its wattage by its operating voltage (110 or 220). For example, a 1000-watt blow dryer operating on 110 volts will use just over 9 amperes. Many salon and home power lines are fused at 15 amperes, so you **cannot use** two 1000-watt blow dryers on the same line. If you try to do so, the fuse will stop the current.

Safety Tips ▶ Another safety feature that is often required is **grounding.** In simple terms, this means that a third wire is used in the cord that connects the electrical appliance to the electrical socket. One end of the third wire is connected to all exposed metal parts of the device. The other end is connected to the ground through the salon wiring in a way that minimizes the possibility of shock.

In recent years, **double-insulated** appliances have begun to be used instead of grounded appliances. Double-insulated appliances are also safe to use because all exposed metal parts have been eliminated and special insulation is used. The development of new plastics that can replace metal parts has made these appliances possible.

The use of electricity to stimulate the body is called **electrotherapy.** By stimulating the muscles under the skin, electrotherapy makes the muscles move and flex. Currently, three types of electrotherapy are used—**galvanic therapy, faradic therapy,** and **sinusoidal therapy.** Before we look at the specific characteristics of each type of electrotherapy, we should examine some of the features of electrotherapy in general and note some of the safety precautions that must be taken with all forms of electrotherapy.

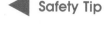 Safety Tip

First of all, it is important for you to know that the current that comes from the wall outlet is **never** applied directly to the client's skin. Since this current has 110 volts, if you applied it directly to the skin, you would **kill your client.** Instead, the 110 volts is reduced to a level the human body can safely tolerate through a device called a **wall plate** (not to be confused with the wall plate around an outlet). The name is a bit misleading because the wall plate is not actually attached to the wall (Figure 34.19). Instead, the wall plate is plugged into the wall outlet. Wall plates come in a variety of sizes and styles and are portable (movable).

Positive and Negative Electrodes

All electrotherapy devices have two poles, one of which is positively charged while the other is negatively charged. The positive electrode (pole) is called the **anode.** It is usually marked in some way—it may be identified with the word **"positive,"** a large "P," or a plus sign (+), or it may be color-coded red. The negative electrode is called the **cathode** (KATH-ohd). It is usually marked with the word **"negative,"** a large "N," or a minus sign (−), or it may be colored black. The type of marking used will depend on the company that manufactured the device.

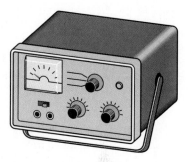
Wall plate

Figure 34.19
Wall plate

Sometimes the electrodes are not marked in any way. If this is the case, you can perform a simple test to determine which is the positive electrode and which is the negative electrode. Place just the tips of the two electrodes in a glass of water **without touching** them together (Figure 34.20). If they touch each other, you will probably blow a fuse or trip a circuit breaker in the machine. Gradually, turn up the current on the machine. The water will "bubble" as the current flows between the electrodes. The current causes the water to break down into gases that produce the bubbles. Although bubbles will appear around both electrodes, **the negative electrode will have more bubbles, and they will be smaller.** The positive electrode will have larger bubbles.

Some of the older machines required the client to hold one of the electrodes. With some newer machines, the electrode is attached to the client using a moistened pad held in place with plastic tape or a strap. More specific precautions will be noted

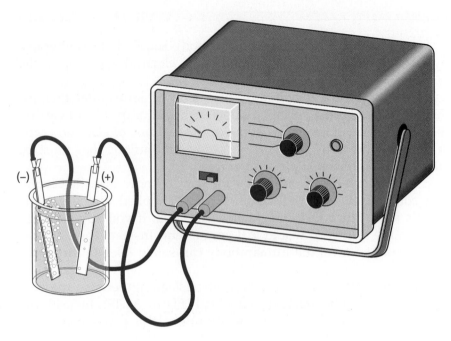

Figure 34.20
Determining which electrode is negative (−)

when we look at the specific types of electrotherapy, but always remember to **read the directions in the operating manual carefully and follow them precisely.**

Caution

Safety Tip

Regardless of the type of electrotherapy you use on your client, **never allow the current to go above 1 milliampere! Larger amounts will cause pain and discomfort to your client.** You can determine the amount of current by looking at the current meter on the machine. The current is easy to regulate if you start at "0" and gradually increase it to a level that is comfortable for your client. The "comfort level" will vary from client to client, so remember to **begin at "0" each time you use electrotherapy.**

Galvanic Electrotherapy

Galvanic electrotherapy is the oldest and most common form of electrotherapy. It is believed to cause a **chemical reaction on the skin** that promotes **beautiful, healthy,** and **youthful** looking skin. Unlike the other types of electrotherapy, which use alternating current, galvanic electrotherapy uses direct current. This current causes the chemical reaction on the skin and is therefore called a **chemical current.** The current can also be used to force chemicals through unbroken skin in a process called **phoresis.**

In addition to these effects, **galvanic electrotherapy causes the muscles to contract and relax.** It also **produces heat** because the current flows through the client's skin, and skin offers some **resistance** to the flow of current.

In galvanic electrotherapy, **the client holds** (or is attached to) the **inactive electrode.** The cosmetologist holds the **active electrode** and applies it to the client's skin. When performing galvanic therapy, **never use the indirect method** in which a part of your body is between the client and the active electrode (the indirect method will be discussed in more detail later in the chapter). Be sure that you **always read and follow the directions in the operating manual very carefully!** If the manual is not available, ask your instructor to be present when you use the device. This is important for your safety as well as for the safety of your client.

Using the Positive Electrode in Galvanic Electrotherapy. The **positive electrode** is believed to produce an **acid reaction** on the skin. This electrode is used to **close the pores** and **firm up skin tissue.** The positive electrode is also a **vasoconstrictor,** which means that it causes the blood vessels to shrink and thus limits the flow of blood through them. Reducing the blood flow also slows down glandular activity, and this has a sedative effect on the skin. Galvanic therapy can even be used on red, irritated skin where it will have a soothing effect. Also note that the positive electrode is believed to have an **astringent** effect, which tends to firm and harden skin tissue.

Using the Negative Electrode for Galvanic Electrotherapy. When the client is in contact with the positive electrode and the cosmetologist touches the negative electrode to the skin, an **alkaline reaction is produced.** This has the opposite effect as the positive electrode. The **negative electrode is believed to soften the skin and increase glandular activity.** It acts as a **vasodilator,** which means that it causes the blood vessels to expand and thus increases the flow of blood. This is irritating to the skin. **Never** apply the negative electrode to red, irritated skin! You would probably use this type of therapy to relax the skin before a facial treatment.

Skin Lightening. **Skin bleaching** is one application of galvanic electrotherapy. As noted earlier, in the process called **phoresis,** the electrotherapy device forces certain substances through the skin without breaking the surface of the skin. There are two forms of phoresis: cataphoresis and anaphoresis.

Cataphoresis is a treatment in which a solution **is pulled** into the skin tissue. In cataphoresis, the client is in contact with the negative electrode, while the cosmetologist uses the positive electrode. The positive electrode is usually wrapped with a cloth that has been soaked in the solution. When you touch the skin with the solution-soaked cloth, the solution is drawn into the skin.

The process of **anaphoresis** is the opposite of cataphoresis. In **anaphoresis,** the solution is **pushed, or forced, into the skin** instead of being "pulled." This is the most effective way to lighten your client's skin. Although a solution-soaked cloth is used in this method, this time the cloth is **wrapped around the negative electrode.** The positive electrode pushes the alkaline lightening solution into the skin.

Electrolytic Suction Cup.   Another skin treatment using galvanic electrotherapy is called the electrolytic-suction-cup treatment. This treatment is said to **soften the skin, open the pores, and increase glandular activity** simultaneously (at the same time). A specially constructed suction cup is brought in contact with the client's skin, causing the pores to open and the skin tissue to soften. At the same time, a very gentle gravity-forced stream of water vapor removes sebum and dirt (Figure 34.21). This leaves the skin looking cleaner and fresher and feeling wonderful.

In this treatment, the special cup is connected to the negative electrode, and the client is attached to the positive electrode. This causes a negative galvanic current to pass through the skin. After you have cleansed the skin, the electrodes are usually reversed. The positive galvanic current will close the pores, firm the tissue, and restore the skin to its natural state of acidity.

Figure 34.21
Electrolytic-suction-cup
treatment

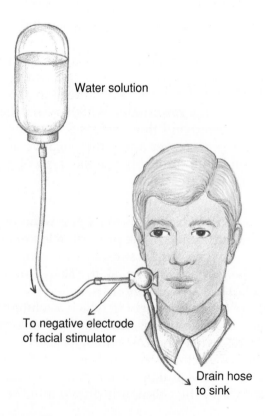

Water solution

To negative electrode
of facial stimulator

Drain hose
to sink

Faradic Electrotherapy

On most electrotherapy machines, the galvanic current can be changed from direct current to alternating current simply by "flipping a switch." The current used in faradic electrotherapy is an alternating current, but it differs from ordinary alternating current in that it is produced from direct current. For this reason, **faradic current** is called an **induced current. Faradic current** is used to exercise the muscles and activate muscle tissue.

Background Information. In an age of wellness and physical fitness, most of us are aware that exercising our muscles is necessary to keep our bodies functioning at their best. This is also true for facial muscles. One way to exercise facial muscles is to stretch them in front of a mirror. Models often do facial exercises to keep their facial muscles in good tone. Unfortunately, few people continue to do these exercises regularly. Instead, many people choose to go to the salon for their facial exercises. Massage and electrical stimulation both aid in preserving facial muscle tone.

   Massage is an excellent way to sooth and relax facial muscles. It is not as effective as electrical stimulation at making the muscles work, but it may do more to protect the skin from "wrinkling" than if you did nothing.

   Faradic electrotherapy is considered the most effective way to make facial muscles work to their potential. It causes the muscles to contract, then relax.

Using Faradic Electrotherapy. When using faradic current, the cosmetologist can choose between the direct method or the indirect method. In the **direct method,** both electrodes are placed on the client's skin. Before being attached to the skin, the felt-covered electrodes are soaked in a conductive solution. **The electrodes should never touch each other.** The current should be set at "0" at first, then gradually increased until the client's comfort/tolerance level has been reached. For the best results, apply the electrodes to the motor points of the face to stimulate the muscles (Figure 34.22). The current traveling between the electrodes through the motor nerves causes the muscles to flex for part of a second. The setting on the machine determines how long the current flows through the muscle before it is automatically turned off.

   In the **indirect method** of faradic electrotherapy, the cosmetologist is between the electrotherapy device and the client, so the current flows through the client to the cosmetologist's fingers. In this method, you usually wear a wrist band, which is one of the electrodes. The other electrode is a solution-soaked pad, which is attached to the client's neck (usually between the shoulders) or is held by the client. After the electrodes are in place, put your fingers

◀ Safety Tip

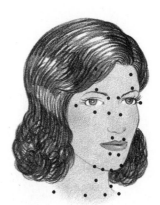

Figure 34.22
Facial motor points

on the client's face, and adjust the current to a comfortable level. Then massage the motor points according to the procedure taught in your school.

Safety Tip ▶ **Safety Considerations.** Whether you use the direct or indirect method, it is important to check your meter to make sure the current is set at "0." If not, the client will get a small shock when touched. Remember to remain in contact with the client's face once the current has been turned "on." Reach over with one hand and turn the current to "0" before removing your other hand from the client's face.

Sinusoidal Electrotherapy

Sinusoidal electrotherapy is similar to faradic electrotherapy. In both modes of operation, alternating current causes the muscles to contract and relax. Some cosmetologists prefer faradic current because they believe it is the **most soothing** and least irritating type of therapy. The 110-volt alternating current used in all salons is sinusoidal. The word **sinusoidal** describes how the current changes from positive polarity to negative polarity. As we have seen, the power company generally regulates the frequency (how often) with which current changes its polarity, so that it changes 60 times per second (60 hertz). Most sinusoidal devices change the frequency of the current to something other than 60 hertz. Some devices allow you to control the frequency as well as the amount of current.

Usually, a slightly modified (changed) sinusoidal wave is used rather than a pure wave. The modified waves produce longer muscle contractions and are believed to massage the muscles more effectively.

Using a Sinusoidal Electrotherapy Device. Sinusoidal electrotherapy is applied in the same way as faradic electrotherapy. The same electrodes are used, and the therapy may be applied directly or indirectly. It produces very smooth, repeated contractions of the facial muscles. Because sinusoidal therapy is able to affect both voluntary and involuntary muscles, it may be used for scalp treatments as well as facial treatments. It is considered to be especially good for stimulating **deep muscles** because **it penetrates more than faradic current.** Thus, sinusoidal therapy is used on middle-aged clients who have facial wrinkles.

Safety Tip ▶ A word of caution is necessary. **The treatment period should be no longer than 30 minutes.** If the muscles become fatigued, the benefits of the treatment will be lost. Never give sinusoidal facial treatments to unhealthy skin. **For example, refuse a service on skin with open cuts or red, open sores!**

High-Frequency Therapy

Another type of electrotherapy is **high-frequency therapy,** which is not used to stimulate muscles. High-frequency treatments use alternating current that changes **thousands of times per second.** Because the frequency change is so fast, no muscular reaction is produced. Instead, these high-frequency currents **produce heat** as they move through the skin. When used correctly, heat can have a definite therapeutic effect on the skin.

The high-frequency treatment is believed to stimulate the nerves in the skin and promote the circulation of blood through the vessels. These treatments are also thought to increase circulation in the lymph system, stimulate overall glandular activity, and improve the general metabolism of the body. Another benefit is that high-frequency treatments have a germicidal effect on the skin, so disorders such as blackheads or simple acne tend to clear up when treated regularly. Tesla high-frequency therapy can also be used to remove warts, moles, or other tissue growths, but this should **not be done by the cosmetologist!**

Although several high-frequency currents are used, the most popular is called **tesla current.** High-frequency tesla currents have a very high voltage, but the current is very small (low). Tesla devices vary considerably in size and style, depending on the manufacturer. Some devices have one electrode while others have two. Small, hand-held, one-electrode units are the most popular because of their low cost. Sometimes these devices are called **violet rays** because the electrode emits a violet-colored light. Many of these devices come with a selection of plug-in electrodes, which are often made of clear glass. The electrodes are available in several sizes and shapes, which allow them to be used on different parts of the body. For example, a rake-shaped, glass electrode is used for the scalp (Figure 34.23).

Indirect Treatments.   Indirect high-frequency treatments are given to clients who have dry skin or scalp. **The indirect treatment is intended to prevent the skin from becoming drier.** As in the indirect method for faradic therapy, the electrode is held by the client or is

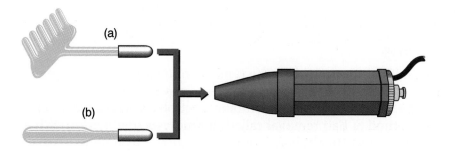

Figure 34.23
A high-frequency unit with glass electrode attachments: (a) hair rake; (b) facial disk (hand-held electrode).

attached to the client. In high-frequency indirect treatments, the current flows through the client's skin to the massaging fingertips of the cosmetologist (Figure 34.24). Heat is produced where the fingertips come in contact with the client. The cosmetologist will have a tingling sensation in his or her fingertips. As a safety precaution, **make sure the machine is set at "0" to start,** and **then** adjust the current to the comfort/tolerance level of the client as well as your own comfort/tolerance level.

Safety Tip ▶

Direct Treatments. Most of the safety rules used in galvanic and faradic therapy also apply to direct high-frequency treatments. Always start with the current at the lowest possible setting, then gradually increase it **after the current** is applied to the skin. When the current has been adjusted to a comfortable level, the glass electrode is moved slowly across the skin. Before using the glass electrode, some cosmetologists like to apply an emollient skin cream, which transfers the heat and distributes it more evenly across the skin. The cream also makes the glass electrode slide across the skin more easily during the treatment. Special care should be taken when using cream on the scalp or skin. **Be sure that the cream does not contain alcohol,** which can be **flammable.** If a cream with a flammable base were used, a spark from the high-frequency unit could ignite the alcohol and start a fire!

When a high-frequency treatment is being given, there will be an odd smell in the air. The odd smell is **ozone,** which is created as the tesla current "breaks down" the air around the electrode. As the ozone drifts up to your nose from the electrode, you will notice a different odor in the air. Ozone is also believed to have a therapeutic effect.

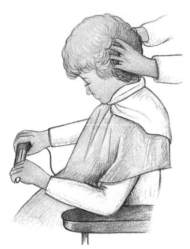

Figure 34.24
Indirect high-frequency treatment

Theory Objective 4
Electrolysis and Thermolysis (Diathermy)

Because cosmetologists are often asked to recommend a treatment that will remove unwanted hair, they should be familiar with the options available to the client. Although a cosmetologist is not licensed to remove unwanted hair with electrical methods in most states, knowing how some of these methods work can often be helpful.

Electrolysis

By definition, **electrolysis** is the removal of unwanted hair using an electrical method. The person who performs this service is an **electrologist.** Electrologists may combine electrolysis with another electrical method of hair removal called **thermolysis** (diathermy). When electrolysis and thermolysis are combined, the technique is called the **blend,** or **dual method.** When used individually, both electrolysis and thermolysis have advantages and disadvantages. The blend, or dual method, tends to take the advantages of both techniques along with the disadvantages.

Electrolysis uses a low-frequency **galvanic** current (Figure 34.25). It is thought that the current breaks down body salts and water in the skin and causes a chemical reaction between the water, salt, and the skin. During this reaction, chlorine, hydrogen, hydroxyl ions, and sodium compounds are formed in the hair follicle. These chemicals combine to form **lye (sodium hydroxide)** and hydrochloric acid at the bottom of the hair follicle. The lye destroys the hair bulb over a period of time by causing the **papilla** (nerve and blood supply) to die. As a result, the hair stops growing. No more hair can grow from that follicle.

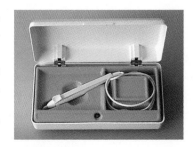

Figure 34.25
An electrolysis machine

It is believed that **the negative electrode causes an alkaline reaction** within the skin, forming sodium hydroxide. When the electrologist's needle is withdrawn from the hair follicle, the sodium hydroxide remains at the bottom of the follicle where it dissolves the tissue and prevents the regrowth of hair. Although this method is considered quite effective, it can be somewhat painful because the treatment of an individual follicle may take from 50 seconds to one and one-half minutes, depending on the resistance of the skin and the moisture content of the tissue. So, the process is very time-consuming. Increasing the galvanic current can speed up the process, but the pain may be too uncomfortable for the client.

Thermolysis (Diathermy)

Thermolysis uses high-frequency current to produce heat in the tissue rather than producing a chemical reaction as electrolysis does. The high-frequency current used in thermolysis is in the megahertz range. A megahertz is a million alternations per second.

The setting for the thermolysis needle before it is inserted into the follicle will depend on how much tissue is to be destroyed. Often the device will have both a manual control for the time the current remains "on" and an automatic timer. The automatic setting is good because it prevents the current from being left on accidentally for too long a time. Thermolysis seldom requires a time period longer than 30 seconds in the manual mode or 1/2 second in the automatic mode. The disadvantage of this method is that if the angle at which the needle is inserted is slightly out of line with the walls of the follicle, the destroyed tissue will not be in the area necessary to stop hair from regrowing (Figure 34.26). Another disadvantage is that determining how long to leave the current on can be difficult. Therefore, if the needle is inserted at the wrong angle or the current is left on for too short a time, the unwanted hair will grow again. In addition, the skin can easily be scarred if you're not extremely careful.

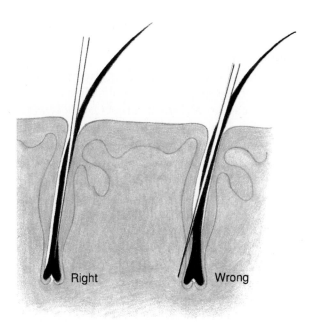

Figure 34.26
A needle inserted into the hair follicle at the right angle and the wrong angle

Blend or Dual Method

The **blend** or **dual method** combines galvanic current with low-level high-frequency current. The result is a method considered to be as effective as electrolysis and as fast and painless as thermolysis.

The addition of high-frequency current improves electrolysis in four ways: (1) The heating action of the electrode applied to the tissue around the follicle makes the tissue porous so that it can more readily absorb the lye produced by the galvanic current. (2) High-frequency current causes the lye to liquify, so it moves around and fills up the follicle cavity. (3) High-frequency current heats up the sodium hydroxide trapped under the skin, which speeds up the dissolving action of the hair-growing tissue. (4) High-frequency current reduces the pain felt during long periods of electrolysis because the current has a numbing, anesthetic effect on the skin.

Theory Objective 5
Benefits of a
High-Frequency Scalp
Treatment

Scalp treatments are an important application of high-frequency electrotherapy. High-frequency scalp treatments may be given after silking but before the curling service as well as in other situations. Consult your instructor about other applications of this type of scalp treatment.

The high-frequency scalp treatment is considered to be beneficial in several ways:

1. It **normalizes** the activity of the sebaceous glands and the apocrine and eccrine sweat glands.

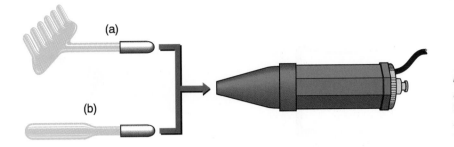

Figure 34.27
(a) The glass rake and (b) the facial disk are used in high-frequency scalp treatments.

2. It increases the circulation of the blood by **stimulating** the scalp.

3. It destroys germs by causing the air bubbles to release ozone and nitrous oxide.

4. It **relaxes** the muscles of the scalp to relieve itchiness, tightness, or falling hair.

The high-frequency appliance is used either directly or indirectly. In the **direct method,** the glass scalp rake or glass facial disk is applied directly to the scalp (Figure 34.27).

The **indirect method** can be used for both skin and scalp applications. The client holds the metal electrode, and the current travels through the client's body and through the hands of the cosmetologist, who acts as a ground for the current. This method is seldom used. If the indirect method is used, the client should not touch any metal object, such as the frame of a metal chair.

Practical Objective 6
High-Frequency Scalp Treatment

Supplies

- high-frequency unit (Figure 34.28)
- 1 glass-rake electrode attachment (direct treatment) or
- 1 glass-rod electrode attachment (indirect treatment)
- timer

Direct Method

Procedure

1. You and your clients should remove all jewelry. Place the client's valuables in a safe place, not on the styling station.

Rationale

1. As a safety precaution, remove all jewelry because it is a good conductor of electrical current. It could cause a shock.

◀ Safety Tip

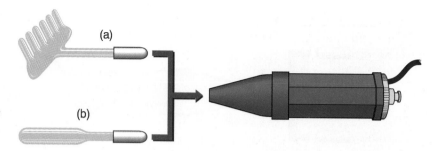

Figure 34.28
A high-frequency unit with (a) a glass rake and (b) a facial disk (hand-held electrode)

2. Attach a glass-covered electrode to the power unit: then plug it into the electrical outlet.

3. Set the timer for 3 minutes.

4. Turn the knob at the end of the power unit very slowly so that you start with the smallest possible amount of current through the glass rake.

Safety Tip

5. **Place your index finger on the top of the glass rake;** then lower the rake to the crown area of the client's head, and remove your finger (Figure 34.29).

2. To prevent electrical shocks, adjust the electrode attachment before you plug the unit in.

3. Overexposure to high-frequency current can burn the skin.

4. This is safe procedure.

5. Placing your index finger on the rake decreases the sparking effect and grounds the electrical current.

Figure 34.29
Placing your index finger on the glass rake as you lower it to the client's head reduces sparking and grounds the current.

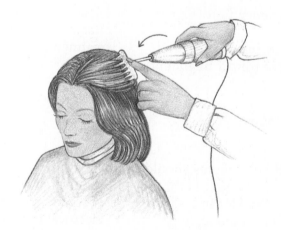

6. Move the glass rake back and forth on the scalp. Work from the forehead to the nape and side to side until the entire scalp area has been stimulated. Move the rake lightly all over the scalp for a small amount of time. Do not break contact.

6. If you are going to give several treatments, the first one should take 2 or 3 minutes; gradually increase the treatments **to a maximum of 5 minutes.** This treatment improves circulation and produces a healthier scalp.

Indirect Method

Procedure

1. Give the glass- or metal-rod electrode to the client. Advise the client to hold it in both hands.

2. Turn on the unit slowly.

3. Give scalp manipulations without breaking contact with the client (Figure 34.30).

Rationale

1. This is standard procedure.

2. This is standard procedure.

3. Give scalp manipulations while the client holds the electrode. The electrical current passes through the client's body and through your hands and body; since you are standing on the floor, the current is grounded.

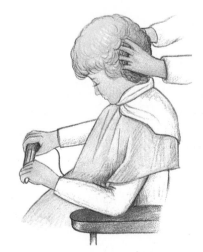

Figure 34.30
The client holds the electrode while you give scalp manipulations.

AC See **Alternating current.**
Alternating current An intermittent flow of electricity that moves first in one direction and then in the opposite direction.
Ampere A measure of electrical current.
Anaphoresis An electrotherapy process in which a solution is pushed into the skin (for lightening).
Anode The positive electrode of an electrotherapy device.
Blend A hair removal technique that combines electrolysis with thermolysis; also called the dual method.
Cataphoresis An electrotherapy process in which a solution is pulled into the skin (for lightening).
Cathode The negative electrode of an electrotherapy device.
Circuit breaker A safety device that stops the flow of current.
Complete circuit The route that an electrical circuit travels from

its source of generation via conductors and back to the source.

Conductor A material that allows electrons to move through it.

Converter A mechanical device used to change direct current so it can be used to power alternating appliances. (This term is now obsolete.)

Current Moving electrons.

Cycle See **Hertz.**

DC See **Direct current.**

Diathermy See **Thermolysis.**

Direct current Current that moves in only one direction, such as that produced by a battery.

Direct method A faradic electrotherapy technique in which both electrodes are placed on the client's skin.

Double-insulated appliance A type of appliance that is not grounded, but is safe to use because of the type of insulation used around its wiring.

Dry cell A type of battery.

Dual method See **Blend.**

Electrologist A person who permanently removes unwanted facial and body hair by using different kinds of electrical current that travels through a very fine needle.

Electrolysis The removal of unwanted hair through an electrical method.

Electrolyte A nonmetallic electrical conductor.

Electrolytic-suction-cup treatment A skin treatment using the galvanic electrotherapy device.

Electron A particle that rotates around the nucleus of an atom.

Electrotherapy The use of electricity to stimulate the body.

Faradic current Alternating current used to exercise the muscles through electrotherapy.

Faradic therapy A type of electrotherapy used on the skin and muscles.

Fuse A safety device that stops electrical current.

Galvanic electrotherapy A therapy that uses direct current; it produces heat and causes muscles to contract and relax.

Galvanic therapy See **Galvanic electrotherapy.**

Generator A device that produces alternating voltage.

Grounding A wiring safety procedure that minimizes the possibility of getting a shock from electrical appliances.

Hertz A unit that measures the alternation of current.

High-frequency treatments Therapy using alternating current to produce heat.

Indirect method A faradic electrotherapy technique in which the cosmetologist is placed between the device and the client.

Insulator Material that will not allow current to pass through.

Nucleus The center of an atom.

Ohm The measurement of resistance in a conductor.

Phoresis A process in which substances are forced through the skin without breaking the surface of the skin.

Photoelectric cells Cells made of materials that will produce a voltage when exposed to any light.

Piezoelectric crystals Crystals that will develop a voltage if pressure is applied in the form of twisting or bending.

Power Voltage multiplied by current in a circuit.

Rectifier A device that changes alternating current into direct current (now usually an electronic device).

Resistance Opposition (measured in ohms) to electrical flow.

Short circuit The condition created when a conductor interferes with a circuit.

Sinusoidal See **Sinusoidal therapy.**

Sinusoidal therapy A treatment using alternating current to contract and relax muscles.

Skin lightening A technique in which galvanic electrotherapy is used to lighten the skin.

Sodium hydroxide A chemical compound also known as lye.

Tesla current A high-frequency current sometimes used in therapy.

Thermocouple A junction between two dissimilar metals that generates a voltage when heated.

Thermolysis (diathermy) A technique that uses high-frequency current to produce heat in the tissue.

Transformer A device that can raise or lower alternating current voltages; normally used to lower voltage down to 110 or 220 volts.

Vasoconstrictor Something that reduces the flow of blood in the blood vessels.

Vasodilator Something that increases the flow of blood in the blood vessels.

Violet ray A small hand-held electrode device used in high-frequency therapy.

Volt A unit of electrical potential.

Voltage Electrical potential.

Wall plate A portable appliance used in electrotherapy that can produce galvanic, faradic, or sinusoidal currents (not to be confused with the wall plate around an outlet).

Watt A unit of electrical power.

Wattage A designation sometimes used to refer to the electrical power of appliances.

Wet cell A type of battery.

1. What term is used to indicate how much electrical potential is available for use?
2. Are 110 volts and 220 volts of electricity used in North America?
3. What electrical term is abbreviated AC?
4. Is copper a good conductor of electricity?
5. Name the center of an atom.
6. Name the rotating particle of an atom.
7. What term means opposition to the flow of electrical current?
8. What device lowers the power line voltage so it is suitable for household use?
9. If you try to draw too much current through a wire, what "blows" or is "tripped"?
10. Is galvanic current an alternating or direct current?
11. Does galvanic current produce a chemical reaction as well as heat?
12. What is the positive electrode called?
13. What is the negative electrode called?
14. Name the process that causes chemicals to be forced through unbroken skin.
15. Is the positive electrode believed to produce an acidic reaction on the skin?
16. Is the negative electrode thought to produce an alkaline reaction on the skin?
17. Does the positive electrode appear to harden and firm up the skin?
18. Is it usually best to begin a treatment with the meter set at 5 milliamperes?
19. Does cataphoresis pull the solution into the skin?
20. Does anaphoresis push, or force, the solution into the skin?
21. Does faradic therapy exercise the facial muscles?
22. Describe the direct and indirect methods of electrotherapy.
23. Is high-frequency therapy a form of galvanic current?
24. Is it thought that indirect treatments prevent the skin from becoming drier?
25. Is removal of unwanted hair using an electrical method called the blender?
26. In electrolysis, does using galvanic current cause lye to form in the hair follicle?
27. Does thermolysis involve the use of high-frequency current to produce heat in the skin tissue?
28. Is it thought that the use of high-frequency current improves the effectiveness of electrolysis?

29. True or false. High-frequency scalp treatments are considered to be beneficial because they normalize the activity of the sebaceous glands and the apocrine and eccrine sweat glands.
30. True or false. It is not necessary to remove all jewelry before giving your client a high-frequency scalp treatment.

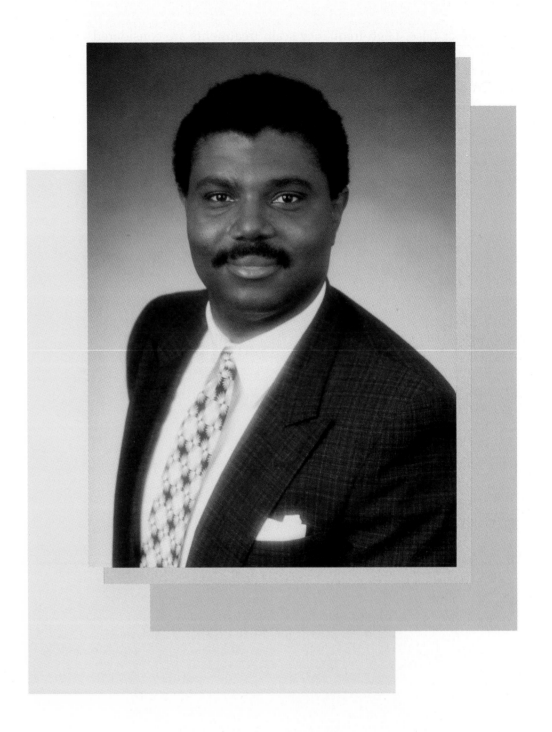

Chemistry of Cosmetology

Provided with the information in this chapter, identify and describe the basic principles of chemistry related to the practice of cosmetology. Score 85 percent or better on a multiple-choice exam on the information in this chapter.

In order to achieve the above level of competence, you should master the following chapter objectives.

Theory Objectives

1. Define matter, substance, and organic and inorganic chemistry, and explain how matter can be changed.
2. Explain what elements, compounds, atoms, ions, and molecules are.
3. Define physical and chemical properties.
4. Identify and describe the kinds of mixtures: solutions, colloids, and suspensions.
5. Describe acids, bases, salts, and pH.

Chemistry is involved in all of the services a cosmetologist provides. Therefore a good cosmetologist should have a working knowledge of the basics of chemistry.

Have you ever had a course in chemistry or do you know someone who has? Did you or your friend find the course difficult? If you think chemistry is hard, you are right—at least to a certain extent. Chemistry can be a very complicated field—some people spend many years learning to become chemists.

But before you start worrying about mastering this chapter, you should keep a few things in mind: (1) Chemistry always has been an important part of cosmetology. (2) Chemistry has become even more important in recent years as new products have been developed from complex chemical formulas. (3) You or your friend may have had **no particular** reason for studying chemistry; it may have just been one of several courses you took along with English, history, and math. This situation is different, because now you will be able to apply what you learn. You have a **specific** reason for learning the basics of chemistry because you will use chemical principles both as a student and later as a cosmetologist.

Does this mean that you must be a chemist? No! But it would be a good idea for you to learn the basic principles of chemistry that are explained in this chapter. Give this chapter a chance, and you will be surprised by how quickly you will learn the chemistry you need for your career. You may even become interested in chemistry once you understand how it applies to cosmetology.

From time to time, you may find that the material is hard to understand. Stick to it! Chemistry can be difficult, but once you have learned it, you will have mastered a very important part of cosmetology.

Theory Objective 1
Matter, Substance, and Organic and Inorganic Chemistry, and the Ways Matter Can Be Changed

Chemistry is a science concerned with matter and the way it changes. This definition sounds simple, but the rest of this chapter will be devoted to showing just what this statement means.

Matter

It is a hot summer day. The room is stuffy, so you open the window. A cool breeze blows in, and the room feels much more comfortable. But now you are thirsty, so you go into the kitchen for a nice, cold glass of ice water. You turn on the faucet and fill a glass with water. Then you add a few ice cubes from the refrigerator.

In these actions, you have just come in contact with all three forms of **matter.** Matter is everywhere around us. In chemistry, **matter** is defined as anything that has **weight** and takes up **space.** Matter takes three forms, all of which you experienced on that hot summer day: **solid** (the ice cubes), **liquid** (the water), and **gas** (the air). A solid (ice cubes or powders) has definite shape and volume. A liquid (water or shampoos) has definite volume but indefinite shape. A gas (hydrogen peroxide evaporating) has indefinite shape and indefinite volume.

As a cosmetologist, you will work with all three forms of matter every day. You probably have already realized that you will be working with solids (a client's hair, fingernails, and skin), but the various products that you will use are also examples of matter. They come in all forms—solids, liquids, and gases—and it is very important to know which form you are using because they act differently.

Another important term that is related to matter is **substance.** A **substance** is a unit or part of matter that has a particular set of qualities that define what it is. Elements and compounds are pure substances (elements and compounds are explained in the next objective). In cosmetology, cosmetics are often made from organic substances, but an **antioxidant** must be added to prevent them from spoiling.

Organic and Inorganic Chemistry

Scientists usually talk about two branches of chemistry: organic and inorganic. Until a little over a hundred years ago, scientists defined **organic chemistry** as the study of matter that comes from life processes; that is, matter that is either alive or was once alive. **Inorganic chemistry** is the study of matter that is not alive and never has been alive (Figure 35.1).

The old phrase "animal, vegetable, or mineral" is an easy way to remember this distinction. In a sense, the phrase includes all matter. **Animal** and **vegetable** describe everything that is or was alive. (In addition to obvious examples, these categories include a wooden desk, which came from a tree, and the oil in your car—oil was formed millions of years ago from dead plants and animals.) The last part of the phrase, mineral, describes inorganic matter. Rocks and metals are examples of inorganic matter.

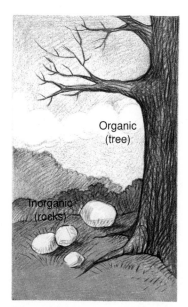

Figure 35.1
Organic and inorganic matter

This distinction we have made between **organic** (living) and **inorganic** (nonliving) matter is convenient and useful, but it is not entirely accurate in a scientific sense. Scientists have been able to make many combinations of organic matter in laboratories, which somewhat blurs the distinction between organic and inorganic. Nevertheless, the definition presented here should be suitable for your purposes, as long as you keep in mind that the difference between organic and inorganic matter is much more complicated than the difference between trees and rocks.

Scientists also have another way of explaining the difference between organic and inorganic chemistry. They say that **organic chemistry** is concerned with combinations of carbon in matter; in particular, it is concerned with hydrocarbons, a special type of carbons. Most combinations of **carbon are organic.** They can be found in all types of living things (plants and animals) or in products made from living things, such as soft coal, petroleum, and natural gas. In general, carbons will burn and are soluble (will dissolve) only in organic solvents, such as alcohol. They are not soluble in water.

Inorganic chemistry is concerned with the study of matter that does not have carbon in it. Minerals are a good example (remember the phrase "animal, vegetable, or mineral" that we mentioned earlier?). Many minerals occur in nature, and scientists have learned to make new combinations of inorganic matter in the laboratory as well. Sodium hydroxide, silver, and water are all examples of inorganic matter.

A few forms of inorganic matter do contain carbon. One is carbon dioxide, which is what you exhale when you breathe. Diamonds and the lead in your pencil are other examples.

Physical and Chemical Changes

Matter can be changed in two ways: physically and chemically. If you make a **physical change** in matter, you may change the way it looks, but you will not change its makeup. For example, you may change the way an ice cube looks by letting it sit in the open air, but you will not change the fact that it is water: the ice will become liquid water instead of frozen water, but it will still be water (Figure 35.2). In this case, heat caused the physical change.

A physical change does not have to change the way something looks. For example, when you open the window to let a cool breeze into your house, you create a physical change: you lower the temperature inside the house. Note again that the physical change affects only the form—in this case, the temperature—not the makeup of the matter.

Chemical changes are different. Matter is changed chemically when another kind of matter is added to or taken away from it. The result of a chemical change is something new and different. In

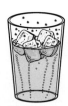

Figure 35.2
When ice melts, only a physical change occurs, not a chemical change.

a sense, when you chemically change something, you destroy it. You will still have matter, but it will not be the same as when you started. If you enjoy cooking, you may have some very complicated combinations of chemicals in your kitchen in the seasonings you use. But even if you are not a cook, your kitchen probably contains a simple example of a chemical change: salt. Salt is made of sodium (a metal) and chloride (a gas). These two substances are very different, but when they are combined, the result is something completely different from either sodium or chlorine: sodium chloride (salt). In this case, a chemical change has occurred: the actual makeup of the substances has changed. For another example of a chemical change, think of what happens when you combine hydrogen and oxygen in the proper proportions. You create hydrogen peroxide, which is very different from either hydrogen or oxygen alone.

Heat plays an important part in many chemical changes. Some chemical changes need heat to take place. Others give off heat when they take place.

Theory Objective 2
Elements, Compounds, Atoms, Ions, and Molecules

Elements and Compounds

As we have seen, salt is a simple combination of sodium and chlorine. This kind of combination is called a **compound.** Compounds can be very complicated and include many more substances than salt does, but all of them are made from **elements.**

Stop for a minute and think of the thousands and thousands of words that we can make with only 26 letters in the alphabet. The same is true for elements. Elements are the basic units of substances. Although there are only 105 elements (92 can be found in the natural world; 13 have been created by scientists), they can be combined to form an almost limitless number of compounds.

Atoms, Ions, and Molecules

At one time, scientists thought that elements were the smallest kind of matter that existed, but later they learned differently. Elements are made up of atoms, which are much smaller than elements and cannot be seen by the unaided eye. An **atom** is the basic unit of an element. An element, such as hydrogen or oxygen, has only **one kind** of atom.

An atom can be broken into smaller parts, but then it is no longer an element. For example, if you broke up an atom of sodium, you would no longer have an atom of sodium. You would have a sodium **ion.**

Basically, an atom has three kinds of particles—**protons, electrons,** and **neutrons** (Figure 35.3). Protons and electrons have

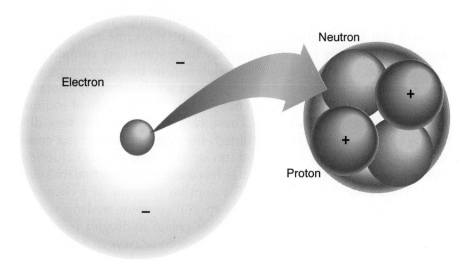

Figure 35.3
An atom of helium

power that scientists call an electrical charge. Protons have a positive (plus) charge, and electrons have a negative (minus) charge.
The core of the atom sometimes contains neutrons, which do not
have a charge. Normally, an atom has the same number of positive
and negative charges, so they balance each other off. When the
number of protons and electrons is not equal, you have an ion. The
number of electrons an atom has is what gives it the ability to combine with other atoms in chemical reactions.

Sometimes an atom gains an electron from an atom of another element. When this occurs, the atom that gained the electron
is called a negatively charged ion (it now has one more electron—
negative charge—than protons). The atom that lost an electron is
called a positively charged ion (it now has one more proton—
positive charge—than electrons).

This gain or loss of electrons is the chemical process that
goes into making a compound. Atoms gain or lose electrons and
become joined to each other and form a **molecule.** A molecule is a
combination of atoms that forms the basic unit of a compound. An
atom is to an element as a molecule is to a compound. If you break
up an atom of an element, you no longer have an element;
similarly, if you break up a molecule of a compound, you no longer
have a compound.

Let's return to our earlier example of salt. As you know,
sodium and chlorine are the two elements in this compound. An
atom of sodium gives up one of its electrons to an atom of chlorine
as shown in Figure 35.4. The result is two ions—one sodium, the
other chlorine. The sodium ion does not have all the characteristics
of the element sodium because it is not a complete atom. The same
is true of the chlorine ion. Together they form a molecule of the

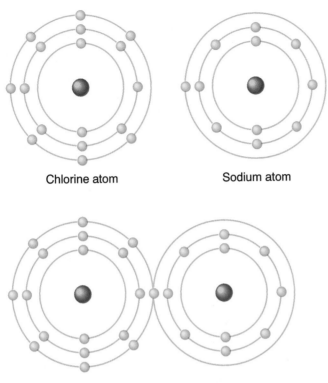

Chlorine atom   Sodium atom

Sodium Chloride molecule

Figure 35.4
Sodium has only one electron in its outer shell and tends to give it up easily. Chlorine, on the other hand, has seven electrons in its outer shell and needs one more electron to complete that shell. Chlorine therefore borrows one electron from a sodium atom to complete its outer shell. Both ions then have complete outer shells that are held together by strong electric forces. Together the sodium and chlorine ions form a sodium chloride (salt) molecule.

compound sodium chloride, which is totally different from both sodium and chlorine. If you separate the sodium and chlorine ions, the compound will be destroyed.

Another way atoms combine is by **sharing** electrons. In a water molecule, for example, two atoms of hydrogen share their single electrons with an atom of oxygen, which has six electrons in its outer shell (Figure 35.5). In any atom, the first (innermost shell) can contain only two electrons, and the second shell can contain only eight electrons. Therefore, in a water molecule, the oxygen atom completes its second shell by adding the two hydrogen electrons to its own six electrons, and each hydrogen atom completes its first shell by adding one electron to the electron it already has.

The process we have just described can also be discussed in terms of chemical changes. These changes can take two forms: synthesis and decomposition (analysis). In **synthesis,** a compound is created by combining elements or simpler compounds. Thus, the formation of salt from sodium and chlorine and the formation of water from hydrogen and oxygen are examples of synthesis. In **decomposition** (analysis), a compound is broken down into its parts.

Another example of a chemical change that leads to the formation of a compound is what happens when sulfur is burned

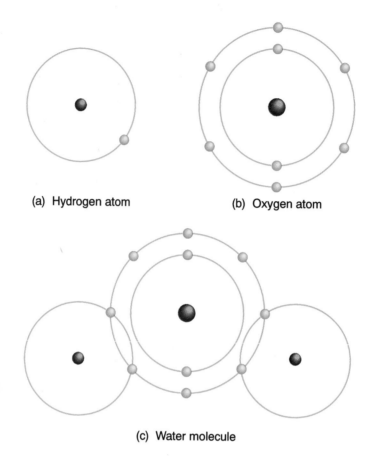

(a) Hydrogen atom   (b) Oxygen atom

(c) Water molecule

Figure 35.5
(a) Two hydrogen atoms share electrons with (b) an oxygen atom to form (c) a water molecule.

(Figure 35.6). Each atom of carbon in the sulfur combines with two atoms of oxygen from the air. This cluster of three atoms forms one molecule of carbon dioxide. The chemical symbol for carbon dioxide is CO_2, which corresponds to the 1 atom of carbon and the 2 atoms of oxygen that make up the carbon dioxide molecule. Note that when sulfur is burned, it also undergoes a physical change. The physical change is easier to see, but the chemical change is taking place as well.

Another familiar example in which both physical and chemical changes occur is the use of hydrogen peroxide. When you apply peroxide to the hair, it oxidizes or gives up an atom (ion) of oxygen. The chemical formula of hydrogen peroxide is H_2O_2. When peroxide loses oxygen, it becomes H_2O, which is water.

Theory Objective 3
Physical and Chemical
Properties

Substances look different and undergo different physical and chemical changes as a result of their **properties** (characteristics). The physical condition of a substance is one of its properties. Others

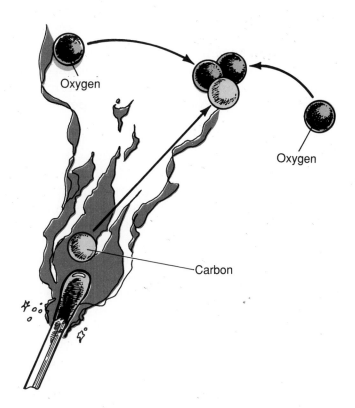

Oxygen

Oxygen

Carbon

Figure 35.6
The formation of carbon dioxide from one carbon atom and two oxygen atoms

include its color and odor. As you have seen, physical changes do not change the chemical makeup of a substance. Therefore they can be reversed.

A substance's **chemical properties** are the way it reacts when it is combined with another substance. For example, one of hydrogen's chemical properties is its ability to **attract** or **draw** oxygen atoms from other elements.

Theory Objective 4
Kinds of Mixtures:
Solutions, Colloids, and
Suspensions

As we noted earlier in this chapter, compounds are combinations of elements that are joined by chemical means. **Mixtures** are also combinations of elements or compounds or both, but unlike compounds, the parts of a mixture are only joined **physically.** This means that the individual parts of a mixture keep their own properties and can be separated easily by physical or mechanical means. Face powders are mixtures as are the various oils on the human skin.

Many important cosmetic preparations are mixtures, so you should be familiar with their characteristics. Mixtures can be found in all the basic forms of matter—solids, liquids, and gases. In addition, mixtures can be divided into three types: solutions, colloids, and suspensions.

Solutions

True **solutions** are **homogeneous mixtures** of two or more elements or compounds. This means that the same proportion of the elements or compounds can be found throughout the mixture. For example, if a solution contains 35 percent hydrogen, 35 percent oxygen, and 30 percent formaldehyde, you will find those exact percentages of the ingredients at any place in the solution. The particles are so small that they cannot be seen separately—even through a microscope.

Two **examples** of **solutions** in different physical states are air and formalin. In air, gases (oxygen, hydrogen, and so on) are dissolved in a gas (nitrogen); and in formalin, a gas (formaldehyde) is dissolved in a liquid (water). Most solutions used in the salon are either liquids dissolved in other liquids or solids dissolved in liquids.

The substance in which the particles are dissolved is called the **solvent.** The particles that dissolve are called the **solutes** (SAHL-yoots). Water, alcohol, acetone, and glycerine are the solvents most commonly used in salon products, although many other solvents may also be found.

Solutions can be divided into three types, depending on the amount of solute used (Figure 35.7). **Diluted** solutions contain only a small percentage of solute; **concentrated** solutions have a much larger percentage; and **saturated** solutions have as much of a solute as a solvent can dissolve at a particular temperature (heat can affect the ability of a solvent to dissolve a solute).

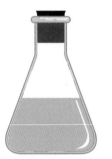

Figure 35.7
A saturated solution

Colloids

Colloids are mixtures containing particles that are larger than those in a solution. These particles have only a **slight** tendency to settle.

The particles of the colloid are called **colloidal particles;** the substance in which the particles are distributed is called the **dispersing medium.** Colloids can be found in any of the three physical states. The following are some examples of colloids in various physical states:

1. Liquid aerosol—a liquid dispersed in a gas.
2. Solid aerosol—a solid dispersed in a gas
3. Liquid emulsion—a liquid dispersed in a liquid
4. Solvent—a solid dispersed in a liquid

It is especially important to know about **liquid emulsions,** since many preparations are in this form. Emulsions contain tiny droplets of one liquid suspended in another liquid. Salon emulsions are usually oil-in-water mixtures. If emulsions are allowed to stand, the two types of ingredients may separate into layers. The emulsions sold by cosmetics manufacturers, however, usually contain an **emulsifying agent,** which breaks the oil into very small droplets and keeps them from coming together again. Thus, the agent makes the mixture smoother and more stable. Many salon creams and lotions are emulsions.

Suspensions

Suspensions are mixtures of a solid and a liquid or a solid and a gas. The solid particles in suspensions will **settle** out (separate) when the preparation is allowed to stand. Because these particles are rather large, suspensions have a cloudy appearance. Calamine lotion is an example of a suspension.

Theory Objective 5
Acids, Bases, Salts, and pH

Acids and **bases** are compounds. They are used in many hair-care products because their effects on the hair are predictable.

The way acids and bases work can be understood by looking at the structure of compounds. As we pointed out earlier in this chapter, an atom is the basic unit of an element, and a molecule—a combination of atoms—is the smallest basic unit of a compound. An ion is a particle that has an electric charge. Whether the charge is positive or negative depends on the makeup of the ion.

Cosmetologists are especially concerned with two types of ions: hydrogen and hydroxyl (hydroxide). **Hydrogen ions** are positively (+) charged particles (one or a group of atoms) of hydrogen. **Hydroxyl ions** are negatively (−) charged hydrogen ions that also have oxygen attached to them (hydroxyl radical). If a solution has more hydrogen ions than hydroxyl ions, it is an acid. If a solution has more hydroxyl ions than hydrogen ions, it is a base.

The term **pH** refers to the **concentration** (percentage) of hydrogen ions in a solution. This concentration determines whether the solution has acidity (an acid) or alkalinity (a base). If a solution is not an acid, it may be a base or it may be **neutral.** A solution in which the **concentrations** of hydrogen and hydroxyl are the same is neutral because the acid and the base balance each other.

The pH scale (0–14) shows the degree of acidity or alkalinity of a solution or substance. The middle of the scale, 7, is the neutral point. The numbers 0 to 6.9 indicate acidity; 7.1 to 14 represent alkalinity.

Certain substances, such as litmus paper, are **indicators.** They turn a certain color in the presence of an acid and a different color in the presence of a base. You can use them to find out if a solution is alkaline or acid. Many other kinds of indicators are also available from dealers.

When acids and bases react, they form water and a **salt.** This reaction is called **neutralization.** Salts contain both a metal and a nonmetal because they are formed by a combination of an acid and a base. Some salts also contain oxygen.

Acid and alkaline products affect the hair differently. **Acid products** shrink and harden the imbrications (scales) of the shaft of the hair. They also neutralize the alkalinity of hair products that have a pH over 7 (bases). Acid rinses, for example, are used to neutralize alkaline shampoos.

Alkaline products swell and soften the hair strand, opening the imbrications. Ammonia, for example, is an alkali that is used in permanent hair colors to open the imbrications of the hair so that the color molecules can pass into the inner layers of the hair. Alkaline products can neutralize acid products, but this is not a common application in cosmetology.

Skin and hair are acid. They have a pH of 4.5 to 5.5. Salon products that have a pH of 4.5 to 5.5 are said to be **acid-balanced in respect to skin and hair.** Thus, using an acid-balanced product does not change the natural pH of the skin or hair.

Glossary

Acid Any substance that has a pH rating under 7.

Alkaline Any substance that has a pH rating over 7.

Antioxidant An additive used in cosmetics that are made from organic substances to prevent spoilage.

Atom The basic unit of an element.

Chemical change A change in a substance made by adding or removing another kind of matter.

Chemical properties The way a substance behaves when it reacts to other substances, compounds, or forms of energy.

Chemistry The study of matter and the way it changes.

Colloid A mixture containing particles that are larger than those of a solution.

Compound A chemical combination of elements.

Concentrated solutions Solutions that contain a large percentage of solute.

Dilute solutions Solutions that contain only a small percentage of solute.

Elements The basic units of substances; they are made up of atoms.

Emulsion A mixture containing tiny droplets of one liquid suspended in another liquid.

Gas A form of matter having indefinite shape and indefinite volume.

Inorganic chemistry The branch of chemistry that is concerned with the study of matter that does not contain carbons (inorganic substances).

Inorganic matter Anything that is not alive and has never been alive.

Liquid A form of matter that has definite volume but indefinite shape.

Matter Anything that has weight and takes up space.

Mixture A physical combination of elements or compounds or both.

Molecule A combination of atoms that is the smallest basic unit of a compound.

Organic chemistry A branch of chemistry concerned with combinations of carbons, especially hydrocarbons.

Physical change A change in a substance brought about by a physical force, such as a change in temperature or pressure.

Physical properties Characteristics such as a substance's physical state, color, and odor.

Salt A compound formed when acids and bases (alkalis) react.

Saturated solutions Solutions that contain as much of a solute as a solvent can dissolve at a particular temperature.

Solid A form of matter having definite shape and definite volume.

Solute (SAHL-yoot) The particles that are dissolved in a solvent, making a solution.

Solution A homogeneous mixture of two or more substances or compounds.

Solvent A substance that dissolves particles, making a solution.

Substance A unit or part of matter that has a particular set of qualities that define what it is.

Suspension A mixture of a solid and a liquid or a solid and a gas.

Questions

1. What is something that takes up space and has weight?
2. In what kind of chemistry might a rock be studied?
3. In what kind of chemistry might a dead tree limb be studied?
4. What science is concerned with matter and the way it changes?
5. Are carbons organic?
6. When two or more elements are joined chemically, what is formed?
7. Does a solid have a definite shape and volume?
8. Does a liquid have a definite volume and a definite shape?

9. True or false. A gas has an indefinite shape and an indefinite volume.
10. Are elements and compounds pure substances?
11. What is formed when different elements are combined together?
12. What is the smallest and most basic part of an element?
13. Name the three particles found in an atom.
14. True or false. Breaking down a compound into its parts is known as decomposition.
15. Give four examples of solvents used in the beauty salon.
16. Are hydrogen ions positively charged?
17. Are hydroxyl ions negatively charged?

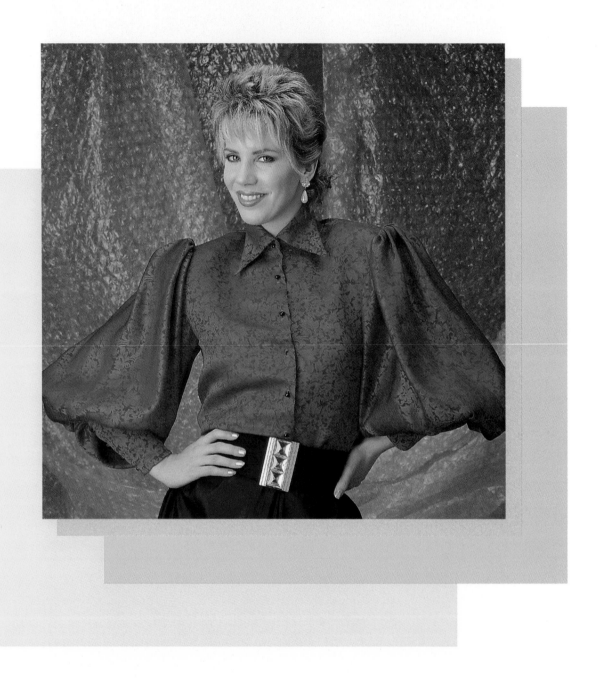

Anatomy and Physiology in Cosmetology

Provided with the information in this chapter and classroom instruction, define anatomy and physiology, and identify important bone structures, muscles, and nerves. Score 85 percent or better on a multiple-choice exam on the information in this chapter.

In order to achieve the above level of competence, you should master the following chapter objectives.

Theory Objectives

1. Define the terms physiology and anatomy, describe physiological cells and tissues, and list the systems of the body that may be affected by school and salon services.
2. Define osteology, and explain the structure and function of bones, cartilage, ligaments, joints, and synovial fluid.
3. Describe the major bones of the head, neck, trunk, arm, and hand.
4. Define myology; describe the functions of the muscles and identify three types of muscles; and explain muscle contraction, origin, and insertion.
5. Describe the muscles of the head, face, trunk, and arm.
6. Define neurological terms and explain the divisions of the nervous system and the brain.
7. Explain the types and functions of nerves found in the head, face, neck, arm, hand, and fingers, and describe the arc reflex.

Introduction

Anatomy and physiology are concerned with the structure and functions of the body. The bones, muscles, and nerves of the body are often affected by the services you will perform as a cosmetologist, so you should understand the basics of these subjects.

Theory Objective 1

Physiology and Anatomy, Physiological Cells and Tissues, and Systems of the Body Affected by School and Salon Services

The study of the body may be divided into two very broad categories: **physiology,** which is the study of **body functions,** and **anatomy,** which is the study of the **structure of the body.**

The study of physiology begins with the smallest, most basic unit of the body: the **cell.** Cells have several structures that can be seen through a microscope. The outside of the cell is called the **cell membrane.** Inside the membrane is the **cytoplasm** (SIGH-tah-plaz-uhm), which is a jelly-like substance. The **nucleus** (NOO-klee-uhs) is like the brain (center) of the cell. It directs the cell's activities. When a cell becomes fully grown, it splits to make two cells from one. In other words, the parent cell becomes two equal cells. This process is called mitosis. The **centrosome** (SEN-treh-sohm) of the cell helps the cell divide.

Each cell of the body can take in nutrients (food). Cells use food for **energy** and **growth** and can also **store** nutrients to be used later. These processes are called **metabolism** (meh-TAB-eh-liz-uhm). **Anabolism** (ah-NAB-eh-liz-uhm) refers to processes that build up the cell, and **catabolism** (keh-TAB-eh-liz-uhm) refers to the processes that supply energy.

Thousands of similar cells working together to accomplish a specialized function form a **tissue.** You should be concerned with four types of tissue: connective, muscular, nervous, and epithelial. Each type serves a particular function:

- **Connective tissue** binds, supports, protects, and nourishes the body. Bones, cartilage, ligaments, tendons, blood, and adipose (fatty) tissue are all examples of connective tissue.

- **Muscular tissue** forms the muscles, which give the body its ability to **move.**

Table 36.1
Anatomical Terms

Term	Meaning
Superior	Above, upper
Inferior	Below, lower
Anterior	In front of, frontal
Posterior	In back of, behind
Medial	Toward the midline of the body
Lateral	Away from the midline, toward the edge of the body
Proximal	Closer to center
Distal	Away from center

- **Nervous tissue** makes up the nerves and brain. Nerve tissue is the body's communication system.

- **Epithelial** (ep-eh-THEE-lee-ehl) **tissue** lines all the surfaces of the body.

Two or more different types of tissues **working together** to perform a particular function form an **organ.** For example, the liver is an organ. A **group of organs** working together to accomplish a major function is called a **system.**

You will find that certain terms are used frequently in anatomy to indicate the location of the organ or tissue being discussed. Table 36.1 lists some of these terms and their meaning.

Some Important Systems of the Body

Several systems of the body may be **directly affected** by the practice of cosmetology. They include the **skeletal, muscular, nervous, vascular** (blood and blood vessels), and **endocrine** (glands) systems. There are other systems, but they are not directly related to cosmetology.

Theory Objective 2
Osteology and the Structure and Function of Bones, Cartilage, Ligaments, and Joints, and Synovial Fluid

Osteology (ahs-tee-AHL-eh-jee) is the scientific study of **bone.** The bones of the body **protect the organs** (for example, the rib cage protects the heart and lungs), support the body, and provide the leverage necessary for body movement (Figure 36.1). As a group, the bones are called the **skeletal system.** The skeletal system is made up of three kinds of connective tissue—bone, ligament, and cartilage.

Although bone is considered a living tissue (though it does contain nonliving matter), it is both rigid enough to support the body and flexible enough to remain intact despite the jarring of

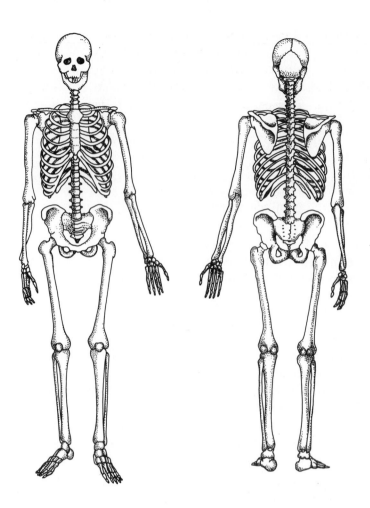

Figure 36.1
The skeletal system

everyday life. Living bone tissue is made up of cancellous and compact tissue.

Cancellous (spongy) tissue can be found at each end of the shafts of the **long bones,** such as the leg bones. It also makes up most of the inside of the **flat bones,** such as those of the skull.

Compact, or dense, **bone tissue** makes up the shafts of the long bones and forms the outside of the flat bones. Blood vessels pass through canals in this layer.

The shafts of the long bones contain yellow, fatty **marrow.** The cancellous tissue at the ends of the long bones contains **red marrow.** All blood cells are produced in this red marrow.

Each bone is covered with a fiber known as the **periosteum** (per-ee-AHS-tee-uhm). This outer covering forms new bone tissue and contains blood vessels and nerves that extend to the bone; muscles, ligaments, and tendons attach to the bone at the periosteum.

Bones are held together by ligaments, cushioned by cartilage, and lubricated by the synovial fluid.

Cartilage (KAHR-tah-lij) is basically the same as bone tissue, but it does not contain inorganic matter. It has a smooth surface that protects the bones from stress. Bones normally rub against each other, and cartilage keeps this from being painful. Cartilage also aids in shaping the external features of the face, such as the ends of the nose and ear.

Ligaments (LIG-eh-mehnts) are bands or sheets of connective tissue that hold the bones together. They allow bones to move without slipping out of place.

The place at which two or more bones are joined is commonly called a joint. There are three kinds of joints: immovable (such as those in the skull), slightly movable (such as the spine), and freely movable (such as the knee).

The synovial (seh-NOH-vee-ahl) fluid is a special type of tissue that helps to lubricate and cushion the bones at the joints. It cuts down on friction and makes movement easier.

Theory Objective 3
Major Bones of the Head, Neck, Trunk, Arm, and Hand

The **skull** is the skeleton of the entire head (Figure 36.2). It protects the brain and gives the head its shape. The following are the major bones of the skull:

- **Cranium.** The bones that encase the brain. One of the two main parts of the skull.

- **Ethmoid (ETH-moid) bone**. The upper part of the bony structure that divides the nasal cavity in half.

- **Frontal bone.** The front of the skull, including the forehead and the roof of the eye sockets.

Figure 36.2
Bones of the head and neck

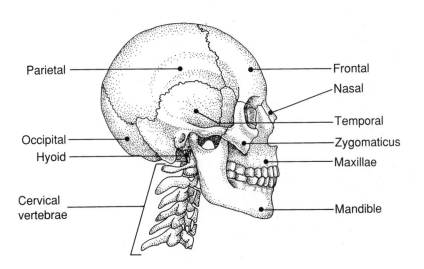

Parietal — Frontal
Nasal
Temporal
Occipital — Zygomaticus
Hyoid — Maxillae
Cervical vertebrae — Mandible

- **Occipital (ahk-SIP-eh-tehl) bone.** The rearmost bone of the skull and cranium.
- **Parietal (peh-RIGH-eht-ehl) bones.** The top and sides of the cranium.
- **Sphenoid (SFEE-noid) bone.** A butterfly-shaped bone located almost at the exact center of the head. It is a connecting bone.
- **Temporal bones.** The bones that form the bony part of the skull above and in front of the ears.

The face is the other main part of the skull. The facial bones include the following:

- **Conchae or turbinals.** The bones located at the side walls of the nasal cavity and protruding into it. They warm and clean the air.
- **Lacrimals (LAK-rih-mehlz).** The bones on the inner sides of the eye sockets. They form the part of the canal through which the lacrimal (tear) duct joins the eye socket with the nasal cavity.
- **Mandible.** The jawbone. It forms the entire lower portion of the face and holds the teeth.
- **Maxillae (mak-SIL-ee).** The two bones that form the hard palate, the lower portion of the eye sockets, and the upper portion of the jaw.
- **Nasal bones.** The bones that shape the bridge of the nose.
- **Palatines (PAL-eh-tynes).** The two bones that form part of the hard palate, which is the roof of the mouth.
- **Zygomaticus (zigh-goh-MAT-i-kus) or malars (MAY-lahrz).** The two bones that form the outer, lower portion of the eye sockets and the cheekbones.

The neck and trunk contain the following bones:

- **Cervical vertebrae (SER-vi-kehl VEHRT-eh-bray).** The first seven cervical vertebrae are in the back of the neck.
- **Hyoid (HIGH-oid).** The U-shaped bone situated above the larynx (Adam's apple).
- **Ribs.** A bony cage of 24 bones that protects the heart, lungs, and other organs.
- **Sternum (STEHR-nuhm).** The breastbone. It forms the front attachment for the ribs.

The bones of the arm and hand include the following:

- **Carpals (KAHR-puhlz).** The eight bones of the wrist.

- **Clavicles (KLAV-i-kehlz).** The collarbones.

- **Humerus (HYOOM-eh-ruhs).** The large bone of the upper arm.

- **Metacarpals (met-ah-KAHR-puhlz).** The five bones of the palm. They connect the wrist with the fingers in this order: first metacarpal (thumb); second metacarpal (index finger); third metacarpal (middle finger); fourth metacarpal (ring finger); fifth metacarpal (little finger).

- **Phalanges (FAY-lanj-eez).** The bones of the fingers (digits).

- **Radius (RAY-dee-uhs).** One bone of the forearm. It is on the thumb side.

- **Scapulae (SKAP-yeh-lee).** The shoulder blades.

- **Ulna (UHL-nah).** One of the two bones of the forearm. It is on the little-finger side.

Theory Objective 4
Myology, the Functions and Types of Muscles, and Muscle Contraction, Origin, and Insertion

Myology (migh-AHL-eh-jee) is the study of the muscular system, including both the muscles (over 500 of them) and the specialized connective tissue associated with them.

A **muscle** is a bundle of elastic fibers surrounded by a tough membrane known as the **fascia** (FASH-yah). The fascia separates the muscles and helps to hold them in place. Muscles vary in size, length, and shape according to their function and the area they affect. Muscle pressure on bones causes the body to grow or results in body movement.

The cells that make up muscle tissue have several qualities: **extensibility** (ability to stretch); **contractibility** (ability to shorten); **elasticity** (ability to return to the original shape); and **excitability** (ability to respond to stimulus). In the muscular system, this stimulus is provided by the nerves.

Three different types of muscle tissue are found in the body. They are striated, smooth, and cardiac muscles.

Striated (STRIGH-ay-tehd) muscles, also called voluntary muscles and skeletal muscles, look striped if you look at them under a microscope (Figure 36.3a). The nerves in striated muscle come from the **cerebrospinal tract** of the **nervous system**. These muscles can be controlled by the individual; that is, the individual can move them as he or she wishes.

Parts of the body that function automatically, such as the internal organs and the blood vessels, are lined with **smooth** (involuntary) muscles (Figure 36.3b). The nerves in smooth muscle come

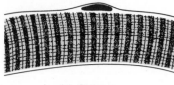

(a) Striated

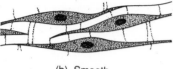

(b) Smooth

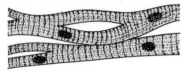

(c) Cardiac

Figure 36.3
Types of muscle tissue

from a special branch of the nervous system known as the **autonomic** (aw-teh-NAHM-ik) **nervous system.**

Cardiac muscle tissue is found only in the heart (Figure 36.3c). It has some of the characteristics of both of the other types. Cardiac muscle is the **only type** of muscle tissue that can contract on its own at regular intervals at all times. It is influenced by the autonomic nervous system.

You cannot move if your muscles do not contract. Absolutely all body movements result from the contraction of one or more muscles.

A muscle is attached to the skeleton at two points. One is called the **origin,** or **proximal** point; the other is called the **insertion,** or **distal** point. The proximal point is **closer** to the center of the body than the distal point. When a muscle is stimulated, it contracts and becomes shorter and thicker than when it was relaxed. The contraction draws the two points of the muscle closer together, but the insertion moves much more than the origin. Thus, when the muscle contracts, the insertion moves toward the origin, and when the muscle relaxes, the insertion moves away from the origin.

Theory Objective 5
Muscles of the Head,
Face, Trunk, and Arm

When you massage a client's head and face, the following muscles are affected (Figure 36.4):

- **Buccinator (BUK-si-nay-tehr).** The muscle that extends from the mandible and maxilla to the orbicularis oris muscle and the skin of the lips. It draws in the cheeks.

- **Corrugator (kor-uh-GAY-tehr).** The muscle located on the frontal bone between the eyebrows and extending to the middle of the eyebrow. Named for its zigzag edge, it draws the eyebrows together and down.

- **Depressor anguli oris (di-PRES-ehr AN-gyoo-ligh OR-iss) triangularis.** The muscle from the mandible to the lower corners of the mouth.

- **Depressor labii inferioris (LAY-bee-igh in-FIHR-ee-or-iss).** The muscle from the mandible to the lower lip. It lowers the corner of the mouth.

- **Epicranius (ep-i-KRA-nee-uhs).** The epicranius muscle has two bellies of muscle joined by a sheet of connective tissue, called an **aponeurosis** (ap-oh-nyoo-ROH-siss). The two bellies are called the **frontalis** and the **occipitalis.**

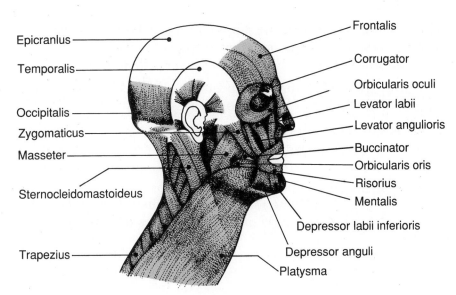

Epicranlus

Temporalis

Occipitalis

Zygomaticus

Masseter

Sternocleidomastoideus

Trapezius

Frontalis

Corrugator

Orbicularis oculi

Levator labii

Levator angulioris

Buccinator

Orbicularis oris

Risorius

Mentalis

Depressor labii inferioris

Depressor anguli

Platysma

Figure 36.4
Muscles of the head and neck

- **Frontalis (fruhn-TAL-iss).** The muscle along the eyebrows to the aponeurosis. It raises the eyebrows and wrinkles the forehead.

- **Levator anguli oris (le-VAT-ehr AN-gyoo-ligh OR-iss).** The muscle of the upper lip that raises the corner of the mouth.

- **Levator labii (LAY-bee-igh) superioris.** The muscle from the maxilla to the upper lip. It raises the upper lip.

- **Levator palpebrae (PAL-peh-bree) superioris.** The muscle that raises the upper eyelid.

- **Masseter (mah-SEET-ehr).** The muscle extending from the bony prominence in front of the ear to the angle of the jaw. It is used to clench the teeth.

- **Procerus.** The muscle that covers the nose. It wrinkles the nose.

- **Mentalis (men-TAL-iss).** The muscle from the point of the chin to the base of your front teeth. It is used to pout.

- **Nasalis (nas-SAL-iss).** The muscles of the nose. They can be used to wrinkle the nose.

- **Occipitalis (ohk-sip-eh-TAL-iss).** The muscle that extends from the occipital bone to the aponeurosis. It draws the scalp backward.

- **Orbicularis oculi (or-bik-yoo-LAY-riss AHK-yeh-lye).** The bands of circular muscle in the eye socket that close the eyelids.

- **Orbicularis oris (OH-riss).** Muscles surrounding the mouth and running into the lip. They cause the mouth to pucker.

■ **Platysma (pla-TIZ-mah).** A muscle running from the chest to the entire length of the mandible. It pulls the corner of the mouth down.

■ **Risorius (ri-SAH-ri-uhs).** A subcutaneous muscle extending to the skin at the corner of the mouth. It is used to smile.

■ **Temporalis (tem-peh-RA-liss).** A muscle on the flat part of the side of the head above the ear to the mandible. It is used to bite.

■ **Zygomaticus (zigh-goh-MAT-i-kuhs) major.** A muscle extending from the zygomatic bone to the corner of the orbicularis oris muscle. It draws the angle of the mouth back and up.

The trunk muscles include the following (Figures 36.5 and 36.6):

■ **Latissimus dorsi (la-TIS-seh-muhs DOR-sigh).** A muscle covering the lower half of the thoracic vertebrae, all lumbar vertebrae, and the iliac crest to the humerus. It draws the arm to the body and rotates the arm outward.

■ **Sterno-cleido-mastoideus (ster-noh-KLYE-doh-mas-toyd-ee-ahs).** A muscle extending from the clavicle and sternum to the bony prominence behind the ear. It flexes the head toward the shoulder on one side and turns the face to the opposite side.

■ **Trapezius (tra-PEE-see-uz).** Muscles covering the occipital bone, the vertebrae of the neck and throat to the clavicle, and the scapulae. They rotate the shoulder blades and draw the head backward or to one side.

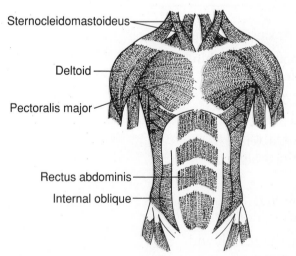

Figure 36.5
Muscles of the trunk (front view)

Sternocleidomastoideus

Deltoid

Pectoralis major

Rectus abdominis

Internal oblique

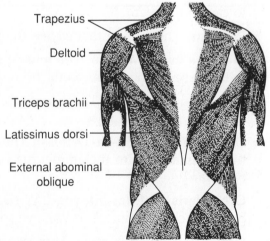

Figure 36.6
Muscles of the trunk (back view)

Trapezius

Deltoid

Triceps brachii

Latissimus dorsi

External abominal oblique

The following are the main muscles of the arm:

- **Biceps brachii (BIGH-seps BRAK-ee-igh).** A muscle that extends from the scapula to the radius and the aponeurosis in the forearm. It flexes the forearm.

- **Deltoid (DEL-toyd).** A muscle extending from the clavicle and scapula to the humerus. It extends and rotates the arm.

- **Triceps brachii (TRIGH-seps BRAK-ee-igh).** A muscle extending from the scapula and back of the humerus to the ulna. It extends the forearm.

Theory Objective 6
Neurological Terms and the Divisions of the Nervous System and Brain

Neurology (noo-RAHL-eh-jee) is the study of the nervous system. The nervous system covers the entire body and enables the parts of the body to communicate with each other.

The basic structural unit of the nervous system is the **neuron** (NOO-rahn). It is composed of a cell body called the **axon** (AK-sahn), which carries nervous impulses away from the cell body, and the **dendrite(s)** (DEN-dright), which carries impulses to the cell body. A single nerve contains many neurons and may vary in diameter from microscopic to almost the size of a clothesline.

Sensory, or **afferent,** neurons carry nervous impulses such as smell, hearing, sight, taste, and touch toward the brain. **Motor,** or **efferent,** neurons carry nervous impulses away from the brain to the body.

The nervous system is divided into three parts, the **central, peripheral,** and **autonomic** systems:

- The **central nervous system** consists of the brain and spinal cord. It carries all of the incoming and outgoing messages of the body.

- The **peripheral nervous system** includes all nerves branching into the body from the central nervous system.

- The **autonomic (or automatic) nervous system** controls all automatic processes, such as circulation, digestion, and respiration. Although the autonomic nervous system is physically part of the central and peripheral system, it operates as a separate unit.

The autonomic nervous system is subdivided into the **sympathetic** and the **parasympathetic** nervous systems. The parasympathetic nervous system controls quiet activities, such as digestion, while the sympathetic nervous system controls reactions to stress, such as fear.

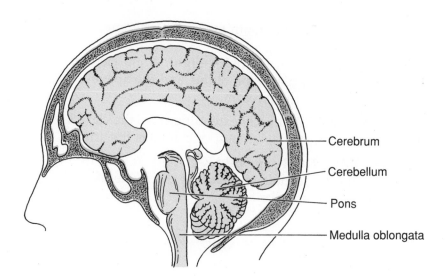

Cerebrum

Cerebellum

Pons

Medulla oblongata

Figure 36.7
Main parts of the brain

The following are the four major parts of the brain (Figure 36.7):

- **Cerebrum (seh-REE-bruhm).** The large, uppermost portion of the brain. It receives and interprets sensory and motor information and controls memory and reasoning.

- **Cerebellum (ser-eh-BEL-uhm).** The portion of the brain inside the occipital bone. It makes coordinated movement possible.

- **Pons (PAHNZ).** The part of the brain that serves as a relay station between the spinal cord, the cerebrum, and the cerebellum.

- **Medulla oblongata (meh-DUHL-ah ahb-lon-GAHT-ah).** Some of the parasympathetic and sympathetic nerves start in this part of the brain. It regulates some of the activities controlled by the autonomic nervous system.

Theory Objective 7
Types and Functions of Nerves in the Head, Face, Neck, Arm, Hand, and Finger; Reflex Arc

In addition to the brain, portions of the nervous system that are of interest to the cosmetologist include the 12 pairs of cranial nerves. These nerves, which start in the brain, reach and affect the head, face, and neck. The most important cranial nerves are briefly described here.

The **fifth cranial** nerve, also called the **trifacial** or **trigeminal** (trigh-JEM-i-nal) nerve, is a mixed nerve; its motor impulses control chewing, while its sensory neurons carry impulses from the face (Figure 36.8). The major branches of the trigeminal nerve include the following:

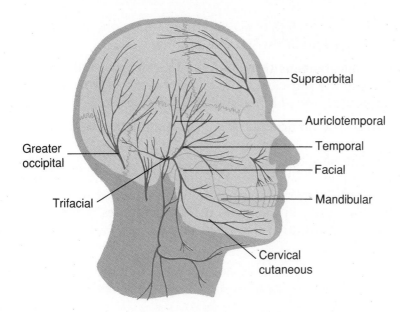

Figure 36.8
Nerves of the head and neck

- **Ophthalmic (ahf-THAL-mik) branch.** Sensory to the skin of the forehead, eyes, and nose. The **supratrochlear** (soo-prah-TROK-lee-ar) nerve, which is involved in facial massage, is part of the ophthalmic branch.

- **Maxillary (MAK-seh-ler-ee) branch.** Sensory to the skin covering the maxillae. The **nasal nerve,** which is involved in facial massage, is a subdivision of the maxillary branch.

- **Mandibular (man-DIB-yeh-lehr) branch.** Sensory to the skin covering the mandible and the teeth of the lower jaw, and motor to the muscles of chewing. The **auriculotemporal** (aw-RIK-yeh-loh-TEM-peh-rehl) and **mental nerves,** which are involved in facial massage, are part of this branch.

The **seventh** cranial, or **facial,** nerve is the main motor nerve of the face. It is also sensory to **taste.**

The **eleventh** cranial nerve (or **accessory,** or **spinal accessory**) is the motor nerve that serves the sterno-cleido-mastoideus and the trapezius muscles, both of which are found in the trunk.

The cervical nerves emerging at the neck supply nerves to the back of the head and neck.

The nerves that supply the arm and hand include the following (Figure 36.9):

- **Ulnar.** A nerve that starts on the little-finger side of the forearm and goes to that side of the hand and forearm.

- **Radial.** A nerve that starts on the thumb side of the arm and goes to the back of the arm and the back and lateral sides of the forearm and hand.

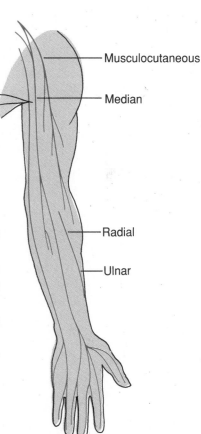

Figure 36.9
Nerves of the arm and hand (front view, palm)

■ **Median.** A nerve that is very deep in the arm and goes to the middle portion of the forearm and hand.

■ **Musculocutaneous (MUHS-kyoo-loh-TAY-nee-uhs).** A nerve that is in the muscles of the anterior arm and goes to the muscles (i.e., the biceps) that flex the forearm.

■ **Digital.** The branches that supply the **phalanges** (fingers).

The simplest nerve pathway an impulse can travel is the **reflex arc.** It brings together information that individuals respond to automatically. For example, the reflex arc causes you to pull away from a hot stove. In this case, the digital nerves that extend to the fingers cause you to withdraw your hand.

Glossary

Afferent (AF-eh-rent) neurons See **Sensory neurons.**

Anabolism (ah-NAB-eh-liz-uhm) The process of building up the cell.

Anatomy The study of the structure of the body.

Aponeurosis (ap-oh-nyoo-ROH-sis) A connective tissue that joins two muscles.

Auriculotemporal (aw-RIK-yeh-loh-TEM-peh-rehl) A subdivision of the mandibular branch of the fifth cranial nerve; involved in facial massage.

Autonomic (aw-teh-NAHM-ik) nervous system The portion of the nervous system that controls a person's automatic functions, such as breathing, heartbeat, and so on.

Axon (AK-sahn) The part of the neuron that carries impulses away from the cell body.

Biceps brachii (BIGH-seps BRAK-ee-igh) A muscle that flexes the forearm.

Buccinator (BUK-si-nay-tehr) A muscle that draws in the cheeks and is used to suck.

Cancellous (KAN-seh-luhs) tissue The spongy tissue found at each end of the shafts of the long bones and inside the flat bones.

Carpals (KAHR-puhlz) The bones of the wrist.

Cartilage (KAHR-tah-lij) A tissue similar to bone tissue that protects the bones from stress; it acts like a cushion for bones.

Catabolism (keh-TAB-eh-liz-uhm) The processes that supply energy to the body.

Cell The basic unit of the body. The entire body structure is made of cells.

Cell membrane The outside of the cell.

Central nervous system The brain and spinal cord.

Centrosome (SEN-treh-sohm) The part of the cell that helps the cell divide and reproduce.

Cerebellum (ser-eh-BEL-uhm) The portion of the brain inside the occipital bone that makes coordinated movement possible.

Cerebrum (seh-REE-bruhm) The large, uppermost portion of the brain that receives and interprets sensory and motor information and controls memory and reasoning.

Cervical vertebrae (SER-vi-kehl VEHRT-eh-bray) The seven bones in the back of the neck. The first two vertebrae enable the head to move.

Clavicles (KLAV-i-kehlz) The two bones commonly called the collarbones.

Compact bone tissue The tissue that makes up the shafts of long bones and forms the outside of flat bones. Blood vessels are contained in this layer.

Conchae The bones located at the side walls of the nasal cavity and protruding into it.

Connective tissue The tissue that binds, supports, or helps protect the body, such as bone, cartilage, ligament, tendon, and adipose (fatty) tissue.

Corrugator (kor-uh-GAY-tehr) The muscle that draws the eyebrows down and together.

Cranial nerves The 12 pairs of nerves that start in the brain and reach and affect the head, face, and neck.

Cranium The bones that encase the brain.

Cytoplasm (SIGH-tah-plaz-uhm) A jelly-like substance inside the cell membrane that contains the nucleus of the cell.

Deltoid (DEL-toyd) A muscle that extends and rotates the arm.

Dendrite (DEN-dright) The part of the neuron that carries impulses to the cell body.

Depressor anguli oris (di-PRES-ehr AN-gyoo-ligh OR-iss) A muscle that depresses the corner of the mouth and is used to frown. Also called the triangularis.

Depressor labii inferioris (di-PRES-ehr LAY-bee-igh in-FIHR-ee-or-iss) The muscle that lowers the lower lip.

Digital nerves Branches of the arm nerves that serve the fingers.

Distal point See **Insertion.**

Efferent (EF-eh-rent) neurons See **Motor neurons.**

Eleventh cranial nerve The motor nerve that serves the sterno-cleido-mastoideus and trapezius muscles. Also called the accessory or spinal accessory.

Epicranius (ep-i-KRA-nee-uhs) A two-part muscle joined by a sheet of connective tissue. The two parts are called the frontalis and the occipitalis.

Epithelial (ep-eh-THEE-lee-ehl) tissue The tissue that lines all the surfaces of the body.

Ethmoid (ETH-moid) bone The bone forming the upper part of the bony structure that divides the nasal cavity in half.

Facial nerve See **Seventh cranial nerve.**

Fascia (FASH-yah) A tough membrane that separates the muscles and helps to hold them in place.

Fifth cranial nerve The nerve that controls chewing and carries impulses from the face. Also called the trifacial or trigeminal nerve.

Frontal bone The bone that forms the front of the skull.

Frontalis (fruhn-TAL-iss) The muscle along the eyebrows that raises the brows and wrinkles the forehead. Part of the epicranius muscle.

Humerus (HYOOM-eh-ruhs) The large bone of the upper arm.

Hyoid (HIGH-oid) The U-shaped bone above the larynx to which the muscles of the tongue are attached.

Insertion The point of muscle attachment that is farther away from the center of the body. Also called the distal point.

Joint The place where two or more bones are joined.

Lacrimal (LAK-rih-mehl) bones The two bones on the inner sides of the eye sockets.

Latissimus dorsi (la-TIS-seh-muhs DOR-sigh) A muscle that draws the arm in toward the body, extends the elbow to the back, and rotates the arm outward.

Levator anguli oris (le-VAT-ehr AN-gyoo-ligh OR-iss) The muscle that raises the corner of the mouth.

Levator labii superioris (le-VAT-ehr LAY-bee-igh soo-PIHR-ee-or-iss) The muscle that raises the upper lip.

Levator palpebrae superioris (le-VAT-ehr PAL-peh-bree soo-PIHR-ee-or-iss) The muscle that raises the upper eyelid.

Ligaments (LIG-eh-mehnts) Bands or sheets of connective tissue that hold the bones together.

Malar (MAY-lahr) bones See **Zygomatic bones.**

Mandible (MAN-deh-behl) The jawbone.

Mandibular (man-DIB-yeh-lehr) nerve branch A part of the fifth cranial nerve that is sensory to the skin covering the mandible and the teeth of the lower jaw, and motor to the muscles of chewing.

Marrow A yellow, fatty tissue found in the shafts of long bones, and a red tissue in the cancellous tissue of long bones that produces the blood cells.

Masseter (mah-SEET-ehr) A muscle of the jaw used to clench the teeth.

Maxillae (mak-SIL-ee) The two bones that, together with the palatines, form the hard palate. They also form the lower portion of the eye sockets and the upper portion of the jaw.

Maxillary (MAK-seh-ler-ee) nerve branch A branch of the fifth cranial nerve sensory to the skin covering the maxillae.

Median nerve One of the nerves of the forearm and hand.

Medulla oblongata (meh-DUHL-ah ahb-lon-GAHT-ah) The part of the brain that regulates some of the activities controlled by the autonomic nervous system.

Mentalis (men-TAL-iss) A chin muscle that makes the lower lip protrude; used to frown.

Metabolism (meh-TAB-eh-liz-uhm) The processes of taking in nutrients and processing them for use in the body.

Metacarpals (met-ah-KAHR-puhlz) The five bones of the palm.

Motor neurons The neurons that carry impulses away from the brain. Also called efferent neurons.

Muscle A bundle of elastic fibers surrounded by fascia that enables the body to move.

Muscular tissue The tissue that forms the muscles.

Musculocutaneous (MUHS-kyoo-loh-TAY-nee-uhs) One of the nerves of the arm.

Myology (migh-AHL-eh-jee) The study of the muscular system.

Nasal bones The two bones that shape the bridge of the nose.

Nasal nerve A part of the maxillary branch of the fifth cranial nerve; involved in facial massage.

Nervous tissue The tissue that makes up the nerves and brain.

Neurology (noo-RAHL-eh-jee) The study of the nervous system.

Neuron (NOO-rahn) The basic structural unit of the nervous system; composed of an axon and dendrite(s).

Nucleus (NOO-klee-uhs) The center of the cell; the portion of the cell that directs the cell's activities.

Occipital (ahk-SIP-eh-tehl) bone The rearmost bone of the skull.

Occipitalis (ohk-sip-eh-TAL-iss) The muscle that draws the scalp backward. Part of the epicranius muscle.

Ophthalmic (ahf-THAL-mik) nerve branch A branch of the fifth cranial nerve that is sensory to the skin of the forehead, eyes, and nose.

Orbicularis oculi (or-bik-yoo-LAY-riss AHK-yeh-lye) The bands of circular muscle in the eye sockets that close the eyelids.

Orbicularis oris (or-bik-yoo-LAY-riss OH-riss) A circular band of muscle surrounding the mouth that causes the lips to pucker.

Origin The point of muscle attachment that is closer to the center of the body. Also called the proximal point.

Osteology (ahs-tee-AHL-eh-jee) The scientific study of bone.

Palatines (PAL-eh-tynes) The two bones that form part of the hard palate, which is the back portion of the roof of the mouth.

Parasympathetic (par-eh-sim-peh-THET-ik) nervous system All nerves branching into the body from the central nervous system.

Parietal (peh-RIGH-eht-ehl) bones The bones that form the top and sides of the skull.

Periosteum (per-ee-AHS-tee-uhm) The outer fiber covering of the bone; it connects the bone to the muscles, ligaments, and tendons.

Peripheral (peh-RIF-eh-rehl) nervous system All nerves branching into the body from the central nervous system.

Phalanges (FAY-lanj-eez) The bones of the fingers.

Physiology The study of body functions.

Platysma (pla-TIZ-mah) A muscle that pulls the corner of the mouth down; used to frown.

Pons (PAHNZ) The part of the brain that serves as a relay station between the spinal cord, the cerebrum, and the cerebellum.

Proximal point See **Origin**.

Radial nerve One of the nerves of the arm.

Radius (RAY-dee-uhs) The bone of the arm located on the thumb side.

Reflex arc The simplest nerve pathway a nerve impulse can travel.

Ribs The 24 bones of the chest that protect the heart, lungs, and other internal organs.

Risorius (ri-SAH-ri-uhs) A mouth muscle that is used to smile.

Scapulae (SKAP-yeh-lee) The two bones that, with the clavicles, hold the arm in place. Commonly called the shoulder blades.

Sensory neurons The neurons that carry impulses toward the brain. Also called afferent neurons.

Seventh cranial nerve The main motor nerve to the face, also sensory to taste.

Skeletal system All the bones in the body.

Smooth muscle The type of muscle tissue that makes up the involuntary muscle system and is not under the control of the individual; the muscles of internal organs are an example. Called smooth because it looks smooth under a microscope.

Sphenoid (SFEE-noid) bone A butterfly-shaped bone located almost at the center of the head.

Sterno-cleido-mastoideus (ster-noh-KLYE-doh-mas-toyd-ee-ahs) A muscle that flexes the head toward the shoulder on the same side and turns the face to the opposite side.

Sternum (STEHR-nuhm) The breastbone; it is located in the
    center of the chest.

Striated (STRIGH-ay-tehd) muscle A muscle that is controlled by
    the individual, such as the arm or leg muscles. It is called
    striated because it looks striped under a microscope.

Supratrochlear (soo-prah-TROK-lee-ar) nerve A nerve that is part
    of the ophthalmic branch of the fifth cranial nerve and is
    involved in facial massage.

Sympathetic (sim-peh-THET-ik) nervous system The part of the
    autonomic nervous system that reacts to stress, such as
    fear.

Synovial (seh-NOH-vee-ahl) fluid A tissue that helps lubricate
    and cushion the joints.

System A group of organs working together to accomplish a
    major function of the body.

Temporal bones The bones that form the bony part of the skull
    around the ears.

Temporalis (tem-peh-RA-liss) A muscle on the side of the head;
    used for biting.

Tissue A group of similar cells that work together to accomplish
    a specialized function.

Trapezius (tra-PEE-see-uz) A muscle that draws the head back
    and to the side, raises the shoulder, and rotates the
    shoulder blades.

Triceps brachii (TRIGH-seps BRAK-ee-igh) A muscle that
    extends the forearm.

Trifacial nerve See **Fifth cranial nerve.**

Trigeminal (trigh-JEM-i-nal) nerve See **Fifth cranial nerve.**

Turbinals See **Conchae.**

Ulna (UHL-nah) The bone of the forearm on the little-finger side.

Ulnar nerve One of the nerves of the arm.

Zygomatic (zigh-goh-MAT-ik) bones The two bones that form
    the outer, lower portion of the eye sockets and the
    cheekbones.

Zygomaticus (zigh-goh-MAT-i-kuhs) major A muscle that draws
    the angle of the mouth backward and upward.

Questions

1. Define physiology.
2. What is the study of the overall structure of the body called?
3. What is the outside of the cell called?
4. Define cytoplasm.
5. What is the cycle of cell energy, growth, and storage called?
6. What is tissue?
7. Define connective tissue.

8. What is epithelial tissue?
9. What is formed when two or more different types of tissue work together to perform a certain function?
10. What term is used to refer to a group of organs working together to perform a major function?
11. What is the scientific name for the study of bones?
12. Is the cranium located in the head?
13. Does synovial fluid lubricate body joints where the bones meet?
14. Does the mandible form the lower jaw?
15. What is the scientific study of muscles called?
16. Is the deltoid muscle located in the forehead?
17. Where is the occipital bone located?

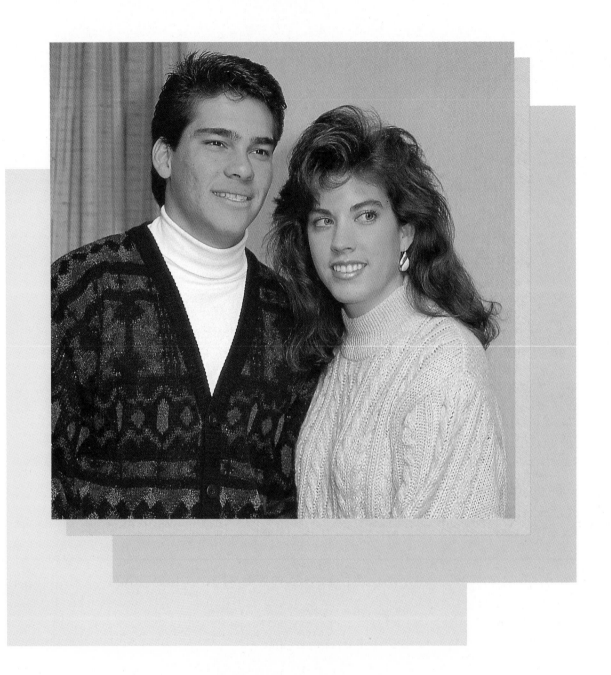

Anatomy and Physiology in Cosmetology: Vascular and Endocrine Systems

Learning Objective

Provided with the information in this chapter and classroom instruction, identify the vascular system of the body, and describe and classify its parts. Identify the endocrine system and its major parts. Score 85 percent or better on a multiple-choice exam on the information in this chapter.

In order to achieve the above level of competence, you should master the following chapter objectives.

Theory Objectives

1. Define angiology, and identify the three subdivisions of the vascular system, the parts and functions of the heart and blood vessels, and the function of pulmonary circulation.
2. Identify the arteries and veins of the head, face, neck, arm, and hand, and describe the composition of blood and the lymphatic system.
3. Describe the endocrine system and its five major glands.

Blood circulates through the body through the **vascular system.** Services involving massage, heat, chemicals, and light therapy increase blood circulation, so you need to have a basic knowledge of this system.

Introduction

Theory Objective 1

Angiology and the Three Subdivisions of the Vascular System, Parts and Functions of the Heart and Blood Vessels, and the Function of Pulmonary Circulation

Angiology (an-jee-AHL-eh-jee) is the study of the vascular system, which includes the **circulatory system** and the **lymphatic system.**

The **circulatory system** consists of the **heart** and **blood vessels.** (Thus, the three subdivisions of the vascular system are the heart, blood vessels, and lymphatic system.) It brings food and oxygen to all cells of the body, removes the waste and carbon dioxide from cells, guards the body against infection, and regulates body temperature.

Unlike the circulatory system, the **lymphatic** (lim-FAT-ik) **system** circulates fluids in only one direction—from the tissues **toward the heart.** The open-ended vessels of the lymphatic system collect a fluid that comes from the blood and return it to the general circulation.

The heart is a major part of the circulatory system (Figure 37.1). It is made up of cardiac muscle tissue and is about the size of a closed fist. It is located in the chest cavity, between the lungs, and is surrounded by a tough membranous sac called the **pericardium** (per-he-KAHRD-ee-uhm)—pericardium means **surrounding the heart.**

The heart is divided into four chambers: the two upper chambers, or **auricles** (AWR-i-kehlz), receive the blood from the rest of the body, and the two lower chambers, or **ventricles** (VEN-tri-kehlz), send the blood back to the body (Figure 37.2). The heart has four major valves, two of which separate the auricles from the ventricles. These are known as **bicuspid** (bigh-KUHS-pehd) and **tricuspid** (trigh-KUHS-pehd) valves. The other two valves separate the ventricles from the arteries, which carry blood away from the heart. Normally, these valves close very tightly, allowing no blood to seep

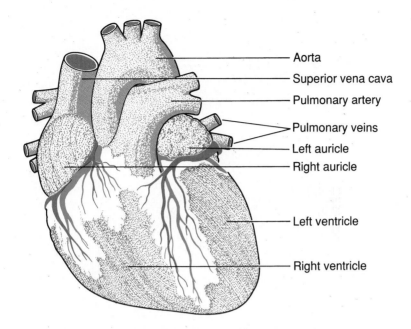

Aorta
Superior vena cava
Pulmonary artery
Pulmonary veins
Left auricle
Right auricle
Left ventricle
Right ventricle

Figure 37.1
The heart

from the auricles to the ventricles or from the ventricles to the arteries. This causes a great buildup of pressure that helps the heart pump blood through the body.

Arteries are vessels that carry blood away **from the heart** to the body. This blood carries oxygen from the lungs and nutrients that will be used by the cells. Although the arteries vary in size, they all have three layers of tissue—an outer layer, an inner layer, and a middle layer of smooth muscle, which can make the circumference of the artery larger or smaller.

From the arteries, the blood moves into the **capillaries.** These blood vessels are much smaller than the arteries. Capillaries can be seen only with the aid of a microscope and contain just one layer of tissue. They carry nutrients (food) and oxygen to the cells and take waste products and carbon dioxide away.

This exchange of nutrients for waste products and oxygen for carbon dioxide is accomplished in two ways. One is **pressure.** The force of the blood flow (the pulse) pushes food through the capillary walls at the arterial end of a capillary bed (a group of capillaries).

The other method by which material is exchanged is **osmosis** (ahz-MOH-sis). Simply stated, osmosis involves the tendency of substances (in this case, the nutrients) to equalize on either side of a membrane (the capillary wall). In other words, since there are more nutrients inside the capillary than outside at the beginning of the process, the nutrients will tend to move through the capillary

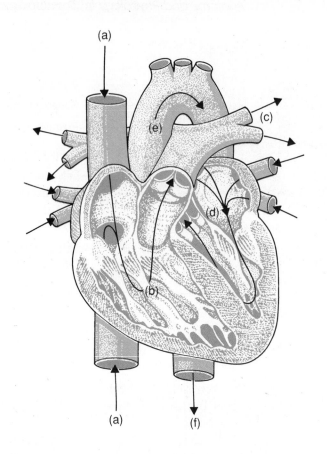

Figure 37.2

The flow of blood through the heart. (a) The blood enters the right auricle from the veins and (b) passes through a valve to the right ventricle. (c) The ventricle pumps the blood to the lungs through the pulmonary artery. (d) From the lungs, the blood returns to the left auricle and (e) passes through a valve to the left ventricle. (f) The ventricle pumps the blood into the aorta, which distributes it to the body.

wall into the cells. This process continues until there are equal amounts of nutrients on both sides of the wall.

After the blood leaves the capillaries, it goes on to the **veins,** which will carry it back **to the heart.** Note that now the blood is carrying waste products and carbon dioxide from the cells. The veins, which are only two layers thick, do not go directly to the heart. Instead, they carry the blood to a point where the waste products and carbon dioxide can be removed. The kidneys and liver remove the metabolic waste products, excess water, salts, and dead cells. The lungs rid the body of carbon dioxide.

After it passes through the kidneys and liver, the blood is returned **to the heart** primarily through the activity of the contracting skeletal muscles. The veins also help keep the blood moving toward the heart.

The process by which carbon dioxide is removed from the blood and replaced by oxygen is known as **pulmonary** (PUHL-mah-ner-ee) **circulation.** As we have seen, veins carry blood that has carbon dioxide in it from the body to the heart. Then the heart sends the blood through the pulmonary artery to the lungs, where the carbon dioxide is replaced with oxygen. The fresh blood, which now contains oxygen, comes back from the **lungs to the heart** in the pulmonary veins. Then the heart sends this fresh blood to the rest of the body.

Blood reaches the head, face, and neck through a series of arteries (Figure 37.3). The blood flows out of the heart through the **aorta** (ay-ORT-ah), **the largest artery in the body.** Branching off from the aorta is the **common carotid** (keh-RAHT-ehd) **artery,** which is the main supplier of blood to the head, face, and neck, as well as to the area on either side of the throat. The common carotid branches into the **internal** and **external carotid arteries.**

The **internal carotid artery** supplies the brain and the eye sockets, eyelids, and forehead via the **ophthalmic** (ahf-THAL-mik) **artery.** The **external carotid artery** supplies blood to the superficial tissues of the head, face, and neck. Its branches include the **facial,** or **external maxillary** (MAX-seh-ler-ee), **artery,** which supplies the lower portion of the face, the mouth, and the nose; the **occipital** (ahk-SIP-eh-tahl) **artery,** which supplies the scalp and the back of the head up to the crown; the **posterior auricular artery,** which is the source of blood for the scalp behind and above the ear; and the **transverse facial artery,** which supplies the muscles, skin, and scalp of the sides, front, and top of the head.

The veins in these regions follow the arteries and have the same names. For instance, the **transverse facial vein** is near the **transverse facial artery.** There is one exception to this rule. The veins that drain the area supplied by the internal and external carotid arteries are called the **internal** and **external jugular** (JUHG-yeh-lehr) **veins.**

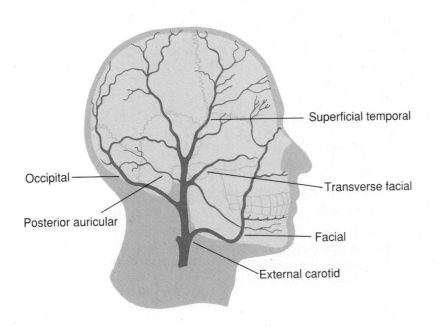

Figure 37.3
Arteries of the head and neck

Superficial temporal

Occipital

Transverse facial

Posterior auricular

Facial

External carotid

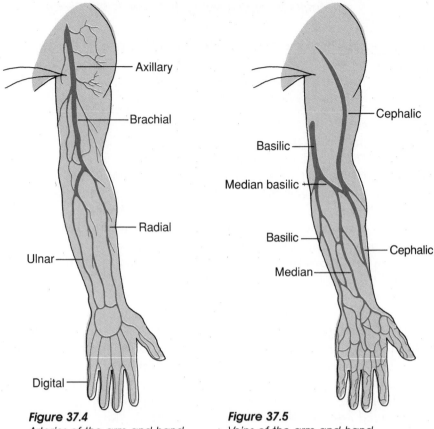

Figure 37.4
*Arteries of the arm and hand.
An exterior view of the arm
and hand is included as a
reference point.*

Figure 37.5
Veins of the arm and hand

The **brachial** (BRAK-ee-ehl) **artery** supplies the arm and hand (Figure 37.4). It comes from the aorta and divides into the **radial** and **ulnar arteries.**

The veins in the deeper body tissues follow the same pattern and have the same names as the arteries, but the superficial (close to the surface) veins do not (Figure 37.5). They are on the anterior side of the forearm (inner arm).

Composition of Blood

Now that we have seen how the exchange system works and have examined the major blood vessels of the body, it's time to look at the blood itself.

The body contains 8 to 10 pints of **blood,** one-half to two-thirds of which is held by the skin. The temperature of blood is approximately 98.6° F (37° C). It ranges in color from **bright red or scarlet in the arteries** to a **deep red, almost purple, in the veins.** Blood is considered a specialized connective tissue. The main components of blood are as follows:

- **Plasma** (PLAZ-mah) is a **yellow liquid** that accounts for approximately two-thirds of the volume of blood. Plasma is mostly water, but it also contains food elements, waste products, and dissolved salts.

- **Red blood cells,** or **erythrocytes** (i-RITH-rah-sights), give blood its color. They are shaped like discs, are highly flexible, and contain a substance called **hemoglobin** (HEE-mah-gloh-behn), which enables them to exchange oxygen for carbon dioxide in the body. In adults, red blood cells are manufactured primarily by the marrow of flat bones.

- **White blood cells,** or **leukocytes** (LOO-koh-sights), are much larger than red blood cells. They fight infection in the body.

- **Blood platelets,** or **thrombocytes,** are colorless cells. They **help blood clot** and thus form a scab over a wound. This process, together with the activity of the **leukocytes,** is how the circulatory system **protects the body against disease.**

Lymphatic System

The **lymphatic** (lim-FAT-ik) **system** is closely related to the circulatory system. It is a one-directional vascular system that collects excess fluid from the spaces between the cells and puts it back into the body's circulation.

Lymph (LIMF) itself is a colorless liquid that comes from plasma. It contains white blood cells and a few red blood cells. Lymph obtains leukocytes from the blood and makes its own kind of leukocytes called **lymphocytes** (LIM-feh-sights) at the lymph nodes.

The lymphatic system has only one kind of vessel, which varies in size. Some vessels are very small, such as the minute lymphatic vessels that collect the excess fluid. Other vessels are larger, such as those that eventually empty into the **vena cava** (VAY-nah KAY-vah), the large vein that empties into the right auricle of the heart.

A specialized set of lymphatic vessels are called **lacteals** (LAK-tee-ehlz). They absorb fat **(chyle)** from the intestine and carry it to the main lymphatic vessel, which in turn drains into the veins.

Theory Objective 3
Endocrine System and Its Five Major Glands

The **endocrine** (EN-deh-krehn) **system** is a system of **ductless glands** that release chemicals called **hormones** (HOR-mohnz) into the blood (Figure 37.6). The hormones affect, among other things, the skin, hair, and scalp. The endocrine system helps control such bodily functions as growth, general health, and reproduction.

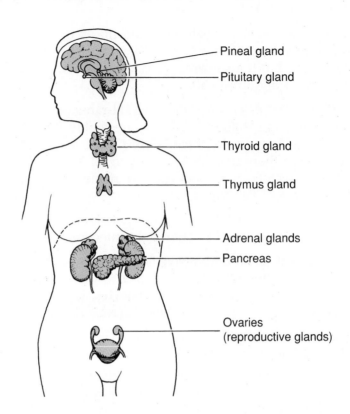

Figure 37.6
Endocrine system

The following are the major glands of the endocrine system:

- **Pituitary (peh-TOO-eh-ter-ee) gland.** This gland is located **at the base of the brain.** It **regulates** the functions of **all other endocrine glands** and also regulates the water balance in the body. The **hypothalamus** (high-poh-THAL-eh-muhs)—the part of the brain to which the pituitary is connected—regulates the activities (secretions) of the pituitary gland. The hypothalamus, in turn, can be regulated by higher centers in the brain.

- **Thyroid (THIGH-roid) gland.** The thyroid gland located **on either side of the larynx (throat) controls** the body's **metabolism,** which affects the individual's weight. An underactive thyroid results in a condition known as hypothyroidism, which is characterized by excessive weight gain. An overactive thyroid results in hyperthyroidism, which leads to severe weight loss.

- **Pancreas (PAN-kree-uhs).** This gland, which is located **behind the stomach, affects** the **amount of sugar the body uses.** Specialized cells in a pancreas produce the **hormone insulin** (IN-suh-lehn). If the pancreas does not produce enough insulin, diabetes results.

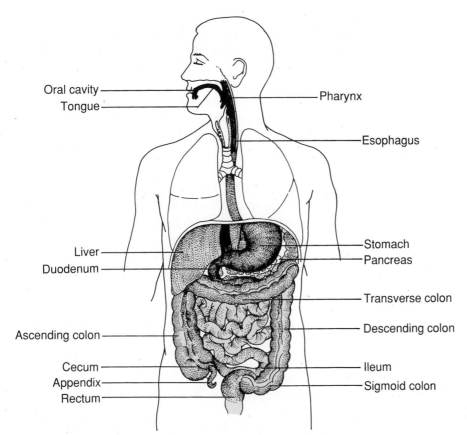

Oral cavity
Tongue
Pharynx
Esophagus
Liver
Duodenum
Stomach
Pancreas
Transverse colon
Descending colon
Ascending colon
Cecum
Appendix
Rectum
Ileum
Sigmoid colon

Figure 37.7
The digestive tract

- **Adrenal (ah-DREEN-ehl) glands.** These glands are located **above the kidneys.** They **produce** the hormone **adrenaline,** which improves the body's ability to withstand stress.

- **Reproductive glands.** The reproductive glands include both **ductless (endocrine)** and **ducted (exocrine)** glands.

Glossary

Adrenal (ah-DREEN-ehl) glands Endocrine glands located just above the kidneys that help the body cope with stress by producing the hormone adrenaline.

Angiology (an-jee-AHL-eh-jee) The study of the vascular system, which includes the circulatory system and the lymphatic system.

Aorta (ay-ORT-ah) The largest artery in the circulatory system of the body.

Arteries (AHRT-eh-reez) The vessels that carry blood from the heart to the body.

Auricles (AWR-i-kehlz) The two upper chambers of the heart.

Bicuspid (bigh-KUHS-pehd) valve One of the major valves of the heart; it separates the auricles from the ventricles.

Blood platelets (PLAYT-lehts) Colorless cells in the blood that help the blood clot.

Brachial (BRAK-ee-ehl) artery The artery that supplies blood to the arms and hands. It comes from the aorta and divides into the radial and ulnar arteries.

Capillaries (KAP-eh-ler-eez) The microscopic blood vessels that carry nutrients and oxygen to the cells from the arteries and take waste products to the veins.

Chyle (KYLE) The fat in the intestine absorbed by the lacteals.

Circulatory system The heart and the blood vessels. This system brings food and oxygen to all the cells of the body, removes the waste and carbon dioxide from the cells, guards the body against infection, and regulates body temperature.

Common carotid artery The artery that is the main supplier of blood to the head, face, and neck; it also supplies blood to the area on either side of the throat.

Endocrine (EN-deh-krehn) system A system of ductless glands that release hormones into the blood.

Erythrocytes (i-RITH-rah-sights) See **Red blood cells.**

External carotid artery The artery that supplies blood to the superficial tissues of the head, face, and neck.

External maxillary (MAX-seh-ler-ee) artery See **Facial artery.**

Facial artery A branch of the external carotid artery that supplies the lower portion of the face, the mouth, and the nose. Also called the external maxillary artery.

Hemoglobin (HEE-mah-gloh-behn) A substance found in red blood cells.

Hormones (HOR-mohnz) The chemicals that help control growth, general health, and reproduction.

Hypothalamus (high-poh-THAL-eh-muhs) The part of the brain that regulates the activities of the pituitary gland.

Insulin (IN-suh-lehn) The hormone produced by the pancreas that affects the amount of sugar used by the body.

Internal carotid artery The artery that supplies the brain, eye sockets, eyelids, and head via the ophthalmic artery.

Jugular (JUHG-yeh-lehr) veins The veins that drain the area supplied by the internal and external carotid arteries.

Lacteals (LAK-tee-ehlz) A specialized set of lymphatic vessels that absorb fat from the intestine and carry it to the main lymphatic vessel, which drains into the veins.

Leukocytes (LOO-koh-sights) See **White blood cells.**

Lymph (LIMF) A colorless liquid that comes from plasma and makes lymphocytes.

Lymphatic (lim-FAT-ik) system The part of the circulatory system that collects excess fluid from the spaces between the cells and puts it back into the body's circulation.

Lymphocytes (LIM-feh-sights) A white blood cell manufactured by the lymph nodes.

Occipital (ahk-SIP-eh-tehl) artery The artery that supplies blood to the scalp and the back of the head up to the crown.

Ophthalmic (ahf-THAL-mik) artery A subdivision of the internal carotid artery.

Osmosis (ahz-MOH-sis) A process of exchange in the capillaries that provides nutrients to the cells and removes waste products.

Pancreas (PAN-kree-uhs) An endocrine gland located behind the stomach that produces the hormone insulin, which affects the amount of sugar used by the body.

Pericardium (per-eh-KAHRD-ee-uhm) The tough membrane that surrounds the heart.

Pituitary (peh-TOO-eh-ter-ee) gland A gland located at the base of the brain that regulates the functions of all other endocrine glands and regulates the water balance in the body.

Plasma (PLAZ-mah) A yellow liquid found in the blood that contains water, food elements, waste products, and dissolved salts.

Posterior auricular (pah-STIR-ee-ehr aw-RIK-yeh-lehr) artery The artery that supplies blood to the scalp behind and above the ear.

Pulmonary (PUHL-mah-ner-ee) circulation The process of removing carbon dioxide from the blood and replacing it with oxygen.

Radial (RAY-dee-ehl) artery A subdivision of the brachial artery.

Red blood cells Red, disc-shaped cells in the blood that give blood its color and exchange oxygen for carbon dioxide in the body.

Thyroid (THIGH-roid) The endocrine glands located on either side of the throat that control the body's metabolism.

Transverse facial artery The artery that supplies blood to the masseter muscle.

Tricuspid (trigh-KUHS-pehd) valve One of the major valves of the heart; it separates the auricles from the ventricles.

Ulnar (UHL-nahr) artery A subdivision of the brachial artery.

Veins The blood vessels that carry blood, waste products, and carbon dioxide to a point of removal.

Vena cava (VAY-nah KAY-vah) The large vein that empties into the right auricle of the heart.

Ventricles (VEN-tri-kehlz) The two lower chambers of the heart.

White blood cells Large, white blood cells that fight infection in the body. Also called leukocytes.

Questions (Objective 1)

1. What topic is studied in angiology?
2. What is another name for the vascular system?
3. What is another name for the cardiac muscle tissue that surrounds the heart?
4. What is the function of the circulatory system?
5. In what part of the body is the heart located?
6. Are the upper chambers of the heart called auricles?
7. Are the lower chambers of the heart called ventricles?
8. Do arteries carry blood from the heart?
9. Do veins carry blood to the heart?
10. Are capillaries large or small blood vessels?
11. To which organ do the pulmonary blood vessels carry the blood from the heart?

Questions (Objective 2)

1. Which is the largest artery in the human body?
2. What artery in the neck is a major branch of the aorta?
3. What main artery divides into two branches to become the radial and ulnar arteries?
4. How many pints of blood does the human body contain?
5. Would blood in an artery look bright red/scarlet?
6. Are red blood cells called erythrocytes?
7. What is another name for white blood cells?
8. Which component of the blood causes it to clot?

Questions (Objective 3)

1. It is true that the endocrine system is made up of ductless glands?
2. Does the endocrine system have something to do with hormones in the body?
3. Where is the pituitary gland located?
4. Does the pituitary gland regulate all other endocrine glands?
5. Does the hypothalamus regulate the pituitary gland?
6. What gland located in the throat regulates body metabolism?
7. What gland makes insulin in the body?

Using the Glossaries in this Book

The terms in the glossaries at the end of each chapter are defined only as they relate to the practice of cosmetology.

Entries are alphabetized using the letter-by-letter rather than the word-by-word system. This means that the words have been alphabetized through the first mark of punctuation, disregarding hyphens and spaces between words. For example:

- Acid

- Acid-balanced

- Acidity

- Acid rinse

Prepositions have been ignored in alphabetizing the glossary entries.

Pronunciations are indicated by respellings, according to sounds shown in familiar words (see the Pronunciation Key). The accented (stressed) syllable is in capital letters.

Pronunciation Key

Symbol for a Sound	Key Word and Respelling	Symbol for a Sound	Key Word and Respelling
a	sat (SAT), paddle (PAD-l)	n	notice (NOH-tiss)
*ah	bar (BAHR)	ng	ring (RING), singer
ai	pair (PAIR)		(SING-gehr)
ar	fare (FARE)	o	dot (DOT)
aw	saw (SAW)	oh	goat (GOHT), go (GOH)
ay	day (DAY)	oi	soil (SOIL)
b	bob (BOB)	oo	scoot (SKOOT)
ch	chin (CHIN)		yule (YOOL), leukemia
d	did (DID)		(loo-KEE-mee-ah)
e	set (SET)	or	nor (NOR)
ee	see (SEE)	ow	tower (TOW-ehr)
ehr	merry (MEHR-ee)	p	pep (PEP)
er	fern (FERN), turn (TURN)	ph	phy (fee), phone (fone)
f	fifty (FIF-tee)	r	reed (REED)
g	gig (GIG)	s	sips (SIPS)
h	hat (HAT)	sh	ship (SHIP)
hw	wheel (WHEEL)	ss	base (BAYSS)
i	sit (SIT)	t	tent (TENT)
igh	might (MIGHT)	th	thank (THANK)
ihr	tier (TIHR)	*th*	than (*THAN*)
ism	organism (OR-gehn-iz-uhm), patriotism (PAY-tree-ah-tiz-uhm)	u	shut (SHUT), hook (HUK)
		*uh	but (BUHT)
		v	vivid (VIV-id)
j	jam (JAM)	w	wag (WAG)
k	kid (KID)	y	yes (YESS)
ks	six (SIKS)	The y sometimes replaces (igh); example:
kw	quack (KWAK)	childish (CHYL-dish).
l	let (LET), battle (BAT-l)	z	zoos (ZOOZ)
m	mom (MOM)	zh	measure (MEZH-ehr)

*The symbols ah, eh, and uh are sometimes used to show syllables containing vowel sounds that are muted (stressed very little).

Glossary Index

Photo credits continued

of 3M Company; **72** (a-c) Courtesy of the Wella Corporation, (b) Scanning electron micrograph courtesy of Scruples Professional Salon Products, (d, e) Helene Curtis Ind. Inc.; **73** (f, g, h, i, j) Courtesy of the Wella Corporation; **82** Tony Evans; **84, 85** @ David Young-Wolff/PhotoEdit; **90** John Dalton; **99–101** Tony Evans; **112, 126, 134** Courtesy of Scruples Professional Salon Products; **146** @ Bold Images, 248 N. Fairview Ave., Roseville, MN 55113, makeup by Brian L. DuChien; **149, 156, 157** Tony Evans; **174** Courtesy of Scruples Professional Salon Products; **177, 181, 183** Tony Evans; **194, 206** Courtesy of Scruples Professional Salon Products; **209, 210, 211, 212** Tony Evans; **214** (both) Courtesy of 3M Company; **215** Tony Evans; **240, 241, 242, 243** David Hanover Photography; **260** Courtesy of Scruples Professional Salon Products; **264, 265** Tony Evans; **270** Courtesy of Scruples Professional Salon Products; **272, 273** Tony Evans; **288, 291, 293** Courtesy of Scruples Professional Salon Products; **293** Tony Evans; **298–99** Courtesy of Roux, Revlon Professional Products Group; **302** Courtesy of Scruples Professional Salon Products; **308** @ David Young-Wolff/PhotoEdit; **314** Courtesy of Scruples Professional Salon Products; **328–29** Chart courtesy of Framesi USA, Inc.; **330–31** Color charts supplied by Matrix, © 1991 Matrix Essentials, Inc.; **344** Courtesy of Scruples Professional Salon Products; **347** (both) Courtesy of 3M Company; **350** @ David Young-Wolff/PhotoEdit; **356, 372** Courtesy of Scruples Professional Salon Products; **382, 384, 386** Tony Evans; **408** Courtesy of Scruples Professional Salon Products; **412** Tony Evans; **413** Scanning electron micrograph courtesy of Scruples; **416, 417** Tony Evans; **424, 426** David Hanover Photography; **430** Courtesy of Dudley Products, Inc.; **432, 433, 435, 439, 440** Tony Evans; **446** David Hanover Photography; **449** Tony Evans; **464, 490** Courtesy of Scruples Professional Salon Products; **497, 508** Tony Evans; **512** David Hanover Photography; **514** Tony Evans; **525–27** David Hanover Photography; **530** @ David Young-Wolff/PhotoEdit; **546** Courtesy of Dudley Products, Inc.; **550**(all), **551, 566** Tony Evans; **572, 582** Courtesy of Scruples Professional Salon Products; **592** @ Bold Images; makeup by Brian L. DuChien; **595** @ Frank Siteman/Stock Boston; **596** @ David Young-Wolff/PhotoEdit; **599** (top) @ David Young-Wolff/PhotoEdit, (bottom) Tony Evans; **604** Thomas K. Perry; **606, 611** @ David Young-Wolff/PhotoEdit; **626** Courtesy of Scruples Professional Salon Products; **629, 631, 632, 633, 634, 635** @ David Young-Wolff/PhotoEdit; **642** @ Bold Images, makeup by Brian L. DuChien; **661** @ David Young-Wolff/PhotoEdit; **670** @ Bold Images, makeup by Brian L. DuChien; **686, 708** Courtesy of Scruples Professional Salon Products.